Ophthalmic Oncology

M. D. ANDERSON SOLID TUMOR ONCOLOGY SERIES

Series Editor: Raphael E. Pollock, M.D., Ph.D.

PUBLISHED VOLUMES

Liver Cancer
Edited by STEVEN A. CURLEY, M.D.

Breast Cancer
Edited by S. EVA SINGLETARY, M.D.

Pancreatic Cancer
Edited by DOUGLAS B. EVANS, M.D., PETER W.T. PISTERS, M.D., and JAMES L. ABBRUZZESE, M.D.

Bita Esmaeli
Editor

Ophthalmic Oncology

Springer

Editor
Bita Esmaeli
The University of Texas
M.D. Anderson Cancer Center
Section of Ophthalmology
Department of Head and Neck Surgery
Houston, TX 77030, USA
besmaeli@mdanderson.org

Series Editor
Raphael E. Pollock
The University of Texas
M.D. Anderson Cancer Center
Houston, TX, USA

ISBN 978-1-4419-0373-0 e-ISBN 978-1-4419-0374-7
DOI 10.1007/978-1-4419-0374-7
Springer New York Dordrecht Heidelberg London

Library of Congress Control Number: 2010934256

Printed on acid-free paper

Springer is part of Springer Science+Business Media (www.springer.com)

Preface

A little over a decade ago, I had the privilege of helping to establish the first full-time ophthalmic oncology service based at a Comprehensive Cancer Center in the United States. Our Ophthalmic Oncology Service at The University of Texas M.D. Anderson Cancer Center has grown to include 4 subspecialty areas of ophthalmology: orbital oncology/oculoplastic surgery, ocular oncology, ocular surface diseases, and neuro-ophthalmology. *Ophthalmic Oncology* grew from faculty's unique experiences and observations in their ophthalmology subspecialty areas at M.D. Anderson. The book highlights the unique aspects of ophthalmic oncology as a surgical and medical discipline practiced at a Comprehensive Cancer Center. The multidisciplinary management of ocular, orbital, and ocular adnexal (eyelid, conjunctival, and periocular soft tissues) cancers is emphasized, as well as the current recommendations and practices at our institution. In addition, ocular conditions caused as a direct result of cancer treatment are reviewed using illustrative photographs and case presentations. The authors include ophthalmology faculty members, current and former M.D. Anderson fellows, and experts in complementary disciplines such as radiation oncology, dermatopathology, ophthalmic pathology, radiology, plastic surgery, and other surgical subspecialties.

With an abundance of clinical photographs, clinicians will be able to correctly diagnose cancers of the orbit, eye, and ocular adnexal structures.

I appreciate the contributions of each of the authors who took time out of their busy schedules to meet the deadlines for this project. I particularly thank my three ophthalmology colleagues at M.D. Anderson, Dr. Dan Gombos, Dr. Stella Kim, and Dr. Jade Schiffman, who not only have helped put together some of the sections in this book as section editors and authors but also because of their unique contributions to the growth of our program in Ophthalmic Oncology at M.D. Anderson. My special gratitude goes to Stephanie Deming and Sue Moreau from the Department of Scientific Publications at M.D. Anderson for their tireless long hours of editing for this book. I also would like to thank Dr. Raphael Pollock for the opportunity to organize and lead this effort and the privilege to edit this book in the M.D. Anderson Solid Tumor Oncology Series. Finally, I am grateful for the support provided by the dedicated staff at Springer—Stacy Lazar, Maureen Tobin, and Laura Walsh.

Bita Esmaeli
Houston, Texas

Contents

Contributors

Syed Mehdi Ahmad Department of Ophthalmology, Baylor University Medical Center at Dallas, Dallas, TX, USA, sma967@gmail.com

M. Amir Ahmadi Department of Ophthalmology, University of Illinois at Chicago, Chicago, IL, USA, mamirahmadi@yahoo.com

Alessandro Bonanno Department of Sociology, Sam Houston State University, Huntsville, TX, USA, soc_aab@shsu.edu

Christopher J. Calvano Division of Ophthalmic Plastic Surgery, Kresge Eye Institute, Wayne State University, Detroit, MI, USA, chris_calvano@yahoo.com

Gerardo D. Camoriano Department of Ophthalmology and Visual Sciences, The University of Texas Medical Branch, Galveston, TX, USA, gdcamori@utmb.edu

Heather Chang Jules Stein Eye Institute, UCLA Medical Center, Los Angeles, CA, USA, hkwon88@yahoo.com

Patty Chevez-Barrios Retinoblastoma Center of Houston, The Methodist Hospital, Houston, TX, USA, pchevez-barrios@tmhs.org

Murali Chintagumpala Department of Pediatrics, Section of Hematology and Oncology, Baylor College of Medicine, Texas Children's Hospital, Houston, TX, USA, muralic@txccc.org

Jin Young Choi Department of Sociology, Sam Houston State University, Huntsville, TX, USA, jyc002@shsu.edu

Garvin H. Davis Department of Ophthalmology, The University of Texas at Houston, Houston, TX, USA, gdavis@uth.tmc.edu

J. Matthew Debnam Section of Neuroradiology, Department of Radiology, The University of Texas M.D. Anderson Cancer Center, Houston, TX, USA, matthew.debnam@mdanderson.org

Sheri L. DeMartelaere Ophthalmology Service, Department of Surgery, Brooke Army Medical Center, Fort Sam Houston, TX, USA, sheri.l.demartelaere@us.army.mil

Vikram Durairaj Departments of Ophthalmology, Otolaryngology, Head and Neck Surgery, University of Colorado School of Medicine, Denver, CO, USA, vikram.durairaj@ucdenver.edu

Jonathan J. Dutton Department of Ophthalmology, Kittner Eye Center, University of North Carolina School of Medicine, Chapel Hill, NC, USA, jonathan_dutton@med.unc.edu

George K. Escaravage Department of Ophthalmology, University of North Carolina School of Medicine, Chapel Hill, NC, USA, george.escaravage@gmail.com

Bita Esmaeli Section of Ophthalmology, Department of Head and Neck Surgery, The University of Texas M.D. Anderson Cancer Center, Houston, TX, USA, besmaeli@mdanderson.org

Meghan S. Flemmons Department of Ophthalmology and Visual Sciences, The University of Texas Medical Branch, Galveston, TX, USA, meghan.flemmons@duke.edu

Steven J. Frank Department of Radiation Oncology, The University of Texas M.D. Anderson Cancer Center, Houston, TX, USA, sjfrank@mdanderson.org

Adam S. Garden Department of Radiation Oncology, The University of Texas M.D. Anderson Cancer Center, Houston, TX, USA, agarden@mdanderson.org

Maurizio L. Ghisoli Department of Hematology and Oncology, Medical City Children's Hospital, Texas Oncology, Dallas, TX, USA, maurizio.ghisoli@usoncology.com

Bernard F. Godley Department of Ophthalmology and Visual Sciences, The University of Texas Medical Branch, Galveston, TX, USA, bgodley@utmb.edu

Dominick Golio Departments of Surgery and Ophthalmology, State University of New York, Downstate Medical Center, Brooklyn, NY, USA, dominickgoliomd@pol.net

Dan S. Gombos Section of Ophthalmology, Department of Head and Neck Surgery, The University of Texas M.D. Anderson Cancer Center, Houston, TX, USA, dgombos@mdanderson.org

Miguel Gonzalez-Candial Department of Orbital and Ophthalmic Plastic Surgery, Universitat Autonoma de Barcelona, I.M.O. Barcelona, Barcelona, Spain, mgcandial@mac.com

Matthew M. Hanasono Department of Plastic Surgery, The University of Texas M.D. Anderson Cancer Center, Houston, TX, USA, mhanasono@mdanderson.org

Brent Hayek Section of Oculoplastics, Orbital and Cosmetic Surgery, Department of Ophthalmology, Emory University Eye Center, Atlanta, GA, USA, bhayek@me.com

Cindy Herzog Children's Cancer Hospital, The University of Texas M.D. Anderson Cancer Center, Houston, TX, USA, cherzog@mdanderson.org

Eric M. Hink Oculofacial Plastic and Orbital Surgery, Department of Ophthalmology, University of Colorado School of Medicine, Denver, CO, USA, eric.hink@ucdenver.edu

Hao H. Ho Jefferson Medical College, Philadelphia, PA, USA, hao.huy.ho@gmail.com

Viet H. Ho Danville San Ramon Eye Medical Corp., Danville, CA, USA, viethuyho@yahoo.com

Adam Hsu Section of Ophthalmology, Department of Head and Neck Surgery, The University of Texas M.D. Anderson Cancer Center, Houston, TX, USA, ayhsu@yahoo.com

Winston W. Huh Division of Pediatrics, The University of Texas M.D. Anderson Cancer Center, Houston, TX, USA, whuh@mdanderson.org

Richard L. Hurwitz Retinoblastoma Center of Houston and Center for Cell and Gene Therapy, Baylor College of Medicine, Texas Children's Cancer Center, Houston, TX, USA, rhurwitz@txccc.org

Doina Ivan Department of Pathology, The University of Texas M.D. Anderson Cancer Center, Houston, TX, USA, doivan@mdanderson.org

Thomas E. Johnson Department of Ophthalmology, Bascom Palmer Eye Institute, University of Miami Miller School of Medicine, Miami, FL, USA, tjohnson@med.miami.edu

Kapil G. Kapoor Department of Ophthalmology and Visual Sciences, The University of Texas Medical Branch, Galveston, TX, USA, kgkapoor@utmb.edu

Gibran S. Khurshid Department of Ophthalmology and Visual Sciences, The University of Texas Medical Branch, Galveston, TX, USA, sk.gibran@utmb.edu

Stella K. Kim Section of Ophthalmology, Department of Head and Neck Surgery, The University of Texas M.D. Anderson Cancer Center, Houston, TX, USA, skim@mdanderson.org

Michelle Ludwig Department of Radiation Oncology, The University of Texas M.D. Anderson Cancer Center, Houston, TX, USA, mludwig@mdanderson.org

Anita Mahajan Department of Radiation Oncology, The University of Texas M.D. Anderson Cancer Center, Houston, TX, USA, amahajan@mdanderson.org

Tanuj Nakra Ophthalmic Plastic and Orbital Surgery, Texas Oculoplastic Consultants, Austin, TX, USA, tnakra@tocaustin.com

John D. Ng Departments of Ophthalmology and Otolaryngology and Head and Neck Surgery, Casey Eye Institute and Devers Eye Institute, Oregon Health Sciences University, Portland, OR, USA, ngj@ohsu.edu

Anitha Raghunath Section of Ophthalmology, Department of Head and Neck Surgery, The University of Texas M.D. Anderson Cancer Center, Houston, TX, USA, anitha.raghunath@gmail.com

Aaron Savar Section of Ophthalmology, Department of Head and Neck Surgery, The University of Texas M.D. Anderson Cancer Center, Houston, TX, USA, asavar@gmail.com

Jade S. Schiffman Section of Ophthalmology, Department of Head and Neck Surgery, The University of Texas M.D. Anderson Cancer Center, Houston, TX, USA, jschiffm@mdanderson.org

Frank W. Scribbick III Department of Ophthalmology, Lions Eye Pathology Laboratory, The University of Texas Health Science Center, San Antonio, TX, USA, scribbick@uthscsa.edu

Roman Shinder Section of Ophthalmology, Department of Head and Neck Surgery, The University of Texas M.D. Anderson Cancer Center, Houston, TX, USA, romanshinder@hotmail.com

Sonali Singh Department of Ophthalmology, Veterans Hospital, Temple, TX, USA, sonalis25@gmail.com

John M. Slopis Department of Neuro-Oncology, The University of Texas M.D. Anderson Cancer Center, Houston, TX, USA, jmslopis@mdanderson.org

Mehryar Taban Department of Orbito-Facial Surgery, Jules Stein Eye Institute, University of California, Los Angeles, Los Angeles, CA, USA, tabanmd@yahoo.com

Rosa Ana Tang Department of Neurology, The University of Texas Health Science Center at Houston, Houston, TX, USA, rtang@neuroeye.com

Michelle D. Williams Department of Pathology, The University of Texas M.D. Anderson Cancer Center, Houston, TX, USA, mdwillia@mdanderson.org

Peter E. Zage Department of Pediatrics, The University of Texas M.D. Anderson Cancer Center, Houston, TX, USA, pezage@mdanderson.org

Part I
Orbital and Adnexal Oncology

Section Editor: Bita Esmaeli

Chapter 1
Primary Orbital Cancers in Adults

Roman Shinder and Bita Esmaeli

Abstract Neoplasms of the orbit in adults may be primary tumors, secondary tumors extending from adjacent structures, or metastatic tumors. The incidence of primary malignant orbital neoplasms is low. A computed tomography scan is usually the initial radiographic modality employed to investigate suspicious lesions. Biopsy is usually undertaken to establish a diagnosis and formulate a treatment plan. Prognosis depends on the type of tumor and extent of local or systemic disease at presentation. This chapter is not intended to provide an exhaustive discussion of all possible primary orbital cancers; rather, it focuses on the management of tumors most commonly encountered at a tertiary cancer center. Benign tumors of the orbit in adults, lacrimal gland tumors, and pediatric orbital tumors are also covered in Chapters 2, 7, and 3, respectively.

1.1 Lymphoproliferative Disorders

Lymphoproliferative disorders, a heterogeneous group of neoplasms of the lymphoid system, account for greater than 20% of all orbital masses and are the most common orbital malignancies in adults [1, 2]. The majority of primary orbital lymphomas are B-cell non-Hodgkin lymphomas. The incidence of orbital lymphomas has been increasing in recent years, although the factors responsible for this rise are poorly understood. Recognized risk factors include chronic autoimmune diseases and occupations that involve exposure to bioactive solvents and reagents.

R. Shinder (✉)
Section of Ophthalmology, Department of Head and Neck Surgery, The University of Texas M.D. Anderson Cancer Center, Houston, TX, USA
e-mail: romanshinder@hotmail.com

B. Esmaeli (ed.), *Ophthalmic Oncology*, M.D. Anderson Solid Tumor Oncology Series 6, DOI 10.1007/978-1-4419-0374-7_1,

1.1.1 Presenting Signs and Symptoms, Histopathologic and Molecular Genetic Characteristics, and Diagnosis

Over the past 20 years, our understanding of orbital lymphoproliferative lesions has undergone profound change. This is primarily due to the development of increasingly sophisticated and specific immunodiagnostic and molecular techniques in tissue pathology. Historically, lymphoid tumors were classified as either benign reactive lymphoid hyperplasias or malignant lymphomas. More recently, it has been accepted that lymphoproliferative lesions represent a spectrum and that ultimate behavior is challenging to predict. Patients with microscopically benign lymphoid infiltrates eventually may develop systemic lymphoma, while malignant lymphomas may be well circumscribed and respond to local therapy without subsequent extraorbital involvement. At present, 70–80% of lymphoproliferative lesions are considered malignant on the basis of monoclonal cell-surface markers, whereas 90% are found to be malignant through molecular genetic testing [2]. With further advances in diagnostic techniques, the proportion of cases classified as benign reactive lymphoid hyperplasia is likely to continue to diminish.

Typically, lymphoproliferative lesions of the orbit present as progressive, painless masses in the sixth to eighth decades of life [1]. The tumors are often located anteriorly in the extraconal orbital space and may present as a palpable, rubbery mass. Lesions typically mold themselves around orbital structures rather than invading them; therefore, disturbances of extraocular motility or vision are unusual. Orbital lymphomas may be associated (22% of cases) with a salmon-colored, fleshy, subconjunctival extension that molds to the shape of the globe, commonly referred to as a salmon patch (Fig. 1.1) [2]. There is usually a history of slow growth over

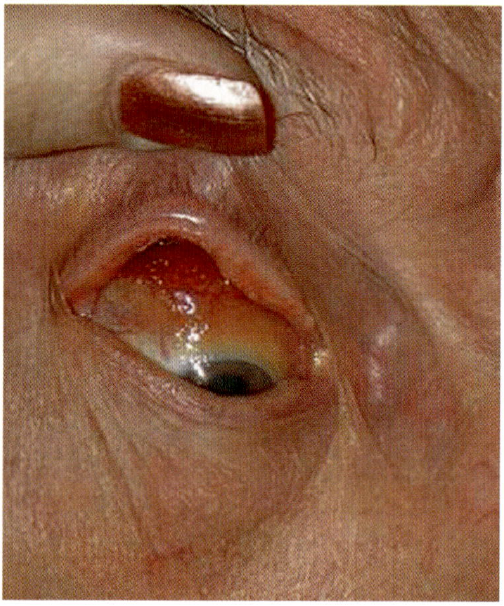

Fig. 1.1 Orbital and conjunctival MALT lymphoma with a "salmon patch" infiltrate on the ocular surface

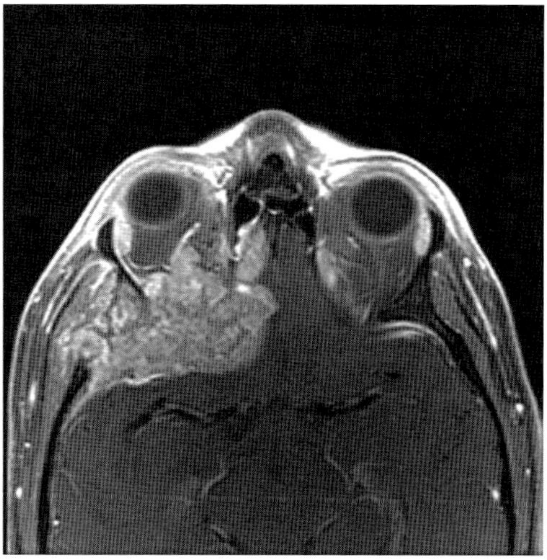

Fig. 1.2 Unusual presentation of diffuse large B-cell lymphoma of orbit with bony invasion in the orbital apex and extension intracranially

a period of months to years. Orbital imaging displays a characteristic, cohesive, putty-like molding of the tumor around structures, and bone erosion or infiltration is unusual except in high-grade malignant lymphomas (Fig. 1.2). The most common site involved is the lacrimal fossa, where up to 50% of lymphoproliferative lesions occur [3]. Approximately 17% of lymphoid lesions occur bilaterally in the orbits; while bilateral involvement markedly increases the risk for systemic disease, it does not, by itself, signify systemic involvement [3].

An open biopsy is recommended for all lesions confined to the orbit to obtain adequate tissue to establish a diagnosis. If systemic disease is present, biopsy of an accessible lymph node is preferred over orbital biopsy because nodal architecture is helpful in diagnosis and the procedure may be safer [4]. The majority of the specimen should be sent fresh to the laboratory for flow cytometry and immunohistochemistry; the remainder of the specimen may be fixed for microscopic analysis. Histologically, a continuum is seen ranging from benign reactive hyperplasia to atypical lymphoid hyperplasia to low-grade lymphoma to high-grade lymphoma. All variants are characterized by a hypercellular lymphoid proliferation with a scant stromal component; thus, it is difficult to categorize a lesion solely by light microscopy. Immunopathology and molecular studies are therefore used as aids in tumor categorization.

It is thought that malignant lymphomas represent clonal expansions of abnormal precursor cells. Immunologic studies of lymphocyte cell-surface markers may be used to classify tumors as containing B or T cells and as being monoclonal (malignant) or polyclonal (benign). DNA hybridization is more sensitive than cell-surface marker typing in assessing clonality, but the DNA hybridization technique is more time consuming and expensive [5]. Importantly, monoclonality established by either immunophenotyping or molecular genetic testing does not predict which tumors will lead to systemic disease. Approximately 90% of lymphomas show monoclonality by molecular genetic studies.

Marginal zone lymphomas, also known as mucosa-associated lymphoid tumor (MALT), represent the largest group of orbital lymphomas, accounting for 40–60% [6]. It was previously thought that low-grade MALT-type lymphomas rarely undergo systemic spread. However, recent studies demonstrate that at least 50% of patients will develop systemic disease within 10 years [6]. MALT lymphomas undergo histologic transformation to a more aggressive lymphoma in 15–20% of patients, usually after several years, and the risk of transformation is unrelated to therapy [7].

Prior, concurrent, or future systemic spread may occur in patients with ocular adnexal lymphomas. In a recent report from our center, more than half of patients with orbital and ocular adnexal lymphoma were found to have extraorbital involvement at the time of diagnosis [8]. This is higher than previously reported rates, in part because of the more aggressive lymphomas seen at our tertiary cancer center and likely because of the uniform staging workup performed here, which included total-body positron emission tomography in the majority of patients and bone marrow biopsies in all patients. The anatomic location of the tumor may help predict the risk of developing systemic disease; risk is lowest for conjunctival lymphomas (20% of cases), greater for orbital lymphomas (35% of cases), and highest for eyelid lymphomas (67% of cases) [9]. Although most cases of primary orbital lymphoma are low grade, secondary orbital lymphomas in patients with prior or concurrent disease are typically intermediate or high grade [10]. Secondary orbital lymphoma may appear at any time after initial diagnosis of non-Hodgkin's lymphoma and may occur as either a manifestation of disseminated relapse or the only site of active recurrence [10].

An important option to consider in the differential diagnosis of patients with orbital lymphoproliferative lesions is idiopathic orbital inflammation. Inflammatory disorders can be differentiated from lymphoma on the basis of their acute presentation, rapid response to steroids, and polymorphic infiltrate on histopathology.

1.1.2 Treatment

Important determinants of the optimal management of orbital lymphoma are the stage at presentation, histologic classification, extent of disease, patient comorbidities, and potential ocular toxicity of treatment. Proper initial staging is critical and should include total-body positron emission tomography, bone marrow biopsy, and, for MALT lymphoma and mantle cell lymphoma, gastrointestinal endoscopy [9].

Radiation therapy has classically been the treatment of choice for patients with localized low-grade ocular adnexal lymphoma as it achieves local control in greater than 90% of cases [11]. However, radiation therapy is a form of local therapy and thus does not address the risk of systemic relapse. Also, it may cause immediate and delayed ocular side effects, including dry-eye syndrome, keratopathy, cataract, and retinopathy. Furthermore, since careful staging proves that more than 50% of patients have systemic disease on presentation, systemic

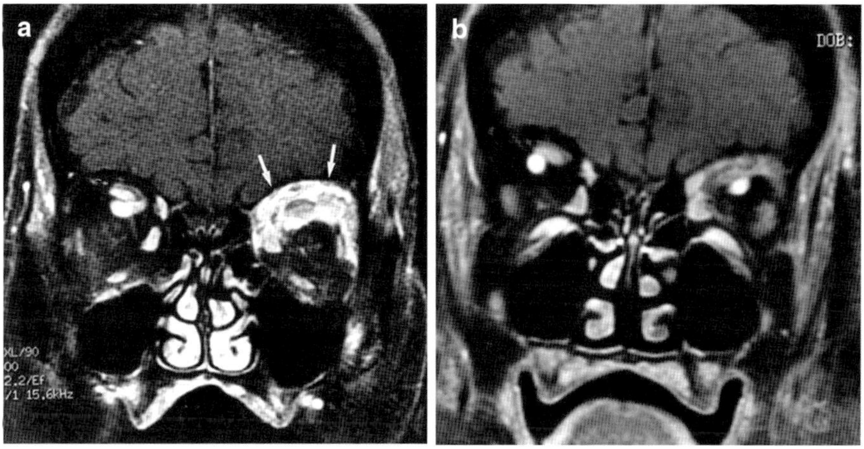

Fig. 1.3 Magnetic resonance imaging of orbital lymphoma before (**a**) and after (**b**) radioimmunotherapy using ibritumomab tiuxetan (Zevalin)

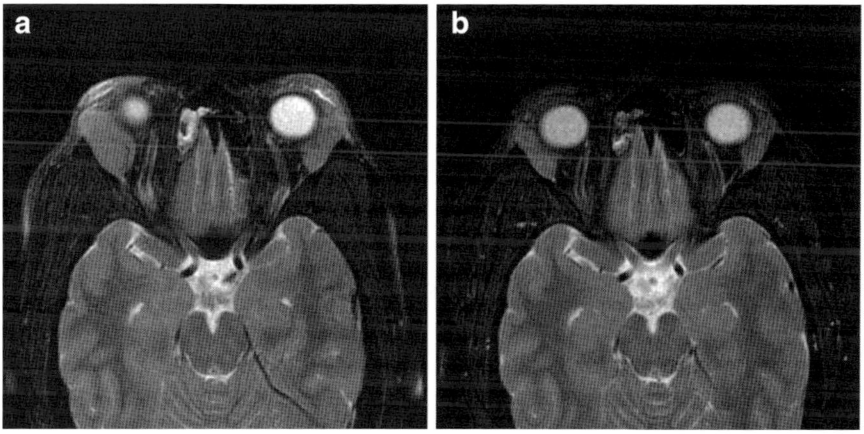

Fig. 1.4 Magnetic resonance imaging of benign lymphoid hyperplasia of orbit before (**a**) and after (**b**) treatment with rituximab. From Hao HH, Savar A, Samaniego F, et al. Treatment of benign lymphoid hyperplasia of the orbit with rituximab. Ophthal Plast Reconstr Surg 2010;26:11–13. Reprinted with permission

therapy, such as monoclonal antibody immunotherapy or radioimmunotherapy, can be considered as an alternative to radiation therapy (Figs. 1.3 and 1.4). Systemic combination chemotherapy regimens, such as cyclophosphamide, doxorubicin, vincristine, and prednisone or similar protocols, are used for more aggressive histologic varieties of lymphoma, such as diffuse large B-cell lymphoma or mantle cell lymphoma [12].

Recently, there has been a trend toward the use of monoclonal antibody therapy or radioimmunotherapy directed against CD20 (rituximab or ibritumomab tiuxetan) to treat not only ocular adnexal lymphoma but also non-Hodgkin's lymphoma in general [8, 13–17]. Being a systemic treatment, monoclonal antibody therapy not only may be effective in local control but also may offer better overall systemic control of lymphoma. It may also be less toxic to the ocular structures compared to radiation therapy [10, 18]. Rituximab alone may yield good initial response but is associated with a 50% chance of distant relapse [17]. Rituximab in combination with chemotherapy or radioimmunotherapy may be associated with a higher durable response rate [17, 19]. Surgical excision is typically not a viable option for orbital lymphoma because of the infiltrative nature of the tumor. Rituximab may also be a good treatment option for orbital benign lymphoid hyperplasia [20].

1.1.3 Follow-up

Regardless of treatment, response to therapy should be monitored via conventional imaging; positron emission tomography could also be used as an adjunct [21]. Because the lymphoproliferative diseases show substantial overlap in terms of clinical behavior, all patients should be followed indefinitely by an oncologist and have periodic systemic workups. Workups should include examination for lymphadenopathy, complete blood cell count with differential, and body imaging.

1.2 Mesenchymal Tumors

Approximately 2% of tumors detected on orbital biopsy are tumors of fibrous connective tissue, cartilage, or bone [22]. The tumors in this group arise from primitive mesenchymal stem cells capable of developing into a variety of cell types.

1.2.1 Fibrous Histiocytoma

Fibrous histiocytoma (fibroxanthoma) may be the most common primary orbital mesenchymal neoplasm in adults. The median age at presentation is 43 years, and the superior nasal orbit is the most common site [23]. Fibrous histiocytoma is usually slow growing and characteristically very firm, displacing normal structures. The most common clinical signs are proptosis and mass effect with decreased vision; less common signs are diplopia, pain, lid edema, tearing, ptosis, and ophthalmoplegia [24]. Both fibroblastic and histiocytic cells in a storiform (mat-like) pattern are found in these locally aggressive tumors [24]. Although most are benign, intermediate and malignant varieties exist, but fewer than 10% have metastatic potential [23]. It is often difficult to distinguish this tumor clinically or microscopically from hemangiopericytoma (see Section 1.2.3). Management is surgical excision supplemented by adjuvant post operative radiation therapy or possibly chemotherapy.

1.2.2 Solitary Fibrous Tumor

A relatively new entity, solitary fibrous tumor, has been described. Unlike fibrous histiocytoma, the other major entity that has to be considered in the differential diagnosis, solitary fibrous tumor is composed of spindle-shaped, strongly CD34-positive cells [24]. Solitary fibrous tumors can occur anywhere in the orbit, are well circumscribed, lack a capsule, and may recur and undergo malignant transformation if incompletely excised. Their characteristic magnetic resonance imaging feature is heterogeneity and low T2 signal intensity [24]. Before the typical immunohistochemical features of solitary fibrous tumors were described, a number of these mesenchymal tumors were likely misclassified as fibrous histiocytoma, hemangiopericytoma, and schwannoma [23]. However, many pathologists believe that solitary fibrous tumor is a very close entity to hemangiopericytoma from the standpoint of its biological and clinical behavior.

1.2.3 Hemangiopericytoma

Hemangiopericytomas are rare, encapsulated, cellular tumors typically located in the superior orbit, which appear in middle-aged adults (median age, 42 years) [25]. Hemangiopericytomas can manifest with proptosis, pain, diplopia, decreased vision, ophthalmoplegia, conjunctival prolapse, and prominent blood vessels in the fornix. These tumors may resemble cavernous hemangiomas on imaging, appearing as homogeneously enhancing, well-defined masses. Histologically, tumors are composed of a rich capillary network in a staghorn pattern surrounded by pericytes. Tumors may be benign, intermediate, or malignant. It is difficult to predict biological activity on the basis of histology; histologically benign lesions may recur and metastasize, whereas malignant lesions may remain localized [25]. Complete excision with long-term patient follow-up is a must as one-third of these tumors recur. Hemangiopericytomas may undergo malignant transformation, and 10–15% metastasize [25]. Tumors with a biologically aggressive behavior are handled with a more radical approach, including preoperative embolization, wider excision, and pre- or post operative radiation therapy [25]. Preoperative radiation therapy may lead to a decrease in the size of the tumor, making complete surgical excision easier and decreasing the risk of recurrence after surgical removal (unpublished observations, Dr. Bita Esmaeli) (Fig. 1.5).

1.2.4 Other Mesenchymal Tumors

Various types of malignant mesenchymal tumors, such as liposarcoma, fibrosarcoma, chondrosarcoma, synovial sarcoma (Fig. 1.6), Ewing sarcoma, and osteosarcoma, can present in the orbit. Combined-modality treatment with a combination of chemotherapy, surgery, and radiation therapy is the most common approach to treatment of these rare but aggressive tumors of the orbit [7].

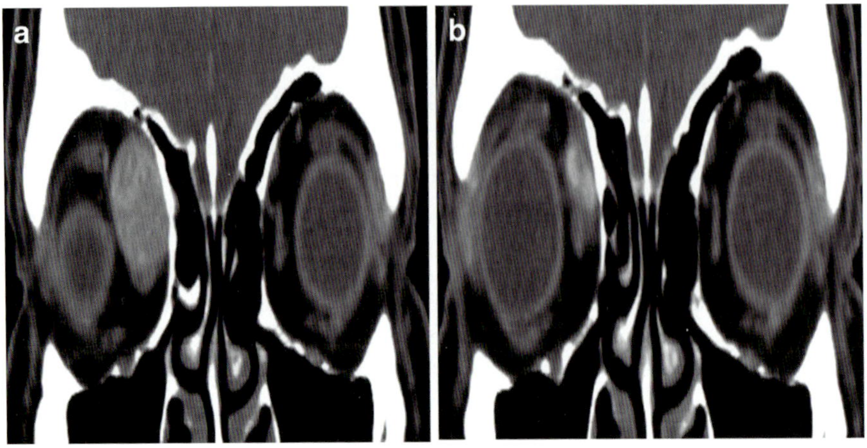

Fig. 1.5 Computed tomography of a recurrent orbital hemangiopericytoma before (**a**) and after (**b**) treatment with neoadjuvant radiation therapy which was administered prior to surgical resection of the mass

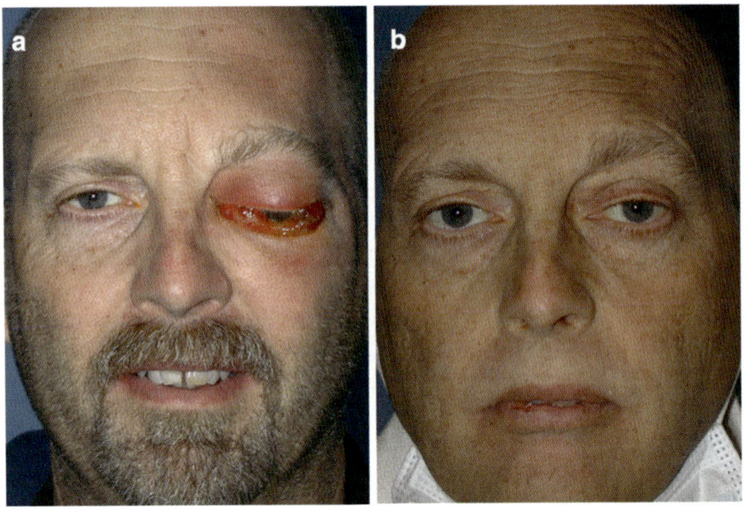

Fig. 1.6 (**a**) Left orbital synovial sarcoma causing proptosis, chemosis, and exposure conjunctivitis (**b**) Improved clinical appearance following treatment with chemotherapy and radiation therapy. From Savar A, Trent J, Al-Zubidi N, et al. Efficay of adjuvant and neoadjuvant therapies for adult orbital sarcomas. Ophthal Plast Reconstr Surg 2010;26:185–189. Reprinted with permission

1.3 Lacrimal Gland Tumors

Lacrimal gland tumors are covered in Chapter 7.

References

1. White WL, Ferry JA. Ocular adnexal lymphoma: a clinicopathologic study with identification of lymphomas of mucosa-associated lymphoid tissue type. Ophthalmology 1995;102: 1994–2006.
2. Rootman J, White VA, Connors JM, et al. Lymphoproliferative, leukemic, and histiocytic lesions of the orbit. In: Rootman J, editor. Diseases of the Orbit: A Multidisciplinary Approach, second edition. Philadelphia, PA: Lippincott Williams & Wilkins, 2003: 385–400.
3. Coupland SE, Krause L, Delecluse H-J, et al. Lymphoproliferative lesions of the ocular adnexa: analysis of 112 cases. Ophthalmology 1998;105:1430–41.
4. Albert DM, Jakobiec FA, editors. Principles and Practice of Ophthalmology. Philadelphia, PA: Saunders, 1994:2005–16.
5. Johnson TE, Tse DT, Byrne GE Jr, et al. Ocular-adnexal lymphoid tumors: a clinicopathologic and molecular genetic study of 77 patients. Ophthal Plast Reconstr Surg 1999;15:171–9.
6. Jenkins C, Rose GE, Bunce C, et al. Histologic features of ocular adnexal lymphoma (REAL classification) and their association with patient morbidity and survival. Br J Ophthalmol 2000;84:907–13.
7. Savar A, Trent J, Al-Zubidi N, Huh W, Anderson P, Shinder R, Esmaeli B. Efficacy of adjuvant and neoadjuvant therapies for adult orbital sarcomas. Ophthal Plast Reconstr Surg. 2010 May-Jun;26(3):185–9.
8. Jakobiec FA, Iwamoto T, Patell M, et al. Ocular adnexal monoclonal lymphoid tumors with a favorable prognosis. Ophthalmology 1986;93:1547–57.
9. Hatef H, Roberts D, McLaughlin P, et al. Prevalence and nature of systemic involvement and stage at initial examination in patients with orbital and ocular adnexal lymphoma. Arch Ophthalmol 2007;125:1663–7.
10. Esmaeli B, Ahmadi A, Manning J, et al. Clinical presentation and treatment of secondary orbital lymphoma. Ophthal Plast Reconstr Surg 2002;18:247–53.
11. Kennerdell JS, Flores NE, Hartsock RJ. Low-dose radiotherapy for lymphoid lesions of the orbit and ocular adnexa. Ophthal Plast Reconstr Surg 1999;15:129–33.
12. Bardenstein DS. Ocular adnexal lymphoma: classification, clinical disease, and molecular biology. Ophthalmol Clin North Am 2005;18:187–97.
13. Esmaeli B, Murray JL, Ahmadi MA, et al. Immunotherapy for low grade non-Hodgkin secondary lymphoma of the orbit. Arch Ophthalmol 2002;120:1225–7.
14. McLaughlin P, Grillo-Lopez AJ, Link BK, et al. Rituximab chimeric anti-CD20 monoclonal antibody therapy for relapsed indolent lymphoma. half of patients respond to a four-dose treatment program. J Clin Oncol 1998;16:2825–33.
15. Davies AJ. Radioimmunotherapy for B-cell lymphoma: Y90 ibritumomab tiuxetan and I (131) tositumomab. Oncogene 2007;26:3614–28.
16. Sullivan TJ, Grimes D, Bunce I. Monoclonal antibody treatment of orbital lymphoma. Ophthal Plast Reconstr Surg 2004;20:103–6.
17. Shome D, Esmaeli B. Targeted monoclonal antibody therapy and radioimmunotherapy for lymphoproliferative disorders of the ocular adnexa. Curr Opin Ophthalmol 2008;19:414–21.
18. Bairey O, Kremer I, Rakowsky E, et al. Orbital and adnexal involvement in systemic non-Hodgkin's lymphoma. Cancer 1994;73:2395–9.
19. Esmaeli B, McLaughlin P, Pro B, et al. Prospective trial of targeted radioimmunotherapy with Y-90 ibritumomab tiuxetan (Zevalin) for front-line treatment of early-stage extranodal indolent ocular adnexal lymphoma. Ann Oncol 2009;20:709–14.
20. Ho HH, Savar A, Samaniego F, et al. Treatment of benign lymphoid hyperplasia of the orbit with rituximab. Ophthal Plast Reconstr Surg 2010; 26:11–3.
21. Gayed I, Eskandari MF, McLaughlin P, et al. Value of positron emission tomography in staging ocular adnexal lymphomas and evaluating their response to therapy. Ophthalmic Surg Lasers Imaging 2007;38:319–25.

22. Rootman J. Neoplasia. In: Rootman J, editor. Diseases of the Orbit: A Multidisciplinary Approach, second edition. Philadelphia, PA: Lippincott Williams & Wilkins, 2003:262.
23. Katz BJ, Nerad JA. Ophthalmic manifestations of fibrous dysplasia – a disease of children and adults. Ophthalmology 1998;105:2207–15.
24. Rootman J. Neoplasia. In: Rootman J, editor. Diseases of the Orbit: A Multidisciplinary Approach, second edition. Philadelphia, PA: Lippincott Williams & Wilkins, 2003:276–8.
25. Rootman J. Neoplasia. In: Rootman J, editor. Diseases of the Orbit: A Multidisciplinary Approach, second edition. Philadelphia, PA: Lippincott Williams & Wilkins, 2003:544–6.

Chapter 2
Nonmalignant Tumors of the Orbit

Eric M. Hink and Vikram Durairaj

Abstract Most orbital tumors are nonmalignant. Nonmalignant orbital tumors can arise from any of the structures within the orbit, including blood vessels, fat, nerves, lacrimal gland, and connective tissue. Nonmalignant orbital tumors can be grouped into cystic lesions, vascular tumors, lymphoproliferative lesions, inflammatory lesions, mesenchymal tumors, neurogenic tumors, and lacrimal gland tumors. Although most orbital tumors are benign, their location may compromise ocular health and function and necessitate treatment with surgery, radiation, or chemotherapy. Patient characteristics, signs, and findings on ophthalmic examination and imaging, including computed tomography and magnetic resonance imaging, guide the clinician in formulating a differential diagnosis.

2.1 Presentation

Orbital tumors often present with a constellation of signs suggestive of a space-occupying lesion in the bony confines of the orbit. These orbital signs include lid edema or fullness; ptosis or retraction; proptosis or nonaxial globe displacement; axial hyperopia or acquired astigmatism; vascular or lymphatic congestion producing conjunctival chemosis; hyperemia or secondary glaucoma; dysmotility or palsy of cranial nerve II, III, IV, V, or VI; chorioretinal folds; optic nerve edema or atrophy; and double vision or loss of vision. In addition to a complete ophthalmic examination, appropriate imaging, including ultrasonography, computed tomography (CT), and magnetic resonance imaging (MRI), provides valuable information regarding the location and radiographic characteristics of the lesion. Often the patient's age, sex, race, clinical course, and radiographic images can narrow the differential diagnosis. Incisional or excisional biopsy may be pursued to confirm the diagnosis.

E.M. Hink (✉)
Oculofacial Plastic and Orbital Surgery, Department of Ophthalmology, University of Colorado School of Medicine, Denver, CO, USA
e-mail: eric.hink@ucdenver.edu

B. Esmaeli (ed.), *Ophthalmic Oncology*, M.D. Anderson Solid Tumor Oncology Series 6, DOI 10.1007/978-1-4419-0374-7_2,

2.2 Cystic Lesions

Almost all orbital cysts are benign. Cystic lesions may arise from developmental abnormalities or from the adjacent sinuses or cranium.

Most congenital orbital cysts are choristomas known as dermoid or epidermoid cysts. These cysts are the most common orbital tumors in children, accounting for 30–46% of all excised orbital tumors in this age group [1]. These cysts arise from nests of ectodermal cells that become trapped in the orbital bony sutures, most commonly the frontozygomatic suture, during closure of the neural tube [2]. Dermoid or epidermoid cysts often present as firm, smooth, partially mobile masses along the superotemporal orbital rim. "Dumbbell" dermoids may have a deep orbital component. Deep orbital dermoids typically present later in life with orbital signs. Imaging of dermoid and epidermoid cysts demonstrates a well-demarcated cystic lesion with surrounding bony sclerosis, erosion, and remodeling. These lesions can frequently be excised without difficulty (Fig. 2.1). Pathological examination will demonstrate a cyst lined with stratified squamous epithelium and filled with keratin. Dermoid cysts contain dermal appendages, including hair and sebaceous glands, whereas epidermoid cysts are devoid of such elements. Dermoid and epidermoid cysts rarely rupture in vivo, but when they do, often as the result of trauma, a vigorous inflammatory reaction occurs, leading to a clinical picture similar to idiopathic orbital inflammation or orbital cellulitis.

Another type of congenital orbital tumor is the orbital teratoma, a rare congenital cystic tumor derived from all three embryonic germ layers that is rarely malignant [3].

Acquired cysts include chocolate cysts, hemorrhagic cysts, and lacrimal gland cysts. Chocolate cysts are most often associated with lymphangiomas. Lacrimal

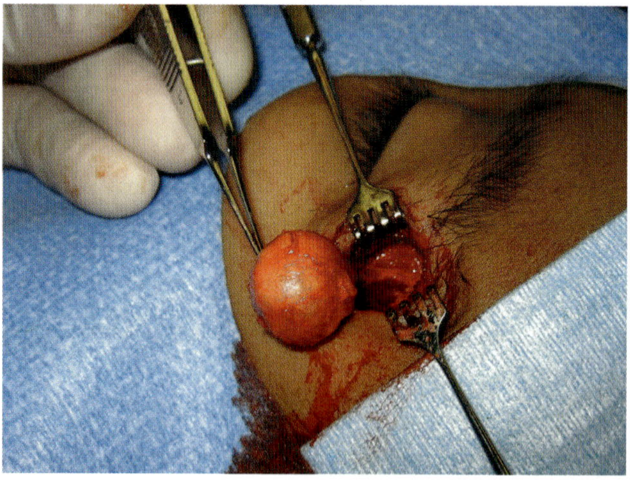

Fig. 2.1 Surgical excision of dermoid cyst in a 2-year-old patient

gland cysts, known as dacryops, form when the excretory ducts of the lacrimal gland become obstructed. In addition, bacterial abscesses or larval cysts may arise in the orbit during infection.

In adults, cystic orbital lesions often arise from the adjacent sinuses and herniate into the orbit. Mucoceles or mucopyoceles arise from an obstructed sinus ostium causing chronic sinusitis. In children, a congenital nasolacrimal duct obstruction, often the result of an imperforate valve of Hasner, can form a cystic tear-filled mass known as a dacryocystocele. These present as a bluish, soft, cystic mass below the medial canthal tendon, and early probing is advocated to prevent dacryocystitis [4]. Dacryocystoceles are often associated with nasal dacryoceles that can cause upper airway obstruction and require immediate surgical marsupialization. Rarely, congenital herniations of intracranial contents known as cephaloceles, including meningoceles and encephaloceles, can involve the orbit via the orbital fissures or bony defects [3].

2.3 Vascular Tumors

Vascular lesions are the second most common orbital tumors in children and the most common orbital tumors in adults [1, 5]. There is some debate as to the classification and naming of these tumors. The traditional nomenclature will be used in this chapter.

Capillary hemangiomas (benign hemangioendotheliomas) are the most common vascular orbital tumor in children. The tumor varies in location and presentation, although it generally appears within the first few months of life, grows for 6–12 months, and then involutes over the next few years [1]. Superficial capillary hemangiomas involving the dermis appear as bright red lesions or "strawberry nevi." Subdermal tumors may appear as a blue mass in the eyelid. The presence of numerous capillary hemangiomas may cause platelet sequestration and thrombocytopenia, a phenomenon known as Kasabach–Merritt syndrome. Because these tumors frequently involute, management typically involves limiting the tumors' amblyogenic (deprivational, strabismic, and astigmatic) effects. Intralesional steroids and limited surgical resection are the mainstays of therapy. Recently the systemic oral administration of propranolol has shown promising results in the treatment of infantile capillary hemangioma (please see a more detailed discussion of this topic in Chapter 3).

Cavernous hemangiomas are the most common benign orbital tumor in adults, with middle-aged women being the most frequently affected [5]. Cavernous hemangiomas typically appear with orbital signs. Imaging demonstrates a well-circumscribed mass with limited systemic vascular communication and poor contrast enhancement. These tumors can be intraconal, and cautious surgical excision may be required if these tumors compromise ocular function (Fig. 2.2) [5].

Hemangiopericytomas are benign pericyte tumors primarily appearing during middle age. They present with orbital signs and appear similar to cavernous

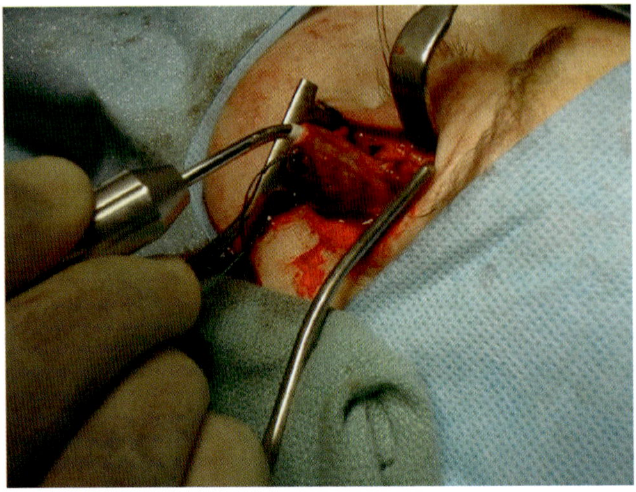

Fig. 2.2 Lateral orbitotomy with bone flap with excision of cavernous hemangioma. Cryoprobe used for assistance in removal

hemangiomas on imaging; however, hemangiopericytomas can undergo malignant transformation and therefore must be completely resected [6]. Please see a more detailed discussion in Chapter 1.

Lymphangiomas are benign lymphatic vascular tumors that usually manifest within the first decade of life. These tumors progress slowly and may involve the conjunctiva, appearing as a multilobulated mass [1]. They can undergo acute enlargement during viral infections. Chocolate cysts can form, most often during infection, when a blood vessel in the lymphangioma spontaneously ruptures and bleeds into the lymphatic channels. Drainage of these chocolate cysts may be required to prevent ocular sequela. Lymphangiomas are infiltrative in nature, and complete excision is not possible, but surgery can be used to debulk large tumors [7].

Orbital varix is an abnormal dilation of an ophthalmic vein that may be congenital or acquired. Proptosis can be exacerbated by the Valsalva maneuver. CT will demonstrate a dilated vein and may show phleboliths [1]. Conservative management is usually advocated, as these lesions can be difficult to remove. Partial resection and embolization may be attempted.

Arteriovenous malformations are congenital abnormalities of the orbital vasculature in which arteries anastomose directly to veins, without an intervening capillary bed. "Corkscrew" episcleral vessels can be observed (Fig. 2.3). Arteriovenous malformations may be embolized or resected [8].

Acquired malformations are typically the result of trauma resulting in carotid cavernous fistulas between the internal carotid artery and the cavernous sinus. Dural sinus fistulas, connecting the small meningeal artery to the cavernous sinus, may spontaneously form in elderly patients with vasculopathy. These lesions may result in pulsatile proptosis, dilated episcleral veins, secondary glaucoma, and cranial

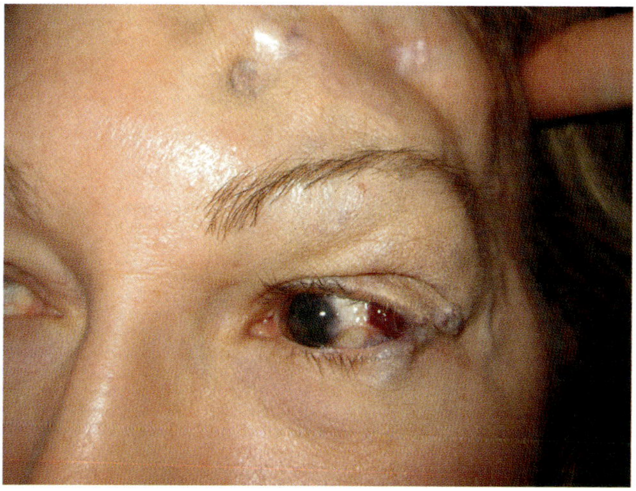

Fig. 2.3 Arteriovenous malformation of the left orbit. Note episcleral involvement

nerve VI palsy. CT demonstrates an enlarged superior ophthalmic vein and possible enlargement of the extraocular muscles. Embolization is the treatment of choice [9].

2.4 Lymphoproliferative Masses

The clinical spectrum of histiocytic, hematopoietic, and lymphoproliferative orbital masses ranges from benign, reactive, inflammatory masses to malignant tumors. Often cytology, immunohistochemistry, and molecular genetic analyses are necessary to distinguish benign from malignant processes.

Langerhans cell histiocytosis is now the preferred term for histiocytosis X, eosinophilic granuloma, Hand–Schüller–Christian disease, and Letterer–Siwe disease. On the relatively benign end of the spectrum, Langerhans cell histiocytosis may present as a unifocal bony orbital mass (Fig. 2.4). These are thought to represent 1–3% of pediatric orbital tumors [1]. Presenting signs may include orbital signs with or without evidence of orbital inflammation. CT will demonstrate an intraosseous lytic lesion. A complete systemic workup is mandatory. Treatment is controversial and may involve observation, excision and curettage, steroids, radiation therapy, and chemotherapy. Systemic chemotherapy may be considered in an effort to decrease the likelihood that the patient will develop diabetes insipidus.

Juvenile xanthogranuloma is a non-Langerhans cell histiocytosis. Although cutaneous and ocular involvement is more common, isolated orbital tumors do occur [10]. There is no systemic involvement. Treatment modalities include observation, steroids, chemotherapy, and radiation therapy.

Reactive lymphoid hyperplasia is a term used to describe benign lymphoproliferative lesions of the orbit. Lymphoproliferative orbital masses can present as a

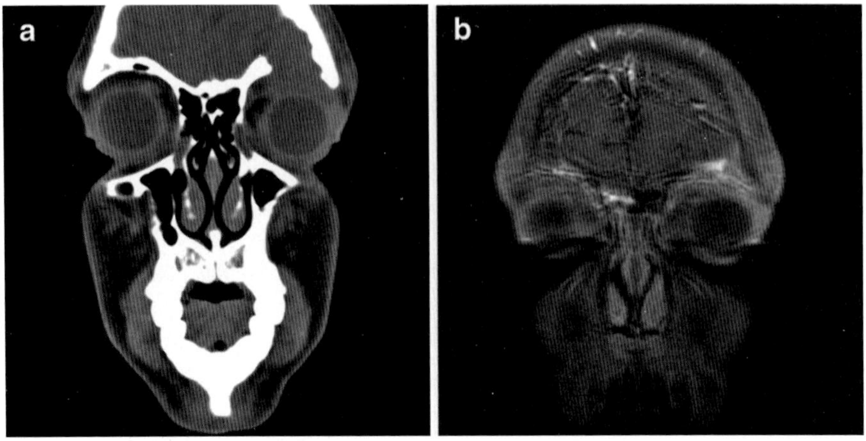

Fig. 2.4 (**a**) Computed tomography of Langerhans cell histiocytosis of orbit with extension into the frontal lobe in a 12-year old. (**b**) There was significant resolution of the mass in the orbit with biopsy and curettage of the lesion through an anterior orbitotomy approach with injection of intralesional steroids

visible mass beneath the conjunctiva, described as a "salmon patch," or with painless proptosis. Imaging will demonstrate a heterogeneous mass molding the adjacent structures without invasion. Biopsy and systemic workups are necessary to establish a diagnosis under the Revised European and American Lymphoma classification [11]. Classifying orbital lymphomas is a complex and rapidly evolving field; however, as our understanding of lymphoma continues to expand, the number of orbital lesions classified under the term "reactive lymphoid hyperplasia" diminishes. For a more detailed discussion of treatment option for benign lymphoid hyperplasia, please refer to Chapter 1.

2.5 Inflammatory Masses

Noninfectious orbital inflammation may affect any orbital structure, including the lacrimal gland, muscles, fat, and optic nerve. Systemic causes include thyroiditis, sarcoidosis, vasculitis, and lupus. Biopsy may be necessary to establish a diagnosis [12].

Idiopathic orbital inflammation can frequently present with edema of orbital structures, causing an orbital pseudotumor. Eyelid edema and erythema, orbital pain, restrictive dysmotility, diplopia, and uveitis may be present. The extraocular muscles, lacrimal gland, orbital fat, or posterior sclera may be involved. If the extraocular muscles are involved, CT will demonstrate enlargement of the muscle belly and tendon, distinguishing this from thyroid orbitopathy. Treatment with oral steroids is often rapidly effective, but rebound inflammation can occur during the tapering off of steroids.

2.6 Mesenchymal Tumors

Benign mesenchymal tumors of the orbit include lipomas, fibrous histiocytomas, solitary fibrous tumor, fibrous dysplasia, and osteomas. Dermolipoma, or lipodermoid, is a benign congenital tumor typically visible lateral to the globe. The tumor is typically unilateral, smooth, and yellow. Histologically, there is a mixture of collagenous and adipose tissue surrounded by a stratified squamous epithelium. These tumors do not typically require excision and may be associated with Goldenhar syndrome [1]. Fibrous histiocytomas are rare orbital tumors that may be benign or malignant. Benign tumors can typically be resected without recurrence [13]. A solitary fibrous tumor is a mesenchymal tumor that rarely involves the orbit; when it does involve the orbit, it is typically indolent [14], is well encapsulated, and can often be resected en bloc. Many pathologists believe that solitary fibrous tumor is closely related to hemangiopericytoma from the standpoint of its biological and clinical behavior. Fibrous dysplasia is a genetic but nonfamilial osteodystrophy that can affect craniofacial bones, including the orbit [15]. Osteomas are benign, slowly progressive bony tumors that can invade the orbit from the paranasal sinus.

2.7 Neurogenic Tumors

Orbital neurogenic tumors arise from the optic nerve or peripheral orbital nerves. Optic nerve gliomas (also known as juvenile pilocytic astrocytomas) are benign, slow-growing optic nerve tumors. Although most often intraorbital, they can affect the optic chiasm and tract. Typically presenting between 2 and 6 years of age, they account for 2–3% of all pediatric orbital tumors. Girls are affected more often than boys at a ratio of 3:2 [1]. Twenty-five percent of patients with optic nerve gliomas have neurofibromatosis type I, and 15% of patients with neurofibromatosis type I will develop an optic nerve glioma [16]. CT or MRI scans will show characteristic fusiform enlargement of the optic nerve. Management involves observation, surgical resection, and radiation therapy or chemotherapy. These tumors are often stable and may involute; thus, observation is often employed. Surgical resection results in a loss of vision but may be necessary when the tumor threatens the chiasm or causes significant proptosis and corneal exposure.

Neurofibromas are benign tumors that arise from peripheral nerves and contain axons, Schwann cells, and fibroblasts. Plexiform neurofibromas can involve the orbit and eyelid and may result in S-shaped ptosis (Fig. 2.5). They have been described as a "bag of worms" on examination and are pathognomonic for neurofibromatosis type I [1]. These tumors are difficult to excise completely. Isolated neurofibromas can usually be excised without recurrence. Malignant transformation is rare, but transformation to sarcoma has been observed and warrants aggressive therapy (Fig. 2.6).

Meningiomas arise from the arachnoid villi and can be invasive. Orbital meningiomas most often arise from the intracranial portion of the sphenoid wing (Fig. 2.7)

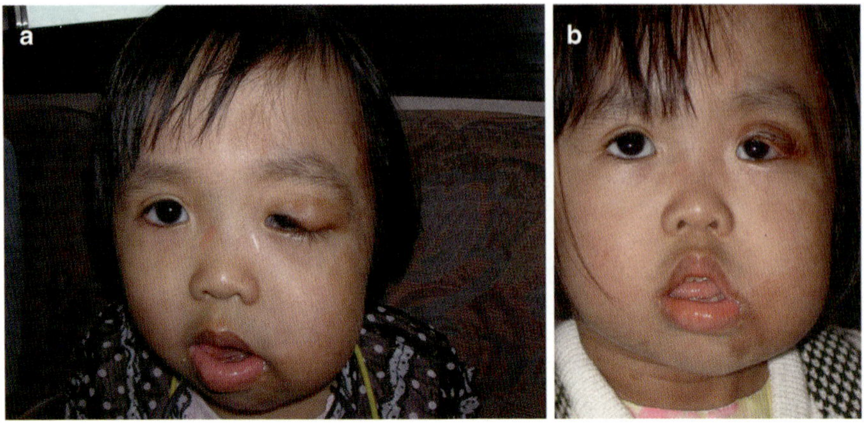

Fig. 2.5 (**a**) Plexiform neurofibroma of upper eyelid causing a secondary mechanical ptosis and amblyopia in a 3-year old with neurofibromatosis. (**b**) Appearance after debulking of the mass and correction of ptosis. Photos are courtesy of Dr. Bita Esmaeli

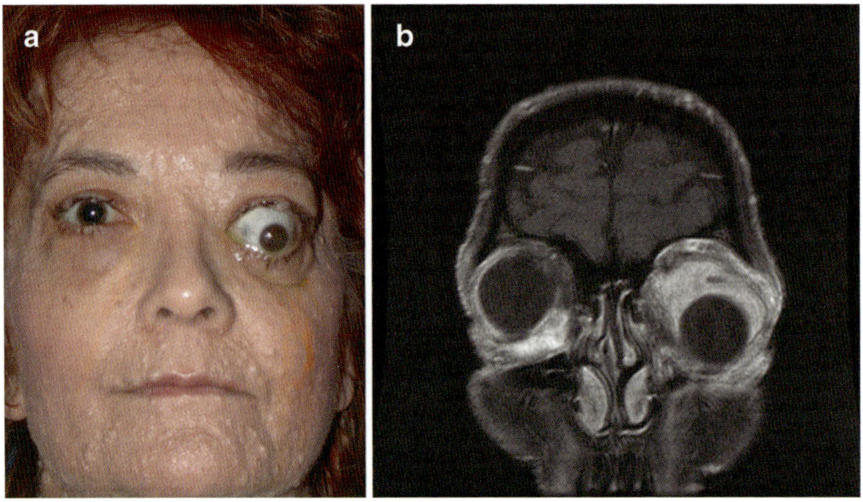

Fig. 2.6 Orbital neurofibroma transformed to sarcoma. (**a**) External photograph of a patient with neurofibromatosis and long-standing bilateral orbital neurofibromas with the right orbital neurofibroma recently transformed to sarcoma. (**b**) MRI of a right orbital sarcoma transformed from a neurofibroma in the same patient. Photos are courtesy of Dr. Bita Esmaeli

and extend into the orbit through the bone, superior orbital fissure, or optic canal. Orbital signs including proptosis and early visual deficits can occur. CT will demonstrate hyperostosis and may show intralesional calcifications. Primary orbital meningiomas are less common and arise from the optic nerve sheath. Compressive

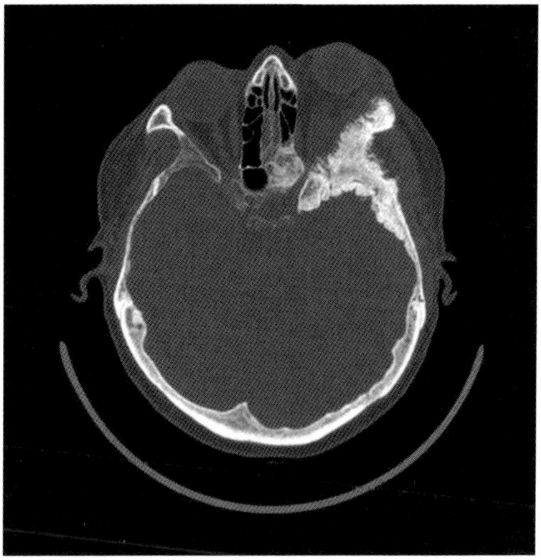

Fig. 2.7 Computed tomography scan demonstrating sphenoid wing meningioma of the right orbit. Note hyperostosis of sphenoid bone. Figure courtesy of Dr. Bita Esmaeli

optic neuropathy and vision loss are often the presenting signs. The clinical triad of proptosis, optic atrophy, and an opto-ciliary shunt vessel has been described but is not pathognomonic. Imaging will demonstrate tubular enlargement of the optic nerve that may have a "tram track" appearance ("tram track" refers to the appearance of the enhancing tumor surrounding the central nonenhancing optic nerve on axial imaging). Treatment options include observation, radiation therapy, and surgical excision [17]. Radiation therapy is offered when there is documented progressive visual loss. Surgical excision of optic nerve sheath meningiomas often results in blindness and should be reserved for cases that threaten the optic chiasm.

Schwannomas, or neurilemomas, arise from Schwann cells on peripheral nerves. In the orbit they arise most often on the first division of the trigeminal nerve. They are typically well encapsulated and have a fusiform appearance on imaging. Schwannomas are typically isodense to brain on CT and MRI. They are often amenable to surgical excision [18].

2.8 Lacrimal Gland Tumors

Most lacrimal gland tumors are inflammatory or lymphoproliferative lesions [7]. Epithelial tumors of the lacrimal gland are divided into benign pleomorphic adenomas and malignant lesions. Pleomorphic adenomas typically present with painless proptosis, and imaging demonstrates a well-defined mass in the lacrimal gland fossa. Complete surgical resection without incisional biopsy is recommended because of the risk of recurrence and malignant transformation [19]. For a more detailed discussion of lacrimal gland neoplasms, please see Chapter 7.

References

1. Castillo BV Jr, Kaufman L. Pediatric tumors of the eye and orbit. Pediatr Clin North Am 2003;50:149–72.
2. Ahuja R, Azar NF. Orbital dermoids in children. Semin Ophthalmol 2006;21:207–11.
3. Shields JA, Shields CL. Orbital cysts of childhood—classification, clinical features, and management. Surv Ophthalmol 2004;49:281–99.
4. Becker BB. The treatment of congenital dacryocystocele. Am J Ophthalmol 2006;142:835–8.
5. Scheuerle AF, Steiner HH, Kolling G, et al. Treatment and long-term outcome of patients with orbital cavernomas. Am J Ophthalmol 2004;138:237–44.
6. Valentini V, Nicolai G, Fabiani F, et al. Surgical treatment of recurrent orbital hemangiopericytoma. J Craniofac Surg 2004;15:106–13.
7. Shields JA, Shields CL, Scartozzi R. Survey of 1264 patients with orbital tumors and simulating lesions: the 2002 Montgomery lecture, part 1. Ophthalmology 2004;111:997–1008.
8. Trombly R, Sandberg DI, Wolfe SA, et al. High-flow orbital arteriovenous malformation in a child: current management and options. J Craniofac Surg 2006;17:779–82.
9. Leibovitch I, Modjtahedi S, Duckwiler GR, et al. Lessons learned from difficult or unsuccessful cannulations of the superior ophthalmic vein in the treatment of cavernous sinus dural fistulas. Ophthalmology 2006;113:1220–6.
10. Vick VL, Wilson MW, Fleming JC, et al. Orbital and eyelid manifestations of xanthogranulomatous disease. Orbit 2006;25:221–5.
11. Coupland SE, Hummel M, Stein H. Ocular adnexal lymphomas: five case presentations and a review of the literature. Surv Ophthalmol 2002;47:470–90.
12. Gordon LK. Orbital inflammatory disease: a diagnostic and therapeutic challenge. Eye 2006;20:1196–206.
13. Bajaj MS, Pushker N, Kashyap S, et al. Fibrous histiocytoma of the lacrimal gland. Ophthal Plast Reconstr Surg 2007;23:145–7.
14. Cerda-Nicolas M, Lopez-Gines C, Gil-Beso R, et al. Solitary fibrous tumor of the orbit: morphological cytogenetic and molecular features. Neuropathology 2006;26:557–63.
15. Hullar TE, Lustig LR. Paget's disease and fibrous dysplasia. Otolaryngol Clin North Am 2003;36:707–32.
16. Liu GT. Optic gliomas of the anterior visual pathway. Curr Opin Ophthalmol 2006;17:427–31.
17. Carrasco JR, Penne RB. Optic nerve sheath meningiomas and advanced treatment options. Curr Opin Ophthalmol 2004;15:406–10.
18. Cantore WA. Neural orbital tumors. Curr Opin Ophthalmol 2000;11:367–71.
19. Bernardini FP, Devoto MH, Croxatto JO. Epithelial tumors of the lacrimal gland: an update. Curr Opin Ophthalmol 2008;19:409–13.

Chapter 3
Pediatric Orbital Tumors

Jonathan J. Dutton and George K. Escaravage

Abstract Though pediatric orbital tumors are rarely encountered outside referral centers, ophthalmologists must maintain a strong familiarity with these entities as efficient diagnosis and treatment are often paramount for optimal outcome. Most pediatric orbital tumors are biologically benign, but depending on their growth rate and anatomic location, benign tumors in the orbit can lead to vision loss, disfigurement, and even death. In this chapter, we review the literature on and discuss the most common benign and malignant orbital tumors in the pediatric population. We discuss tumor presentation, imaging characteristics, histopathologic appearance, treatment, and prognosis. Retinoblastoma and rhabdomyosarcoma are extensively discussed in other chapters in this book.

3.1 Introduction

Pediatric ophthalmic tumors are rare and differ from ophthalmic tumors seen primarily in adulthood. The majority of ophthalmic tumors in children are biologically benign, but some benign tumors can have a major impact on vision and can even result in significant mortality. In addition, a number of malignant ophthalmic tumors occur primarily in childhood. Some pediatric tumors are congenital, presenting at birth or within the first year of life, whereas others do not typically present until later in childhood or during adolescence.

Age at presentation and clinical symptoms depend largely on tumor location and rate of growth. Orbital signs such as proptosis, globe dystopia, strabismus, decreased vision, and optic nerve compression can range from subtle to alarming. Modern imaging modalities such as computed tomography (CT), magnetic resonance imaging (MRI), and orbital ultrasonography are essential for evaluation and management, and an ophthalmic pathologist is often critical for accurate interpretation of the surgical biopsy specimen.

J.J. Dutton (✉)
Department of Ophthalmology, Kittner Eye Center, University of North Carolina School of Medicine, Chapel Hill, NC, USA
e-mail: jonathan_dutton@med.unc.edu

B. Esmaeli (ed.), *Ophthalmic Oncology*, M.D. Anderson Solid Tumor Oncology Series 6, DOI 10.1007/978-1-4419-0374-7_3,

Orbital lesions were previously classified by various methods. As histopathologic and immunohistochemical techniques have advanced, the lines historically drawn between seemingly distinct clinical entities have become blurred, and some lesions have crossed traditional clinical diagnostic boundaries. In Table 3.1, we have

Table 3.1 Most common pediatric orbital tumors

Cystic/developmental
Congenital cystic eye
Dacryocystocele
Dacryops
Dermatolipoma
Dermoid cyst/epidermoid cyst
Encephalocele
Meningocele
Meningoencephalocele
Microphthalmos with cyst
Teratoma
Vascular
Arteriovenous malformation
Capillary hemangioma
Cavernous hemangioma
Lymphangioma
Orbital varix
Infectious
Orbital abscess
Subperiosteal abscess
Histiocytic
Juvenile xanthogranuloma
Langerhans cell histiocytosis (eosinophilic granuloma)
Neural
Neurofibroma (plexiform and solitary)
Optic pathway glioma
Schwannoma
Inflammatory
Idiopathic orbital inflammatory syndrome (orbital pseudotumor)
Thyroid orbitopathy
Orbital involvement of other inflammatory conditions such as Wegener's granulomatosis and sarcoidosis
Mesenchymal tumors
Fibrous histiocytoma
Rhabdomyosarcoma
Ewing sarcoma
Other malignant tumors
Granulocytic sarcoma (chloroma)
Leukemia
Neuroblastoma
Wilms tumor

organized the major pediatric orbital tumors on the basis of pathophysiologic criteria. In the following pages, we briefly discuss the most common of these lesions.

3.2 Cystic Lesions

Collectively, cystic structures are the most commonly encountered orbital lesions in the pediatric population. Orbital cystic lesions can present as congenital or acquired lesions and are most often benign. Most orbital cystic lesions are dermoid cysts. However, other types of orbital cystic lesions are commonly reported, including neural cysts of ocular maldevelopment; neural cysts with associated central nervous system tissue; secondary cysts such as mucoceles and dentigerous cysts; parasitic cysts; and solid tumors with cystic components, such as teratomas, rhabdomyosarcomas, and adenoid cystic carcinomas.

3.2.1 Dermoid Cyst

Dermoid cysts are the most common orbital cystic lesions, accounting for over 40% of all pediatric orbital tumors and up to 89% of all orbital cystic lesions of childhood [1–3]. Typically, dermoid cysts are developmental choristomas arising from ectoderm trapped in bony sutures during embryogenic migration or caused by failure of surface ectoderm to separate from the neural tube. Dermoid cysts slowly enlarge as they fill with sebum and keratin. Growth may be outward into the eyelid, in which case cysts typically present in early childhood, or inward into the orbit, in which case cysts tend to present later in life. Most dermoids arise from keratinized squamous epithelium, but occasionally dermoids can originate from nonkeratinized conjunctival epithelium with goblet cells [4, 5]. Epidermoid cysts present similarly but lack dermal adnexal elements in the cyst wall.

3.2.1.1 Clinical Presentation

Orbital dermoid cysts can present at any age from infancy to old age, though they most commonly present in childhood and the teen years [6]. Fewer than 25% are clinically evident at birth. In 90% of cases, patients present with a slow-growing, painless, subcutaneous mass. Approximately 75% of dermoids are located in the superotemporal orbit associated with the frontozygomatic suture line, though they can also present medially in the frontonasal or frontoethmoid suture lines [7]. Typically, the mass is nontender, is firm to slightly fluctuant, and mimics a lacrimal gland tumor (Fig. 3.1a). Only rarely is the globe displaced or is vision decreased [8]. Deep orbital or intraconal dermoid cysts most often present in later adolescence or early adulthood with proptosis and ocular motility disturbance; this presentation is more common with dermoid cysts of conjunctival origin. Rupture of the cyst wall can result in an intense inflammatory reaction similar to orbital cellulitis. Very

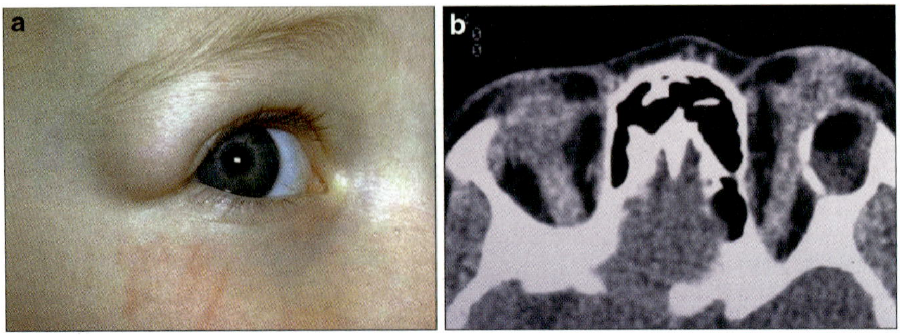

Fig. 3.1 (**a**) Young child with a dermoid cyst at the right frontozygomatic suture line. (**b**) Dermoid cyst expanding into the superolateral orbit, showing a fluid–fat interface

rarely, a dermoid cyst can be located within an extraocular muscle [9]. Particularly for medially located dermoid cysts, differential diagnosis should include various cephaloceles and dacryocystoceles, which underscores the need for orbital imaging.

3.2.1.2 Imaging

The CT appearance of orbital dermoid cysts is a round to oval, well-defined, cystic lesion, typically in the anterior superotemporal orbit (Fig. 3.1b) [10]. The lesion is almost always extraconal and has a cystic center with generally low density [11]. Denser foci within the cyst represent flecks of keratin and sebum. The cyst is surrounded by a thin rim of tissue density that may be partially calcified. Adjacent bone commonly shows remodeling, and the orbital contour can be enlarged. Occasionally, the cystic cavity extends across bones into the temporal fossa, frontal sinus, or intracranial vault [12]. Contrast administration produces enhancement of the cyst rim but not of the lumen.

On MRI with T1-weighted images, the cyst cavity produces a relatively low signal [13]. It is isointense or slightly hyperintense to vitreous and orbital muscles and hypointense to fat [14]. On T2-weighted sequences, the signal is isointense or hypointense with respect to vitreous and hyperintense to fat. Images may be homogeneous to heterogeneous depending on the cyst contents. A fat–fluid level is seen in some cases, with the upper lipid layer giving a brighter signal on T1 and a lower signal on T2 relative to the lower water–keratin layer. Newer sequencing techniques may allow improved visualization. Diffusion-weighted imaging may provide better visualization of the cystic margins and lipid component of cystic contents [15]. With gadolinium, the cyst rim shows moderate enhancement, but the lumen does not enhance.

On B-scan ultrasonography, dermoid cysts are rounded, well-outlined lesions with a smooth contour, whose internal appearance varies with the cyst's contents [16]. Orbital dermoid cysts often produce excavation of adjacent orbital bone and are occasionally associated with a small, solitary bone defect.

3.2.1.3 Histopathology

Dermoid cysts are lined by keratinized, stratified squamous epithelium, identical to that of the epidermis, with adnexal structures including sebaceous and eccrine glands and hair follicles [17]. Epidermoid cysts have a similar stratified squamous epithelium lining; however, the cyst wall lacks dermal structures or other adnexal elements. The cavity of dermoid cysts may contain keratin, hair shafts, and sebaceous secretions. If the cyst ruptures, it incites an intense granulomatous inflammatory response.

3.2.1.4 Treatment

Appropriate management of orbital dermoid cysts is complete surgical excision of the cyst wall and its contents [18]. More than half of cases show histologic evidence of leakage and associated inflammation. The risk of cyst wall rupture increases with cyst size and patient age [19], most likely because of thinning of the cystic wall with growth and increased risk of incidental trauma with increased age. Therefore, early removal is indicated to prevent tissue fibrosis. The lesions can often be bluntly dissected from most surrounding tissues; however, they are often firmly adherent at bony sutures. For deeper orbital cysts and very large cysts for which exposure is difficult, the cyst wall can be carefully opened and the cyst contents aspirated to allow safer complete resection of the cyst wall. Following any expression of cyst contents, the orbital site should be copiously irrigated with a dilute steroid solution to remove particles of lipid and keratin debris. When cysts extend into adjacent sinuses or intracranially, a combined approach with otolaryngology or neurosurgery may be required. For large dermoid cysts, percutaneous drainage and ablation with sclerosing agents under fluoroscopic guidance has been reported, but long-term data regarding recurrence after such treatment are lacking at this time [20].

3.2.1.5 Prognosis

The prognosis of patients with orbital dermoid cysts is usually excellent. The inflammatory reaction to spontaneous cyst capsular rupture can be treated effectively with systemic steroids. In rare cases, however, spontaneous rupture can result in orbital fibrosis and permanent dysfunction.

3.2.2 Teratoma

Teratoma is an extremely rare congenital solid lesion with prominent cystic components [21–23]. By definition, it contains tissue of varying maturity from all three germinal layers and may include skin, bone, cartilage, brain, bowel, lung, and glandular tissue [24]. More commonly affecting the sacrococcygeal region, head and neck, and gonads, teratoma only rarely involves the orbit, either as a primary lesion or as a secondary extension from the intracranial cavity or the paranasal sinus.

It presents unilaterally, is more common in girls, and is generally not associated with other congenital deformities or genetic syndromes [23]. Though proliferation of pluripotential stem cells is thought to contribute, the pathogenesis of teratoma remains unclear.

3.2.2.1 Clinical Presentation

If abnormalities are not noted on prenatal ultrasonography, orbital teratoma generally presents at or shortly after birth with severe, rapidly progressive unilateral proptosis with significant craniofacial distortion. There is marked stretching of the eyelids, extreme chemosis, and exposure keratopathy (Fig. 3.2). Symptoms progress during the first days or weeks of life owing to retained secretions in cystic components of the tumor. Transillumination usually demonstrates the cystic nature of this lesion. The eye is usually normal in structure; however, vision loss may occur because of globe or optic nerve compression, or the globe may rupture because of marked corneal exposure and thinning. Malignant transformation is possible in some teratomas but is extremely rare [25–28]. Orbital teratoma must be differentiated from other rapidly enlarging tumors of childhood, such as rhabdomyosarcoma. Very large tumors may extend intracranially, producing secondary hydrocephalus. Though most orbital teratomas present in children younger than 2 years of age, these lesions may also progress slowly over many years.

3.2.2.2 Imaging

On CT, teratomas appear as irregular, heterogeneous masses with both solid and multilobulated, cystic components. Cystic areas of low-attenuation fat density are seen, and a fat–fluid level may be demonstrated in some of the cyst cavities. Focal spots of internal calcification, representing formed bone elements and even teeth, are common. The orbital contour is usually enlarged, and the lesion may extend into

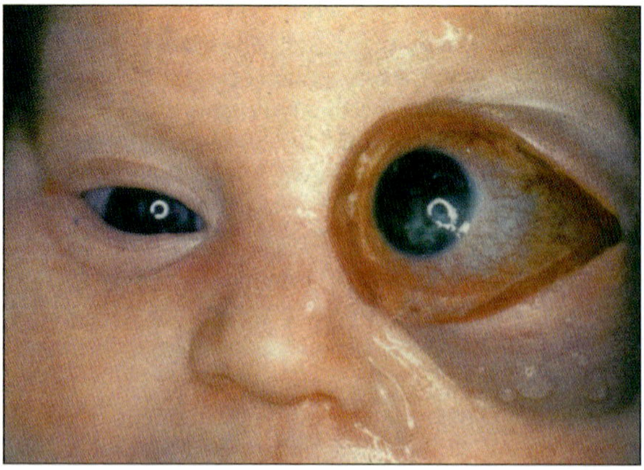

Fig. 3.2 Orbital teratoma of the left orbit displacing the globe forward. From Dutton JJ, Byrne SF, Proia AD, eds. Diagnostic Atlas of Orbital Diseases. Saunders; 2000. Reprinted with permission

adjacent sinuses or intracranially. With contrast administration, the more solid areas show moderate enhancement.

MRI of orbital teratomas shows an orbital mass with heterogeneous signal intensity representing solid and cystic elements. Regions of tissue inflammation show increased signal intensity, especially on T1-weighted images. Fat within cystic cavities, or less commonly within the cyst walls, produces a high signal intensity that is hyperintense to vitreous on T1-weighted images and hypointense to vitreous on T2-weighted images. A fat–fluid level may be seen in some cases, with the upper lipid layer giving a brighter signal on T1 and a lower signal on T2 relative to the lower water–keratin layer. With gadolinium, the solid regions and rim show moderate enhancement, but the cyst cavities do not enhance.

3.2.2.3 Histopathology

Teratomas display well-differentiated structures arising from varying proportions of ectodermal (keratinized squamous epithelium and adnexal structures), mesodermal (bone, cartilage, fat, and fibrous tissue), and endodermal germ layers (gastrointestinal or respiratory mucosa). Retained secretions from mucosal tissue form the cystic component of these lesions.

3.2.2.4 Treatment

For definitive diagnosis of orbital teratoma, fine-needle aspiration is not sufficient. For diagnosis and treatment, surgical excision with preservation of the eye is preferred if at all possible [29, 30]. In some cases, vision may be preserved. Aspiration of the cyst contents can facilitate removal of large lesions through a lateral orbitotomy incision. Advanced cases with a deformed blind eye may require enucleation or a limited exenteration for adequate removal; involvement of surrounding structures may require a combined approach with neurosurgery or otolaryngology.

3.2.2.5 Prognosis

The cosmetic result in patients with orbital teratoma following prompt surgical treatment can be good. Vision is usually decreased but may be preserved in some cases. When a teratoma is advanced or neglected, the prognosis for vision is poor owing to compression and/or exposure of ocular structures. Incompletely resected lesions may recur. Though extremely rare, tumors containing immature cells are associated with malignant degeneration; in these cases, wide surgical excision has been successfully employed. Currently, data regarding adjuvant therapies are insufficient [27].

3.3 Vascular Tumors

Vascular lesions are the second most common type of orbital tumor in the pediatric population. This group of tumors is better understood as a spectrum of disease, as lesions often have multiple components with a predominant morphology and velocity of blood flow. Capillary hemangiomas and lymphangiomas comprise the majority of pediatric orbital vascular tumors and are the focus of this section. Other vascular tumors rarely encountered in the pediatric population include cavernous hemangiomas, arteriovenous malformations, and orbital varices [31].

3.3.1 Capillary Hemangioma

Capillary hemangiomas are congenital hamartomas of vascular channels. In the orbit, they represent the most common vascular tumors of childhood. They may involve the eyelid skin or deep orbit but nearly always include an anterior component. Typically, there is a proliferative phase characterized by a period of rapid growth during the first 6–12 months of life, which is thought to be due to rapid division of immature, incompletely differentiated vascular endothelium and pericytes [32]. This is usually followed by a general involutional phase of slow regression, clinically evident in 75% of cases by 7 years of age. There is a slight female preponderance; the female:male ratio is 3:2.

3.3.1.1 Clinical Presentation

Capillary hemangiomas of the orbit usually present at birth or, less commonly, within the first year of life [33, 34]. The most common location is in the upper eyelid and superior orbit. Lesions vary from small, isolated, and clinically insignificant masses to large and disfiguring masses causing visual impairment (Fig. 3.3). Lesions with eyelid and dermal involvement most often have a nonblanching red color, while anterior lesions are fluctuant to palpation and bluish. About half of cases show tumor enlargement on crying or Valsalva maneuver. Close clinical observation is indicated as more than half of affected patients will develop amblyopia, primarily due to asymmetric astigmatism or visual deprivation because of upper eyelid ptosis.

3.3.1.2 Imaging

On CT, orbital capillary hemangiomas appear as well-defined to infiltrating masses. They may be intraconal or extraconal in location and can extend forward into the eyelids. Rarely, these lesions occur as intraosseous lesions, forming an expansile mass with intact tables. With contrast administration, enhancement is moderate to marked.

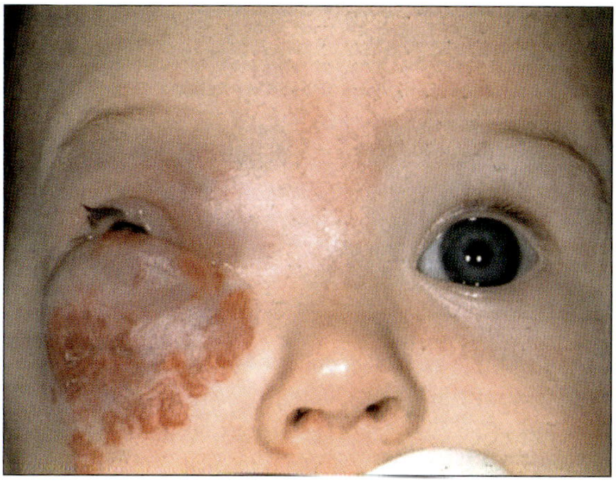

Fig. 3.3 Capillary hemangioma of the right lower eyelid occluding the pupillary axis

On T1-weighted images, capillary hemangiomas give a heterogeneous signal, hyperintense to muscle and hypointense to fat. On T2-weighted sequences, the signal remains heterogeneous with areas of both high and low intensity. Stagnant blood appears as hyperintense to fat, whereas blood with a high flow rate produces a signal void that is hypointense to other orbital tissues. With gadolinium, there is diffuse heterogeneous enhancement, best demonstrated with fat suppression algorithms.

On B-scan ultrasonography, capillary hemangiomas are typically irregular orbital masses with heterogeneous internal echoes [35]. These tumors can be quite poorly outlined, or they may display a relatively distinct posterior border. Kinetic findings include a soft, compressible consistency.

3.3.1.3 Histopathology

Capillary hemangiomas are composed of closely packed, thin-walled capillaries forming lobules. Lobules are separated by thin fibrous septa. The capillaries may be lined by flattened endothelium and contain erythrocytes, or they may have plump endothelial cells, making the vascular lumen inconspicuous [36]. The tumors are usually well circumscribed, though not encapsulated, by fibrous connective tissue.

3.3.1.4 Treatment

In most cases, the appropriate treatment of capillary hemangioma is observation. Glucocorticoid receptor expression is high in these lesions [37]. Therefore, when lesions are large, causing amblyopia, globe exposure, or optic nerve compromise, intralesional or systemic steroids are most commonly used and generally result in dramatic regression [38]. The treatment regimen must be tailored to tumor location and treatment responsiveness as well as to the patient's age and the inherent risks of each modality. For small, localized, noninfiltrative lesions, surgical excision can be effective [39, 40]. For larger lesions not responsive to steroids, recombinant interferon alpha-2a has been used as an alternative treatment with good results [39]. Various types of intralesional laser photocoagulation have also been found to reduce lesion size significantly [40, 41]. After a serendipitous discovery of its effectiveness, propranolol has recently been reported to be highly effective in the treatment of severe, disfiguring lesions; a multicenter trial is currently being organized to study optimal treatment paradigms [42].

3.3.1.5 Prognosis

Most capillary hemangiomas regress spontaneously by the age of 7 years, leaving a remnant of fibrofatty tissue [43, 44]. Intralesional steroid injections are generally safe and effective [45–47] but can be associated with serious complications such as central retinal artery occlusion from intravascular placement and hemodynamic continuity between the hemangioma and systemic circulation. Local steroids have also been associated with skin depigmentation, fat atrophy, eyelid necrosis, and even adrenal suppression [48–51]. Surgery can result in significant bleeding and cosmetic deformity and is often reserved for cosmetically objectionable tumor remnant.

3.3.2 Lymphangioma

Lymphangiomas are congenital lesions of abortive vascular elements that arborize among normal structures in the orbit [52]. They arise from venous anlage with variable proportions of venous and lymphatic components. Although lymphangiomas are hemodynamically isolated from large-flow vessels of the arteriovenous system, they are prone to intralesional hemorrhage from intrinsic capillaries. Such events expand portions of the vascular network into large "chocolate" cysts, leading to clinical urgency. Orbital lesions may be deep or combined with a superficial component. Approximately 65% of lymphangiomas present in the first decade of life, and 92% present by the end of the third decade [53].

3.3.2.1 Clinical Presentation

Generally, deep lesions may not be clinically apparent until there is a sudden hemorrhage, which may be associated with upper respiratory infections. Such events can be associated with motility impairment, compressive optic neuropathy, or exposure keratopathy; in such cases, the lesion must be differentiated from orbital cellulitis or rhabdomyosarcoma. Increased intraocular pressure can cause nausea and vomiting, and excessive vagal stimulation can result in bradycardia and somnolence through the oculocardiac reflex. The eyelids may be infiltrated, and more superficial components in the conjunctiva may appear as clear fluid-filled channels and cysts (Fig. 3.4a). Periorbital and facial cellulitis is sometimes associated with upper respiratory infections [54]. Recurrent hemorrhages are seen in about half of cases, and the interval between events may be weeks to decades. Hemorrhagic cysts

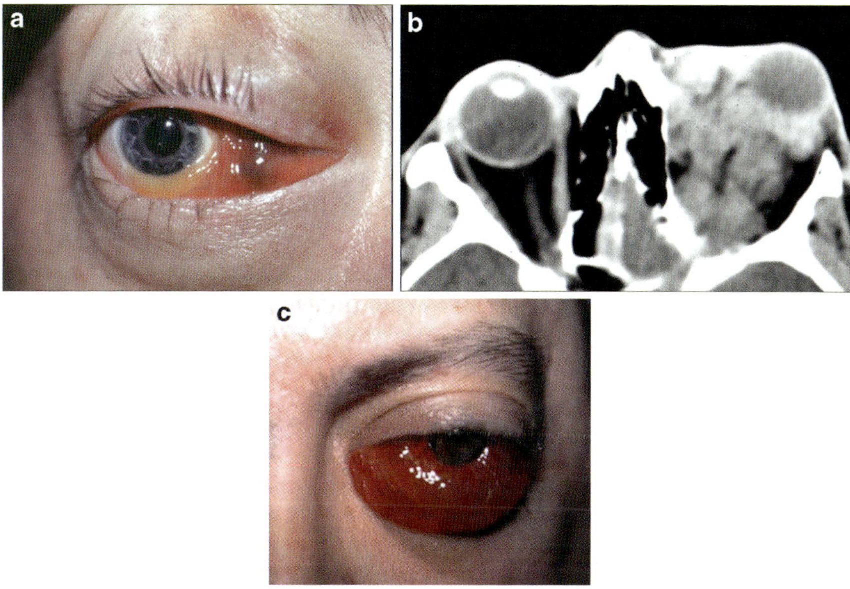

Fig. 3.4 (**a**) Orbital lymphangioma with proptosis and hemorrhagic chemosis. (**b**) CT scan of orbital lymphangioma diffusely infiltrating orbital tissues. (**c**) Massive, acute proptosis and chemosis after acute hemorrhage associated with lymphangioma

usually resolve spontaneously but in some cases require surgical drainage. Large lesions can extend intracranially; in addition, a high proportion of patients with orbital lymphangiomas have associated noncontiguous intracranial vascular anomalies, necessitating concurrent brain imaging [55, 56]. Less commonly, children and some adults present with slowly progressive, painless proptosis.

3.3.2.2 Imaging

CT in a patient with orbital lymphangioma typically shows an irregular, heterogeneous, poorly defined density that infiltrates among normal orbital structures and crosses anatomic boundaries such as the orbital septum and fascial layers (Fig. 3.4b). Low-density cystic areas are present, and occasionally calcified phleboliths may be seen [57]. With contrast administration, enhancement varies from patchy to diffuse. Larger lesions may extend into adjacent sinuses, the middle cranial fossa, or through the inferior orbital fissure into the infratemporal fossa.

MRI delineates lymphangiomas better than does CT and is more definitive in imaging of the cystic components [52, 58]. On MRI, a diffuse infiltrative mass is seen that may have one or more distinct cystic cavities [58, 59]. T1-weighted imaging produces a heterogeneous signal that is mildly hyperintense to muscle and hypointense to fat. The T2-weighted images are highly variable; blood cysts generally show a high signal intensity that is hyperintense to fat. Serpentine zones of signal voids in the orbit represent vessels containing rapidly flowing blood. Within cysts, acute hemorrhage is hypointense to muscle on T1-weighted images; older blood is hyperintense on both T1- and T2-weighted sequences because of the presence of paramagnetic methemoglobin. With further degradation of the blood to ferritin and hemosiderin, low signal intensity is seen on the T1- and T2-weighted images.

Lymphangiomas are typically composed of numerous channels that contain lymph and/or blood and thus produce heterogeneous echoes on B-scan ultrasonography [60]. Hemorrhage produces weak internal echoes, but lymph is echolucent. Endothelial-lined walls of the cystic spaces present dense acoustic interfaces. Lymph-filled channels are more easily compressible on kinetic examination than are blood-filled channels.

3.3.2.3 Histopathology

Orbital lymphangiomas are infiltrative lesions having wide variation in the size of the lymphatic channels. The channels in a given lesion vary from the size of capillaries to cavernous spaces. Attenuated endothelium resembling normal lymphatic endothelium lines the channels. The adventitial coat of the lymphatic spaces is inconspicuous in most orbital lymphangiomas. The lymphatic spaces contain proteinaceous (eosinophilic) fluid with lymphocytes, and erythrocytes may be seen after spontaneous hemorrhage into the tumor. The stroma between lymphatic channels begins as loose fibrous connective tissue with lymphoid aggregates. Older lesions and lesions previously partially resected have a fibrotic stroma, often with hemosiderin deposits from prior bleeding. Platelet-derived growth factor receptors alpha and beta and epidermal growth factor receptor tyrosine kinase are expressed on endothelial and smooth muscle cells of vascular channels [61].

3.3.2.4 Treatment

For most cases, observation is the best course of action as spontaneous hemorrhages most often spontaneously resolve [62, 63]. Close monitoring of relative afferent pupillary defects and extraocular motility is essential. Because of the highly infiltrative nature of orbital lymphangiomas, surgery is hazardous and may lead to significant damage to normal ocular and orbital structures. However, acute hemorrhagic cysts sometimes require urgent surgical evacuation because of visual compromise or corneal exposure (Fig. 3.4c). Drainage with partial resection of the cyst or ligation of feeding vessels should be the goal, rather than complete resection. Parenteral steroids have been reported to expedite resolution of signs and symptoms but are not always effective [64, 65]. Recent alternative interventions with described success include intralesional administration of sclerosing agents [66] and use of tissue adhesives to augment cystic dissection [67]. The role of platelet-derived growth factor receptor inhibitors such as imatinib mesylate is also being studied [61].

3.3.2.5 Prognosis

Except in rare cases, complete resection of orbital lymphangiomas is not possible. Recurrent hemorrhages occur in over half of cases over many years. Severe amblyopia unresponsive to therapy and disfiguring cosmesis are common sequelae. Relentless orbital bleeding with severe pain may require orbital exenteration for palliation. Poor visual outcome and sequelae of orbital scarring are associated with multiple surgeries.

3.4 Histiocytic Lesions

Though much less common than cystic or vascular lesions, histiocytic orbital tumors are also commonly reported in the pediatric population. Histiocytic proliferation in bone and soft tissues can affect any location in the body; however, the pediatric entities of most significance for the ophthalmologist are Langerhans cell histiocytosis (eosinophilic granuloma) and juvenile xanthogranuloma. Juvenile xanthogranuloma, which is caused by macrophage-derived non-Langerhans-cell histiocytes, is rarely encountered in the orbit and most commonly presents as iris lesions or cutaneous nodules. On the other hand, the dendritic histiocytic proliferation of the Langerhans cell histiocytosis spectrum of disease ranges from solitary orbital lesions to disseminated fatal disease. The most common form, eosinophilic granuloma, is the focus of this section.

3.4.1 Eosinophilic Granuloma

Langerhans cell histiocytosis is a spectrum of disease, ranging from solitary bone lesions to acute systemic, life-threatening involvement [68, 69]. It involves the pathologic proliferation of Langerhans cells, which is thought to result from a cytokine-mediated immune dysregulation [70]. Eosinophilic granuloma accounts for up to 70% of cases of Langerhans cell histiocytosis and is unifocal, primarily involving the skull [71, 72]. Orbital involvement is common, predominantly in children and teens. The peak incidence is at 5–10 years of age, and males are affected more than females in a ratio of 2:1.

3.4.1.1 Clinical Presentation

Symptoms of eosinophilic granuloma usually develop rapidly over weeks to months. The most common orbital site of involvement is superotemporal in the zygomatic and frontal bones, the marrow of which is a potential site for Langerhans cell proliferation. Patients typically present with an expanding painful mass, upper eyelid swelling, ptosis, and displacement of the globe (Fig. 3.5a). Local tenderness and erythema of the overlying skin are usually prominent features. In patients with this

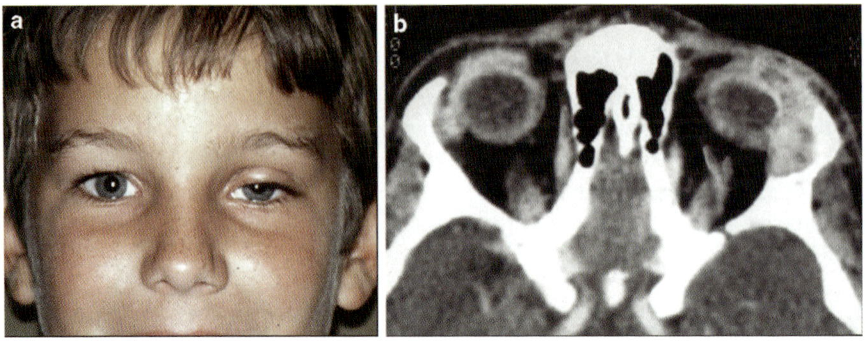

Fig. 3.5 (**a**) Eosinophilic granuloma at the left superotemporal orbital rim, causing ptosis of the upper eyelid. (**b**) CT scan showing the lesion originating in the zygomatic bone

presentation and with bony destruction noted on imaging, dermoid cysts, neuroblastoma, Ewing sarcoma, Wilms tumor, and lacrimal gland malignancies must be considered in the differential diagnosis.

3.4.1.2 Imaging

On CT, a soft-tissue mass of moderate density is characteristically seen near the superotemporal bony orbital rim [73]. The mass occurs within a well-defined osteolytic defect with irregular "punched-out" borders that may extend into the intracranial fossa (Fig. 3.5b). The inner and outer tables are unevenly involved, producing a "beveled edge" appearance. Marginal sclerosis and variable periosteal reaction may be present. With contrast administration, there is mild enhancement.

On MRI, bone destruction appears as an irregular signal void. The soft-tissue component produces a well-circumscribed heterogeneous signal that is hyperintense to muscle and hypointense to fat on T1-weighted images. T2-weighted images demonstrate high-signal areas that are hyperintense to fat. Enhancement with gadolinium is marked and slightly heterogeneous. Intracranial extension is sometimes demonstrated on MRI when it is not seen on CT.

3.4.1.3 Histopathology

Langerhans cells are large histiocytes with grooved or folded nuclei. In eosinophilic granuloma, the Langerhans cells are mixed with mononuclear and multinucleated histiocytes, lymphocytes, plasma cells, and neutrophils. The eosinophilic component of the infiltrate varies from scattered cells to sheets of eosinophils. Classically, intracytoplasmic Birbeck granules can be demonstrated in the Langerhans cells by electron microscopy. However, this diagnostic confirmation has largely been replaced with positive immunohistochemical staining for S100 protein and CD1a [74].

3.4.1.4 Treatment

After diagnostic confirmation with biopsy, management with subtotal surgical curettage has yielded good results with lesion involution and reossification [75]. Intralesional corticosteroids can provide additional benefit [76], likely by inhibition of the cytokine inflammatory mediators interleukin-1 and prostaglandin E2 [68]. Historically, low-dose radiotherapy at 900–1500 cGy has also yielded good results; however, it probably should be reserved for lesions not responsive or not amenable to surgical intervention or intralesional steroids. For patients with multifocal or systemic involvement, a multidisciplinary approach with pediatric oncology is recommended because, particularly in children younger than 1 year of age, these findings significantly raise the risk of recurrence, reactivation, and death [77]. Some studies suggest that administration of systemic chemotherapy may help prevent future onset of diabetes insipidus, orthopedic problems, and hearing and other neurologic sequelae [78]. More aggressive attempts at complete resection and various combinations of chemotherapeutic protocols have been reported [79].

3.4.1.5 Prognosis

In children with eosinophilic granuloma, the prognosis for vision and for life is excellent. Spontaneous resolution with healing of the bony defects has been reported. Treatment with surgery or radiotherapy generally results in a cure. However, these children should be followed with serial examinations and CT in a concerted effort with pediatric oncology.

3.5 Neural Tumors

Pediatric orbital tumors of neural origin may arise from the optic nerve or any of the peripheral nerves in the orbit. Of neuroectodermal origin, these tumors typically present with acquired, progressive proptosis or vision loss in childhood and are most often benign. The most commonly encountered neural orbital tumors, optic nerve gliomas and plexiform neurofibromas, are highly associated with neurofibromatosis type 1 and are described below. Others neural orbital tumors include solitary neurofibroma, schwannoma (neurilemoma), medulloblastoma, and neuroblastoma (usually metastatic to the orbit and discussed later in this chapter).

3.5.1 Optic Nerve Glioma

Optic nerve gliomas are uncommon neoplasms of astrocytic glia located along the visual pathways [80]. They represent 1.5–3.5% of all orbital tumors and 66% of primary optic nerve tumors [81]. Gliomas are seen most commonly in children, with a mean age at presentation of approximately 9 years [82]. Males and females are equally affected. The optic nerve alone is involved in 24% of cases; the chiasm is involved with or without at least one contiguous optic nerve in the remaining 76% of cases. In 46% of patients, invasion of the midbrain or the third ventricle is present. About 29% of optic gliomas are seen in patients with neurofibromatosis type 1, and 15% of patients with neurofibromatosis develop optic gliomas [83]. In patients with neurofibromatosis, the mean age at diagnosis of optic glioma is younger [84], and the tumor tends to involve the chiasm less frequently. The presence of bilateral optic nerve gliomas is virtually diagnostic of neurofibromatosis.

3.5.1.1 Clinical Presentation

Most children with optic nerve glioma present with slowly progressive decreased vision [84]. More than 55% have visual acuity of 20/300 or worse in the affected eye at diagnosis [81]. Proptosis is frequent with gliomas involving the orbital portion of the optic nerve but is uncommon when the lesion primarily involves the chiasm (Fig. 3.6a). Motility disturbance or nystagmus occurs in 25% of cases. Optic atrophy is a typical finding, but one-third of cases present with disc edema. Chiasmal tumors can be associated with increased intracranial pressure and with hypothalamic signs, including precocious puberty, diabetes insipidus, and panhypopituitarism. Sudden enlargement of the tumor can result from mucodegeneration and arachnoid hyperplasia rather than from tumor growth. Normal orbital imaging findings in children with neurofibromatosis do not preclude the future development of optic nerve glioma [85].

3.5.1.2 Imaging

On CT, orbital glioma appears as a well-outlined enlargement of the optic nerve that is usually fusiform but may be more rounded or even multilobulated (Fig. 3.6b). Increased tortuosity or kinking of the nerve is a common finding. The tumor is isodense to brain but typically has a heterogeneous structure. Less dense cystic spaces

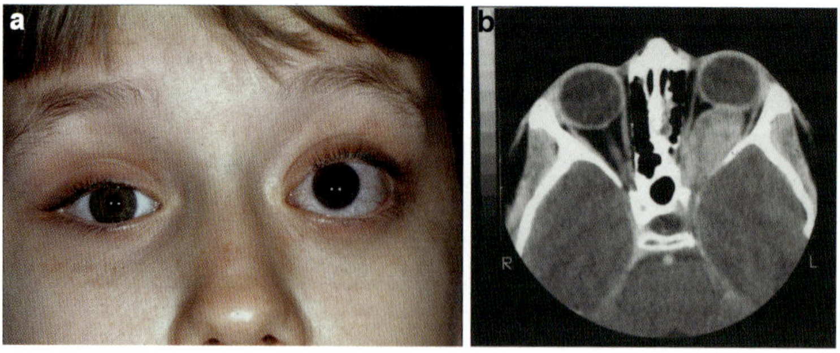

Fig. 3.6 (**a**) Left optic nerve glioma in a child with neurofibromatosis type 1. (**b**) CT scan showing a fusiform lesion of the optic nerve extending from the globe to the orbital apex

correspond to areas of mucinous accumulation. Small high-attenuation foci of calcification are rare. Following contrast administration, enhancement is heterogeneous and varies from imperceptible to moderate.

In general, MRI is regarded as superior to CT in imaging of optic gliomas, and particularly in identifying intracranial extension [86, 87]. On T1-weighted images, gliomas are isointense or slightly hypointense with respect to cortical gray matter. A dilated subarachnoid space filled with cerebrospinal fluid may appear on MRI as a hypointense zone surrounding the tumor. Low-signal hypointense areas within the lesion represent cysts of mucinous degeneration and necrosis. On T2-weighted images, the signal may be more variable. Small fusiform tumors can be homogeneously hyperintense owing to the proton-rich water component and prolonged relaxation time. Larger lesions are usually heterogeneous, with a peripheral zone of hyperintense arachnoidal hyperplasia and cerebrospinal fluid and a hypointense inner zone of optic nerve and glial cells. There is moderate to marked enhancement with gadolinium, but less than with meningiomas. Chiasmal or optic tract enhancement is a sign of intracranial involvement.

3.5.1.3 Histopathology

The histologic picture is that of a low-grade pilocytic ("hair-like") astrocytoma. Elongated spindle-shaped astrocytes with uniform oval nuclei form intersecting bundles that distend the fibrous pial septa of the optic nerve. The astrocytes are cytologically benign, and mitotic figures are not apparent. In most tumors, there are some astrocytes with spherical or cylindrical, swollen cell processes that stain brightly eosinophilic ("Rosenthal fibers"). There are usually pale cystic areas scattered among the astrocytes; these contain mucin (glycosaminoglycans) that can be highlighted using immunohistochemical stains. Mucin may be particularly prominent in long-standing tumors. If the tumor infiltrates the surrounding meninges, the astrocytes are accompanied by fibroblasts and meningothelial cells. Though confirmation is not usually necessary for diagnosis, the astrocytic nature of the neoplasm can be immunohistochemically confirmed in paraffin sections using antibodies against glial fibrillary acidic protein.

3.5.1.4 Treatment

The goal of treatment of optic gliomas is to halt vision loss or tumor growth.

The natural history and the clinical course of optic gliomas are highly variable. As a result, therapeutic options are controversial and must be individualized.

For lesions confined to the orbit in patients with good vision, minimal proptosis, and no signs of progression, observation with serial examination and MRI is appropriate. Advances in therapeutic regimens and the negative sequelae of alternative treatments have brought many authors to recommend chemotherapy as first-line treatment for all children [88]. While chemotherapy may shrink tumors and delay progression, visual acuity typically does not improve, and a high progression rate persists [82, 89]. Traditionally, use of radiotherapy had been limited to advanced cases in older children owing to the risk of neurocognitive effects, secondary malignancies, endocrinopathies, and cerebrovascular disease, such as moyamoya disease; however, newer techniques that limit damage to normal tissues, such as fractionated stereotactic radiotherapy and proton beam radiotherapy, have been reported to be effective in preventing progression and are less likely to cause damage to normal tissues [90]. Surgical debulking is now typically limited to hypothalamic debulking combined with adjuvant therapy and shunting in cases of secondary hydrocephalus. In addition, because of certain loss of vision, resection of orbital optic nerve gliomas is currently limited to scenarios in which proptosis is of cosmetic concern or causing severe exposure.

3.5.1.5 Prognosis

Tumor location determines prognosis for vision and for life. More posterior tumors tend to cause more visual loss [91]. After the initial visual deterioration seen in 80% of patients, vision tends to stabilize. In 26% of cases, vision remains better than 20/40, and in 45% of cases, vision remains better than 20/200. For lesions confined to the orbit, prognosis for life is excellent, and the mortality rate is less than 5%. With chiasmal involvement, the mortality rate remains less than 10% [92]. Tumors associated with midbrain invasion are associated with a 55% mortality rate over 10 years. There is some evidence that sporadic lesions are associated with higher morbidity than neurofibromatosis-associated gliomata [93].

3.5.2 Plexiform Neurofibroma

Plexiform neurofibroma represents 1–2% of all orbital tumors. It is the most common benign peripheral nerve tumor occurring in the eyelid and orbit and is considered pathognomonic for neurofibromatosis. The lesion can arise from and grow along any peripheral nerve, but in the orbit, it most often involves sensory nerves.

A hamartoma of neuroectodermal origin, plexiform neurofibroma typically presents in children during the first decade of life, and one-third of tumors involve the eyelids. Plexiform neurofibroma may be associated with widening of the superior orbital fissure or defects in the greater sphenoid wing. It should be differentiated from solitary neurofibromas, which are isolated, well demarcated on imaging, and typically completely resectable.

3.5.2.1 Clinical Presentation

When the eyelid is involved, plexiform neurofibroma has a characteristic S shape due to thickening, fat deposition, and horizontal redundancy [94]. On palpation, the individual thickened nerve bundles have been described as feeling like a "bag of worms." Mechanical ptosis can be profound and in younger children may result in deprivation amblyopia (Fig. 3.7). With orbital involvement, the globe can be proptotic or enophthalmic, depending on the degree of bony expansion of the

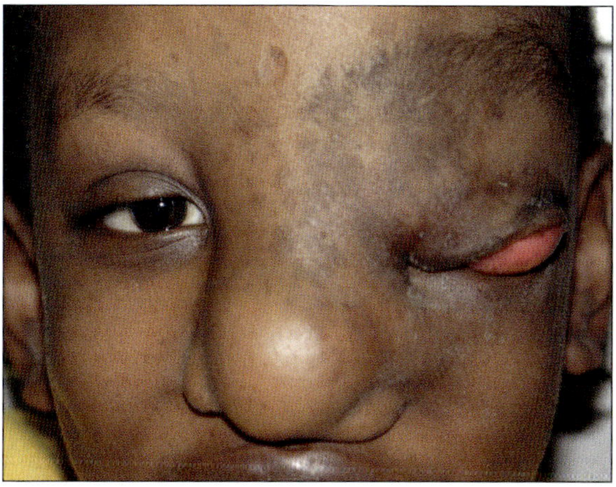

Fig. 3.7 Plexiform neurofibromatosis of the left eyelids and face with typical S-shaped contour of the upper lid

orbit and the degree of greater sphenoid wing dysplasia [95]. With large defects in the sphenoid bone, the temporal lobe may herniate into the orbit, causing pulsatile exophthalmos. The orbital lesion may be associated with uveal neurofibromas (50%), iris nodules (77%), prominent corneal nerves (25%), or optic nerve gliomas (15%). There may also be extensive temporal and facial involvement and intracranial extension [96].

3.5.2.2 Imaging

On CT, plexiform neurofibroma appears as a moderately dense, irregular, diffuse mass that crosses multiple tissue planes. There is thickening of eyelids and periorbital soft tissues. Abnormalities may include increased density of intraconal fat due to involvement of small intraconal nerves; irregular nodular thickening of optic nerve sheath from tumor involvement of posterior ciliary nerves; or thickening of sclera/choroid from tumor within these structures. Plexiform neurofibroma surrounds normal orbital structures and may be inseparable from extraocular muscles. The orbital contour and superior orbital fissure are frequently enlarged. When large regions of the sphenoid bone are absent, a meningoencephalocele may prolapse into the orbit. With contrast administration, the tumor shows moderate enhancement.

The MRI appearance is of an ill-defined and irregular mass in the orbit or the eyelid. On T1-weighted images, the tumor produces a heterogeneous, hypointense signal with respect to muscle. Signal intensity is increased on T2-weighted sequences, where the tumor is hyperintense to muscle and isointense or slightly hyperintense to fat. Tumor is best demonstrated using fat suppression techniques. With gadolinium, enhancement is variably mild to moderate.

3.5.2.3 Histopathology

In plexiform neurofibromas, large segments of peripheral nerve become convoluted and appear like a "bag of worms" macroscopically. Microscopically, there is an unencapsulated tortuous mass of expanded nerve branches, each surrounded by a perineurium. In early lesions, the nerve is swollen by endoneurial accumulation of myxoid (glycosaminoglycan-rich) matrix. As the lesions age, Schwann cells proliferate, and collagen accumulates within the nerves.

3.5.2.4 Treatment

Management is usually frustrating and disappointing for the patient and surgeon because of the infiltrative nature and vascularity of this tumor. Typically, complete resection is uncommon, and recurrences are expected. When the lesion is stable or its enlargement does not cause visual loss or psychosocial concern, observation is prudent [97]. Repeated surgical debulking may be necessary to maintain visual function and for some cosmetic improvement. Concurrent conservative levator resection can aid in ptosis repair. Advances in custom alloplastic implants and computer-aided stereolithography have been described to address pulsatile exophthalmos [98]. In cases of poor vision, severe proptosis, and orbital pain, exenteration may be considered, followed by appropriate reconstruction [99]. There is no role for radiotherapy, and it may increase the risk of secondary malignancies [100].

3.5.2.5 Prognosis

The overall prognosis for life is good. Rarely, the tumor can erode into the cranial cavity with fatal results, and patients with neurofibromatosis have a significant risk of secondary malignant tumors. The prognosis for vision depends on the extent of tumor invasion as well as the potential complications of surgical intervention. Rarely, rhabdomyosarcoma has been reported in association with neurofibromatosis type 1 and should be considered by the clinician if initial presentation or clinical course is atypical [101]. Malignant transformation of neurofibromas into myxoid sarcomas and development of malignant peripheral nerve sheath tumors have also been reported in a small proportion of patients with neurofibromatosis [100, 102]. Please also see Chapter 2 and Fig. 2.6.

3.6 Malignant Lesions

Orbital malignancies comprise a very important minority of pediatric orbital tumors. They may be primary, secondary, or metastatic and more commonly present later in infancy and childhood. Acquired proptosis, motility disturbances, and visual compromise can range from insidious to disquieting. Combinations of therapeutic advances have improved prognosis for patients with many but not all pediatric orbital malignancies. Appropriate diagnosis and treatment requires the cooperative efforts of the orbital surgeon, pediatric oncologist, and radiotherapist. Rhabdomyosarcoma is the most commonly encountered malignant pediatric orbital tumor and is discussed elsewhere in this book (Chapter 4). We focus here on three other less commonly encountered primary malignant tumors of the orbit—Ewing sarcoma, neuroblastoma, and granulocytic sarcoma—and on retinoblastoma with orbital extension.

3.6.1 Ewing Sarcoma

Ewing sarcoma is part of a family of neoplasms characterized by undifferentiated small round cells arising in bone. Though the cell of origin is still controversial, most believe the cell of origin is a mesenchymal cell reprogrammed to a neuroectodermal phenotype [103]. The tumor classically involves the long bones of the limbs, ribs, and pelvis; when the orbit is involved, the tumor usually has arisen as a metastasis from a distant site, though primary osseous and extraosseous orbital lesions have been reported [104–106]. Seventy-five percent of patients are aged 20 years or younger, and 90% are less than 30 years old. Males are more frequently affected than females in a ratio of 1.6:1, and Ewing sarcoma primarily affects Caucasians.

3.6.1.1 Clinical Presentation

Tumor growth is typically insidious. Although the patient often comes to medical attention following an episode of trauma, ophthalmic symptoms usually have been present for months [107]. Ophthalmoplegia and ptosis are followed by proptosis, displacement of the globe, and possibly diplopia (Fig. 3.8). There may also be intermittent pain [108]. A soft nontender mass may be palpable beneath the orbital rim. Hemorrhagic necrosis may cause erythema and local warmth, simulating osteomyelitis. Systemic symptoms of fever, fatigue, anorexia, and weight loss are associated with disseminated metastases, seen in 10–30% of patients at initial diagnosis.

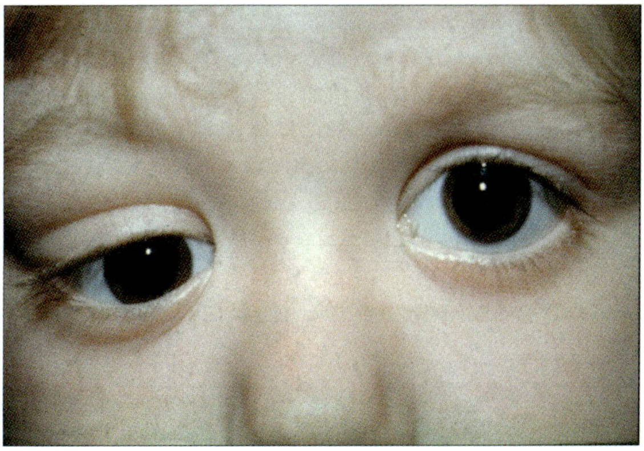

Fig. 3.8 A young child with Ewing sarcoma of the right superior orbital rim displacing the globe downward. From Dutton JJ, Byrne SF, Proia AD, eds. Diagnostic Atlas of Orbital Diseases. Saunders; 2000. Reprinted with permission

3.6.1.2 Imaging

The CT scan reveals an irregular heterogeneous cystic mass [109]. Adjacent bone shows mottled destruction, and the mass frequently extends from the maxillary sinus or mandible. Patchy hypodense areas correlate with old hemorrhage and necrosis. Enhancement with contrast administration is variable.

On MRI, an extraosseous mass is seen contiguous with bone destruction. The T1-weighted signal is low and hypointense to both fat and muscle. On T2-weighted sequences, the signal is high and is isointense to fat and hyperintense to muscle. Heterogeneity is due to areas of necrosis that produce lower signal intensity. There is generally no significant periosteal reaction. With gadolinium, only the cellular areas enhance.

3.6.1.3 Histopathology

The most common pattern of Ewing sarcoma, referred to as diffuse or cohesive, has broad sheets of uniform, small, round cells mixed with dark cells; other malignancies with similar microscopic presentation include rhabdomyosarcoma, neuroblastoma, and lymphoma. Round tumor cells are slightly larger than lymphocytes and have round nuclei (often with indentations), finely dispersed chromatin, one or two small nucleoli, and scant cytoplasm that is pale or vacuolated owing to the presence of glycogen. The cytoplasmic borders are indistinct. The dark cells have denser and more elongated nuclei and tend to form aggregates. Positive immunohistochemical staining for CD99, a cell surface glycoprotein, or for O13, a monoclonal antibody against the *MIC2* gene product, supports the diagnosis of Ewing sarcoma, though neither is specific for this entity [103, 110]. In addition, virtually all Ewing tumor cells demonstrate a translocation involving chromosome 22.

3.6.1.4 Treatment

Ewing sarcoma is typically regarded as a systemic disease until a metastatic evaluation reveals no other lesions. After initial biopsy for diagnosis, aggressive multiagent chemotherapy is initiated, using one of various combinations of vincristine, doxorubicin, cyclophosphamide, and dactinomycin [111]. After initial chemotherapeutic cytoreduction, definitive surgical excision or radiotherapy is performed, followed by consolidation chemotherapy. Regular surveillance is critical. Multiple biological therapies are under investigation [112].

3.6.1.5 Prognosis

Until recently, treatment with surgery and radiotherapy alone yielded a 5-year survival rate of only 10%. Advances in therapy, primarily in adjunctive chemotherapy, have reduced the recurrence rate to about 5% and improved the 5-year survival rate to approximately 65% [112]. However, patients with metastasis at presentation continue to have a poor prognosis, with a 25% survival rate at 5 years, though a concerted effort is under way to advance the understanding and therapeutic options for this subset of the population [113].

3.6.2 *Neuroblastoma*

Representing 8–10% of pediatric cancers, neuroblastoma is the most frequent extracranial solid tumor and the most common tumor metastatic to the orbit in children. It is a malignant neoplasm of primitive neuroblasts—progenitor cells of the sympathetic nervous system. The tumor usually arises during the first 2 years of life, and the primary tumor is usually located in the adrenal medulla or the sympathetic or parasympathetic tissues of the pelvis, chest, or cervical region. The vast majority of orbital involvement is from metastatic disease, and in 90% of these cases, the primary tumor is in the abdomen. In 92–97% of cases involving the orbit, the presence of a primary tumor in the chest or abdomen is known prior to onset of orbital symptoms, and 40% of metastatic neuroblastomas to the orbit are bilateral [114, 115]. Very rarely, neuroblastoma arises as a primary tumor in the orbit [116].

3.6.2.1 Clinical Presentation

Ophthalmic involvement develops in 20% of children with neuroblastoma. These children are often systemically ill-appearing, with fever, weight loss, and irritability. The child typically presents with rapid progression of proptosis and periorbital ecchymosis (due to rapid necrosis of tumor cells) over several weeks (Fig. 3.9). Eyelid edema, ptosis, and displacement of the globe are also common findings. In

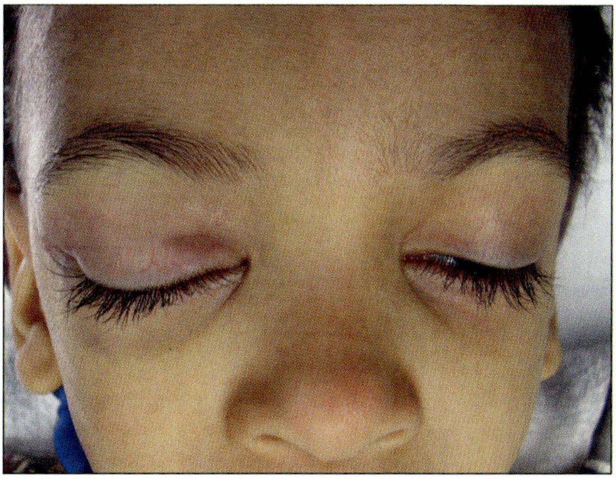

Fig. 3.9 Metastatic neuroblastoma of the right orbit with ecchymosis of the upper eyelid

5% of children, blindness is seen, either as an early finding or as a result of treatment [117]. On funduscopic examination, optic disc edema, choroidal folds, retinal striae, and dilated retinal vessels may be seen. Horner syndrome together with ipsilateral iris heterochromia, secondary to tumor in the cervical sympathetic chain, is the presenting sign in rare cases. Opsoclonus is a paraneoplastic finding that has been reported with systemic as well as localized disease [118]. Increased intracranial pressure and separation of bony sutures can be associated with intracranial metastases. In very rare instances, neuroblastoma can occur as a primary tumor in the orbit of adults.

3.6.2.2 Imaging

On CT, neuroblastoma appears as a large, irregular, poorly defined orbital mass. It may be unilateral or bilateral. Lower-attenuating, more lucent areas within the lesion represent sites of tumor necrosis and hemorrhage. Destruction of adjacent bone may be seen on bone window settings.

The MRI appearance of neuroblastoma is of a mass with ill-defined margins from infiltration into adjacent orbital structures. On T1-weighted images, the resonance signal is heterogeneous or homogeneous and hypointense to cortical gray matter and muscle. On T2-weighted images, the signal is isointense or slightly hyperintense to gray matter and muscle. With gadolinium, enhancement varies from mild to marked.

In addition to CT and MRI, scintigraphic imaging can help with staging and with evaluation of response to treatment. A norepinephrine analog, metaiodobenzylguanidine, with an attached iodine radioisotope can show bony and soft-tissue involvement due to preferential uptake by adrenergic secretory vesicles [119]. In addition, technetium 99 bone scans can further decrease the risk of false-negative imaging findings [120].

3.6.2.3 Histopathology

In neuroblastoma, small regular cells with round deeply staining nuclei, scant cytoplasm, and indistinct cell borders form sheets or vague nodules. One-fourth to one-third of cases have Homer-Wright rosettes with tumor cells around a central area containing fibrillar material. Most tumors exhibit necrosis, which may be extensive, leaving viable tumor cells only around blood vessels. Neuroblastoma cells express neuron-specific enolase, neurofilament protein, peripherin, chromogranin, synaptophysin, and other neural-related antigens. Immunohistochemical staining for neuron-specific enolase and protein gene product 9.5 [117] is often necessary to differentiate neuroblastoma from other small cell tumors such as Ewing sarcoma/primitive neuroectodermal tumor, rhabdomyosarcoma, lymphoma, and retinoblastoma.

3.6.2.4 Treatment

If orbital findings are the presenting signs, then urgent referral to pediatric oncology for systemic evaluation is critical. Systemic evaluation includes measurement of urine catecholamines, various imaging modalities for staging, and possibly bone marrow biopsy. Biopsy of orbital lesions may occasionally be necessary for diagnosis; however, resection is not indicated initially as staging will determine the most appropriate treatment. The principal treatment is chemotherapy, often including vincristine, doxorubicin, carboplatin, dacarbazine, and etoposide. After induction chemotherapy, surgical resection of primary tumors and bulky metastatic disease may be indicated. In cases of low-risk disease, surgical resection without chemotherapy may be recommended. Radiotherapy has been shown to decrease local recurrence but is typically not recommended for early-stage tumors because of the risk of secondary tumors. Autologous bone marrow transplantation is often necessary because of marrow ablation by chemotherapy. Current efforts to advance therapy include immunotherapy and targeting of biological markers of the disease [121].

3.6.2.5 Prognosis

One-third of children with orbital neuroblastoma develop visual loss either as a direct consequence of tumor or secondary to treatment. Prognosis is primarily dependent on risk stratum as determined on the basis of the initial presentation. Age at presentation, stage, histopathologic characteristics, DNA index (ploidy), and N-*myc* amplification status allow disease to be characterized and treated. Recent data reveal 95 and 90% 10-year survival rates for patients with low- and intermediate-risk disease, respectively; however, the 10-year survival rate for patients with high-risk or metastatic disease remains low, at 30–40% [119, 122]. Seventy percent of patients present to the ophthalmologist with metastatic disease, and therefore orbital disease typically portends a poor prognosis. Palliative fractional external-beam radiotherapy ($\geq$2,000 cGy) has been reported to produce good results for symptomatic metastatic lesions [123]. Once orbital metastases develop, the overall prognosis is generally poor. Despite aggressive therapy, recurrence rates of 90% may be seen at 1–2 years. The 3-year survival rate in patients with recurrence is 11%.

3.6.3 Retinoblastoma

Retinoblastoma is the most common intraocular malignancy in childhood. Chapter 14 describes its evaluation and treatment. In this section, primary consideration is given to orbital extension of retinoblastoma and the risk of secondary tumors associated with retinoblastoma.

Orbital involvement by retinoblastoma occurs via extraocular extension along the optic nerve or through scleral emissary canals. The risk of metastasis is greatly increased by orbital disease. Tumor can spread to the central nervous system via the subarachnoid space, to regional lymph nodes via the lymphatics, or hematogenously to bones or viscera.

3.6.3.1 Clinical Presentation

In developed nations, at primary presentation of retinoblastoma, extraocular extension is usually absent or only microscopic, and therefore orbital symptoms are usually absent. However, in developing nations, extraocular extension of tumor and orbital symptoms are much more common at primary presentation [124, 125]. With significant orbital involvement, proptosis or globe displacement may be seen (Fig. 3.10) [126]. Periocular inflammation similar to orbital cellulitis has also been reported [126, 127]. In developed nations, most cases of orbital retinoblastoma present as a recurrence following primary enucleation for ocular tumor. Displacement of the orbital implant, inability to wear an ocular prosthesis, ecchymosis, chemosis, bleeding from the socket, signs of cellulitis, or nondescript constitutional symptoms may be present. Tumor can spread intracranially via the paranasal sinuses or neural foramina.

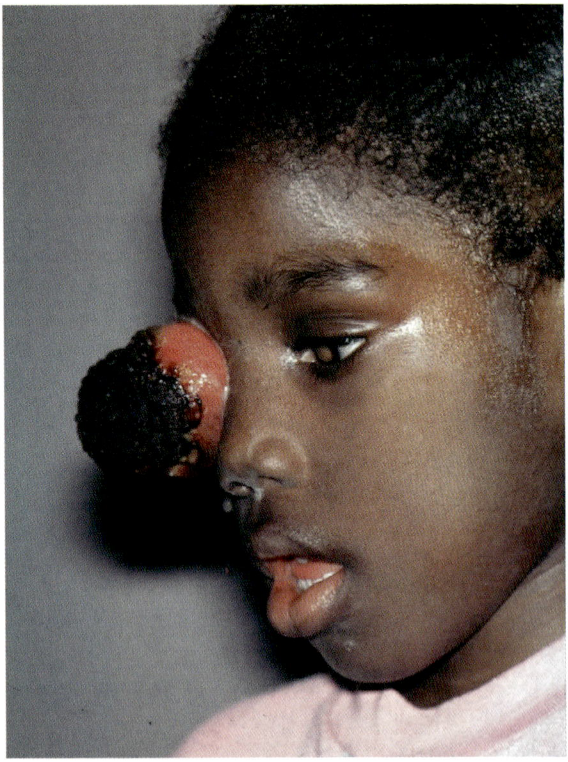

Fig. 3.10 Massive orbital extension of retinoblastoma with surface necrosis. Photograph used with permission courtesy of Dr. Ted Wojno

3.6.3.2 Imaging

On CT, orbital extension of retinoblastoma appears as a contiguous, high-density intraconal mass that may be localized along the optic nerve. Intralesional calcification is present in 90% of tumors. Mild to moderate enhancement is seen with contrast administration.

MRI is the most sensitive method for detection of orbital extension of retinoblastoma. On T1-weighted images, retinoblastoma produces a homogeneous to heterogeneous signal that is hyperintense to vitreous and muscle and hypointense to fat. On T2-weighted images, retinoblastoma is hypointense to vitreous and isointense to fat. Small foci of calcification may not be visible, but larger calcifications appear as dark signal voids on T1- and T2-weighted images. With gadolinium, the tumor shows moderate to marked heterogeneous enhancement, with areas of calcification remaining markedly hypointense [128].

3.6.3.3 Histopathology

Typically associated with an exophytic growth pattern, orbital extension of retinoblastoma or recurrent orbital tumor tends to be much less differentiated than that of the intraocular primary tumor. The tumor cells are small and round with large, deeply staining nuclei of variable size and shape and scant cytoplasm. Rosettes are uncommon and are poorly formed if present in the orbit. It is difficult, and sometimes impossible, to conclusively distinguish a recurrent retinoblastoma from a second primary tumor. Foci of calcification are noted in areas of necrosis.

3.6.3.4 Treatment

Management of orbital retinoblastoma depends on the extent of orbital involvement. For large orbital tumors, excision combined with chemotherapy and radiotherapy offers the best chances for long-term survival [129]. Exenteration should be reserved for massive orbital involvement [130]. Overall, use of external-beam radiotherapy is limited because of the risks of secondary malignancies. When radiotherapy is used in cases of positive surgical margins or massive orbital or metastatic disease, it is combined with chemotherapy to help minimize the radiation dosage [131–133]. Metastatic disease is currently being approached with various combinations of induction chemotherapy; surgery and irradiation to treat bulky disease; high-dose chemotherapy; and autologous stem cell rescue [134, 135].

3.6.3.5 Prognosis

Extraocular extension is one of the most prominent risk factors for metastatic retinoblastoma [136]. With gross orbital invasion, the likelihood of central nervous system extension, systemic metastases, and death is increased considerably, though current therapeutic regimens have resulted in a vast improvement in mortality [137–139]. The risk of secondary malignancies is well described in survivors of hereditary retinoblastomas and necessitates lifelong clinical follow-up; this risk is considerably amplified if initial treatment included irradiation [140]. In one series, rates of second malignancies were reported to be as high as 30% in the radiation field (especially in patients treated before 1 year of age) and 8% in untreated areas [141]. The most common of these secondary tumors are osteosarcoma, soft-tissue sarcomas, melanoma, and extraorbital cancers, including cancers of the brain and nasal cavities, sarcomas, and epithelial carcinomas, particularly of the lung and bladder [134, 142, 143]. Irradiation also carries the risk of cataract, keratopathy, radiation retinopathy, and retarded orbital growth in young children.

3.6.4 Granulocytic Sarcoma

The term "granulocytic sarcoma" is a misnomer—granulocytic sarcoma is an extramedullary solid tumor commonly associated with acute myelogenous leukemia (AML) in children. In adults this tumor is more commonly associated with acute lymphoblastic leukemia, chronic myelogenous leukemia, or myelodysplastic disorders [144–146]. Also referred to as chloroma or myeloid sarcoma, granulocytic sarcoma is the most common form of leukemic infiltrate involving the orbit and affects 30% of patients with AML [147]. In up to 88% of cases, orbital tumor presentation precedes the blast phase of AML by months to years, though it can also occur concurrently with the blast phase, or even during periods of remission [148].

3.6.4.1 Clinical Presentation

The mean age of presentation of granulocytic sarcoma is typically 8–9 years. The disease is unilateral in 90% of cases and presents as a rapidly enlarging orbital mass with diplopia and proptosis (Fig. 3.11a). The lateral orbital wall is most commonly involved, causing medial displacement of the globe. Pain, retinal striae, or optic disk edema may also be present [149]. Myeloperoxidase within the mass often imparts a green hue on examination, which is why granulocytic sarcoma is also referred to as chloroma. Orbital involvement can also be bilateral [150, 151].

3.6.4.2 Imaging

On CT, granulocytic sarcomas typically are irregular, are moderately defined, and have a homogeneous density (Fig. 3.11b). Often lateral in location, they may also encase or invade the lacrimal gland, extraocular muscles, or orbital fat [152]. Bony erosion and subperiosteal reaction have been noted, and contrast enhancement is uniformly minimal to moderate [153]. Brain lesions demonstrate more variability in appearance [154].

On T1-weighted images, the irregular mass is isointense to cortical gray matter and to muscle. On T2-weighted sequences, the lesion is isointense to white matter and muscle. Enhancement is homogeneous and moderate with gadolinium [155].

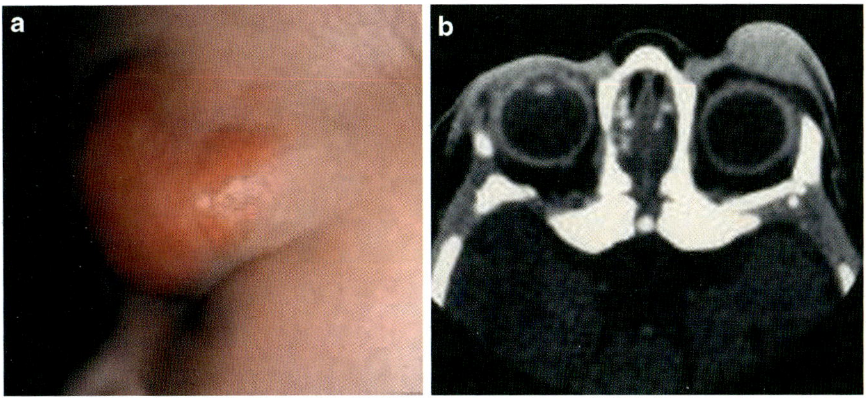

Fig. 3.11 (**a**) Rapidly enlarging granulocytic sarcoma of the superotemporal orbit causing mechanical ptosis. (**b**) CT scan showing an infiltrative, homogeneous lesion in the anterior orbit and subcutaneous eyelid soft tissue. From Dutton JJ, Byrne SF, Proia AD, eds. Diagnostic Atlas of Orbital Diseases. Saunders; 2000. Reprinted with permission

3.6.4.3 Histopathology

Granulocytic sarcomas range from being composed entirely of myeloblasts to demonstrating variable evidence of granulocytic differentiation. Myeloblasts are large cells with ovoid, vesicular nuclei, multiple nucleoli, and scant cytoplasm. With granulocytic differentiation, eosinophilic granules appear in the cytoplasm, cytoplasm increases, and the nuclei are more progressively folded. In highly differentiated tumors, eosinophils are often present. Special staining for myeloperoxidase, lysozyme, and chloracetate esterase (Leder stain) can be used to confirm the granulocytic origin of the cells [150, 156]. However, immunohistochemistry, particularly staining for CD68, is essential to confirm the diagnosis as poorly differentiated tumors are often misdiagnosed as medium- to large-cell lymphoma [157]. Cytogenetic studies demonstrate a high incidence of translocations, particularly *t*(8:21) [158].

3.6.4.4 Treatment

Granulocytic sarcoma in the setting of known systemic AML is treated primarily with chemotherapy, though surgery and radiotherapy can be used in an adjunct role [159, 160]. Bone marrow transplantation may be necessary in aggressive cases [158, 161]. In patients with localized orbital lesions and no evidence of systemic disease, radiotherapy was previously used. However, these lesions are also responsive to intensive induction chemotherapy protocols for AML.

3.6.4.5 Prognosis

The prognosis of patients with AML and granulocytic sarcoma or other forms of extramedullary infiltration was previously described to be poorer than the prognosis of patients with AML only [158, 161, 162]. However, more recently, the prognosis of patients with AML with and without extramedullary infiltration is controversial and under close study [163]. The 5-year event-free survival rates are typically between 30 and 40%, though higher white blood cell counts and central nervous system involvement are reportedly poor prognostic indicators [164, 165]. There may be a role for positron emission tomography in the evaluation of response and relapse [166].

3.6.5 Rhabdomyosarcoma

Rhabdomyosarcoma is the most common soft-tissue mesenchymal tumor and the most common malignancy of the orbit in children, representing about 4% of all childhood orbital mass lesions and 1% of orbital tumors. This topic is addressed extensively in Chapter 4.

References

1. Ohtsuka K, Hashimoto M, Suzuki Y. A review of 244 orbital tumors in Japanese patient during a 21-year period: origins and locations. Jpn J Ophthalmol 2005;49(1):49–55.
2. Shields JA, Augsburger JJ, Donoso LA. Orbital dermoid cyst of conjunctival origin. Am J Ophthalmol 1986;101:726–9.
3. Shields JA, Shields CL. Orbital cysts of childhood—classification, clinical features, and management. Surv Ophthalmol 2004;49(3):281–99.
4. Dutton JJ, Fowler AM, Proia AD. Dermoid cyst of conjunctival origin. Ophthal Plast Reconstr Surg 2006;22(2):137–9.
5. McCollough ML, Glover AT, Grabski WJ, et al. Orbital dermoid cysts showing conjunctival epithelium. Am J Dermatopathol 1991;13:611–15.
6. Sherman RP, Rootman J, LaPointe JS. Orbital dermoids: clinical presentation and management. Br J Ophthalmol 1984;68:642–52.
7. Bonavolonta G, Tranfa F, de Conciliis C, et al. Dermoid cysts: 16-year survey. Ophthal Plast Reconstr Surg 1995;11:187–92.
8. Emerick GT, Shields CL, Shields JA, et al. Chewing-induced visual impairment from a dumbbell dermoid cyst. Ophthal Plast Reconstr Surg 1997;13:57–61.
9. Howard GR, Nerad JA, Bonavolonta G, et al. Orbital dermoid cysts located within the lateral rectus muscle. Ophthalmology 1994;101:767–71.
10. Blei L, Chambers JT, Liotta LA, et al. Orbital dermoid diagnosed by computed tomographic scanning. Am J Ophthalmol 1978;85:58–61.
11. Nugent RA, Lapointe JS, Rootman J, et al. Orbital dermoids: features on CT. Radiology 1987;165:475–8.
12. Sathananthan N, Moseley IF, Rose GE, et al. The frequency and clinical significance of bone involvement in outer canthus dermoid cysts. Br J Ophthalmol 1993;77:789–94.
13. De Potter P, Flanders AE, Shields CL, et al. Magnetic resonance imaging of orbital tumors. Int Ophthalmol Clin 1993;33:163–73.
14. Hakyemez B, Aksoy U, Yildiz H, et al. Intracranial epidermoid cysts: diffusion-weighted, FLAIR, and conventional MR findings. Eur J Radiol 2005;54:214–20.
15. Grove AS Jr. Giant dermoid cysts of the orbit. Ophthalmology 1979;86:1513–20.
16. Traboulsi EI, Azar DT, Khattar J, et al. A-scan ultrasonography in the diagnosis of orbital dermoid cysts. Ann Ophthalmol 1988;20:229–32.

17. Shields JA, Kaden IH, Eagle RC Jr, et al. Orbital dermoid cysts: clinicopathologic correlations, classification, and management. The 1997 Josephine E. Schuleler lecture. Ophthal Plast Reconstr Surg 1997;13:265–76.
18. Kersten RC. The eyelid crease approach to superficial lateral dermoid cysts. J Pediatr Ophthalmol Strabismus 1988;25:48–51.
19. Columbo, F, Holbach LM, Naumann GO. Chronic inflammation in dermoid cysts: a clinicopathologic study of 115 patients. Orbit 2000;19(2):97–107.
20. Golden RP, Shields WE 2nd, Cahill KV, et al. Percutaneous drainage and ablation of orbital dermoid cysts. J AAPOS 2007;11(5):438–42.
21. Appalanarasayya K, Dev OB. Teratoma of the orbit. Int Surg 1970;54:301–3.
22. Berlin AJ, Rich LS, Hahn JF. Congenital orbital teratoma. Child's Brain 1983;10:208–16.
23. Bilgic S, Dayanir V, Kiratli H, et al. Congenital orbital teratoma: a clinicopathologic case report. Ophthal Plast Reconstr Surg 1997;13:142–6.
24 Ferry AP. Teratoma of the orbit: a report of two cases. Surv Ophthalmol 1965;10:434–42.
25. Garden JW, McManis JC. Congenital orbital–intracranial teratoma with subsequent malignancy. Case report. Br J Ophthalmol 1986;70:111–13.
26. Lee GA, Sullivan TJ, Tsikleas GP, et al. Congenital orbital teratoma. Aust N Z J Ophthalmol 1997;25:63–6.
27. Mahesh L, Krishnakumar S, Subramanian N, et al. Malignant teratoma of the orbit: a clinicopathological study of a case. Orbit 2003;22(4):305–9.
28. Soares EJC, Lopes KDS, Andrafe JDS, et al. Orbital malignant teratoma. A case report. Orbit 1983;2:235–42.
29. Chang DF, Dallow RL, Walton DS. Congenital orbital teratoma: report of a case with visual preservation. J Pediatr Ophthalmol 1980;17:88–95.
30. Itami K, Traboulsi EI, Karim FWA, et al. Conservative surgery in orbital teratoma. Orbit 1986;5:61–5.
31. Gundalp I, Gunduz K. Vascular tumors of the orbit. Doc Ophthalmol 1995;89:337–45.
32. Dadras SS, North PE, Bertoncini J, et al. Infantile hemangiomas are arrested in an early developmental vascular differentiation state. Mod Pathol 2004;17(9):1068–79.
33. Haik BG, Jakobiec FA, Ellsworth RM, et al. Capillary hemangioma of the lids and orbit: an analysis of the clinical features and therapeutic results in 101 cases. Ophthalmology 1979;86:760–92.
34. Haik BG, Karcioglu ZA, Goson RA, et al. Capillary hemangioma (infantile periocular hemangioma). Surv Ophthalmol 1994;38:399–426.
35. Byrne SF, Green RL. Ultrasound of the Eye and Orbit. St. Louis, MO: Mosby-Yearbook, 1992:332.
36. Balchunas ER, Quencer RM, Byrne SF, et al. Correlative of the computed tomographic, ultrasonographic, and pathological characteristics of cavernous versus capillary hemangiomas of the orbit. J Clin Neuroophthalmol 1983;6:14.
37. Jiang XW, Wang GH, Li JH, et al. Expression of glucocorticoid receptor isoforms in cutaneous hemangiomas and vascular malformations. Chin Med J 2005;118(12):977–81.
38. Cogen MS, Elsas FJ. Eyelid depigmentation following corticosteroid injection for infantile ocular adnexal hemangioma. J Pediatr Ophthalmol Strabismus 1989;26:35–8.
39. Wilson MW, Hoehn ME, Haik BG, et al. Low-dose cyclophosphamide and interferon alpha 2a for the treatment of capillary hemangioma of the orbit. Ophthalmology 2007;114(5):1007–11.
40. Deans RM, Harris GJ, Kivlin JD. Surgical dissection of capillary hemangiomas. An alternative to intralesional corticosteroids. Arch Ophthalmol 1992;110:1743–7.
41. Burstein FD, Simms C, Cohen SR, et al. Intralesional laser therapy of extensive hemangiomas in 100 consecutive pediatric patients. Ann Plast Surg 2000;44(2):188–94.
42. Léauté-Labrèze CE, Hubiche T, Boralevi F, et al. Propranolol for severe hemangiomas of infancy. N Engl J Med 2008;358(24):2649–51.

43. Verity DH, Rose GE, Restori M. The effect of intralesional steroid injections on the volume and blood flow in periocular capillary haemangiomas. Orbit 2008;27(1):41–7.
44. Kavanagh EC, Heran MK, Peleg A, et al. Imaging of the natural history of an orbital capillary hemangioma. Orbit 2006;25(1):69–72.
45. Egbert JE, Paul S, Engel WK, et al. High injection pressure during intralesional injection of corticosteroids into capillary hemangiomas. Arch Ophthalmol 2001;119(5):677–83.
46. O'Keefe M, Lanigan B, Byrne SA. Capillary haemangioma of the eyelids and orbit: a clinical review of the safety and efficacy of intralesional steroid. Acta Ophthalmol Scand 2003;81(3):294–8.
47. Schwartz SR, Kodsi SR, Blei F, et al. Treatment of capillary hemangiomas causing refractive and occlusional amblyopia. J AAPOS 2007;11(6):577–83.
48. Sutula FC, Glover AT. Eyelid necrosis following intralesional corticosteroid injection for capillary hemangioma. Ophthalmic Surg 1987;18(2):103–5.
49. Ruttum MS, Abrams GW, Harris GJ, et al. Bilateral retinal embolization associated with intralesional corticosteroid injection for capillary hemangioma of infancy. J Pediatr Ophthalmol Strabismus 1993;30(1):4–7.
50. Goyal R, Watts P, Lane CM, et al. Adrenal suppression and failure to thrive after steroid injections for periocular hemangioma. Ophthalmology 2004;111(2):389–95.
51. Weiss AH, Kelly JP. Reappraisal of astigmatism induced by periocular capillary hemangioma and treatment with intralesional corticosteroid injection. Ophthalmology 2008;115(2):390–7.
52. Bilaniuk LT. Vascular lesions of the orbit in children. Neuroimag Clin N Am 2005;15(1):107–20.
53. Selva D, Strianese D, Bonavolonta G, et al. Orbital venous-lymphatic malformations (lymphangiomas) mimicking cavernous hemangiomas. Am J Ophthalmol 2001;131(3):364–70.
54. Brooks SE, Pillai JJ, Bains H. Orbital cellulitis due to occult orbital lymphangioma. South Med J 2001;94(5):532–5.
55. Bisdorff A, Mulliken JB, Carrico J, et al. Intracranial vascular anomalies in patients with periorbital lymphatic and lymphaticovenous malformations. AJNR Am J Neuroradiol 2007;28(2):335–41.
56. Vachharajani A, Paes B. Orbital lymphangioma with non-contiguous cerebral arteriovenous malformation, manifesting with thrombocytopenia (Kasabach–Merritt syndrome) and intracerebral hemorrhage. Acta Paediatr 2002;91(1):98–9.
57. Huckabee RE, Raila FA. MRI and CT comparison of an orbital cavernous lymphangioma. J Miss State Med Assoc 1991;32:371–3.
58. Bond JB, Haik BG, Taveras JL, et al. Magnetic resonance imaging of orbital lymphangioma with and without gadolinium contrast enhancement. Ophthalmology 1992;99: 1318–24.
59. Gelbert F, Riche MC, Reizine D, et al. MR imaging of head and neck vascular malformations. J Magn Reson Imaging 1991;1:579–84.
60. Byrne SF, Green RL. Orbital ultrasound. In: Tasman W, Jaeger EA, editors. Duane's Clinical Ophthalmology. Vol 1. Philadelphia, PA: JB Lippincott, 1991:24.
61. Esmaeli B, Prieto VG, Gonnering R, et al. Growth factor receptor expression in orbital lymphangioma: possible therapeutic implications. Orbit 2004;23(4):263–9.
62. Harris GJ, Sakol PJ, Bonavolonta GT, et al. An analysis of thirty cases of orbital lymphangioma. Pathophysiologic considerations and management recommendations. Ophthalmology 1990;97:1583–92.
63. Wilson ME, Parker PL, Chavis RM. Conservative management of childhood orbital lymphangioma. Ophthalmology 1989;96:484–9.
64. Sires BS, Goins CR, Anderson RL, et al. Systemic corticosteroid use in orbital lymphangioma. Ophthal Plast Reconstr Surg 2001;17(2):85–90.
65. Tawfik HA, Budin H, Dutton JJ. Lack of response to systemic corticosteroids in patients with lymphangioma. Ophthal Plast Reconstr Surg 2005;21(4):302–5.

66. Schwarcz RM, Ben Simon GJ, Cook T, Goldberg RA. Sclerosing therapy as first line treatment for low flow vascular lesions of the orbit. Am J Ophthalmol 2006;141(2):333–9.
67. Boulos PR, Harissi-Dagher M, Kavalec C, et al. Intralesional injection of Tisseel fibrin glue for resection of lymphangiomas and other thin-walled orbital cysts. Ophthal Plast Reconstr Surg 2005;21(3):171–6.
68. de Graaf JH, Egeler RM. New insights into the pathogenesis of Langerhans cell histiocytosis. Curr Opin Pediatr 1997;9(1):46–50.
69. Shields JA, Shields CL. Clinical spectrum of histiocytic tumors of the orbit. Trans Pa Acad Ophthalmol Otolaryngol 1990;42:931–7.
70. Harris GJ. Langerhans cell histiocytosis of the orbit: a need for interdisciplinary dialogue. Am J Ophthalmol 2006;141(2):374–8.
71. Egeler RM, Annels NE, Hogendoorn PC. Langerhans cell histiocytosis: a pathologic combination of oncogenesis and immune dysregulation. Pediatr Blood Cancer 2004;42(5):401–3.
72. Konrad H, Clark BJ, Rose GE. Lymphocytic, plasmacytic, histiocytic, and hematopoietic tumors of the orbit. In: Tasman W, Jaeger EA, editors. Duane's Clinical Ophthalmology. Philadelphia, PA: Lippincott Williams & Wilkins, 2000:30–2.
73. Banna M, Oltuola PS. Orbital histiocytosis on computed tomography. J Comput Tomogr 1983;7:167–70.
74. Leonidas JC, Guelfguat M, Valderrama E. Langerhans cell histiocytosis. Lancet 2003;361(9365):1293–5.
75. Gündüz K, Palamar M, Parmak N, et al. Eosinophilic granuloma of the orbit: report of two cases. J AAPOS 2007;11(5):506–8.
76. Kindy-Degnan NA, Laflamme P, Duprat G, et al. Intralesional steroid in the treatment of an orbital eosinophilic granuloma. Arch Ophthalmol 1991;109:617–8.
77. Jubran RF, Marachelian A, Dorey F, et al. Predictors of outcome in children with Langerhans cell histiocytosis. Pediatr Blood Cancer 2005;45(1):37–42.
78. Haupt R, Nanduri V, Calevo MG, et al. Permanent consequences in Langerhans cell histiocytosis patients: a pilot study from the Histiocyte Society Late Effects Study Group. Pediatr Blood Cancer 2004;42(5):438–44.
79. Binning MJ, Brockmeyer DL. Novel multidisciplinary approach for treatment of Langerhans cell histiocytosis of the skull base. Skull Base 2008;18(1):53–8.
80. Thompson CR, Lessell S. Anterior visual pathway gliomas. Int Ophthalmol Clin 1997;37:261–79.
81. Dutton JJ. Gliomas of the anterior visual pathway. Surv Ophthalmol 1994;38:427–52.
82. Lee AG. Neuro-ophthalmological management of optic pathway gliomas. Neurosurg Focus 2007;23(5):E1.
83. North KN. Neurofibromatosis 1 in childhood. Semin Pediatr Neurol 1998;5(4):231–42.
84. Astrup J. Natural history and clinical management of optic pathway glioma. Br J Neurosurg 2003;17(4):327–35.
85. Zeid JL, Charrow J, Sandu M, et al. Orbital optic nerve gliomas in children with neurofibromatosis type 1. J AAPOS 2006;10(6):534–9.
86. Es SV, North KN, McHugh K, et al. MRI findings in children with neurofibromatosis type 1: a prospective study. Pediatr Radiol 1996;26:478–87.
87. Pungavkar SA, Lawande MA, Patkar DP, et al. Bilateral optic pathway glioma with intracranial calcification: magnetic resonance imaging and magnetic resonance spectroscopy findings. Australas Radiol 2005;49(6):489–92.
88. Liu GT. Optic gliomas of the anterior visual pathway. Curr Opin Ophthalmol 2006;17(5):427–31.
89. Jahraus CD, Tarbell NJ. Optic pathway gliomas. Pediatr Blood Cancer 2006;46(5):586–96.
90. Combs SE, Schulz-Ertner D, Moschos D, et al. Fractionated stereotactic radiotherapy of optic pathway gliomas: tolerance and long-term outcome. Int J Radiat Oncol Biol Phys 2005;62(3):814–9.

91. Balcer LJ, Liu GT, Heller G, et al. Visual loss in children with neurofibromatosis type 1 and optic pathway gliomas: relation to tumor location by magnetic resonance imaging. Am J Ophthalmol 2001;131(4):442–5.
92. Tow SL, Chandela S, Miller NR, et al. Long-term outcome in children with gliomas of the anterior visual pathway. Pediatr Neurol 2003;28:262–70.
93. Czyzyk E, Jóźwiak S, Roszkowski M, et al. Optic pathway gliomas in children with and without neurofibromatosis 1. J Child Neurol 2003;18(7):471–8.
94. Farris SR, Grove AS Jr. Orbital and eyelid manifestations of neurofibromatosis: a clinical study and literature review. Ophthal Plast Reconstr Surg 1996;12:245–59.
95. Jackson IT, Carbonnel A, Potparic Z, et al. Orbitotemporal neurofibromatosis: classification and treatment. Plast Reconstr Surg 1993;92(1):1–11.
96. Tada M, Sawamura Y, Ishii N, et al. Massive plexiform neurofibroma in the orbit in a child with von Recklinghausen's disease. Childs Nerv Syst 1998;14:210–2.
97. Erb MH, Uzcategui N, See RF, et al. Orbitotemporal neurofibromatosis: classification and treatment. Orbit 2007;26(4):223–8.
98. Wu CT, Lee ST, Chen JF, et al. Computer-aided design for three-dimensional titanium mesh used for repairing skull base bone defect in pediatric neurofibromatosis type 1. A novel approach combining biomodeling and neuronavigation. Pediatr Neurosurg 2008;44(2): 133–9.
99. Kwiat DM, Bersani TA, Hodge C, et al. Surgical technique: two-step orbital reconstruction in neurofibromatosis type 1 with a matched implant and exenteration. Ophthal Plast Reconstr Surg 2004;20(2):158–61.
100. Dutton JJ, Tawfik HA, DeBacker CM, et al. Multiple recurrences in malignant peripheral nerve sheath tumor of the orbit: a case report and a review of the literature. Ophthal Plast Reconstr Surg 2001;17(4):293–9.
101. Shome D, Honavar SG, Reddy VA, et al. Orbital embryonal rhabdomyosarcoma in association with neurofibromatosis type 1. Ophthal Plast Reconstr Surg 2007;23(2): 147–8.
102. Schatz H. Benign orbital neurilemoma: sarcomatous transformation in von Recklinghausen's disease. Arch Ophthalmol 1971;86:268–73.
103. Zagar TM, Triche TJ, Kinsella TJ. Extraosseous Ewing's sarcoma: 25 years later. J Clin Oncol 2008;26(26):4230–2.
104. Choi RY, Lucarelli MJ, Imesch PD, et al. Primary orbital Ewing sarcoma in a middle-aged woman. Arch Ophthalmol 1999;117(4):535–7.
105. Guzowski M, Tumuluri K, Walker DM, et al. Primary orbital Ewing sarcoma in a middle-aged man. Ophthal Plast Reconstr Surg 2005;21(6):449–51.
106. Li T, Goldberg RA, Becker B, et al. Primary orbital extraskeletal Ewing sarcoma. Arch Ophthalmol 2003;121(7):1049–52.
107. Dutton JJ, Rose JG Jr, DeBacker CM, et al. Orbital Ewing's sarcoma of the orbit. Ophthal Plast Reconstr Surg 2000;16(4):292–300.
108. Sharma A, Garg A, Mishra NK, et al. Primary Ewing's sarcoma of the sphenoid bone with unusual imaging features: a case report. Clin Neurol Neurosurg 2005;107(6):528–31.
109. Henk CB, Grampp S, Wiesbauer P, et al. Ewing sarcoma. Diagnostic imaging. Radiologe 1998;38:509–22.
110. Wilson DJ, Dailey RA, Griffeth MT, et al. Primary Ewing sarcoma of the orbit. Ophthal Plast Reconstr Surg 2001;17(4):300–3.
111. Frandsen E. Ewing's sarcoma of the orbit. Nord Med 1952;48:1673.
112. Ludwig JA. Ewing sarcoma: historical perspectives, current state-of-the-art, and opportunities for targeted therapy in the future. Curr Opin Oncol 2008;20(4):412–8.
113. Leavey PJ, Collier AB. Ewing's sarcoma: prognostic criteria, outcomes, and future treatments. Expert Rev Anticancer Ther 2008;8:617–24.
114. Belgaumi AF, Kauffman WM, Jenkins JJ, et al. Blindness in children with neuroblastoma. Cancer 1997;80:1997–2004.

115. Musarella M, Chan HSL, DeBoer G, et al. Ocular involvement in neuroblastoma: prognostic implications. Ophthalmology 1984;91:936–40.
116. Mirzai H, Baser EF, Tansug N, et al. Primary orbital neuroblastoma in a neonate. Indian J Ophthalmol 2006;54:206–8.
117. Lau JJ, Trobe JD, Ruiz RE, et al. Metastatic neuroblastoma presenting with binocular blindness from intracranial compression of the optic nerves. J Neuroophthalmol 2004;24(2):119–24.
118. Mortada A. Clinical characteristics of early orbital neuroblastoma. Am J Ophthalmol 1967;63:1787–93.
119. Messina JA, Cheng SC, Franc BL, et al. Evaluation of semi-quantitative scoring system for metaiodobenzylguanidine (mIBG) scans in patients with relapsed neuroblastoma. Pediatr Blood Cancer 2006;47(7):865–74.
120. Park JR, Eggert A, Caron H. Neuroblastoma: biology, prognosis, and treatment. Pediatr Clin North Am 2008;55(1):97–120.
121. Ishola TA, Chung DH. Neuroblastoma. Surg Oncol 2007;16:149–56.
122. Friedman GK, Castleberry RP. Changing trends of research and treatment in infant neuroblastoma. Pediatr Blood Cancer 2007;49(7 Suppl):1060–5.
123. Paulino AC. Palliative radiotherapy in children with neuroblastoma. Pediatr Hematol Oncol 2003;20(2):111–7.
124. Bakhshi S, Singh P, Chawla N. Malignant childhood proptosis: study of 104 cases. J Pediatr Hematol Oncol 2008;30(1):73–6.
125. Menon BS, Alagaratnam J, Juraida E, et al. Late presentation of retinoblastoma in Malaysia. Pediatr Blood Cancer 2009;52(2):215–7.
126. Rootman J, Ellsworth RM, Hofbauer J, et al. Orbital extension of retinoblastoma: a clinicopathologic study. Can J Ophthalmol 1978;13:72–80.
127. Agarwal M, Biswas J, S K, Shanmugam MP. Retinoblastoma presenting as orbital cellulitis: report of four cases with a review of the literature. Orbit 2004;23(2):93–8.
128. Foster BS, Mukai S. Intraocular retinoblastoma presenting as ocular and orbital inflammation. Int Ophthalmol Clin 1996;36:153–60.
129. Antoneli CB, Steinhorst F, de Cassia Braga Ribeiro K, et al. Extraocular retinoblastoma: a 13 year experience. Cancer 2003;98:1292–8.
130. Kiratli H, Bigic S, Ozerdem U. Management of massive orbital involvement of intraocular retinoblastoma. Ophthalmology 1998;105:322–6.
131. Chantada G, Fandiño A, Casak S, et al. Treatment of overt extraocular retinoblastoma. Med Pediatr Oncol 2003;40(3):158–61.
132. Eng C, Li FP, Abramson DH, et al. Mortality from second tumors among long-term survivors of retinoblastoma. J Natl Cancer Inst 1993;85(14):1121–8.
133. Moll AC, Imhof SM, Bouter LM, et al. Second primary tumors in patients with hereditary retinoblastoma: a register-based follow-up study, 1945–1994. Int J Cancer 1996;67(4): 515–9.
134. Chung EM, Specht CS, Schroeder JW. From the archives of the AFIP. Pediatric orbit tumors and tumorlike lesions: neuroepithelial lesions of the ocular globe and optic nerve. Radiographics 2007;27(4):1159–86.
135. Dunkel IJ, Aledo A, Kernan NA, et al. Successful treatment of metastatic retinoblastoma. Cancer 2000;89(10):2117–21.
136. Finger PT, Harbour JW, Karcioglu ZA. Risk factors for metastasis in retinoblastoma. Surv Ophthalmol 2002;47(1):1–16.
137. Bowman RJ, Mafwiri M, Luthert P, et al. Outcome of retinoblastoma in east Africa. Pediatr Blood Cancer 2008;50(1):160–2.
138. Gündüz K, Müftüoglu O, Günalp I, et al. Metastatic retinoblastoma clinical features, treatment, and prognosis. Ophthalmology 2006;113(9):1558–66.
139. Kim JW, Kathpalia V, Dunkel I, et al. Orbital recurrence of retinoblastoma following enucleation. Br J Ophthalmol 2008;115(8):1398–1404.

140. Kleinerman RA, Tucker MA, Tarone RE, et al. Risk of new cancers after radiotherapy in long-term survivors of retinoblastoma: an extended follow-up. J Clin Oncol 2005;23(10):2272–9.
141. Abramson DH, Melson MR, Dunkel IJ, et al. Third (fourth and fifth) non-ocular tumors in survivors of retinoblastoma. Ophthalmology 2001;108(10):1868–76.
142. Wong FL, Boice JD Jr, Abramson DH, et al. Cancer incidence after retinoblastoma. Radiation dose and sarcoma risk. JAMA 1997;278(15):1262–7.
143. Fletcher O, Easton D, Anderson K, et al. Lifetime risks of common cancers among retinoblastoma survivors. J Natl Cancer Inst 2004;96(5):357–63.
144. Porto L, Kieslich M, Schwabe D, et al. Granulocytic sarcoma in children. Neuroradiology 2004;46(5):374–7.
145. Esmaeli B, Medeiros LJ, Myers J, et al. Orbital mass secondary to precursor T-cell acute lymphoblastic leukemia: a rare presentation. Arch Ophthalmol 2001;119(3):443–6.
146. Padillo D, Mencía E, Gutiérrez E, et al. Orbital granulocytic sarcoma in a myelodysplastic syndrome. Orbit 1999;18(4):287–90.
147. Jakobiec FA. Granulocytic sarcoma. AJNR Am J Neuroradiol 1991;12(2):263–4.
148. Watkins LM, Remulla HD, Rubin PA. Orbital granulocytic sarcoma in an elderly patient. Am J Ophthalmol 1997;123(6):854–6.
149. Davis JL, Parke DW 2nd, Font RL. Granulocytic sarcoma of the orbit. A clinicopathologic study. Ophthalmology 1985;92(12):1758–62.
150. Zimmerman LE, Font RL. Ophthalmologic manifestations of granulocytic sarcoma (myeloid sarcoma or chloroma). The third Pan American Association of Ophthalmology and American Journal of Ophthalmology Lecture. Am J Ophthalmol 1975;80(6):975–90.
151. Banna M, Aur R, Akkad S. Orbital granulocytic sarcoma. AJNR Am J Neuroradiol 1991;12:255–8.
152. Chung EM, Murphey MD, Specht CS, et al. From the archives of the AFIP. Pediatric orbit tumors and tumorlike lesions: osseous lesions of the orbit. Radiographics 2008;28(4):1193–214.
153. Bulas RB, Laine FJ, Das Narla L. Bilateral orbital granulocytic sarcoma (chloroma) preceding the blast phase of acute myelogenous leukemia: CT findings. Pediatr Radiol 1995;25(6):488–9.
154. Pomeranz SJ, Hawkins HH, Towbin R, et al. Granulocytic sarcoma (chloroma): CT manifestations. Radiology 1985;155(1):167–70.
155. Pui MH, Fletcher BD, Langston JW. Granulocytic sarcoma in childhood leukemia: imaging features. Radiology 1994;190(3):698–702.
156. Stockl FA, Dolmetsch AM, Saornil MA, et al. Orbital granulocytic sarcoma. Br J Ophthalmol 1997;81(12):1084–8.
157. Audouin J, Comperat E, Le Tourneau A, et al. Myeloid sarcoma: clinical and morphologic criteria useful for diagnosis. Int J Surg Pathol 2003;11(4):271–82.
158. Tallman MS, Hakimian D, Shaw JM, et al. Granulocytic sarcoma is associated with the 8;21 translocation in acute myeloid leukemia. J Clin Oncol 1993;11(4):690–7.
159. Ohta K, Kondoh T, Yasuo K, et al. Primary granulocytic sarcoma in the sphenoidal bone and orbit. Childs Nerv Syst 2003;19(9):674–9.
160. Lee SG, Park TS, Cheong JW, et al. Preceding orbital granulocytic sarcoma in an adult patient with acute myelogenous leukemia with t(8;21): a case study and review of the literature. Cancer Genet Cytogenet 2008;185(1):51–4.
161. Cavdar AO, Babacan E, Gözdaşoğlu S, et al. High risk subgroup of acute myelomonocytic leukemia (AMML) with orbito-ocular granulocytic sarcoma (OOGS) in Turkish children. Retrospective analysis of clinical, hematological, ultrastructural, and therapeutical findings of thirty-three OOGS. Acta Haematol 1989;81(2):80–5.
162. Byrd JC, Weiss RB, Arthur DC, et al. Extramedullary leukemia adversely affects hematologic complete remission rate and overall survival in patients with t(8;21)(q22;q22): results from Cancer and Leukemia Group B 8461. J Clin Oncol 1997;15(2):466–75.

163. Schwyzer R, Sherman GG, Cohn RJ, et al. Granulocytic sarcoma in children with acute myeloblastic leukemia and t(8;21). Med Pediatr Oncol 1998;31(3):144–9.
164. Bisschop MM, Révész T, Bierings M, et al. Extramedullary infiltrates at diagnosis have no prognostic significance in children with acute myeloid leukaemia. Leukemia 2001;15:46–9.
165. Kobayashi R, Tawa A, Hanada R, et al. Japanese childhood AML cooperative study group. Extramedullary infiltration at diagnosis and prognosis in children with acute myelogenous leukemia. Pediatr Blood Cancer 2007;48(4):393–8.
166. Kumar J, Seith A, Bakhshi S, et al. Isolated granulocytic sarcoma of the orbit. Eur J Haematol 2007;78(5):456.

Chapter 4
Multidisciplinary Management of Orbital Rhabdomyosarcoma

Winston W. Huh and Anita Mahajan

Abstract Rhabdomyosarcoma (RMS) is the most common orbital malignancy in childhood. Embryonal RMS and alveolar RMS are the two most common histologic subtypes of RMS, and embryonal RMS is the most common subtype of orbital RMS. The clinical presentation of orbital RMS depends on the tumor location in the orbit. Diagnosis is chiefly made through open biopsy, and complete initial tumor resection is uncommon because of the risk of ocular morbidity. The treatment of orbital RMS requires a coordinated effort by the disciplines of ophthalmology, pathology, pediatric oncology, and radiation oncology. Because of advances in the planning and administration of chemotherapy and radiation therapy, the outcome for patients with orbital RMS has improved; the 3-year failure-free survival rate is greater than 90%, and the 3-year overall survival rate is 100%. Continued improvements in therapy are being investigated in an effort to decrease the risk of treatment-related late effects, such as cataracts and facial asymmetry.

4.1 Introduction

Rhabdomyosarcoma (RMS) is the most common soft tissue sarcoma of childhood. The disease accounts for approximately 50% of soft tissue sarcomas in children and has an incidence of 4.6 cases per million children per year [1]. RMS is generally diagnosed in younger children; 60% of cases are diagnosed in children younger than 5 years of age. Approximately one-third of all RMS cases occur in the head and neck area [2], and approximately 10% of all RMS cases occur in the orbit. Orbital RMS is the most common malignant orbital tumor in children [3].

There are two major subtypes of RMS, alveolar (ARMS) and embryonal (ERMS), of which the embryonal subtype is more common. In 80% of ARMS

W.W. Huh (✉)
Division of Pediatrics, The University of Texas M. D. Anderson Cancer Center, Houston, TX, USA
e-mail: whuh@mdanderson.org

B. Esmaeli (ed.), *Ophthalmic Oncology*, M.D. Anderson Solid Tumor Oncology Series 6, DOI 10.1007/978-1-4419-0374-7_4,

cases, there is a characteristic translocation between the forkhead transcription factor (*FKHR/FOXO1*) gene, located on chromosome 13, and either the *PAX3* transcription factor gene, located on chromosome 2, or the *PAX7* transcription factor gene, located on chromosome 1 [4]. Clinically, ARMS is more aggressive than ERMS and is more often associated with regional or distant metastases. Data from the most recent published RMS clinical trial demonstrate that patients with ARMS have a 3-year failure-free survival rate of 66%, compared to 83% for patients with ERMS [5]. ERMS is the most common RMS subtype in the orbit and accounts for approximately 89% of orbital RMS cases [6].

In 1972, the Intergroup Rhabdomyosarcoma Study Group (IRSG) was formed to study the biology and treatment of RMS [7]. In the decades since then, the results of IRSG clinical trials have reinforced the idea that treatment of orbital RMS requires a coordinated effort by the disciplines of ophthalmology, pathology, medical oncology, and radiation oncology. The continued evolution of multidisciplinary care has led to improved survival for patients with orbital RMS.

4.2 Clinical and Radiological Presentation

The most common presentation of orbital RMS is rapid growth of a painless mass that eventually leads to proptosis (Fig. 4.1). The superomedial quadrant is the most

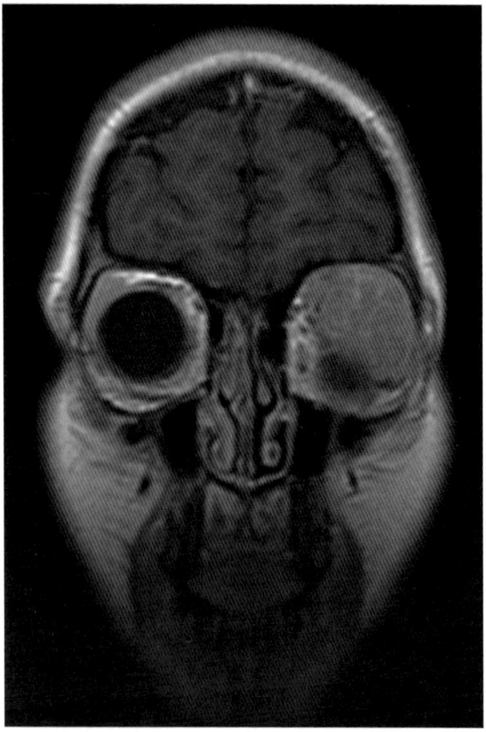

Fig. 4.1 Magnetic resonance images of a 10-year-old girl with a large orbital rhabdomyosarcoma that initially presented with proptosis and periorbital swelling

common location, but tumors can appear anywhere in the orbit [8]. The symptoms depend on the tumor location in the orbit. Anterior tumors result in eyelid edema and sometimes chemosis, while posterior tumors may result in vision changes, especially if there is compression of the optic nerve.

The differential diagnosis includes a variety of malignant and benign disorders, including cystic lesions, orbital cellulitis, granulocytic sarcoma, lymphoma, inflammatory pseudotumor, Langerhans cell histiocytosis, lacrimal gland lesions, peripheral nerve sheath lesions, and metastatic infiltrate from other solid tumors of childhood, such as neuroblastoma [3].

On computed tomography scans, tumors tend to appear isodense to extraocular muscles but enhance with contrast [8, 9]. On magnetic resonance imaging scans, tumors tend to appear isodense to extraocular muscles and hypointense to orbital fat on T1-weighted images [10]. The tumors can be intraconal, extraconal, or both [8]. Bony involvement with erosion can be seen, but invasion of the globe or direct intracranial extension is very uncommon [8].

4.3 Staging

Imaging of the primary tumor site should be done with either computed tomography or magnetic resonance imaging; this imaging should also include the entire neck in order to fully assess nodal status. Although regional lymph node involvement is uncommon, it is encountered occasionally, particularly with the more aggressive histologic subtypes. The posterior orbit lacks lymphatic vessels, but the anterior orbit and eyelids contain lymphatic vessels, by which cancer cells can spread to form regional lymph node metastases. Any clinically or radiographically suspicious nodes should be removed and subjected to histopathologic evaluation since positive nodes would have an impact on the radiation treatment field and dose. The standard evaluation for metastatic disease includes a computed tomography scan of the chest, a bone scan, and bilateral bone marrow aspiration and core biopsies of the iliac crests. Because of the potential for intracranial extension, a lumbar puncture and cytologic analysis of cerebrospinal fluid is part of the standard evaluation. However, distant metastasis of orbital RMS is uncommon [11].

In the first IRSG study, IRS-I, tumors were grouped clinically on the basis of extent of surgical resection [12]. However, subsequent clinical trials demonstrated that other factors, such as histology, anatomic site, and tumor size, were also important [13, 14] Thus, the current staging system combines the classification system of the IRSG with the TNM staging system (Tables 4.1 and 4.2). Because it is difficult to achieve complete tumor resection at the time of presentation because of the risk of damage to surrounding vital ocular structures, orbital RMS is typically diagnosed through open biopsy. In an international review of 306 patients with orbital RMS, only 3% of the patients were able to undergo complete tumor resection at initial surgery, resulting in clinical group I status, whereas 72% of patients had biopsy without attempt at resection as initial surgery and 25% had partial excision as initial surgery [15]. Thus, most orbital RMS cases are classified as stage 1, clinical group III (Tables 4.1 and 4.2).

Table 4.1 Pretreatment TNM staging system for rhabdomyosarcoma

Stage	Site	T	Tumor diameter	N	M
1	Orbit; head and neck (excluding parameningeal); genitourinary—nonbladder and nonprostate; biliary tract	T1 or T2	a or b	N0 or N1 or Nx	M0
2	Bladder or prostate; extremity; cranial parameningeal; other (includes trunk, retroperitoneum, etc.)	T1 or T2	a	N0 or Nx	M0
3	Bladder or prostate; extremity; cranial parameningeal; other (includes trunk, retroperitoneum, etc.)	T1 or T2	a	N1	M0
			b	N0 or N1 or Nx	M0
4	All	T1 or T2	a or b	N0 or N1	M1

Definitions: T1, confined to site of origin; T2, extension and/or fixation to surrounding tissue; a, ≤5 cm in diameter; b, >5 cm in diameter; N0, regional nodes not clinically involved; N1, regional nodes clinically involved by neoplasm; Nx, clinical status of regional nodes unknown; M0, no distant metastasis present; M1, metastasis present

Table 4.2 Clinical grouping classification for rhabdomyosarcoma

Group	Definition
I	Localized disease, completely resected
II	Total gross resection with evidence of regional spread
	Grossly resected tumor with microscopic residual disease
	Regional disease with involved nodes, completely resected with no microscopic residual disease
	Regional disease with involved nodes, grossly resected but with evidence of microscopic residual disease and/or histologic involvement of the most distal regional node (from the primary site) in the dissection specimen
III	Incomplete resection with gross residual disease
IV	Distant metastatic disease present at onset

4.4 Surgery

Prior to the 1970s, orbital exenteration was a standard procedure for achieving local control of orbital RMS. However, now that it has been established that radiation therapy can also provide local control, exenteration is largely reserved for patients with progressive disease or recurrence within a previously irradiated field. It is often difficult to achieve complete surgical resection at the time of initial diagnosis because of the close proximity of the tumor to vital ocular structures and the high risk of unacceptable ocular morbidity or loss of function. However, in patients with ERMS, if complete surgical resection can be performed without undue morbidity and the patient does not have clinically suspicious lymph nodes, surgery is recommended since complete surgical local control obviates the need for radiation therapy. In patients with ARMS, a more aggressive subtype, radiation therapy is always recommended regardless of surgical margin status.

4.5 Chemotherapy

All RMS cases require chemotherapy, and the standard chemotherapeutic regimen is a three-drug combination of vincristine, dactinomycin, and cyclophosphamide. The IRS-II study demonstrated an excellent outcome for patients treated with this regimen: the overall survival rate at 5 years was 92% [16]. Thus, the next two clinical trials of the IRSG, IRS-III and IRS-IV, examined the effect of decreasing the amount of chemotherapy given to patients with orbital RMS, especially those with clinical group I or II disease. The strategy was to exclude cyclophosphamide since it has been associated with late effects such as infertility, secondary malignancies, and osteoporosis [16, 17]. In IRS-III and IRS-IV, patients with group I or II disease received only vincristine and dactinomycin; the main difference between the trials was that in IRS-IV, the duration of therapy was shortened from 50 to 36 weeks [5, 14]. The results were similar to those of IRS-II: the 3-year failure-free and overall survival rates were 91 and 100%, respectively, for IRS-IV with IRS-III having similar results.

Most orbital RMS patients have clinical group III disease. In IRS-III, patients with group III disease received only vincristine and dactinomycin, but in IRS-IV, patients with group III disease received the three-drug regimen. The 3-year failure-free survival rate was significantly better with the three-drug combination (94 versus 80%), but overall survival was not significantly different [13, 17]. In the most recently completed IRSG trial, IRS-V, the two-drug strategy was used: patients with group I, II, or III orbital RMS were treated with a 45-week regimen of vincristine with dactinomycin. The results of the IRS-V trial have not yet been published. The current Children's Oncology Group study for patients with low-risk RMS is attempting to determine if 22 weeks of treatment with vincristine, dactinomycin, and cyclophosphamide is feasible. Only four doses of cyclophosphamide are given, and the dose is 1.2 g/m^2 rather than the 2.2-g/m^2 dose used in prior trials.

4.6 Radiation Therapy

Radiation therapy is a key component in the treatment of RMS. Earlier IRSG studies demonstrated good local control rates with doses of 50.4 Gy. However, the potential late side effects of radiation therapy in orbital RMS survivors need to be recognized. One study of 94 orbital RMS survivors noted that 82% of the patients had a unilateral cataract and 59% of the patients had orbital hypoplasia due to delayed bone growth [18]. Other described effects include dry eye, keratitis, and hormone insufficiency [18, 19]. Thus, there has been great interest in reducing the delivered radiation dose while maintaining the excellent cure rate for orbital RMS. The recently completed IRS-V study and the current Children's Oncology Group study for patients with low-risk RMS employ a strategy in which the dose is dependent upon clinical group and nodal status. Group I patients do not receive radiation therapy. Group II patients receive 36 Gy if there are no clinically involved nodes and 41.4 Gy if there are proven clinically involved lymph nodes. Group III patients, who account for the vast majority of patients with orbital RMS, receive 45 Gy.

Currently, most patients are treated using external-beam photons; however, there has recently been interest in other modalities, such as proton beam therapy, which have the theoretical advantage of an improved dose distribution with greater sparing of surrounding normal tissues [20]. Orbital tumors may be an excellent indication for proton therapy because of the reduced dose to the surrounding brain, neuroendocrine structures, and contralateral eye. Although there are some early data indicating safety and feasibility of proton therapy for orbital RMS in pediatric patients, there are scant long-term data regarding local control and the rate of late effects [21].

4.7 Conclusions and Future Directions

The survival outcome for orbital RMS has improved significantly over the years because of advances in multidisciplinary care. However, long-term survivors of orbital RMS are now experiencing a new set of challenges in terms of late-onset side effects as a result of their cancer therapy. Improvements in all facets of care must continue to be attempted in an effort to lessen the long-term effects of therapy while maintaining the rate of cure.

References

1. Gurney JG, Young JL, Roffers SD, et al. Soft tissue sarcomas. In: Ries LAG, Smith MA, Gurney JG, Linet M, Tamra T, Young JL, Bunin GR, editors. Cancer Incidence and Survival among Children and Adolescents: United States SEER Program 1975–1995. Bethesda, MD: National Cancer Institute SEER Program, 1999. NIH Pub. No. 99-4649.
2. Arndt CAS, Crist WM. Common musculoskeletal tumors of childhood and adolescence. N Engl J Med 1999;341:342–52.
3. Shields JA, Shields CL, Scartozzi R. Survey of 1264 patients with orbital tumors and simulating lesions. The 2002 Montgomery lecture, part 1. Ophthalmology 2004;111:997–1008.
4. Sorensen PHB, Lynch JC, Qualman SJ, et al. PAX3–FKHR and PAX7–FKHR gene fusions are prognostic indicators in alveolar rhabdomyosarcoma: a report from the Children's Oncology Group. J Clin Oncol 2002;20:2672–9.
5. Crist WM, Anderson JR, Meza JL, et al. Intergroup Rhabdomyosarcoma Study—IV: results for patients with nonmetastatic disease. J Clin Oncol 2001;19:3091–102.
6. Kodet R, Newton WA, Hamoudi AB, et al. Orbital rhabdomyosarcomas and related tumors in childhood: relationship of morphology to prognosis—an Intergroup Rhabdomyosarcoma Study. Med Pediatr Oncol 1997;29:51–60.
7. Raney RB, Anderson JR, Barr FG, et al. Rhabdomyosarcoma and undifferentiated sarcoma in the first 2 decades of life: a selective review of Intergroup Rhabdomyosarcoma Study Group

experience and rationale for Intergroup Rhabdomyosarcoma Study V. J Pediatr Hematol Oncol 2001;23:215–20.
8. Sohaib SA, Moseley I, Wright JE. Orbital rhabdomyosarcoma—the radiological characteristics. Clin Radiol 1998;53:357–62.
9. Karcioglu ZA, Hadjistilianou D, Rozans M, et al. Orbital rhabdomyosarcoma. Cancer Control 2004;11:328–33.
10. Park K, van Rijn R, McHugh K. The role of radiology in pediatric soft tissue sarcomas. Cancer Imaging 2008;8:102–15.
11. Breneman JC, Lyden E, Pappo AS, et al. Prognostic factors and clinical outcomes in children and adolescents with metastatic rhabdomyosarcoma—a report from the Intergroup Rhabdomyosarcoma Study IV. J Clin Oncol 2003;21:78–84.
12. Maurer HM, Beltangady M, Gehan EA, et al. The Intergroup Rhabdomyosarcoma Study—I. A final report. Cancer 1988;61:209–20.
13. Maurer HM, Gehan EA, Beltangady M, et al. The Intergroup Rhabdomyosarcoma Study—II. Cancer 1993;71:1904–22.
14. Crist W, Gehan EA, Ragab AH, et al. The third Intergroup Rhabdomyosarcoma Study. J Clin Oncol 1995;13:610–30.
15. Oberlin O, Rey A, Anderson J, et al. Treatment of orbital rhabdomyosarcomas: survival and late effects of treatment—results of an international workshop. J Clin Oncol 2001;19: 197–204.
16. Punyko JA, Mertens AC, Gurney JG, et al. Long-term medical effects of childhood and adolescent rhabdomyosarcoma: a report from the Childhood Cancer Survivor Study. Pediatr Blood Cancer 2005;44:643–53.
17. Sung L, Anderson JR, Donaldson SS, et al. Late events occurring five years or more after successful therapy for childhood rhabdomyosarcoma: a report from the Soft Tissue Sarcoma Committee of the Children's Oncology Group. Eur J Cancer 2004;40:1878–85.
18. Raney RB, Anderson JR, Kollath J, et al. Late effects of therapy in 94 patients with localized rhabdomyosarcoma of the orbit: report from the Intergroup Rhabdomyosarcoma Study—III, 1984–1991. Med Pediatr Oncol 2000;34:413–20.
19. Fiorillo A, Migliorati R, Vassallo P, et al. Radiation late effects in children treated for orbital rhabdomyosarcoma. Radiother Oncol 1998;53:143–8.
20. Schulz-Ertner D, Tsujii H. Particle radiation therapy using proton and heavier ion beams. J Clin Oncol 2007;25:953–64.
21. Timmermann B, Schuck A, Niggli F, et al. Spot-scanning proton therapy for malignant soft tissue tumors in childhood: first experiences at the Paul Scherrer Institute. Int J Radiat Oncol Biol Phys 2007;67:497–504.

Chapter 5
Metastatic Orbital Tumors

Syed Mehdi Ahmad and Bita Esmaeli

Abstract Orbital metastasis is uncommon, accounting for only 1–13% of all orbital tumors reported. The approach to metastatic orbital tumors has dramatically changed in recent decades. The improved life expectancy of patients with common cancers, such as breast cancer and prostate cancer, together with aging of the population and the resultant increase in the number of patients at risk for cancer, has led to a higher incidence of patients living with metastatic disease in unusual sites such as the orbit. Furthermore, vigilant surveillance and advances in diagnostic testing have led to increased detection of orbital metastases. Because of the poor prognosis for patients with metastatic orbital disease, treatment is usually palliative and may include radiotherapy, chemotherapy, hormonal therapy, surgery, or a combination of these modalities. The ophthalmologist may play a pivotal role in the detection and management of these lesions in patients with and without a primary cancer diagnosis.

5.1 Introduction

Orbital metastases were first documented by Horner in 1864 and Perl in 1872. Though many cases have been described in the literature, metastasis to the orbit is rare and occurs less frequently than metastasis to uveal tissue [1]. With emerging novel therapies, the longevity of cancer patients has risen and so has the frequency with which metastases in the orbit are detected [2–4]. Generally, orbital metastases reflect multisystem, end-stage cancer and patients with orbital metastases have a poor prognosis.

S.M. Ahmad (✉)
Department of Ophthalmology, Baylor University Medical Center at Dallas, Dallas, TX, USA
e-mail: sma967@gmail.com

B. Esmaeli (ed.), *Ophthalmic Oncology*, M.D. Anderson Solid Tumor Oncology Series 6, DOI 10.1007/978-1-4419-0374-7_5,

5.2 Incidence

Metastatic orbital lesions have been estimated to account for 1–13% of all orbital tumors reported, and the prevalence of these lesions in cancer patients is estimated to range from 2 to 4.7% [2–13]. With the increase in the median survival time of cancer patients, the true incidence of these metastatic lesions is likely to be higher than reported in the literature. Patients with small orbital lesions are more likely to remain asymptomatic and undiagnosed than patients with similarly sized ocular lesions [6]. For example, subclinical metastatic orbital lesions are estimated to be present in 10–30% of breast cancer patients [2–4, 8]. The presence of debilitating systemic symptoms may overshadow orbital symptoms, thus leading to a lower rate of referral to the ophthalmologist. Another factor suggesting that the true incidence of metastatic orbital lesions may be underestimated is that rates of orbital evaluation at autopsy are low [7].

5.3 Anatomical Considerations

Unilateral presentation is common; bilateral presentation is highly unusual. Some studies have suggested that metastatic disease is more common in the left orbit [10, 11], while other studies have shown no greater prevalence of metastasis to the left orbit [3, 8, 12]. Recent cumulative data have shown the following distribution of involvement: lateral quadrant, 39%; superior, 32%; medial, 20%; and inferior, 12% [3, 12]. Another report of 68 patients with orbital metastasis found that the main

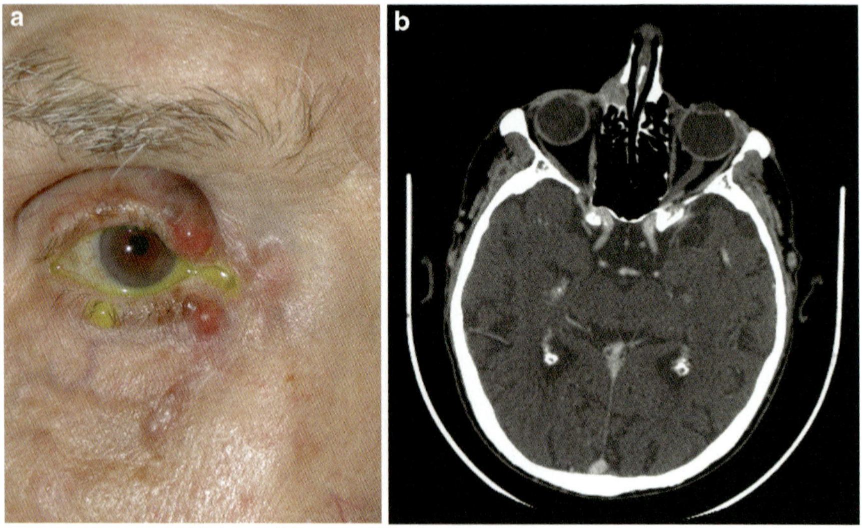

Fig. 5.1 (**a**) Melanoma metastatic to the lacrimal sac and periorbital soft tissue in a 90-year-old man with stage IV cutaneous melanoma. (**b**) Computed tomography scan in the same patient demonstrating the metastatic melanoma lesion in the lacrimal sac

component of the metastatic lesion lay in the anterior orbit in 41 cases and in the posterior orbit in 27 cases [8]. Although different tumor types have a propensity to metastasize to different tissues in the orbit, the overall distribution of metastases within the orbit seems to be in a bone to fat to muscle ratio of 2:2:1 [3].

Isolated metastasis to the eyelid and periocular skin is less common and has been reported mainly in single case reports, most describing cutaneous melanoma nodules [14, 15, 29] in the eyelid or eyelid metastasis in the background of widespread metastatic disease (Fig. 5.1) [16].

5.4 Presentation and Clinical Features

Orbital metastasis is predominantly a condition of adulthood and usually arises from carcinomas [4]. In children, the most common tumor metastatic to the orbit is neuroblastoma. Most orbital metastases present in patients with widespread cancer, although in 19–25% of cases there is no preexisting cancer [2–4]. Orbital metastases are usually associated with a rapid onset of symptoms that may be progressive over weeks to months. Typical manifestations of orbital metastases include mass effect, causing displacement or proptosis of the globe, pain, inflammation, bone involvement, chemosis, and eyelid swelling. Infiltration of soft tissue structures can lead to ptosis, diplopia, or enophthalmos. Because the signs and symptoms of orbital metastases are nonspecific and provide no clinical framework for categorization of lesions, Goldberg et al. [3, 9] suggested categorization into five generalized syndromes of presentation, frequencies of which were as follows: infiltrative (53%); mass (37%); inflammatory (5%); functional (3%); and silent (very rare) [3].

5.5 Diagnosis

A thorough patient history and detailed examination are a must and should be done in conjunction with a prompt referral to an oncologist for a simultaneous evaluation for systemic disease. Computed tomography and magnetic resonance imaging are the primary imaging modalities in evaluating any suspected orbital lesion. Though computed tomography is usually the first choice in evaluating the orbit, magnetic resonance imaging provides the best resolution of orbital soft tissues. A computed tomography scan may be more appropriate for lesions that are known to metastasize to the orbital bony walls, such as metastatic prostate cancer.

Findings on imaging may range from a diffuse infiltrative pattern (Fig. 5.2) with obscuration of normal anatomical landmarks to a focal lesion in which a discrete, well-defined mass is seen; orbital metastatic lesions can be extraconal or intraconal. Enlargement of one or more of the extraocular muscles may be seen, particularly in patients with metastatic cutaneous melanoma (Fig. 5.3). Involvement of the bony orbital walls suggests that prostate cancer is the primary tumor. It is unusual to see cystic changes or calcification within metastatic lesions of the orbit.

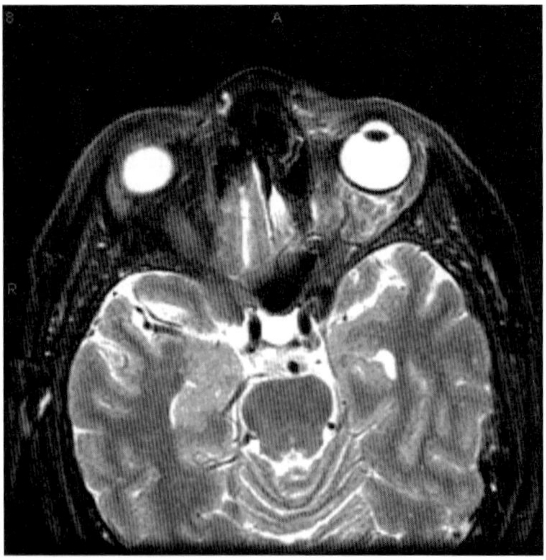

Fig. 5.2 Magnetic resonance imaging demonstrates left orbital infiltration from a metastatic breast carcinoma

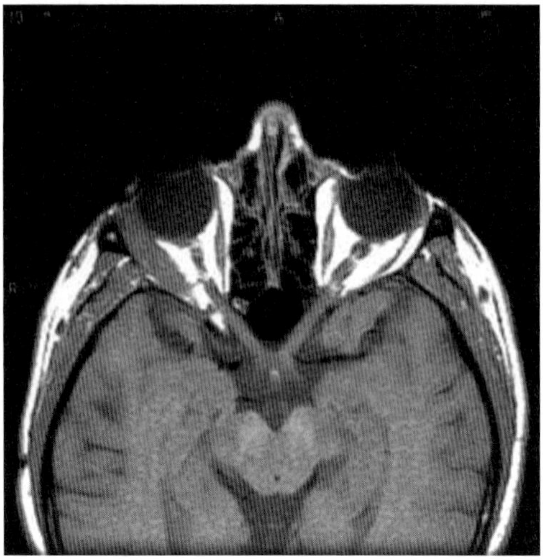

Fig. 5.3 Magnetic resonance imaging of the orbit shows a metastasis to the right lateral rectus muscle from cutaneous melanoma

The definitive diagnosis of an orbital lesion requires a tissue diagnosis. In patients with widespread metastatic disease and/or an established diagnosis of cancer, an orbital biopsy may be forgone and the inherent risks of biopsy—such as visual loss, bleeding, and diplopia—avoided. Fine-needle aspiration biopsy has been advocated by many authorities as an excellent diagnostic modality [3, 17–19]. However, there have been reports of dissemination of tumor cells and risk of globe injury with this procedure, although the probability of such problems is low. Other limitations of fine-needle aspiration biopsy for orbital lesions include lack of opportunity to assess tissue architecture and limited volume of tissue, both of which may limit ability to make a diagnosis in some cases [17–19].

In the case of suspected but undiagnosed breast malignancy, estrogen receptor expression should be measured in the orbital biopsy specimen, not only to aid in diagnosis but also to determine the value of hormonal therapy.

5.6 Treatment

Treatment for orbital metastases is palliative in the sense that the presence of these lesions suggests a hematogenous spread of cancer even if no other metastases are identifiable. Various treatment modalities exist, including radiotherapy, chemotherapy, hormonal therapy, surgery, and combinations of these. The goals of treatment for orbital metastases are to maximize the patient's quality of life and maximize the patient's visual function. Each treatment modality should always be carefully considered in the context of the patient's general state of health, life expectancy, and anticipated effects of treatment.

Radiotherapy is the mainstay of treatment for orbital metastases and is usually administered to control tumor growth, preserve vision, decrease proptosis and exposure keratopathy, and/or improve patient comfort. The recommended dose is 20–40 Gy delivered in fractions over 1–2 weeks [3–9, 20]. Radiotherapy alleviates symptoms in 80% of cases and in some cases restores vision [5]. Shielding of the globe may lessen the risk of radiation-induced side effects, such as radiation retinopathy and cataract formation, in some situations [21].

Systemic chemotherapy may be helpful in the treatment of orbital metastases, especially for chemosensitive tumors, such as small-cell lung cancer and neuroblastoma [22]. Hormonal therapy plays an important role in the treatment of metastases from hormone-sensitive tumors, such as breast cancer and prostate cancer.

Generally, orbital surgery to remove the tumor mass is not curative and may be associated with significant ocular morbidity [2–5, 7–9]. However, in selected cases, partial resection may improve the patient's symptoms and help restore visual function. Orbital exenteration or other radical measures offer no advantage in terms of slowing disease progression or increasing survival time and should be used only in cases of intractable ocular pain or unmanageable local hygiene because of rapid tumor growth.

5.7 Types of Cancer Metastatic to the Orbit

5.7.1 Breast Carcinoma

Breast cancer is the most common primary source of orbital metastases, and the median age of patients with newly diagnosed breast cancer is in the fifth or sixth decade of life [23]. Various large studies show that a breast primary accounts for

28.5–58.8% of cases of orbital metastasis [4, 8, 13]. Most patients, 89% in one series, have an established diagnosis prior to presentation [4]. The mean interval from the diagnosis of breast cancer to the detection of orbital metastasis has been reported to range from 4.5 to 6.5 years [4].

The characteristic presentation of orbital metastases from breast cancer consists of infiltration of the extraocular muscles and surrounding orbital fat, causing motility deficits, proptosis, globe dystopia, and enophthalmos. The association between an enophthalmic presentation and scirrhous adenocarcinoma is well known, but it is important to recognize that breast cancer metastasis to orbit may also produce proptosis rather than enophthalmos.

The histologic features of adenocarcinoma of the breast differ, and the histology of orbital metastases may vary from that of the primary tumor. Orbital metastatic cells are usually undifferentiated anaplastic cells showing single-file infiltration of fat or dense lakes of cellular lobules [4]. In a report by Garrity et al. [4], 94.6% of cases (35/37) were anaplastic grade 3 or grade 4 tumors.

Regardless of the primary tumor, the presence of orbital metastases portends a poor prognosis; the mean survival after diagnosis of such metastases is 31 months (range, 1–116 months) [4, 24]. The only appropriate surgical intervention for breast carcinoma metastatic to the orbit is biopsy to establish the diagnosis, after which external-beam radiotherapy is the mainstay therapy used to stabilize the disease. Chemotherapy or hormonal therapy may also be administered, depending on the overall disease burden.

5.7.2 *Lung Carcinoma*

Lung cancer remains the leading cause of cancer-related mortality in the Western world and is the second most common carcinoma to metastasize to the orbit. It accounts for 8–12% of cases of orbital metastasis. Patients have an aggressive presentation reflecting the degree of mass effect and extraocular muscle infiltration. Compared to breast carcinoma, lung carcinoma metastasizes to the orbit earlier after diagnosis and has a poorer prognosis, with a shorter median survival time (188 vs. 666 days) [4, 25].

Treatment is guided by cancer type and tumor histology. Though there are four principal variants, non-small-cell lung cancer accounts for 80% of thoracic malignancies. The types most likely to metastasize to the orbit are large-cell undifferentiated carcinoma and small-cell carcinoma; squamous cell carcinoma and adenocarcinoma have a low incidence of orbital metastasis [2, 4].

As the majority of patients with metastatic lung carcinoma succumb to disease within a relatively short period, palliative orbital radiotherapy is the only real therapeutic option for patients with orbital metastatic lesions. Debulking surgery or orbital exenteration is reserved for severe cases of intractable orbital pain and should be avoided if at all possible.

5.7.3 Prostate Carcinoma

Despite being the second most common malignant neoplasm in men, prostate carcinoma accounts for only 3–10% of all orbital metastases reported [4, 26]. Several studies report that prostate cancer is the third most common tumor to metastasize to the orbit [3, 4, 7, 9]; however, in some other series it is reported to metastasize to the orbit less frequently than melanoma [3, 8, 15].

Common symptoms include proptosis, diplopia, eyelid swelling, decreased vision, ptosis, and red eye. Because bone metastasis is common in prostate cancer, pain is also a more common symptom in patients with prostatic orbital metastases. Ninety percent of metastatic lesions are predominantly or entirely osteoblastic [27]. When an osteoblastic lesion presents, one must keep the differential diagnosis of meningioma in mind, especially if the sphenoid bone is affected. The rapid development of osteoblastic orbital lesions in an elderly man is highly suggestive of metastatic prostate carcinoma [4].

If metastatic prostate cancer is suspected, the clinician must also inquire about nocturia, weight loss, and pain. Most prostate cancers are adenocarcinomas and range from well to very poorly differentiated. When such tumors are poorly differentiated, the primary site may remain unknown; in such cases, immunohistochemical stains can be used as a diagnostic tool. Specifically, immunoperoxidase stains should be used for prostatic-specific acid phosphatase as these levels are abnormal in more than 80% of patients with metastatic prostate cancer. The prostate-specific antigen level will often be high. Prostate cancer metastatic to the orbit can be managed safely and effectively because it is a radiosensitive malignancy; treatment for orbital disease usually consists of radiotherapy combined with hormonal therapies.

5.7.4 Melanoma

Orbital metastases from cutaneous melanoma represent 5.3–15% of all metastatic tumors of the orbit [3, 8, 15]. These are usually seen in patients with a preexisting diagnosis and disseminated end-stage disease. The primary site of origin is usually the dermis but can also be a mucosal site or the uveal tract [4, 28].

The clinical signs of orbital metastatic melanoma are similar to those of other orbital metastases; however, metastasis to extraocular muscles was seen in more than half of patients [3, 15]. This affinity for muscle would be consistent with the main presenting symptom of diplopia. Imaging studies show smooth enlargement of the muscle rather than a pattern of infiltration into the orbit (Fig. 5.3).

The survival of patients with melanoma metastatic to the orbit depends on the extent of metastatic disease and overall disease burden but generally does not exceed 12 months. However, the mean survival in one series was 19.7 months, much longer than the 5.75 and 8.4 months reported in two other published series [9, 15].

In certain cases, surgical resection to debulk the mass, even incomplete resection, may be appropriate as a palliative measure. In the case of an isolated eyelid or orbital soft tissue metastasis with no other detectable sites of metastasis, complete surgical resection of the mass followed by radiotherapy with doses of 30–60 Gy would be appropriate to achieve local control [25, 26, 29]. In patients with high disease burden and multiple metastatic sites with poor life expectancy, radical surgery is generally not indicated. Though melanoma has traditionally been considered a chemoresistant tumor, various trials of immunotherapy or standard chemotherapy for metastatic melanoma are available and should be considered for these patients.

5.7.5 *Carcinoid Tumors*

Carcinoid tumors are unusual tumors that arise from enterochromaffin cells and account for 4–5% of all orbital metastases [3, 30, 31]. Two-thirds of carcinoid tumors originate from the gastrointestinal tract; other sites of origin include the lung, ovary, thymus, and breast [30]. The peak incidence of such metastases occurs in the sixth decade, and there is a slight female predominance.

Metastatic orbital lesions from carcinoid tumors are usually slow growing and may present with a mass causing proptosis, diplopia, or less commonly inflammatory symptoms. A search for coexisting disorders should be conducted as carcinoid tumors can be associated with multiple endocrine neoplasia (either type 1 or 2) and neurofibromatosis type 1.

Standard treatment is local radiotherapy with combination chemotherapy. External-beam radiotherapy has been reported to be helpful in palliative local control of solitary orbital carcinoids [31]. Novel targeted treatments may play a greater role as standard chemotherapy has a variable degree of efficacy. The 5-year survival rate for patients with orbital metastasis from carcinoid tumors is 72% [31]. Death is usually secondary to cardiac toxicity rather than the cancer itself.

5.7.6 *Other Cancers*

Virtually any cancer that can metastasize through the hematogenous route can gain access to the orbit. Gastrointestinal cancers are a common cause of metastasis to the orbit in Japan [4, 13, 32]. Renal cell carcinoma is the most common urologic malignancy to metastasize to the orbit [4, 33]. In the pediatric population, neuroblastomas and rhabdomyosarcomas have been reported to metastasize to the orbit [4].

5.8 Conclusion

Orbital metastasis is rare. An orbital metastatic lesion may be the initial presentation of cancer in up to 25% of patients. The leading causes of orbital metastasis are breast, lung, and prostate carcinomas and cutaneous melanoma. Clinical manifestations of orbital metastases include rapid onset of orbital symptoms, including mass effect with displacement of the globe or proptosis, diplopia, orbital pain, inflammation, and bony destruction. Orbital metastasis from lung cancer tends to occur early in the disease course, whereas there is generally a long latency period between initial diagnosis and discovery of the orbital metastasis in patients with breast cancer or melanoma. Imaging studies may be helpful in diagnosing orbital metastases but are nonspecific. Fine-needle aspiration or open biopsies provide the best means to obtain a definitive diagnosis, but these procedures should be done only in patients with no known previous history of cancer, in whom the orbit is the only site of suspected metastasis, and for whom having a definitive diagnosis would change the overall management of the disease. The goal of treatment for orbital metastatic lesions is palliative, and the mainstay of treatment is external-beam radiotherapy, which is combined with chemotherapy or hormonal therapy when appropriate. Surgical resection of an orbital or an eyelid metastatic lesion is appropriate only in selected patients with metastatic cutaneous melanoma, in some patients with metastatic sarcoma for whom the ocular adnexa is the only site of detectable metastasis, and in patients with very slow-growing cancers with potential for prolonged survival, such as patients with carcinoid tumors in whom the orbital metastasis cause significant morbidity in the orbit.

References

1. Shields CL, Shields JA, Gross N, et al. Survey of 520 uveal metastases. Ophthalmology 1997;104:1265–76.
2. Ahmad SM, Esmaeli B. Metastatic tumors of the orbit and ocular adnexa. Curr Opin Ophthalmol 2007;18:405–13.
3. Goldberg RA, Rootman J, Cline R. Tumors metastatic to the orbit: a changing picture. Surv Ophthalmol 1990;35:1–24.
4. Garrity JA, Henderson JW, Cameron JD, et al. Metastatic carcinomas. In: Henderson's Orbital Tumors, fourth edition. New York, NY: Raven Press, 2007:313–26.
5. Char DH, Miller T, Kroll S. Orbital metastasis: diagnosis and course. Br J Ophthalmol 1997;81:386–90.
6. Fenton S, Kemp SE, Harnett AN. Screening for ophthalmic involvement in asymptomatic patients with metastatic breast carcinoma. Eye 2004;18:38–40.
7. Ferry AP. Tumors metastatic to the eye and ocular adnexa. In: Jakobiec FA, editor. Ocular and Adnexal Tumors. Birmingham, AL: Aesculapius, 1978:862–92.
8. Shields JA, Shields CL, Brotman HK, et al. Cancer metastatic to the orbit: the 2000 Robert M. Curtis lecture. Ophthal Plast Reconstr Surg 2001;17:346–54.
9. Goldberg RA, Rootman J. Clinical characteristics of metastatic orbital tumors. Ophthalmology 1990;97:620–4.
10. Hart WM. Metastatic carcinoma to the eye and orbit. Int Ophthalmol Clin 1962;2:465–82.
11. Castro PA, Albert DM, Wang WJ, et al. Tumors metastatic to the eye and adnexa. Int Ophthalmol Clin 1982;22:189–223.
12. Font RL, Ferry AP. Carcinoma metastatic to the eye and orbit. III. A clinicopathologic case of 28 cases metastatic to the orbit. Cancer 1976;38:1326–35.
13. Gunalp I, Gunduz K. Metastatic orbital tumors. Jpn J Ophthalmol 1995;39:65–70.
14. Hartstein ME, Beisman B, Kincaid MC. Cutaneous malignant melanoma metastatic to the eyelid. Ophthalmic Surg Lasers Imaging 1998;29:993–5.

15. Zografos L, Ducrey N, Beati D, et al. Metastatic melanoma in the eye and orbit. Ophthalmology 2003;110:2245–56.
16. Esmaeli B, Cleary KL, Ho L, et al. Leiomyosarcoma of the esophagus metastatic to the eyelid: a clinicopathologic report. Ophthal Plast Reconstr Surg 2002;18:159–61.
17. Liu D. Complications of fine needle aspiration biopsy of the orbit. Ophthalmology 1985;92:1768–71.
18. Arora R, Rewari R, Betharia SM. Fine needle aspiration cytology of orbital and adnexal masses. Acta Cytol 1992;36:483–91.
19. Kennerdell JS, Dekker A, Johnson SL, et al. Fine needle aspiration: its use in orbital tumors. Arch Ophthalmol 1979;97:1315–17.
20. Capone A Jr, Slamovits TL. Discrete metastases of solid tumors to extraocular muscles. Arch Ophthalmol 1990;108:237–43.
21. Glassburn JR, Klionsky M, Brady LW. Radiation therapy for metastatic disease involving the orbit. Am J Clin Oncol 1984;7:145–8.
22. Ahmed S, Goel S, Khandwala M, et al. Neuroblastoma with orbital metastasis: ophthalmic presentation and role of ophthalmologists. Eye 2006;20:466–70.
23. Dieing A, Schulz CO, Schmid P, et al. Orbital metastases in breast cancer: report of two cases and review of the literature. J Cancer Res Clin Oncol 2004;130:745–48.
24. Torres JJ, Medel R, Alonso T. Orbital metastases from male breast cancer in two cases. Ophthal Plast Reconstr Surg 2007;23:154–6.
25. Macedo JE, Machado M, Araujo A, et al. Orbital metastasis as a rare form of clinical presentation of non-small cell lung cancer. J Thorac Oncol 2007;2:166–7.
26. Boldt HC, Nerad JA. Orbital metastases from prostate carcinoma. Arch Ophthalmol 1988;106:1403–8.
27. Carriere VM, Karcioglu ZA, Apple DJ, et al. A review of prostate carcinoma with bilateral metastasis and a review of the literature. Ophthalmology 1982;89:402–6.
28. Hutchison BM, Damato BE, Kyle PM, et al. Choroidal melanoma metastatic to the contralateral orbit. Orbit 1994;13:85–9.
29. Ramirez R, Ivan D, Prieto VG, et al. Cutaneous melanoma metastatic to the eyelid and periocular skin. Ophthal Plast Reconstr Surg. 2010;26:88–94.
30. Modlin IM, Lye KD, Kidd M. A 5-decade analysis of 13,715 carcinoid tumors. Cancer 2003;97:934–59.
31. Mehta JS, Abou-Rayyah Y, Rose GE. Orbital carcinoid metastases. Ophthalmology 2006;113:466–72.
32. Amemiya T, Hayashida H, Dake Y. Metastatic orbital tumors in Japan: a review of the literature. Ophthalmic Epidemiol 2002;9:35–47.
33. Shome D, Honavar SG, Gupta P, et al. Metastasis to the eye and orbit from renal cell carcinoma: a report of three cases and review of literature. Surv Ophthalmol 2007;52:213–23.

Chapter 6
Secondary Orbital Tumors Extending from Ocular or Periorbital Structures

Roman Shinder and Bita Esmaeli

Abstract Secondary orbital tumors are those that extend into the orbit from contiguous structures, such as the globe, eyelids, lacrimal sac, bone, sinuses, nasopharynx, and brain. They account for approximately one-quarter of orbital neoplasia. A computed tomography or magnetic resonance imaging scan is used to investigate suspicious lesions, and biopsy is typically undertaken to establish a tissue diagnosis and help construct a treatment plan. Prognosis is often poor owing to significant extension of the tumor at presentation.

6.1 Tumors of Intraocular and Ocular Adnexal Origin

6.1.1 Eyelid Tumors

Eyelid cancers such as basal cell carcinoma, squamous cell carcinoma, and sebaceous gland carcinoma can invade the orbit if the primary tumor is left untreated; such cancers can also appear in the orbit as recurrent disease. Basal cell carcinoma is the most common eyelid cancer to invade the orbit, and basal cell carcinoma arising from the medial canthus is particularly prone to orbital invasion. Ocular adnexal cancers represent the most common indication for orbital exenteration [1], and in some cases, exenteration must be followed by adjuvant radiation therapy. In a large case series reported by Günalp et al. [1], 25% of basal cell carcinomas requiring exenteration represented recurrent disease. The mortality rates after orbital exenteration due to causes related to basal and squamous cell carcinomas were 8 and 12%, respectively, with approximately 2-year follow-up [1].

R. Shinder (✉)
Section of Ophthalmology, Department of Head and Neck Surgery, The University of Texas M.D. Anderson Cancer Center, Houston, TX, USA
e-mail: romanshinder@hotmail.com

B. Esmaeli (ed.), *Ophthalmic Oncology*, M.D. Anderson Solid Tumor Oncology Series 6, DOI 10.1007/978-1-4419-0374-7_6,

6.1.2 Intraocular Tumors

Uveal melanoma and retinoblastoma are intraocular tumors that may display extrascleral spread into the orbit in advanced cases.

Microscopic extension through the sclera and episcleral emissary channels is estimated to be present in 10–40% of enucleated uveal melanoma specimens [2, 3]. Nevertheless, gross orbital extension, which may occur along the optic nerve, remains a rare event in patients with uveal melanoma [4–6]. Optic nerve extension of uveal melanoma is estimated to occur in only 0.6–3.7% of cases (Fig. 6.1) [6]. To decrease the likelihood of orbital recurrence, palliative orbital radiation therapy may be given in cases of uveal melanoma that exhibit microscopic episcleral or optic nerve extension. However, orbital radiation therapy does not reduce the risk of distant organ metastasis from hematogenous spread of uveal melanoma, which can be lethal.

In neglected or untreated cases, retinoblastoma can demonstrate extraocular spread into the orbit, not only through the optic nerve but also through the sclera. Orbital invasion via either route is a risk factor for metastasis. In retinoblastoma, optic nerve involvement is the most important risk factor for central nervous system metastasis [7–10], and extrascleral extension has been reported to be the most significant risk factor for distant metastasis, as the tumor gains access to the vascular and lymphatic channels outside the globe [7].

Treatment modalities for orbital involvement of retinoblastoma or uveal melanoma include combined-modality chemotherapy and radiation therapy and eyelid-sparing exenteration; the mortality rates in patients treated with such modalities are 90 and 71%, respectively [1]. When retinoblastoma cells are present at the cut end of an enucleated optic nerve, adjuvant chemotherapy together with orbital radiation therapy reduces the risk of metastasis [11–13].

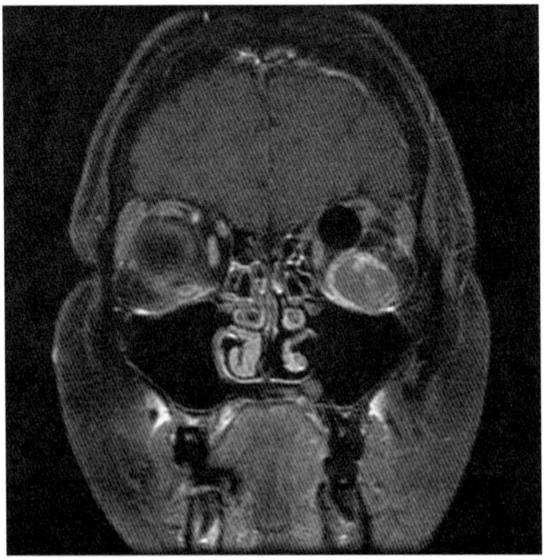

Fig. 6.1 Magnetic resonance image of a left uveal melanoma with extension into the orbit. The patient has undergone enucleation. The uveal melanoma mass in the left orbit is pushing the orbital implant up

6.2 Tumors of Sinus and Nasopharyngeal Origin

Most tumors that secondarily involve the orbit arise from the paranasal sinuses. Such tumors are slightly more common than primary orbital tumors [14, 15]. Epithelial malignancies of the sinuses frequently spread to the orbit; Conley [16] noted that 45% of such tumors invade the orbit. Approximately 80% of sinus and nasopharyngeal tumors with orbital invasion are epithelial [17]. Batsakis [18] divided epithelial malignancies of the nasal cavity and paranasal sinuses into two groups: (1) those arising from metaplastic epithelium, including squamous cell carcinoma and transitional tumors, and (2) those arising from the mucoserous epithelium, including adenocarcinoma and salivary gland neoplasia (e.g., adenoid cystic carcinoma, mucoepidermoid carcinoma, and rare malignant salivary neoplasia). Epithelial tumors occur more frequently in men than women by a ratio of 2:1, and the incidence peaks at 40–60 years [17].

The orbit is at risk of invasion from tumors of sinus or nasopharyngeal origin because it shares three thin, bony walls with the sinuses and nasal cavity: the roof, medial wall, and floor. Tumors can extend into the orbit by bony destruction, through suture lines, or via the perforating blood vessels and nerves that run through the orbital walls. Sinus tumors typically do not show early clinical signs, usually presenting after the tumor has grown to a large size, resulting in a poor prognosis. By definition, orbital invasion of sinus tumors reflects an advanced stage of disease. In these instances, proptosis and globe displacement are common, and the lesion is typically readily visible on orbital computed tomography and magnetic resonance imaging (Fig. 6.2). In the case of suspicious orbital lesions, images should be acquired up to the base of the sinuses to permit adequate evaluation.

6.2.1 Squamous Cell Carcinoma

Squamous cell carcinoma is the most common epithelial tumor secondarily invading the orbit, accounting for 60% of such lesions [19]. Two-thirds of invading squamous cell carcinomas originate within the maxillary sinus, with the ethmoid being the second most common site of origin [17, 19]. In more than 90% of instances, squamous cell carcinomas do not declare themselves clinically until they breach the sinus of origin [17]. Once the orbit is invaded, growth of such tumors may lead to clinical signs including pain and paresthesia in the face or teeth, trismus, a full alveolus, palatal erosion, chronic sinusitis, cheek swelling causing facial asymmetry, nasal obstruction, epistaxis, nasal congestion or discharge, and distortion of the maxilla [17, 20]. Ophthalmic features denoting the maxillary sinus as the site of origin include nonaxial upward globe displacement, infraorbital pain and paresthesia, decreased vision, ophthalmoplegia, diplopia, lower lid fullness, and epiphora [17, 20]. The frequency and the severity of ocular and orbital symptoms in patients with secondary orbital epithelial malignancies attest to the relatively silent origin and late-stage presentation of these tumors. When carcinoma arising in the

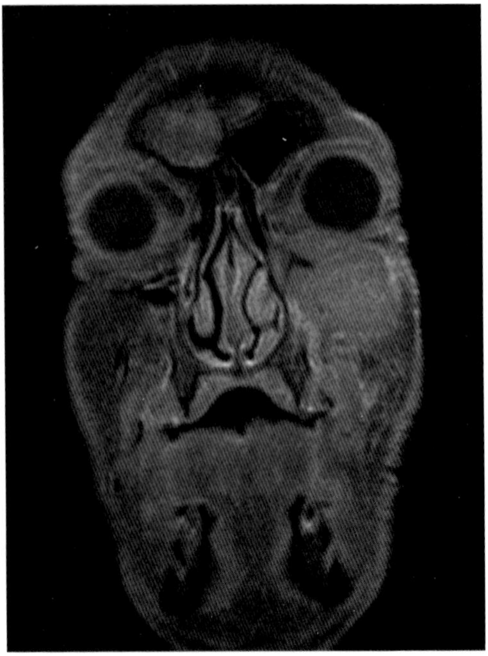

Fig. 6.2 Magnetic resonance image of a left maxillary sinus tumor invading the orbit

ethmoid sinus invades the orbit, lateral and inferior globe displacement may be seen. Nasopharyngeal carcinoma may spread to the orbit through the inferior orbital fissure and have proptosis as a late finding (Fig. 6.3). In all instances of sinus carcinoma invading the orbit, inflammatory signs may be suggested by injection, chemosis, and edema; however, tenderness and significant erythema are unusual [17]. The features that help distinguish secondary epithelial malignancies from practically every other tumefaction of the orbit are chronic, progressive, and relentless facial pain and paresthesia (in 60% of patients) and nonaxial globe displacement (in 48% of patients) [17]. In contrast to secondary epithelial tumors invading the orbit from adjacent structures, metastatic orbital tumors are painful in only about 25% of cases, and proptosis is typically axial [17]. Radiologic findings consist of either focal or widespread destruction of the sinuses, with invasion of adjacent structures by a typically large solid tumor mass, often with extension to the skull base. Histopathologically, the majority of cases consist of moderately well-differentiated keratinizing squamous carcinoma [21].

Treatment of squamous cell carcinoma with orbital invasion is usually a combination of radical surgical excision and radiation therapy and often necessitates exenteration if the periorbita has been invaded [19]. Combined-modality chemotherapy and radiation therapy can also yield nice outcomes in some cases of nasopharyngeal carcinoma with orbital invasion. In addition, patients with regional nodal disease but without distant metastases are potentially curable and should be treated aggressively with neck dissection and postoperative adjuvant irradiation of the nodal

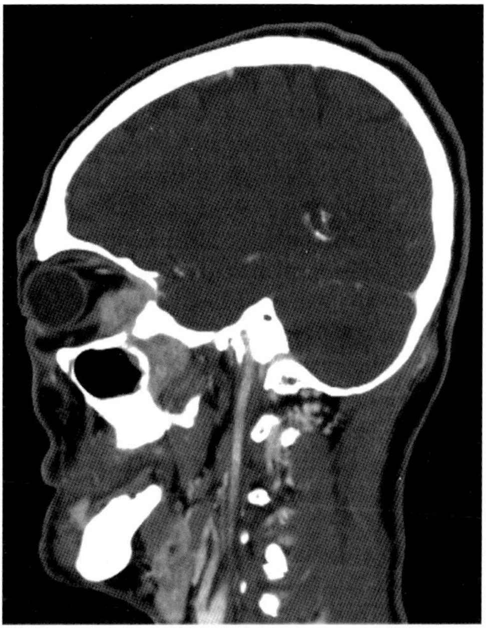

Fig. 6.3 Computed tomography image of a nasopharyngeal carcinoma invading the posterior orbit

basins [17]. In recent years, there has been a shift toward preservation of the ocular structures with reconstruction of surrounding tissues whenever possible. This is particularly true when there is evidence of only minimal orbital invasion or extraperiosteal involvement [17]. Historically, prognosis has been dismal, with a 5-year survival rate of approximately 35% [17]. Tumors arising from the posterior portion of the maxillary sinus are associated with a worse prognosis because of proximity to the orbit, cribriform plate, and pterygoid region [17]. Approximately 10–22% of squamous cell carcinomas have regional lymph node metastases on initial presentation [17]. Mortality is largely linked to the inability to eradicate local disease, with approximately 18% of patients ultimately developing distant metastases [17].

6.2.2 Other Tumors of Sinus and Nasopharyngeal Origin

Transitional carcinomas originate from the epithelium of the nasal cavity and paranasal sinuses, most commonly arising from the ethmoid sinuses or nasopharynx [17]. The majority of lesions are benign papillomas characterized by multiple and multifocal occurrence and local recurrence [17]. Though these lesions may recur, the large majority remain benign. Only 7–9% undergo malignant transformation, and most of these originate in the lateral nasal wall [17]. Treatment is radical surgery, radiation therapy, or both.

Other epithelial paranasal neoplasms that may invade the orbit but occur less frequently include adenoid cystic carcinoma and adenocarcinoma. Both are locally aggressive tumors characterized by a course of indolence, recurrence, and potential mortality.

Nonepithelial paranasal sinus tumors that may invade the orbit include a variety of benign and malignant entities. The most common of these are osteomas, fibrous dysplasia, and sarcomas, while osseous and cartilaginous tumors are rare. Osteoma is the most common of the nonepithelial paranasal sinus tumors; however, its pathogenesis remains unclear, though traumatic, infective, and hamartomatous theories have been proposed [20]. The fact that these tumors were found in 0.42% of plain sinus radiographs reflects their prevalence [22]. Osteomas are benign, slow-growing, well-circumscribed tumors composed of mature bone and can be completely excised in most cases. The most common site of origin is the frontal sinus.

6.3 Tumors of Brain Origin

Meningiomas are the most common intracranial tumor to extend to the orbit, and invasion by any other intracranial tumor is exceedingly rare [17].

6.3.1 Meningioma

Intracranial meningiomas that secondarily invade the orbit are much more common than primary orbital meningiomas. Meningiomas are invasive tumors that arise from arachnoid villi. They commonly (in 18–20% of cases) arise from the dura of the sphenoid wing (i.e., ridge, planum, parasellar region, or optic canal) and may extend into the orbit through bone, the superior orbital fissure, or the optic canal (Fig. 6.4) [17, 23]. Tumor invasion may thus compress the optic nerve or superior orbital fissure. These sphenoid wing meningiomas occur three times more often in women, typically during their fifth decade [22]. Tumors occurring in young patients tend to be more aggressive. Multifocal simultaneous meningiomas may occur, and there is an increased frequency of intracranial and orbital meningiomas in patients with neurofibromatosis type 2 (12% of patients) [22].

Ophthalmic manifestations are dependent on the location of the primary tumor. Medially located meningiomas arising near the sella and optic nerves cause early optic nerve and cavernous sinus compression leading to visual defects, motor and sensory deficits, venous obstructive signs such as edema and chemosis, and papilledema or optic atrophy [23, 24]. Tumors arising near the lateral third of the sphenoid bone, middle cranial fossa, and olfactory groove often produce a temporal fossa mass, chronic proptosis, ophthalmoplegia, and late optic nerve compression [24]. A classic finding in laterally located tumors is fullness in the temporal fossa due to reactive bone thickening (hyperostosis). This may be easily noted in patients

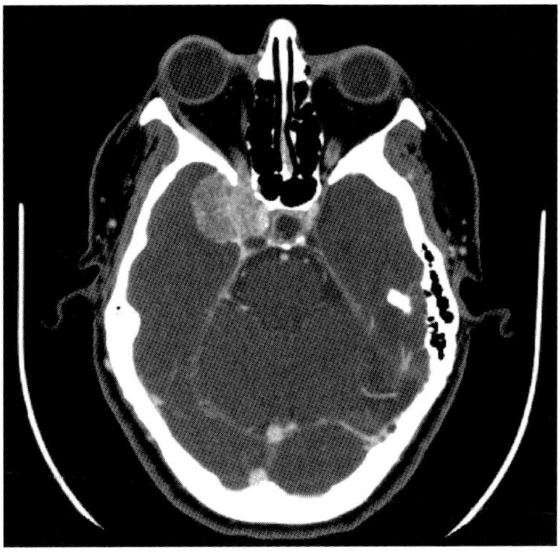

Fig. 6.4 Computed tomography image of a left middle cranial fossa meningioma invading the posterior orbital apex

wearing glasses, as the gap between the temporalis and the temple of the glasses is narrow compared to the gap on the contralateral side. Retrospective review of photographs can also be helpful in this regard. Olfactory groove meningiomas may cause loss of the sense of smell, along with compressive optic neuropathy [24]. Rarely, lower eyelid edema or erythema and chemosis may be present. Overall, half of patients present with progressive unilateral visual loss and half with progressive bilateral visual loss. The exception to this pattern is patients with olfactory groove meningiomas, who have a higher incidence of bilateral visual loss [22].

Computed tomography commonly reveals localized hyperostosis with associated calcifications owing to psammoma bodies in the tumor [25]. At times, bone absorption and destruction are apparent. Magnetic resonance imaging with contrast enhancement can help outline the extent of tumor adjacent to the bone and may prove superior in detecting smaller tumors. The lesion is usually well defined, homogeneous, and characteristically of increased density with uniform postcontrast enhancement [22].

The development of multidisciplinary and microsurgical approaches has substantially improved surgical outcomes for intracranial meningiomas with secondary orbital involvement. Provided the tumor is well defined, excision is very effective. However, invasion of bone and adjacent soft tissues or encasement of vital structures may preclude complete excision. Treatment consists of combined neurosurgical and orbital panoramic orbitotomies with excision or debulking in tandem with postoperative radiation therapy as an adjunct or in cases of incomplete excision, recurrent tumors, or cavernous sinus lesions [22, 26, 27]. Major debulking can be effective in improving cosmesis and alleviating compressive symptoms, leading to reversal or postponement of visual loss [22]. Adjuvant radiation therapy has been proven to reduce overall time to and rates of recurrence [22]. Image-guided techniques may play a role in the future surgical or stereotactic radiosurgical treatment of meningiomas [22, 28]. Because recurrence rates are significant, long-term follow-up of surgical patients is key.

6.3.2 Other Intracranial Tumors

Intracranial glioblastoma multiforme is highly malignant and may enter the orbit by gross destruction of orbital bone, extension through the optic canal and superior orbital fissure, or growth through a previous craniotomy site into the scalp and forehead and then over the superior rim into the anterior orbit [29—31]. Pituitary tumors and craniopharyngiomas have been described as invading the orbit in rare cases, but such invasion usually reflects malignancy and skull-based invasion [17, 32].

References

1. Günalp I, Gündüz K, Dürük K. Orbital exenteration: a review of 429 cases. Int Ophthalmol 1995–1996;19:177–84.
2. Shammas HF, Blodi FC. Orbital extension of choroidal and ciliary body melanomas. Arch Ophthalmol 1977;95:2002–5.
3. Sambuelli R, Luna JD, Reviglio VE, et al. Small choroidal melanoma with massive extraocular extension: invasion through posterior scleral emissary channels. Int Ophthalmol 2001;24:213–8.
4. Shields CL, Shields JA, Yarian DL, et al. Intracranial extension of choroidal melanoma via the optic nerve. Br J Ophthalmol 1987;71:172–6.
5. Saadati H, Calvano C, Diba R, et al. Orbital and optic chiasmal extension of uveal melanoma. Ophthal Plast Reconstr Surg 2004;20:387–90.
6. Wilder HC, Paul EV. Malignant melanoma of the choroid and ciliary body: a study of 2535 cases. Mil Surg 1951;109:370–8.
7. Finger PT, Harbour JW, Karcioglu ZA. Risk factors for metastasis in retinoblastoma. Surv Ophthalmol 2002;47:1–16.
8. Khelfaoui F, Validire P, Auperin A, et al. Histopathologic risk factors in retinoblastoma: a retrospective study of 172 patients treated in a single institution. Cancer 1996;77:1206–13.
9. Shields CL, Shields JA, Baez KA, et al. Choroidal invasion of retinoblastoma: metastatic potential and clinical risk factors. Br J Ophthalmol 1993;77:544–8.
10. Shields CL, Shields JA, Baez K, et al. Optic nerve invasion of retinoblastoma: metastatic potential and clinical risk factors. Cancer 1994;73:692–8.
11. Honavar SG, Singh AD, Shields CL, et al. Postenucleation adjuvant therapy in high-risk retinoblastoma. Arch Ophthalmol 2002;120:923–31.
12. Zelter M, Damel A, Gonzales G, et al. A prospective study on the treatment of retinoblastoma in 72 patients. Cancer 1991;68:1685–90.
13. Doz F, Neuenschwander S, Plantaz D, et al. Etoposide and carboplatin in extraocular retinoblastoma: a study by the Societe Francaise d'Oncologie Pediatrique. J Clin Oncol 1995;13:902–9.
14. McLean IW, Burnier MN, Zimmerman LE, et al. Tumors of the Eye and Ocular Adnexa. Washington, DC: Armed Forces Institute of Pathology, 1994:215–98.
15. Shinder R, Al-Zubidi N, Esmaeli B. Survey of orbital tumors at a comprehensive cancer center in the United States. Head Neck. In Press.
16. Conley J. Concepts in Head and Neck Surgery. New York, NY: Grune & Stratton, 1970:5.
17. Rootman J, Katz SE. Secondary tumors of the orbit. In: Rootman J, editor. Diseases of the Orbit: A Multidisciplinary Approach, second edition. Philadelphia, PA: Lippincott Williams & Wilkins, 2003:304–11.
18. Batsakis JG. Pathology of tumors of the nasal cavity and paranasal sinuses. In: Thawley SE, Panje WR, editors. Comprehensive Management of Head and Neck Tumors, Vol 1. Philadelphia, PA: WB Saunders, 1987:327.

19. Johnson LN, Krohel GB, Yeon EB, et al. Sinus tumors invading the orbit. Ophthalmology 1984;91:209–17.
20. Kanski JJ. Orbit. In: Kanski JJ, editor. Clinical Ophthalmology: A Systematic Approach, fifth edition. London: Butterworth Heinemann, 2003:588.
21. Batsakis JG, Rice DH, Solomon AR. The pathology of head and neck tumors: squamous and mucous-gland carcinomas of the nasal cavity, paranasal sinuses, and larynx, part 6. Head Neck Surg 1980;2:497–508.
22. Rootman J, Selva D. Primary bone tumors of the orbit. In: Rootman J, editor. Diseases of the Orbit: A Multidisciplinary Approach, second edition. Philadelphia, PA: Lippincott Williams & Wilkins, 2003:280–3.
23. Rootman J. Neurogenic tumors. In: Rootman J, editor. Diseases of the Orbit: A Multidisciplinary Approach, second edition. Philadelphia, PA: Lippincott Williams & Wilkins, 2003:228–33.
24. Kanski JJ. Neuro-ophthalmology. In: Kanski JJ, editor. Clinical Ophthalmology: A Systematic Approach, fifth edition. London: Butterworth Heinemann, 2003:645–6.
25. Terstegge K, Schorner W, Henkes H, et al. Hyperostosis in meningiomas: MR findings in patients with recurrent meningioma of the sphenoid wings. AJNR Am J Neuroradiol 1994;15:555–60.
26. McDermott MW, Durity FA, Rootman J, et al. Combined frontotemporal–orbitozygomatic approach for tumors of the sphenoid wing and orbit. Neurosurgery 1990;26:107–16.
27. Peele KA, Kennerdell JS, Maroon JC, et al. The role of postoperative irradiation in the management of sphenoid wing meningioma. A preliminary report. Ophthalmology 1996;103:1761–6.
28. Barnett GH, Steiner CP, Weisenberger J. Intracranial meningioma resection using frameless stereotaxy. J Image Guid Surg 1995;1:46–52.
29. Aoyama I, Makita Y, Nabeshima S, et al. Extradural nasal and orbital extension of glioblastoma multiforme without previous surgical intervention. Surg Neurol 1980;14:343–7.
30. Hoyt WF, Piovenetti E, Malmud N, et al. Cranio-orbital involvement in glioblastoma multiforme. Neurochirurgia 1972;15:1–8.
31. Lawton AW, Karesh JW. Intracranial glioblastoma invading the orbit. Arch Ophthalmol 1986;104:806.
32. Demaerel P, Mosley IF, Scaravilli F. Recurrent craniopharyngioma invading the orbit, cavernous sinus and skull base: a case report. Neuroradiology 1993;35:261–3.

Chapter 7
Lacrimal Gland Tumors

Brent Hayek and Bita Esmaeli

Abstract This chapter outlines the clinical presentation and management of tumors that affect the lacrimal gland. Lacrimal gland tumors can be categorized as lymphoproliferative lesions, benign epithelial tumors, and malignant epithelial tumors. Lymphomas are the most common primary cancers of the orbit in adults, and the lacrimal gland is a frequent site of involvement. Benign epithelial tumors of the lacrimal gland include pleomorphic adenomas, oncocytomas, and spindle cell myoepitheliomas. Adenoid cystic carcinoma is the most common primary malignant epithelial tumor of the lacrimal gland; others include mixed tumor, adenocarcinoma, mucoepidermoid carcinoma, squamous cell carcinoma, oncocytoma, and acinic cell carcinoma. The American Joint Committee on Cancer staging system, which is used to classify many malignant epithelial tumors of the head and neck, can provide objective criteria for staging of lacrimal gland tumors. Because tumor stage at presentation may be associated with prognosis, it should be considered when treatment is planned.

7.1 Introduction

A wide variety of tumors can develop in the lacrimal gland and lacrimal gland fossa (Table 7.1). Lacrimal gland tumors can be categorized as lymphoproliferative lesions, benign epithelial tumors, and malignant epithelial tumors. Overlapping clinical presentations of mass lesions in this region are common, but findings on history as well as specific findings on clinical examination and imaging can help distinguish between different types of lesions [1–6]. Radiographic modalities, particularly computed tomography (CT) and magnetic resonance imaging, are useful in delineating the type of lacrimal gland lesion [7–9].

B. Hayek (✉)
Section of Oculoplastics, Orbital and Cosmetic Surgery, Department of Ophthalmology, Emory University Eye Center, Atlanta, GA, USA
e-mail: bhayek@me.com

B. Esmaeli (ed.), *Ophthalmic Oncology*, M.D. Anderson Solid Tumor Oncology Series 6, DOI 10.1007/978-1-4419-0374-7_7,

Table 7.1 Types of lacrimal gland lesions

Lymphoproliferative diseases
Benign lymphoid hyperplasia
Atypical lymphoid hyperplasia
Malignant lymphoma
Benign tumors
Pleomorphic adenoma (benign mixed tumor)
Benign fibrous histiocytoma
Oncocytoma
Myoepithelioma
Cystadenoma
Malignant tumors
Adenoid cystic carcinoma
Malignant mixed tumor (carcinoma ex pleomorphic adenoma)
Adenocarcinoma
Mucoepidermoid carcinoma
Squamous cell carcinoma
Acinic cell carcinoma
Malignant oncocytoma
Other localized lesions
Dacryops
Dermoid cysts
Hemangioma
Amyloid
Lung and breast metastases

This chapter will outline the clinical presentation and management of the various types of tumors that affect the lacrimal gland. The chapter will also review the American Joint Committee on Cancer (AJCC) staging system for lacrimal gland tumors.

7.2 Lymphoproliferative Lesions of the Lacrimal Gland

Lymphomas are the most common primary cancers of the orbit in adults, representing 20% of orbital masses [4, 10–12]. Almost all lymphomas of the orbit, lacrimal gland, or conjunctiva are of the non-Hodgkin B-cell types; the lacrimal gland is a frequent site of involvement and is estimated to be involved in about 50% of all cases of orbital lymphoma (Fig. 7.1a) [13]. Extranodal marginal-zone B-cell lymphoma (low-grade B-cell lymphoma of the mucosa-associated lymphoid tissue type) is the most common histologic subtype seen in the orbit (Fig. 7.1b) [4, 5, 10, 13, 14]; the next most common subtypes, in decreasing order of frequency, are follicular lymphoma, diffuse large-cell lymphoma, and mantle cell lymphoma.

Clinically, both primary and secondary lymphoproliferative lesions of the lacrimal gland tend to grow slowly and be associated with minimal pain and minimal acute swelling [5, 6]. Most patients are elderly, have unilateral disease, and

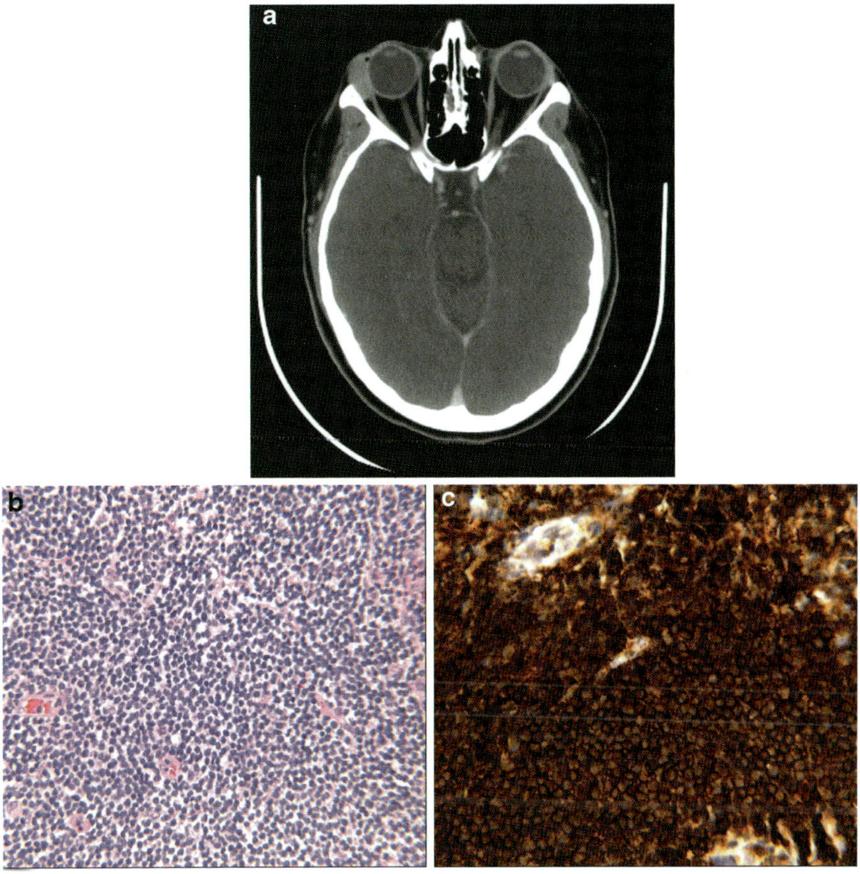

Fig. 7.1 Lymphoma of the lacrimal gland. (**a**) Computed tomography image of a 75-year-old patient with a right lacrimal gland lymphoma. (**b**) Histologic findings indicating low-grade non-Hodgkin B-cell lymphoma. (**c**) The lymphocytes are CD-20 positive, as shown in this photomicrograph. Figures courtesy of Dr. Bita Esmaeli

present with symptoms less than 1 year in duration. The overall rate of systemic involvement associated with orbital lymphoma is reported to be 30–50% [15]. Once the diagnosis of lymphoma of the lacrimal gland is established via a biopsy, a thorough workup is warranted to look for systemic sites of involvement. A total-body positron emission tomography scan is a way to rule out areas of hypermetabolic activity throughout the body and serves as a complement to conventional imaging for staging of lymphomas [15]. Positron emission tomography scans can also be used to evaluate response to therapy [16].

Treatment of lacrimal gland lymphoma depends on the histologic subtype and stage at diagnosis and may include radiation therapy, systemic chemotherapy, monoclonal antibody therapy, or a combination of these [11, 17].

7.3 Benign Epithelial Tumors of the Lacrimal Gland

7.3.1 Pleomorphic Adenoma

The most common epithelial tumor of the lacrimal gland is pleomorphic adenoma (a benign mixed-cell tumor) [18, 19], which accounts for approximately 50% of all epithelial lacrimal gland tumors [5]. Pleomorphic adenoma most commonly presents in the fourth to fifth decades of life and is rare in children [5, 19–21]. Actuarial estimates indicate that the risk of malignant transformation if pleomorphic adenoma is left untreated is 10% in 20 years and 20% in 30 years [19].

Pleomorphic adenoma commonly presents as a slowly progressive, painless mass in the lacrimal gland fossa. Most pleomorphic adenomas affect the orbital lobe, so the most common finding is axial proptosis with downward and medial displacement. However, pleomorphic adenoma may present solely with eyelid ptosis [3]. Patients may complain of diplopia from globe dystopia and restricted eye movement. This tumor affects males slightly more frequently than females and is usually symptomatic for more than a year before diagnosis [5, 19–21].

Examination typically demonstrates a firm, mobile mass just inferior to the superolateral orbital rim. CT and magnetic resonance imaging often show a roundish mass of varying homogeneity, with evidence of bony excavation and remodeling correlating with the slow growth of this lesion. Bony excavation and remodeling is the classic finding on imaging but is not always present. In their review of patients with lacrimal gland pleomorphic adenomas, Garrity et al. [3] found that only 44% of patients had bony abnormalities. Also, atypical presentations of this tumor are not uncommon. Patients may present with signs mimicking orbital cellulitis, chalazion, or dacryoadenitis [22–26].

Pleomorphic adenoma is so named because of its mixed histologic features. The tumor is a lobular, grossly yellowish-white lesion with a thin pseudocapsule. It is solid when cut open (Fig. 7.2) but commonly has areas of cystic degeneration. Histologically, the tumor contains myxoid areas, benign epithelium in nests, and ductal structures. There may also be fibrosis and formation of hyaline cartilage and bone [26]. Immunohistochemical studies indicate that this tumor is derived from ductal epithelium and certain cells in the stroma and myoepithelium. Various reports have demonstrated increased S-100 and glial fibrillary acidic protein expression in pleomorphic adenomas [27–30]. Management involves complete resection of the tumor, the pseudocapsule, and a small margin of normal lacrimal gland/orbital tissue if possible, en bloc without a preliminary incisional biopsy or piecemeal excision (Fig. 7.2a and b) [1, 6, 31–33]. Therefore, the likelihood that the tumor is a benign pleomorphic adenoma must be determined on the basis of clinical and radiographic findings. The rate of correlation between the clinical and histopathologic diagnosis varies from 50 to 87% [3, 6, 34]. The pseudocapsule represents adjacent compressed lacrimal gland/orbital tissue and contains microscopic fenestrations, so excising a margin of normal tissue around the pseudocapsule is advised. In their 1978 series,

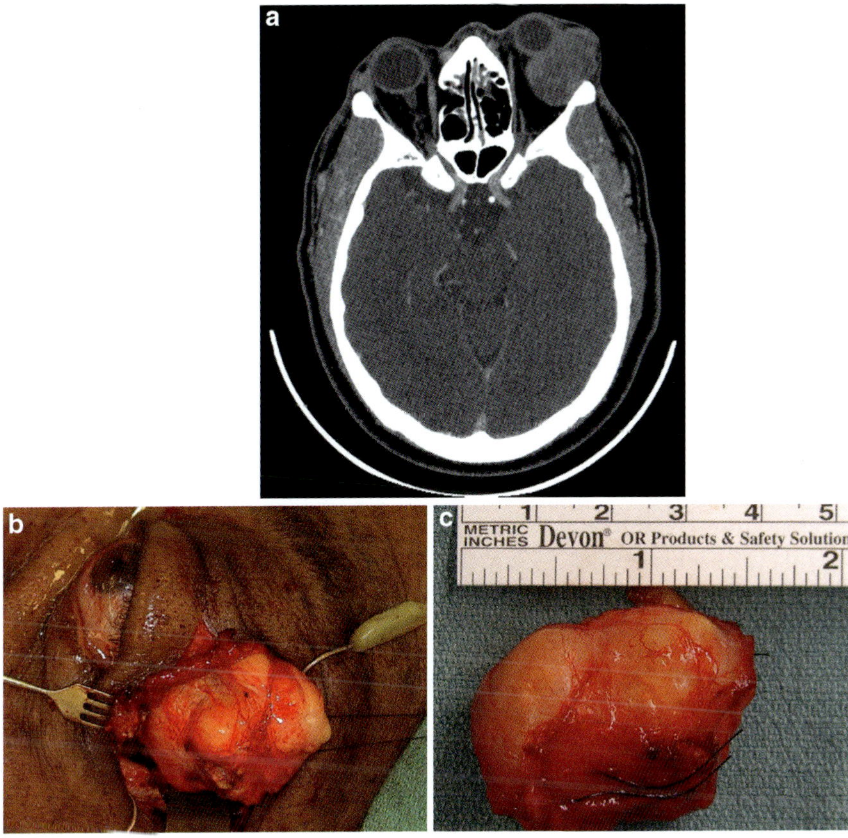

Fig. 7.2 (**a**) Computed tomography image of a patient with a large pleomorphic adenoma of the lacrimal gland. (**b**) En bloc surgical resection of a pleomorphic adenoma of the lacrimal gland through a lateral orbitotomy and bone flap. (**c**) The lesion was excised with its pseudocapsule intact. Figures courtesy of Dr. Bita Esmaeli

Font and Gamel [19] reported a 5-year recurrence rate of 3% for completely excised lesions and 32% for incompletely excised adenomas. An anterolateral orbitotomy will allow for enough exposure to resect the majority of these tumors. Ni et al. [35] reported that all 15 patients who underwent an anterolateral complete resection with a rim of adjacent lacrimal gland/orbital tissue were free of recurrence at a mean follow-up time of 9.7 years (range, 3–21 years).

Long-term surveillance is advised since recurrence has been documented years after excision. Recently, Currie and Rose [36] retrospectively reviewed 72 patients who underwent excision of pleomorphic adenoma and had more than 5 years of follow-up. They stratified patients according to the degree to which the tumor was likely to seed the orbit and found that only one patient, who had a prior incisional biopsy, had a recurrence of benign disease, 12.5 years after excision.

7.3.2 Other Benign Epithelial Tumors

Other benign epithelial lacrimal gland tumors include oncocytoma and spindle cell myoepithelioma. Non malignant tumor lesions simulating clinical presentations similar to those of lacrimal gland lesions include congenital dermoid cysts, dacryops, and cavernous hemangioma.

Oncocytoma (oxyphilic adenoma) refers to a tumor of oncocytes. Oncocytes are found in numerous mucous membranes, including the caruncle, conjunctiva, lacrimal sac, and lacrimal glands. Oncocytoma of the lacrimal gland is rare and has been described as either malignant or benign in a few case reports [37–41]. Oncocytomas tend to grow slowly, have variable symptoms, and can be clinically mistaken for hemangiomas, nevi, or cysts [38]. Histologically, the large epithelial cells of oncocytomas contain a granular eosinophilic cytoplasm and small nuclei without atypia and can form cords and tubular structures [41]. Complete resection of oncocytomas is advised.

Primary spindle cell myoepitheliomas of the lacrimal gland are also rare, but numerous cases of this tumor have been reported in the literature since 1990 [42–44]. Grossniklaus et al. [44] were the first to report a case of non-spindle cell myoepithelioma, which was identified on the basis of immunohistochemistry and ultrastructural features. Myoepitheliomas of the lacrimal gland mimic benign pleomorphic adenomas in that they are associated with a long period of painless proptosis. Myoepitheliomas are encapsulated lesions, and complete resection is possible and advocated [3].

7.4 Malignant Epithelial Tumors of the Lacrimal Gland

7.4.1 Adenoid Cystic Carcinoma

The most common primary malignant epithelial tumor of the lacrimal gland is adenoid cystic carcinoma (ACC). It accounts for 1.6% of all orbital tumors and 20–35% of primary epithelial neoplasms of the lacrimal gland [1–3, 45]. This tumor presents most commonly in the fourth to fifth decades of life and is less common in children and teenagers. ACC has been histologically documented in individuals ranging from 6 to over 70 years, and a number of case reports have been published on this tumor occurring in children [46–50]. It occurs with equal frequencies in males and females. It is known to have an indolent and persistent course with a high risk of local and regional recurrence and late distant metastasis.

For ACC and other epithelial malignancies, the clinical history and presentation may include a palpable mass in the superior lateral quadrant, with associated pain or dysesthesia, and proptosis directed inferomedially. The duration of symptoms is typically less than 1 year. CT imaging may show bony erosion or destruction of the orbital roof and/or lateral wall. ACCs, similar to benign pleomorphic adenomas, are round or ovoid expansible masses (Fig. 7.3a), mainly originating in the orbital

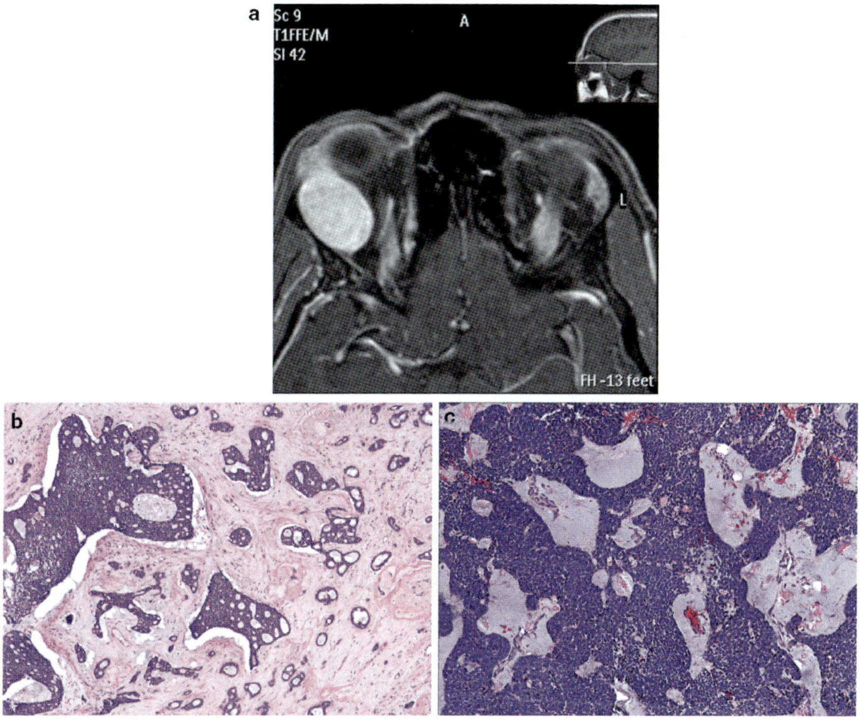

Fig. 7.3 Adenoid cystic carcinoma of the lacrimal gland. (**a**) Magnetic resonance imaging demonstrates a large lobular adenoid cystic carcinoma of the lacrimal gland. Typical histologic findings of adenoid cystic carcinoma of the lacrimal gland with predominantly cribriform pattern ("Swiss cheese" appearance) (**b**) and solid (basaloid) pattern (**c**). Figures courtesy of Dr. Bita Esmaeli

lobe, that displace and may indent the globe. Other signs noted on funduscopic examination may include choroidal striae and, less commonly, optic nerve swelling or decreased vision [6, 14, 26].

ACC of the lacrimal gland has a worse prognosis than ACC of the salivary glands. Lacrimal gland ACC has a tendency for early perineural spread and bony invasion. Even after treatment, rates of recurrence and distant metastasis are high, and death occurs in 50% of patients [51–58].

There are five histologic subtypes of ACC: cribriform ("Swiss cheese" appearance) (Fig. 7.3b), solid (basaloid), sclerosing, comedocarcinomatous, and tubular (ductal). Combinations of different subtypes are not uncommon, but typically one subtype predominates. The cribriform pattern is associated with a more favorable prognosis (particularly in children), and the solid subtype is associated with the worst prognosis [51, 52].

Treatment varies among different institutions, and standard treatments for different stages of the tumor are not well established [1, 52–57]. The most common surgical treatment is an orbital exenteration, usually with removal of the bony walls of the lacrimal gland fossa, and this is usually followed by postoperative radiation therapy. Given the propensity for perineural invasion (seen in about 75% of cases), various forms of adjuvant postoperative radiation therapy have been advocated, including external-beam, proton, and brachytherapy [1, 49, 52–57]. More recently, a regimen of preoperative intraarterial chemotherapy, orbital exenteration followed by radiation therapy, and then intravenous chemotherapy has been employed at one center in an effort to enhance long-term overall survival [55, 56]. The preliminary results of this trial seem promising [56], although the historical control group in this study had an unusually high death rate (close to 100%), which makes the conclusions of this study potentially skewed. The other reason intraarterial chemotherapy and adjuvant chemotherapy have not been more widely used is that standard chemotherapy is quite ineffective in the treatment of metastatic ACC; thus, use of a drug or combination of drugs in the adjuvant setting is not well accepted by the majority of medical oncologists. Another approach that has been advocated at some centers is conservative surgery (globe-preserving surgery) followed by proton radiation therapy.

Given the rarity of ACC of the lacrimal gland, prospective trials comparing different treatment modalities are not practical. In addition, such trials would require long-term follow-up to be meaningful, as late recurrences and death have been reported [14, 52–57]. In a recent retrospective multicenter study, we concluded that AJCC stage at initial diagnosis of lacrimal gland ACC impacts the rates of local recurrence and survival [58]. In this study, we found that an AJCC classification of T3 or greater correlated with poorer survival outcomes in patients with ACC [58].

7.4.2 Other Malignant Epithelial Tumors

Other primary malignant epithelial tumors of the lacrimal gland include malignant mixed tumor (carcinoma ex pleomorphic adenoma), adenocarcinoma, mucoepidermoid carcinoma, squamous cell carcinoma, malignant oncocytoma, and acinic cell carcinoma [1, 19, 38, 59–62].

A malignant mixed tumor of the lacrimal gland may arise out of a long-standing or incompletely resected benign pleomorphic adenoma. Malignant mixed tumors represent 4–19% of lacrimal gland epithelial neoplasms and can be further subclassified on the basis of the malignant elements predominant in the tumor [1–3, 45, 63]. The four most often encountered malignant subtypes are adenocarcinoma, ACC, squamous cell carcinoma, and spindle cell carcinoma. An epithelial–myoepithelial carcinoma subtype has also been described [64]. The adenocarcinoma subtype may be more common in men, and the ACC subtype may be more common in women [19]. Imaging may reveal both benign- and malignant-appearing components [65]. All subtypes of malignant mixed tumors are highly malignant tumors. In light of this fact and the reality that malignant mixed tumors can arise from pleomorphic adenoma, when a benign pleomorphic adenoma is resected, it is critically important to perform a complete resection with an intact capsule and a margin of surrounding normal tissue.

Adenocarcinomas occur with about the same frequency as malignant mixed tumors and are also very malignant [66]. Adenocarcinoma most often affects men in their fourth to sixth decades and is prone to recurrence and early lymphatic and distant metastatic spread [19]. Because of the possibility of early dissemination, it is prudent to perform sonography of the neck and chest radiography at presentation. The clinical presentation and CT appearance of adenocarcinoma are similar to those of ACC. Management of lacrimal gland adenocarcinoma is challenging because of the rarity of this tumor. On the basis of retrospective reviews, some authors advocate orbital exenteration with postoperative radiation therapy for high-grade tumors, whereas others suggest en bloc craniofacial orbitectomy combined with regional lymph node dissection [3, 66]. In cases of low-grade adenocarcinoma of the lacrimal gland, complete surgical resection with preservation of globe and postoperative adjuvant radiation therapy may also be a reasonable option. Four cases have been reported of a subtype of adenocarcinoma of the lacrimal gland, termed primary ductal adenocarcinoma [67–71].

Mucoepidermoid carcinoma of the lacrimal gland is rare [59]. Histologically, the tumor is composed of epidermoid and mucous-secreting cells. Eviatar and Hornblass [59] subclassify these tumors as either low grade (grade 1 or 2) or high grade (grade 3) on the basis of histopathologic features. On the basis of histopathologic review and follow-up of 14 patients, they recommend simple resection with or without radiation therapy for low-grade tumors and orbital exenteration with radiation therapy for high-grade tumors [59].

Primary lacrimal gland squamous cell carcinoma is also a rare tumor and represents fewer than 2% of primary lacrimal gland carcinomas [67]. Most squamous cell carcinomas of the lacrimal gland are the subtype associated with malignant mixed tumors. It is thought that squamous cell carcinoma of the lacrimal gland can also arise from preexisting metaplasia in a dacryops or from choristomatous epithelium-lined cysts [72, 73].

Malignant oncocytoma and acinic cell carcinoma of the lacrimal gland are very rare, and there are only a few case reports in the literature [19, 62].

7.5 AJCC Staging for Lacrimal Gland Tumors

Until recently no uniform classification system had been used to classify lacrimal gland tumors for purposes of reporting outcomes or for selecting treatment algorithms. The AJCC staging system is used to classify many malignant epithelial tumors of the head and neck and can provide objective criteria for management of such tumors [74]. However, there is little information in the literature on the value of AJCC staging for orbital tumors. Most studies and textbooks on orbital tumors make no mention of AJCC stage as a predictor of outcome for cancers of the orbit and ocular adnexa.

In a retrospective analysis of ACC of the lacrimal gland at our institution and several other centers, we found that a tumor size of T3 or greater is associated with a higher rate of local recurrence and poorer prognosis [58]. Thus, incorporation of AJCC stage at presentation as the basis for choosing treatment modalities in multi-institutional clinical trials for epithelial tumors of the lacrimal gland may make sense. This might ultimately lead to a more selective approach to surgical treatment of epithelial tumors of the lacrimal gland, including the use of more conservative surgery with globe preservation followed by radiation therapy for selected patients with smaller tumors and less aggressive histologic subtypes at presentation.

References

1. Wright JE, Rose GE, Garner A. Primary malignant neoplasms of the lacrimal gland. Br J Ophthalmol 1992;76(7):401–7.
2. Ashton N. Epithelial tumours of the lacrimal gland. Mod Probl Ophthalmol 1975;14:306–23.
3. Garrity JA, Henderson JW, Cameron JD. Primary epithelial neoplasms. In: Henderson's Orbital Tumors, fourth edition. Philadelphia, PA: Lippincott, Williams & Wilkins, 2007: 279–96.
4. Lazzarino M, Morra E, Rosso R, et al. Clinicopathologic and immunologic characteristics of non-Hodgkin's lymphomas presenting in the orbit. A report of eight cases. Cancer 1985;55(9):1907–12.
5. Shields CL, Shields JA, Eagle RC, et al. Clinicopathologic review of 142 cases of lacrimal gland lesions. Ophthalmology 1989;96(4):431–5.
6. Hurwitz JJ. A practical approach to the management of lacrimal gland lesions. Ophthalmic Surg 1982;13(10):829–36.
7. Jung WS, Ahn KJ, Park MR, et al. The radiological spectrum of orbital pathologies that involve the lacrimal gland and the lacrimal fossa [review]. Korean J Radiol 2007;8(4):336–42.
8. Lemke AJ, Hosten N, Grote A, et al. Differentiation of lacrimal gland tumors with high resolution computerized tomography in comparison with magnetic resonance tomography [in German]. Ophthalmology 1996;93(3):284–91.
9. Gündüz K, Shields CL, Günalp I, et al. Magnetic resonance imaging of unilateral lacrimal gland lesions. Graefes Arch Clin Exp Ophthalmol 2003;241(11):907–13.
10. Ellis JH, Banks PM, Campbell RJ, et al. Lymphoid tumors of the ocular adnexa. Clinical correlation with the working formulation classification and immunoperoxidase staining of paraffin sections. Ophthalmology 1985;92(10):1311–24.
11. Esik O, Ikeda H, Mukai K, et al. A retrospective analysis of different modalities for treatment of primary orbital non-Hodgkin's lymphomas. Radiother Oncol 1996;38(1):13–18.
12. Freeman C, Berg JW, Cutler SJ. Occurrence and prognosis of extranodal lymphomas. Cancer 1972;29(1):252–60.
13. Jakobiec FA, Font RL. Lymphoid tumors. In: Spencer WH, editor. Ophthalmic Pathology: An Atlas and Textbook. Philadelphia, PA: WB Saunders, 1986:2663–712.
14. White V, Rootman J, Quenville N, et al. Orbital lymphoproliferative and inflammatory lesions. Can J Ophthalmol 1987;22(7):362–73.
15. Hatef E, Roberts D, McLaughlin P, et al. Prevalence and nature of systemic involvement and stage at initial examination in patients with orbital and ocular adnexal lymphoma. Arch Ophthalmol 2007;125(12):1663–7.
16. Gayed I, Eskandari MF, McLaughlin P, et al. Value of positron emission tomography in staging ocular adnexal lymphomas and evaluating their response to therapy. Ophthalmic Surg Lasers Imaging 2007;110:809–15.

17. The Non-Hodgkin's Lymphoma Classification Project. A clinical evaluation of the International Lymphoma Study Group classification of non-Hodgkin's lymphoma. Blood 1997;89(11):3909–18.
18. Yeo JH, Jakobiec FA, Abbott GF, et al. Combined clinical and computed tomographic diagnosis of orbital lymphoid tumors. Am J Ophthalmol 1982;94(2):235–45.
19. Font RL, Gamel JW. Epithelial tumors of the lacrimal gland: analysis of 265 cases. In: Jakobiec FA, editor. Ocular and Adnexal Tumors. Birmingham: Aesculapius, 1978:787–805.
20. Sanders TE. Mixed tumor of the lacrimal gland. Arch Ophthalmol 1939;21:239–60.
21. Faktorovich EG, Crawford JB, Char DH, et al. Benign mixed tumor (pleomorphic adenoma) of the lacrimal gland in a 6-year-old boy. Am J Ophthalmol 1996;122(3):446–7.
22. Vagefi MR, Hong JE, Zwick OM, et al. Atypical presentations of pleomorphic adenoma of the lacrimal gland. Ophthal Plast Reconstr Surg 2007;23(4):272–4.
23. Ramlee N, Ramli N, Tajudin LS. Pleomorphic adenoma in the palpebral lobe of the lacrimal gland misdiagnosed as chalazion. Orbit 2007;26(2):137–9.
24. Halhal M, Meyer A, Morel X, et al. Pleomorphic adenoma mimicking dacryoadenitis [in French]. J Fr Ophthalmol 2004;27(10):1200–3.
25. Stefko ST, DiBernardo C, Green WR, et al. Pleomorphic adenoma of the lacrimal gland with extensive calcification. Arch Ophthalmol 2004;122(5):778–80.
26. Jakobiec FA, Font RL. Lacrimal gland tumors. In: Spencer WH, editor. Ophthalmic Pathology: An Atlas and Textbook. Philadelphia, PA: WB Saunders, 1986:2496–525.
27. Grossniklaus HE, Abbuhl MF, McLean IW. Immunohistologic properties of benign and malignant mixed tumor of the lacrimal gland. Am J Ophthalmol 1990;110(5):540–9.
28. Tosaka Y. Immunohistochemical study of pleomorphic adenoma of lacrimal gland. Jpn J Ophthalmol 1991;35(4):367–76.
29. Nakazato Y, Ishizeki J, Takahashi K, et al. Localization of S-100 protein and glial fibrillary acidic protein-related antigen in pleomorphic adenoma of the salivary glands. Lab Invest 1982;46(6):621–6.
30. Stead RH, Qizilbash AH, Kontozoglou T, et al. An immunohistochemical study of pleomorphic adenomas of the salivary gland: glial fibrillary acidic protein-like immunoreactivity identifies a major myoepithelial component. Hum Pathol 1988;19(1):32–40.
31. Wright JE, Stewart WB, Krohel GB. Clinical presentation and management of lacrimal gland tumours. Br J Ophthalmol 1979;63(9):600–6.
32. Wright JE. Factors affecting the survival of patients with lacrimal gland tumours. Can J Ophthalmol 1982;17(1):3–9.
33. Stewart WB, Krohel GB, Wright JE. Lacrimal gland and fossa lesions: an approach to diagnosis and management. Ophthalmology 1979;86(5):886–95.
34. Rose GE, Wright JE. Pleomorphic adenoma of the lacrimal gland. Br J Ophthalmol 1992;76(7):395–400.
35. Ni C, Cheng SC, Dryja TP, et al. Lacrimal gland tumors: a clinicopathological analysis of 160 cases. Int Ophthalmol Clin 1982;22(1):99–120.
36. Currie ZI, Rose GE. Long-term risk of recurrence after intact excision of pleomorphic adenomas of the lacrimal gland. Arch Ophthalmol 2007;125(12):1643–6.
37. Biggs SL, Font RL. Oncocytic lesions of the caruncle and other ocular adnexa. Arch Ophthalmol 1977;95(3):474–8.
38. Riedel K, Stefani FH, Kampik A. Oncocytoma of the ocular adnexa [in German]. Klin Monatsbl Augenheilkd 1983;182(6):544–8.
39. Calle CA, Castillo IG, Eagle RC, et al. Oncocytoma of the lacrimal gland: case report and review of the literature. Orbit 2006;25:243–7.
40. Eglen DE. Ocular adnexal oncocytoma. Am J Clin Pathol 1982;78:566–8.
41. Economou MA, Seregard S, Sahlin S. Oncocytoma of the lacrimal gland. Acta Ophthalmol Scand 2007;85(5):576–7.
42. Heathcote JG, Hurwitz JJ, Dardick I. A spindle-cell myoepithelioma of the lacrimal gland. Arch Ophthalmol 1990;108(8):1135–9.

43. Font RL, Garner A. Myoepithelioma of the lacrimal gland: report of a case with spindle cell morphology. Br J Ophthalmol 1992;76(10):634–6.
44. Grossniklaus HE, Wojno TH, Wilson MW, et al. Myoepithelioma of the lacrimal gland. Arch Ophthalmol 1997;115(12):1588–90.
45. Font RL, Smith SL, Bryan RG. Malignant epithelial tumors of the lacrimal gland: a clinicopathologic study of 21 cases. Arch Ophthalmol 1998;116(5):613–6.
46. Lorenz B, Stefani FH, Theopold M. Local excision of an adenoid cystic carcinoma of the lacrimal gland in a 12-year-old girl: case report (author's translation) [in German]. Klin Monatsbl Augenheilkd 1982;180(2):164–5.
47. Galliani CA, Faught PR, Ellis FD. Adenoid cystic carcinoma of the lacrimal gland in a six-year-old girl. Pediatr Pathol 1993;13(5):559–65.
48. Tellado MV, McLean IW, Specht CS, et al. Adenoid cystic carcinomas of the lacrimal gland in childhood and adolescence. Ophthalmology 1997;104(10):1622–5.
49. Shields JA, Shields CL, Eagle RC Jr, et al. Adenoid cystic carcinoma of the lacrimal gland simulating a dermoid cyst in a 9-year-old boy. Arch Ophthalmol 1998;116(12):1673–6.
50. Boitte JP, Traoré J, Boukhet F, et al. Adenoid cystic carcinoma of the lacrimal gland in a 14-year-old girl [in French]. J Fr Ophthalmol 2006;29(8):937–40.
51. Gamel JW, Font RL. Adenoid cystic carcinoma of the lacrimal gland: the clinical significance of a basaloid histologic pattern. Hum Pathol 1982;13:219–25.
52. Lee DA, Campbell RJ, Waller RR, et al. A clinicopathologic study of primary adenoid cystic carcinoma of the lacrimal gland. Ophthalmology 1985;92(1):128–34.
53. Esmaeli B, Golio D, Kies M, et al. Surgical management of locally advanced adenoid cystic carcinoma of the lacrimal gland. Ophthal Plast Reconstr Surg 2006;22(5):366–70.
54. Esmaeli B, Ahmadi MA, Youssef A, et al. Outcomes in patients with adenoid cystic carcinoma of the lacrimal gland. Ophthal Plast Reconstr Surg 2004;20(1):22–6.
55. Meldrum ML, Tse DT, Benedetto P. Neoadjuvant intracarotid chemotherapy for treatment of advanced adenocystic carcinoma of the lacrimal gland. Arch Ophthalmol 1998;116(3):315–21.
56. Tse DT, Benedetto P, Dubovy S, et al. Clinical analysis of the effect of intraarterial cytoreductive chemotherapy in the treatment of lacrimal gland adenoid cystic carcinoma. Am J Ophthalmol 2006;141(1):44–53.
57. Henderson JW, Neault RW. En bloc removal of intrinsic neoplasms of the lacrimal gland. Am J Ophthalmol 1976;82(6):905–9.
58. Ahmad SM, Esmaeli B, Williams M, et al. American Joint Committee on Cancer classification predicts outcome of patients with lacrimal-gland adenoid cystic carcinoma. Ophthalmology 2009;116(6):1210–15.
59. Eviatar JA, Hornblass A. Mucoepidermoid carcinoma of the lacrimal gland: 25 cases and a review and update of the literature [review]. Ophthal Plast Reconstr Surg 1993;9(3):170–81.
60. Dithmar S, Wojno TH, Washington C, et al. Mucoepidermoid carcinoma of an accessory lacrimal gland with orbital invasion. Ophthal Plast Reconstr Surg 2000;16(2):162–6.
61. Henderson JW, Farrow GM. Primary malignant mixed tumors of the lacrimal gland. Report of 10 cases. Ophthalmology 1980;87(6):466–75.
62. De Rosa G, Zeppa P, Tranfa F, et al. Acinic cell carcinoma arising in a lacrimal gland. First case report. Cancer 1986;57(10):1988–91.
63. Ni C, Ma X. Primary epithelial lacrimal gland tumors: the pathologic classification of 272 cases. Yan Ke Xue Bao 1994;10(4):201–5.
64. Ostrowski ML, Font RL, Halpern J, et al. Clear cell epithelial–myoepithelial carcinoma arising in pleomorphic adenoma of the lacrimal gland. Ophthalmology 1994;101(5):925–30.
65. Font RL, Patipa M, Rosenbaum PS, et al. Correlation of computed tomographic and histopathologic features in malignant transformation of benign mixed tumor of the lacrimal gland. Surv Ophthalmol 1990;34(6):449–52.
66. Heaps RS, Miller NR, Albert DM, et al. Primary adenocarcinoma of the lacrimal gland. A retrospective study. Ophthalmology 1993;100(12):1856–60.

67. Shields JA, Shields CL, Epstein JA, et al. Primary epithelial malignancies of the lacrimal gland: the 2003 Ramon L. Font lecture. Ophthal Plast Reconstr Surg 2004;20:10–21.
68. Katz SE, Rootman J, Dolman PJ, et al. Primary ductal adenocarcinoma of the lacrimal gland. Ophthalmology 1996;103:157–62.
69. Nasu M, Haisa T, Kondo T, et al. Primary ductal adenocarcinoma of the lacrimal gland. Pathol Int 1998;48:981–4.
70. Krishnakumar S, Subramanian N, Mahesh L, et al. Primary ductal adenocarcinoma of the lacrimal gland in a patient with neurofibromatosis [letter]. Eye 2003;17:843–5.
71. Milman T, Shields JA, Husson M, et al. Primary ductal adenocarcinoma of the lacrimal gland. Ophthalmology 2005;12(11):2048–51.
72. Su GW, Patipa M, Font RL. Primary squamous cell carcinoma arising from an epithelium-lined cyst of the lacrimal gland. Ophthal Plast Reconstr Surg 2005;21(5):383–5.
73. Hotta K, Arisawa T, Mito H, et al. Primary squamous cell carcinoma of the lacrimal gland. Clin Exp Ophthalmol 2005;33(5):534–6.
74. Patel SG, Shah JP. TNM Staging of cancers of the head and neck: striving for uniformity among diversity. CA Cancer J Clin 2005;55:242–5.

Chapter 8
Optic Nerve Sheath Fenestration in Cancer Patients: Indications and Surgical Technique

Thomas E. Johnson

Abstract Optic nerve sheath fenestration (ONSF) entails cutting a window or making linear fenestrations in the retrobulbar optic nerve sheath, which releases pressure and often allows stabilization or improvement of vision. Indications for ONSF include visual loss due to pseudotumor cerebri, optic nerve sheath hemorrhage, dural sinus thrombosis, subdural hematoma, intradural arteriovenous malformation, arachnoiditis with increased intracranial pressure, and cryptococcal meningitis with papilledema due to AIDS. Indications for ONSF in cancer patients are not well established, but a few case reports have shown success of ONSF in patients with perineural metastasis of breast cancer, increased intracranial pressure with papilledema due to a brain tumor, lymphomatous infiltration of the optic nerve, and optic nerve sheath meningioma. ONSF can be performed with a medial orbitotomy approach with disinsertion of the medial rectus muscle, a superomedial eyelid crease incision without extraocular muscle disinsertion, a lateral orbitotomy approach with bone removal, or a lateral canthotomy incision without bone removal. ONSF is considered relatively safe when performed carefully; serious complications occur in about 1% of patients.

8.1 Introduction

The surgical technique of optic nerve sheath fenestration (ONSF) is used most often in the treatment of progressive optic neuropathy in patients with idiopathic increased intracranial pressure (pseudotumor cerebri) in whom medical management has failed. Pseudotumor cerebri is characterized by elevated intracranial pressure and papilledema (Fig. 8.1) in the context of normal neuroimaging studies and cerebrospinal fluid analysis and is a diagnosis of exclusion. Typically, affected patients

---

T.E. Johnson (✉)
Department of Ophthalmology, Bascom Palmer Eye Institute, University of Miami Miller School of Medicine, Miami, FL, USA
e-mail: tjohnson@med.miami.edu

B. Esmaeli (ed.), *Ophthalmic Oncology*, M.D. Anderson Solid Tumor Oncology Series 6, DOI 10.1007/978-1-4419-0374-7_8,

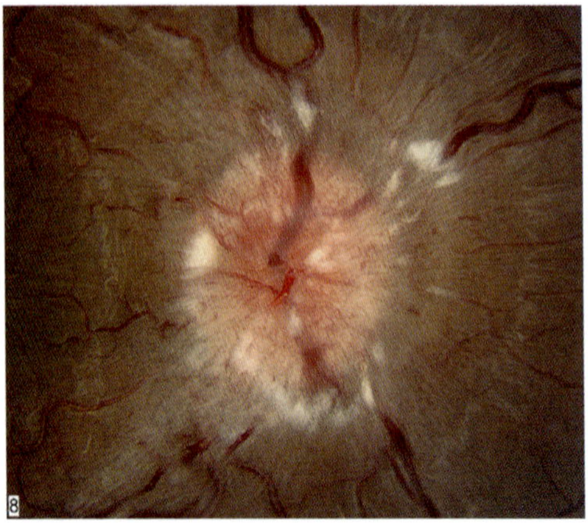

Fig. 8.1 Photograph of optic nerve head swelling in a patient with increased intracranial pressure

are obese females of child-bearing age who present with headache and visual obscuration. In severe cases, patients may report diplopia secondary to cranial nerve VI palsy. The increased nerve sheath pressure can result in progressive visual field loss and even blindness in advanced cases.

Medical treatment includes encouragement of weight loss and oral administration of a carbonic anhydrase inhibitor (e.g., acetazolamide). Furosemide and systemic corticosteroids may also be used. If maximal medical therapy fails or if patients develop intolerance to the medications, surgery is often required. Options include neurosurgical cerebrospinal fluid shunting, using either a ventriculoperitoneal or a lumboperitoneal shunt, and ONSF.

Cutting a window or making linear fenestrations in the retrobulbar optic nerve sheath releases pressure and often allows stabilization or improvement of vision. The mechanism of action is unknown but most likely relates to filtration resulting from successful creation of a meningeal space–orbital fistula [1]. Hamad and coauthors demonstrated cyst-like structures contiguous with the fenestration sites after ONSF on magnetic resonance imaging and echography. They concluded that the procedure creates a filtration apparatus that controls the pressure in the subarachnoid space surrounding the intraorbital segment of the optic nerve [2]. Many patients—in some series, over 50%—experience bilateral resolution of papilledema after unilateral ONSF [3, 4]. ONSF stabilizes or improves vision in the majority of patients with pseudotumor cerebri and visual loss, but the procedure may fail any time after the surgery, and patients need to be followed up routinely [5].

8.2 Indications

In addition to pseudotumor cerebri and visual loss, indications for ONSF include visual loss secondary to optic nerve sheath hemorrhage, dural sinus thrombosis, subdural hematoma, intradural arteriovenous malformation, and arachnoiditis with increased intracranial pressure. Dural sinus occlusion can produce a clinical picture similar to pseudotumor cerebri with elevated intracranial pressure and papilledema [6]. Additionally, ONSF has been employed in the treatment of visual loss in patients with AIDS and cryptococcal meningitis with papilledema [7]. ONSF was not found to be helpful and was found to be possibly harmful in patients with nonarteritic ischemic optic neuropathy [8].

The indications for ONSF in cancer patients are not well established, but a few case reports have shown success of ONSF in patients with neoplastic disease, including patients with perineural metastasis of breast cancer [9], lymphomatous infiltration of the optic nerve [10, 11], increased intracranial pressure with papilledema due to a brain tumor [12], and optic nerve sheath meningioma [13].

8.3 Surgical Techniques

The first optic nerve sheath decompression was described by De Wecker in 1872 [14]. Since then, many different surgical techniques have been described. The optic nerve can be approached through a medial orbitotomy with disinsertion of the medial rectus muscle, a superomedial eyelid crease incision without extraocular muscle disinsertion, a lateral orbitotomy with bone removal, and a lateral canthotomy incision without bone removal. The nerve sheath can be opened either by excising a window of dura and arachnoid or by making multiple linear incisions in the nerve sheath. Most cases are performed under general anesthesia. Preoperative testing usually includes visual acuity measurement, color vision assessment, visual field evaluation using quantitative perimetry, and fundus examination with attention to the optic disks. Most patients require a magnetic resonance imaging scan and/or a computed tomography scan of the brain and orbits to rule out hydrocephalus, space-occupying masses, or vascular malformations that can also cause papilledema. A magnetic resonance venogram is helpful in evaluating patients suspected of having a venous sinus thrombosis.

Instrumentation for ONSF includes surgical loupes and/or an operating microscope, Freer periosteal elevators, ribbon malleable retractors, neurosurgical microforceps, bayonet neurosurgical scissors (e.g., Yasargil bayonet scissors), neurosurgical cottonoids, and a headlight. Four main surgical approaches have been described for ONSF.

8.3.1 *Medial Orbitotomy Approach*

For the medial orbitotomy approach, a 270° medial conjunctival peritomy is made using Westcott scissors. The quadrants between the medial rectus and the superior rectus and between the medial rectus and the inferior rectus are cleared with Stevens scissors. The medial rectus muscle is isolated on a muscle hook, and a double-armed 5-0 polyglactin (Vicryl) suture is passed through the muscle insertion and locked on each end. The medial rectus is disinserted, allowing access to the medial orbital space. Gentle dissection is carried out with blunt Freer elevators or thin ribbon malleable retractors. Slightly dampened neurosurgical cottonoids are used to gently retract the orbital fat. Attention is carefully paid to the pupil, and all pressure is removed if pupillary dilation occurs. The nerve sheath is exposed just behind the globe, where it is most bulbous (Fig. 8.2). Often, there is a fine vascular plexus on the epidural sheath, and these vessels should be avoided when a nerve sheath window is excised. Either an adjacent area of the sheath can be excised or the vessels can be gently moved using the blunt end of a Freer elevator. A neurosurgical microforceps is used to grasp the dural sheath just behind the globe, and a window of approximately 3 mm × 5 mm is cut using bayonet microsurgical scissors. Care is taken to cut through both the dural and the arachnoid sheaths to allow egress of cerebrospinal fluid, and the surgeon should carefully avoid touching the optic nerve within the sheath. A gush of clear cerebrospinal fluid is usually noted when the sheath is adequately opened. After careful inspection to assure meticulous hemostasis, the medial rectus muscle is reattached using the 5-0 Vicryl sutures, and the conjunctiva is closed using 6-0 fast-absorbing plain sutures. An antibiotic–steroid ophthalmic ointment is applied to the eye, and an eye pad is placed over the closed eyelids. No pressure is applied to the eye. Postoperative icepacks are helpful to reduce swelling. The ointment is applied three times per day for a week, and the patient is instructed to avoid any blood thinners, such as aspirin and nonsteroidal anti-inflammatory medications, as well as herbal medications for 1 week.

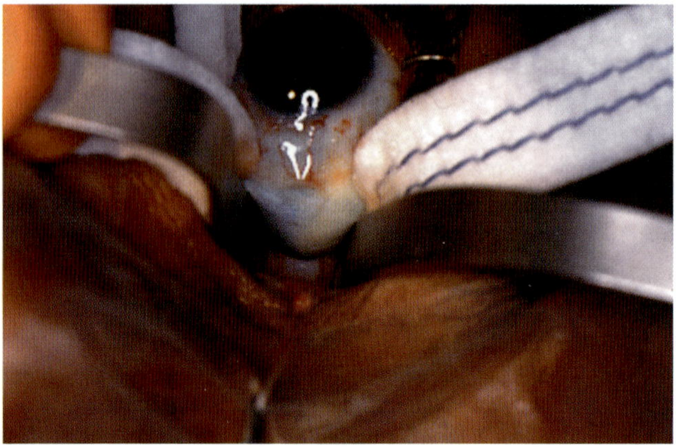

Fig. 8.2 Medial orbitotomy approach to ONSF with disinsertion of the medial rectus muscle and use of neurosurgical cottonoids and malleable retractors

8.3.2 Medial Eyelid Crease Approach

Pelton and Patel [15] described using a medial eyelid crease approach to ONSF without the need for disinsertion of a rectus muscle. A 1-cm eyelid-crease incision is made over the medial third of the upper eyelid, and the incision is carried through skin and orbicularis muscle. Scissors are used to open the orbital septum, and blunt dissection is used to open fascial septi in the superomedial compartment. The medial intraconal space is exposed using gentle retraction with Sewall orbital retractors, and the standard fenestration instruments are used to open a rectangular window in the nerve sheath. Stated advantages include ease of dissection, short incision-to-nerve distance, and angle of approach to the optic nerve.

8.3.3 Lateral Orbitotomy Approach

Tse and coauthors [16] described using a traditional lateral orbitotomy approach with elevation of a bone flap to perform ONSF. They used an operating microscope after adequate exposure of the nerve sheath was accomplished. The lateral rectus muscle was isolated from the bulbar conjunctiva with a 4-0 silk suture, and the globe was adducted in order to move the optic nerve closer to the lateral wall. A window was excised from the bulbous lateral aspect of the retrobulbar nerve sheath. Stated advantages of this approach are that it allows a direct, perpendicular view of the optic nerve using an approach well known to the orbital surgeon and does not require the disinsertion of a rectus muscle. Disadvantages include the need for general anesthesia, longer operating time than the other approaches to ONSF, and greater risk of damage to the ciliary ganglion with resultant pupillary dilation.

8.3.4 Lateral Canthotomy Approach

Kersten and Kulwin [12] described a technique of approaching the optic nerve laterally without elevating a bone flap. A lateral canthotomy and inferior cantholysis exposes the lateral orbital rim. A 4-0 silk suture is placed under the lateral rectus muscle insertion from the bulbar conjunctiva to adduct the globe and bring the nerve closer to the lateral wall. The periosteum on the rim is cut, and the periorbita is elevated 2 cm posterior to the rim. After opening of the periorbita, Sewell retractors are used to retract the lacrimal gland superiorly and the lateral rectus inferiorly. Orbital dissection is gently carried out to expose the nerve, and a fenestration is performed using the operating microscope and standard fenestration instruments. Reported advantages of this technique include ease of operation, as with the medial eyelid crease approach, and a more direct perpendicular view of the nerve, as with the standard lateral orbitotomy approach with bone removal.

8.4 Possible Indications for ONSF in Cancer Patients

As mentioned earlier in the chapter, information about possible indications for ONSF in cancer patients comes mainly from case reports.

8.4.1 Metastatic Breast Cancer

Gasperini and coauthors [9] reported a 36-year-old woman with bilateral anterior optic neuropathy and orbital and central nervous system metastasis of breast cancer. She had progressive bilateral visual loss and bilateral optic disc swelling. ONSF on the left optic nerve by the medial eyelid crease approach resulted in bilateral visual improvement and resolution of disc edema in both eyes. The etiology of bilateral optic neuropathy in this patient was thought to be due to papilledema caused by perineural infiltration by the metastatic breast cancer. The authors concluded that ONSF should be considered as a treatment option for optic neuropathy caused by perineural or intrasheath metastasis [9].

8.4.2 Lymphomatous Optic Neuropathy Diagnosed by Optic Nerve Biopsy

ONSF has been used to diagnose cancer. Dayan and coauthors [10] diagnosed a 74-year-old woman with lymphomatous optic neuropathy by performing an optic nerve biopsy using an ONSF approach. Gross examination of the optic nerve sheath was not diagnostic, but the optic nerve substance showed infiltration with a low-grade B-cell non-Hodgkin lymphoma. The patient had temporary visual deterioration after biopsy but later showed improvement to at least prebiopsy vision. The authors concluded that optic nerve biopsy using an ONSF approach should be considered in enigmatic cases with signs or symptoms suggestive of optic neuropathy even when visual function remains [10].

Kitzmann and coauthors [11] reported a 39-year-old man with T-cell non-Hodgkin lymphoma and bilateral optic nerve infiltration. ONSF was performed, and pathologic examination showed only meningeal dural tissue with no lymphocytes. After dramatic initial visual improvement, the patient's vision decreased to no light perception by postoperative day 17. The authors concluded that ONSF does not appear to be helpful in restoring vision in patients with lymphomatous infiltration of the optic nerve [11].

8.4.3 Adjuvant Therapy in Optic Nerve Sheath Meningioma

Turbin and coauthors used ONSF as adjuvant therapy in two patients with optic nerve sheath meningioma and progressive visual loss. One had received fractionated stereotactic radiotherapy before surgery, and the second patient received radiotherapy after ONSF. In both patients, the visual loss was thought to be due to nerve compression within a tight sheath. Both patients experienced improvement of vision and resolution of disc edema after ONSF. The authors concluded that in selected patients with optic nerve sheath meningioma, severe disc edema, rapid visual loss, and few treatment options, ONSF may have an important but restricted role as an adjuvant to radiotherapy [13].

8.4.4 Papilledema Associated with Brain Tumors

Kersten and Kulwin reported that one of the patients in their series of patients who underwent ONSF had papilledema and visual loss due to an intracranial glioblastoma. That patient's vision improved after ONSF performed using a lateral canthotomy approach. Disk edema cleared in both eyes after unilateral ONSF [12].

8.4.5 Radiation-Induced Optic Neuropathy

Radiation-induced optic neuropathy is a well-recognized complication of external-beam radiotherapy and can result in progressive unilateral or bilateral visual loss months to years after radiotherapy has been completed. Radiation can cause edema and increased perineural pressure in the optic nerve. Mohamed and coauthors treated three patients with pending anterior radiation-induced optic neuropathy with ONSF by a medial orbitotomy with disinsertion of the medial rectus, and all three patients experienced resolution of edema and restoration of vision [17]. ONSF was used proactively in these three cases of impending radiation-induced optic neuropathy to relieve the swelling and increased pressure within the confines of the nerve sheath [17].

8.5 Complications of ONSF

ONSF is considered a relatively safe surgery when performed carefully; serious complications occur in about 1% of patients [18, 19]. Possible complications include partial or complete visual loss due to central retinal artery occlusion, branch retinal artery occlusion, traumatic optic neuropathy due to excessive traction on the nerve, and hemorrhage within the optic nerve sheath. Blindness has been reported in about 1% of ONSF cases. Ocular motility disorders can be transitory or permanent and may be due to medial or lateral rectus muscle damage or a lost muscle. Anisocoria can occur because of injury to the ciliary ganglion or to the ciliary nerves lying along the lateral optic nerve, especially when the nerve is approached from the lateral aspect. Complete blindness with slow recovery of vision has been reported following ONSF performed by the medial approach. The mechanism was thought to be sustained rotational traction on an already compromised optic nerve with resulting axonal demyelination from stretch injury, followed by remyelination of affected axons [20].

8.6 Future Research

Joos and coauthors reported the experimental use of an endoscopic surgical approach to ONSF with the use of the free electron laser in a goat model [21]. Their work creates the potential for performing minimally invasive ONSF in the future [21].

References

1. Keltner JL. Optic nerve sheath decompression: how does it work? Has its time come? Arch Ophthalmol 1988;106:1365–9.
2. Hamad LM, Tse DT, Glaser JS, et al. Neuroimaging of the optic nerve after fenestration for management of pseudotumor cerebri. Arch Ophthalmol 1992;110:636–9.
3. Sergott RC, Savino PJ, Bosley TM. Modified optic nerve sheath decompression provides long-term visual improvement for pseudotumor cerebri. Arch Ophthalmol 1988;106:1384–90.
4. Corbett JJ, Nerad JA, Tse DT, et al. Results of optic nerve sheath fenestration for pseudotumor cerebri: the lateral orbitotomy approach. Arch Ophthalmol 1988;106:1391–7.
5. Spoor TC, McHenry JG. Long-term effectiveness of optic nerve sheath decompression for pseudotumor cerebri. Arch Ophthalmol 1993;111:632–5.
6. Horton JC, Seiff SR, Pitts LH, et al. Decompression of the optic nerve sheath for vision-threatening papilledema caused by dural sinus occlusion. Neurosurgery 1992;31: 203–12.
7. Garrity JA, Herman DC, Imes R, et al. Optic nerve sheath decompression for visual loss in patients with acquired immunodeficiency syndrome and cryptococcal meningitis with papilledema. Am J Ophthalmol 1993;116:472–8.
8. Ischemic Optic Neuropathy Decompression Trial Research Group. Optic nerve decompression surgery for nonarteritic ischemic optic neuropathy (NAION) is not effective and may be harmful. JAMA 1995;273:625–32.
9. Gasperini J, Black E, Van Stavern G. Perineural metastasis of breast cancer treated with optic nerve sheath fenestration. Ophthal Plast Reconstr Surg 2007;23:331–3.
10. Dayan MR, Elston JS, McDonald B. Bilateral lymphomatous optic neuropathy diagnosed on optic nerve biopsy. Arch Ophthalmol 2000;188:1455–7.
11. Kitzmann AS, Pulido JS, Garrity JA, et al. Histologic findings in T-cell lymphoma infiltration of the optic nerve. Ophthalmology 2008;115:e1–6.
12. Kersten RC, Kulwin DR. Optic nerve sheath fenestration through a lateral canthotomy incision. Arch Ophthalmol 1993;111:870–4.
13. Turbin RE, Wladis EJ, Frohman LP, et al. Role for surgery as adjuvant therapy in optic nerve sheath meningioma. Ophthal Plast Reconstr Surg 2006;22:278–82.
14. De Wecker L. On incision of the optic nerve in cases of neuroretinitis. Int Ophthalmol Congr Rep 1872;4:11–14.
15. Pelton RW, Patel BC. Superomedial lid crease approach to the medial intraconal space: a new technique for access to the optic nerve and central space. Ophthal Plast Reconstr Surg 2001;17:241–53.
16. Tse DT, Nerad JA, Anderson RL, et al. Optic nerve sheath fenestration in pseudotumor cerebri: a lateral orbitotomy approach. Arch Ophthalmol 1988;106:1458–62.
17. Mohamed IG, Roa W, Fulton D, et al. Optic nerve sheath fenestration for a reversible optic neuropathy in radiation oncology. Am J Clin Oncol 2000;23:401–5.
18. Banta JT, Farris BK. Pseudotumor cerebri and optic nerve sheath decompression. Ophthalmology 2000;107:1907–12.

19. Hupp SL, Glaser JS, Frazier-Byrne S. Optic nerve sheath decompression: review of 17 cases. Arch Ophthalmol 1987;105:386–9.
20. Brodsky MC. Protracted postsurgical blindness with visual recovery following optic nerve sheath fenestration. Arch Ophthalmol 1998;116:107–9.
21. Joos KM, Shah RJ, Robinson RD, et al. Optic nerve sheath fenestration with endoscopic accessory instruments versus the free electron laser (FEL). Lasers Surg Med 2006;38:846–51.

Chapter 9
Management of Primary Eyelid Cancers

Aaron Savar and Bita Esmaeli

Abstract A number of different cancers can affect the eyelid. Basal cell carcinoma is the most common; squamous cell carcinoma, melanoma, and sebaceous cell carcinoma are less common. Management of these tumors is most commonly surgical, although chemotherapy and radiation therapy play a role in some cases. Complex tumors require a multidisciplinary approach and long-term follow-up.

9.1 Introduction

The spectrum of cancers affecting the eyelids is wide. Primary eyelid malignancies can arise from virtually any cell type, including epidermal tissues, glandular tissues, connective tissues, or lymphocytes. The management of such lesions depends on the type, location, and size of the tumor.

9.2 Types of Eyelid Malignancies

9.2.1 Basal Cell Carcinoma

Basal cell carcinoma (BCC) is the most common type of cancer and accounts for over 90% of eyelid cancers. A large cohort study of eyelid malignancies found an incidence of 14.35 per 100,000 individuals per year [1]. Sun exposure, increased age, immunosuppression, and decreased skin pigmentation are known risk factors. BCC can also be seen in association with xeroderma pigmentosum and Gorlin–Goltz syndrome.

A. Savar (✉)
Section of Ophthalmology, Department of Head and Neck Surgery, The University of Texas M.D. Anderson Cancer Center, Houston, TX, USA
e-mail: asavar@gmail.com

B. Esmaeli (ed.), *Ophthalmic Oncology*, M.D. Anderson Solid Tumor Oncology Series 6, DOI 10.1007/978-1-4419-0374-7_9,

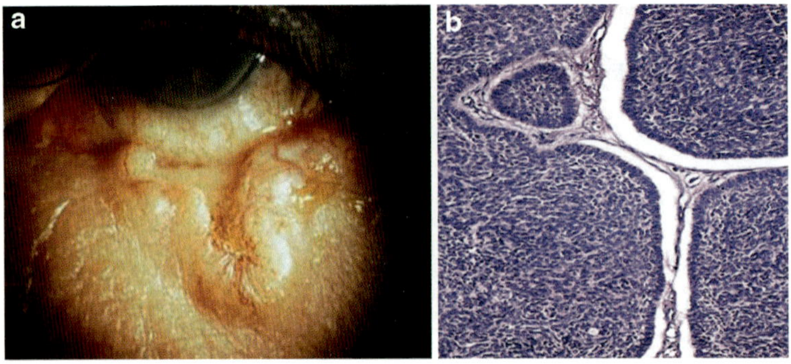

Fig. 9.1 (**a**) Basal cell carcinoma (BCC) of lower eyelid. (**b**) Histologic section of nodular BCC. Note nests of cells with peripheral palisading

BCC lesions can present in a number of ways. Common clinical findings include pearly papules, telangiectatic vessels, and skin ulceration (Fig. 9.1a). The most common periocular locations of BCC are the lower eyelid, the medial canthus, the upper eyelid, and the lateral canthus, in that order. Lesions of the medial canthus have a higher risk of orbital involvement.

Local invasive growth is common if lesions are left untreated. Metastasis is rare and usually occurs only in tumors greater than 3 cm in diameter. In a review of 238 BCCs that metastasized, 12% were in the periocular region [2].

BCCs arise from cells in the stratum basale of the epidermis. Histopathologically, they are characterized by nests of cells with peripheral palisading. There are several pathologic variants described, with nodular BCC being the most common (Fig. 9.1b). Morpheaform BCCs can present with indistinct borders and have more aggressive behavior. Perineural invasion can be observed with BCC and should be treated with postoperative adjuvant radiation therapy.

9.2.2 Squamous Cell Carcinoma

Squamous cell carcinoma (SCC) is the second most common eyelid cancer, accounting for between 5 and 10% of eyelid malignancies in some large studies [3]. As with BCC, sun exposure, increased age, decreased skin pigmentation, and immunosuppression are known risk factors, as is exposure to certain chemicals. SCC is seen more commonly in men than women. SCC is known to arise from actinic keratoses.

SCC can present as an ulcer, a plaque, or a nodule (Fig. 9.2a). Lesions are more common in the lower eyelid. Perineural invasion can be seen with these tumors and can result in pain, paresthesia, or numbness.

The risk of lymph node and distant metastasis is higher than that with BCC. The rate of nodal metastasis has been reported to be as high as 24% with large and

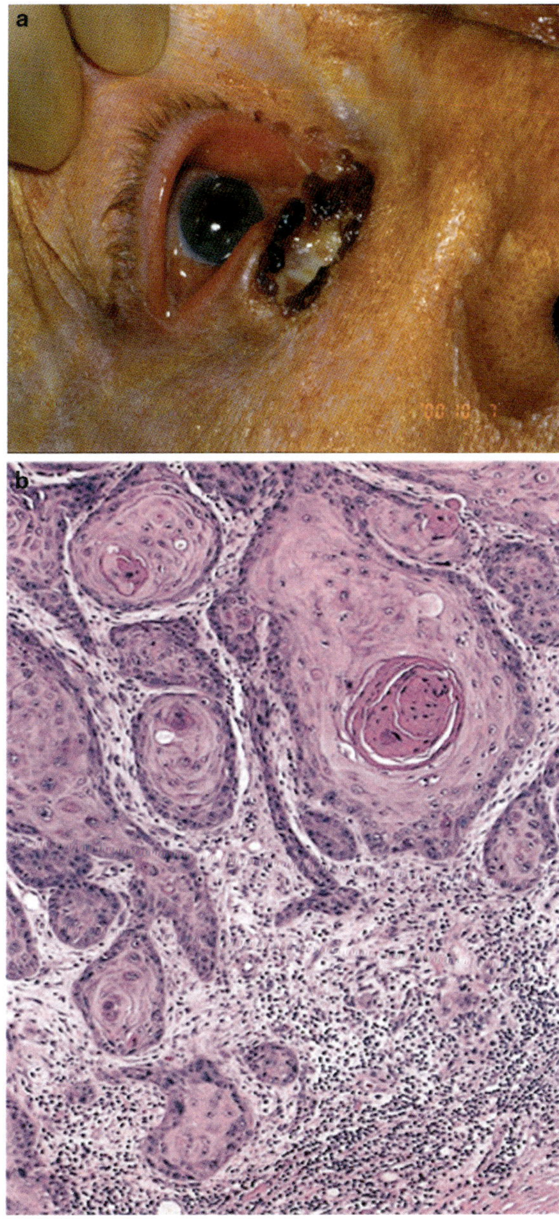

Fig. 9.2 (**a**) Squamous cell carcinoma (SCC) of the lower eyelid. (**b**) Histologic section of invasive SCC

advanced lesions [4]. The risk of nodal metastasis is higher with lesions that are greater than 1 cm in diameter.

SCCs arise from keratinocytes and are characterized by strands and nests of abnormal squamous cells (Fig. 9.2b).

9.2.3 Melanoma

Primary melanomas of the eyelid are rare but potentially lethal. They account for fewer than 1% of eyelid malignancies. They usually present as pigmented lesions with irregular borders and color.

Melanomas arise from melanocytes. In patients with eyelid melanomas, as in patients with melanomas located elsewhere in the body, increased Clark level and Breslow thickness have been shown to be associated with decreased survival [5]. Pathologic subtypes include nodular, superficial spreading, lentigo maligna, and acral lentiginous melanoma and also amelanotic melanoma, a rare variant.

The risk of nodal and systemic metastasis is high and is correlated with Breslow thickness, Clark level, and presence of ulceration, as is the case for cutaneous melanoma in other anatomic sites. A systemic workup for metastasis is recommended for melanomas of intermediate thickness or greater.

9.2.4 Sebaceous Gland Carcinoma

Sebaceous gland carcinoma is a rare, potentially lethal eyelid tumor with a high rate of recurrence and a propensity for metastasis. Prior radiation exposure is a known risk factor. Sebaceous gland carcinoma is also seen in patients with Muir–Torre syndrome.

Diagnosis can often be delayed in sebaceous gland carcinoma as these lesions can be confused with benign lesions. In a series of 60 sebaceous gland carcinomas, over two-thirds were thought initially to be another less serious lesion [6]. Early diagnosis and treatment is critical. In a study of 31 patients, the median time from onset of symptoms to diagnosis was 24 months (range, 1–300 months) [7].

These lesions typically present as a nodule or as diffuse eyelid thickening, and unlike BCC, SCC, and melanoma, sebaceous gland carcinoma is more common in the upper eyelid than the lower eyelid (Fig. 9.3a). Sebaceous gland carcinomas can occur on the bulbar conjunctiva, although this is very rare.

Sebaceous gland carcinoma arises in the eyelids from the meibomian glands or glands of Zeis, or on the caruncle from sebaceous glands present there. Foamy cytoplasm is noted upon histopathologic examination. Special stains, such as

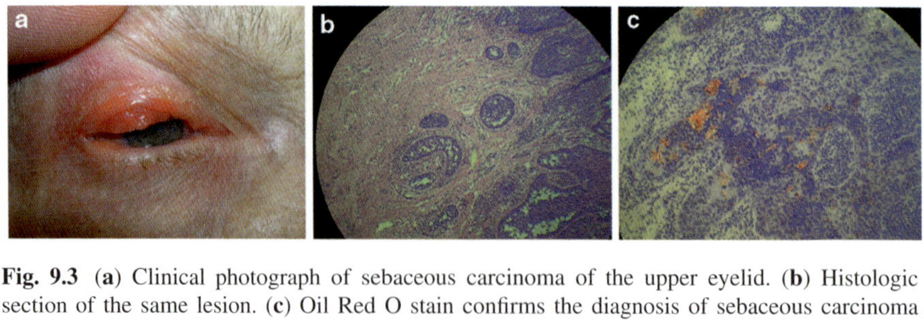

Fig. 9.3 (**a**) Clinical photograph of sebaceous carcinoma of the upper eyelid. (**b**) Histologic section of the same lesion. (**c**) Oil Red O stain confirms the diagnosis of sebaceous carcinoma

Oil Red O, are useful in making this diagnosis and require that surgical specimens be sent for pathological analysis as fresh tissue and not fixed in formalin (Fig. 9.3b, c).

There is a significant risk of metastasis with sebaceous gland carcinoma; therefore, a systemic workup is suggested for most new cases. The estimated risk of nodal metastasis and distant organ metastasis is 10–15%. The most likely sites of metastasis include the lung and the liver. Unlike melanoma, where depth of invasion is correlated with metastatic spread of the cancer, depth of invasion does not appear to correlate with metastatic spread. Rather, tumor size appears to correlate with the metastatic spread of sebaceous gland carcinoma, although to date there are no studies that specifically look at high-risk histologic features that correlate with metastatic behavior.

9.2.5 *Other Primary Eyelid Malignancies*

There are a number of other cancers that can occur in the eyelids, all of which are very uncommon. Because the periocular region is rich with glandular structures, a number of adenocarcinomas can develop in the eyelid in addition to sebaceous gland carcinoma. These include mucinous sweat gland adenocarcinoma [8, 9], adenocarcinoma of the gland of Moll [10–12], and adenoid cystic carcinoma [13].

Lymphomas can present in the eyelid, but this most frequently occurs in cases where there is already systemic involvement [14]. Both B- and T-cell lymphomas can be seen in the eyelid.

Sarcomas of the eyelid are rare. In a study of non-BCC and non-SCC eyelid tumors, sarcomas accounted for 12% of the cases. Kaposi sarcoma is the most common type seen in the eyelid, usually in patients with HIV/AIDS [15] Angiosarcoma is the second most common sarcoma affecting the eyelid [16].

Merkel cell carcinoma is a rare skin cancer thought to arise from mechanoreceptors of the same name. Merkel cell carcinomas exhibit neuroendocrine differentiation and are most commonly seen in the head and neck. Typically they present as firm, purple nodules (Fig. 9.4). These tumors have a high rate of nodal metastasis, with between 15 and 66% having nodal disease at presentation [17, 18]. Recently, a polyomavirus has been implicated as a causative agent in this disease [19].

9.3 Management

Although evaluation and management of some eyelid malignancies is relatively straightforward, a significant proportion of the eyelid cancers seen at a referral cancer center require a comprehensive multidisciplinary approach, often involving consultation with the disciplines of medical oncology, radiation oncology, surgical oncology, radiology, and pathology.

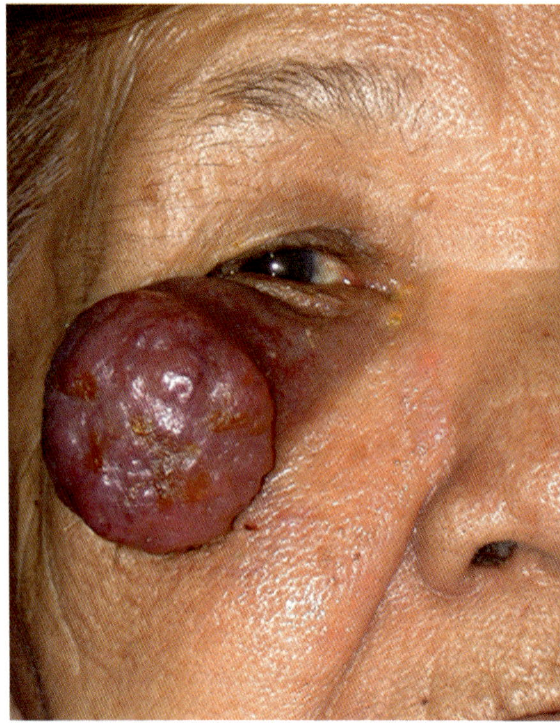

Fig. 9.4 Clinical photograph of Merkel cell carcinoma of the eyelid

9.3.1 Evaluation

Evaluating a patient with an eyelid cancer requires taking a thorough history and performing a complete ophthalmic examination. Prior history of skin cancer and sun exposure are important details to note. Attention to the size and location of the tumor is critical in planning the appropriate treatment. Palpation of the lymph nodes in the preauricular, submandibular, and cervical regions is important in assessing for nodal metastases. The use of American Joint Committee on Cancer staging, while not widely practiced, has been recommended for eyelid carcinomas [20]. The presence of an eyelid skin cancer should prompt the search for skin cancers elsewhere. A full-body skin examination by a dermatologist should be recommended. Orbital imaging, usually magnetic resonance imaging, is necessary for tumors with a propensity for orbital invasion. This modality can also help in identifying perineural invasion, a high-risk characteristic seen in certain tumors.

In cases of more aggressive malignancies, radiologic studies to assess for lymphatic spread and metastases are necessary. Ultrasound evaluation of the neck to assess for suspicious nodes should be performed for most cancers other than BCC, including melanoma and sebaceous gland carcinoma. Any concerning nodes should be subjected to fine-needle aspiration biopsy.

Metastatic workup with a chest X-ray and liver function testing should also be performed for most cancers other than BCC to establish a baseline and assess for lung and liver involvement. In the case of sebaceous gland carcinoma, gastrointestinal and gynecologic evaluations should be performed as well because of the rare association with Muir–Torre syndrome.

9.3.2 Tumor Excision and Eyelid Reconstruction

Surgical excision of eyelid cancers is certainly the most common treatment, but other modalities play a role. Ultimately, the treatment plan depends on the type, location, and extent of disease. If there is uncertainty about the diagnosis, an incisional biopsy, shave biopsy, or punch biopsy can be performed.

The standard treatment for most eyelid malignancies is excision with a margin of normal tissue [21]. This can be accomplished by excision with either intraoperative frozen section analysis or permanent section evaluation to confirm negative margins or by Mohs micrographic surgery. In our practice, the majority of tumors are excised with intraoperative frozen section analysis with review of the sections performed together by the surgeon and an experienced dermatopathologist. For BCC and SCC, typically a 2-mm margin of uninvolved tissue is removed. If necessary, additional tissue is removed until the margins are sufficiently clear. Not surprisingly, incomplete excision is associated with a significantly higher rate of recurrence [21]. In the case of melanomas, wider margins—usually 4 mm— are taken. Additionally, frozen section analysis is not reliable for melanomas. Depending on the situation, either reconstruction of the eyelid is performed immediately after removal of a melanoma, with plans to remove more tissue if necessary when permanent pathology results are available, or the reconstruction is performed the following day once permanent section evaluation of margins is complete.

Mohs micrographic surgery is a technique for excision and analysis of skin cancers employed by specially trained dermatologists. During Mohs surgery the dermatologist excises the tumor and then examines frozen sections of the margin in an *en face* manner. The area is carefully mapped so that additional tissue can be removed from areas with a positive margin. This technique is useful for lesions in certain areas to minimize the amount of tissue removed. It has been shown to be extremely effective in treating periocular BCC, both primary and recurrent lesions [22]. It is not, however, appropriate for excision of melanocytic lesions unless a "slow Mohs" technique with paraffin sections is used. Unlike traditional intraoperative frozen section analysis, in Mohs micrographic surgery the pathologic tissue analysis is performed by the dermatologist.

For advanced eyelid tumors that are invading the orbit or the globe, exenteration may be necessary for local control of disease. In a very large series of 429 orbital exenterations, 40% were performed for eyelid tumors [23]. BCC accounted for 90% of these [24]. Our experience at M.D. Anderson Cancer Center suggests that some invasive eyelid tumors that would typically be treated with an orbital exenteration can be managed with globe-preserving surgery and judicious use of postoperative radiation therapy (Fig. 9.5). This approach would obviously require frequent follow-up clinical examinations and serial imaging to insure that potential local recurrence is identified at the earliest possible time.

While the primary goal of tumor excision is eradication of the cancer, it is important to also consider the functional and cosmetic outcomes. The eyelid and periocular tissues must be reconstructed in a manner that allows for sufficient coverage of the eye while not interfering with vision. Numerous methods of reconstruction have been described for various types of eyelid defects. For small defects,

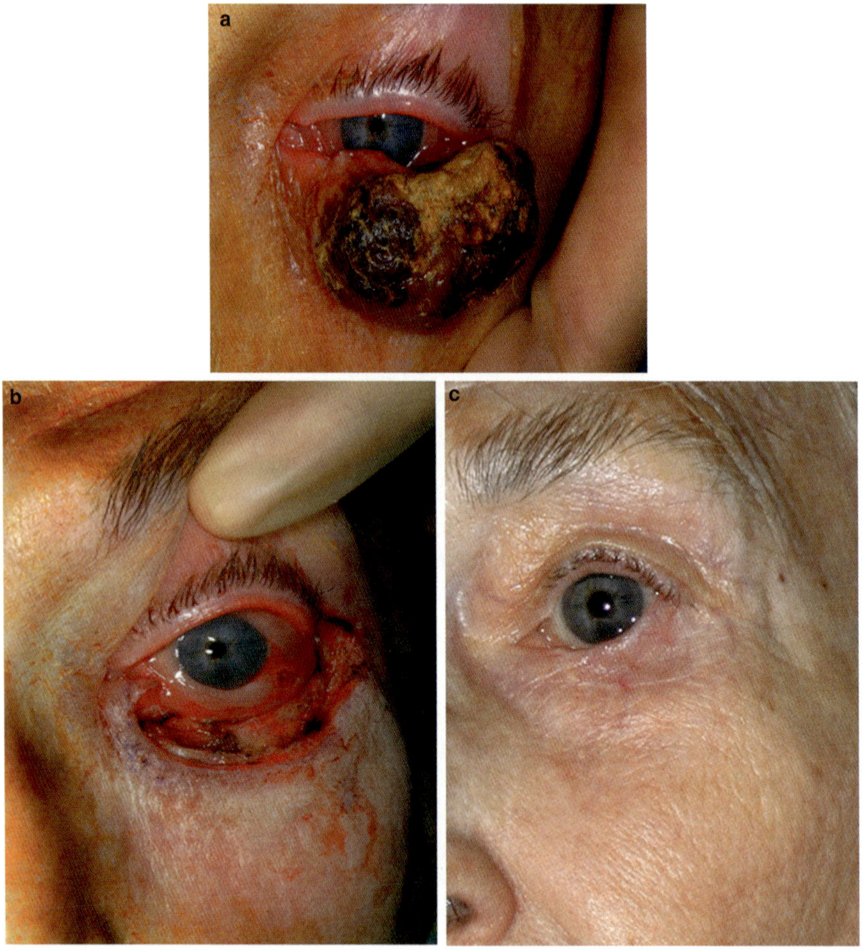

Fig. 9.5 (**a**) Locally advanced squamous cell carcinoma of the lower eyelid. (**b**) Defect size after removal of the mass. (**c**) The lower eyelid was reconstructed with a tarsoconjunctival flap and treated with 60 Gy of postoperative adjuvant radiation therapy. The patient has been recurrence free during the 4 years of follow-up

primary closure is appropriate. Loss of an entire eyelid or a large portion of an eyelid can present a difficult challenge and may necessitate more involved reconstructive techniques [25]. For large lower eyelid defects, our preferred method of reconstruction is a modified Hughes tarsoconjunctival flap. A skin graft is typically taken from one of the upper lids. The flap is usually divided in 4–6 weeks, depending on whether the patient will be receiving postoperative adjuvant radiation therapy. For large upper eyelid defects, a Cutler–Beard technique is used. For more details, please see Chapter 18.

9.3.3 Sentinel Lymph Node Biopsy

Some eyelid malignancies have the potential to spread to the regional lymph nodes in the head and neck prior to systemic metastasis [26]. Sentinel lymph node (SLN) biopsy is a technique for evaluating the nodal status in cancer patients and has been validated in cutaneous melanoma. This technique allows for localization and biopsy of the first draining node, or "sentinel node," of a tumor. It has also been advocated in the management of periocular melanoma, sebaceous gland carcinoma [27–29], and Merkel cell carcinoma. SLN biopsy is recommended for all cutaneous melanomas with a Breslow thickness of greater than 1 mm, Clark level IV, or the presence of ulceration. For conjunctival melanoma, a tumor thickness of 2 mm and the presence of ulceration correlate with a higher risk of having a microscopically positive SLN [29].

Sentinel node biopsy is typically performed at the same time as tumor resection in conjunction with a surgical oncologist or a head and neck surgeon. In our practice, lymphoscintigraphy is performed prior to surgery to identify the expected location of the SLN and allow preoperative planning (Fig 9.6). On the day of

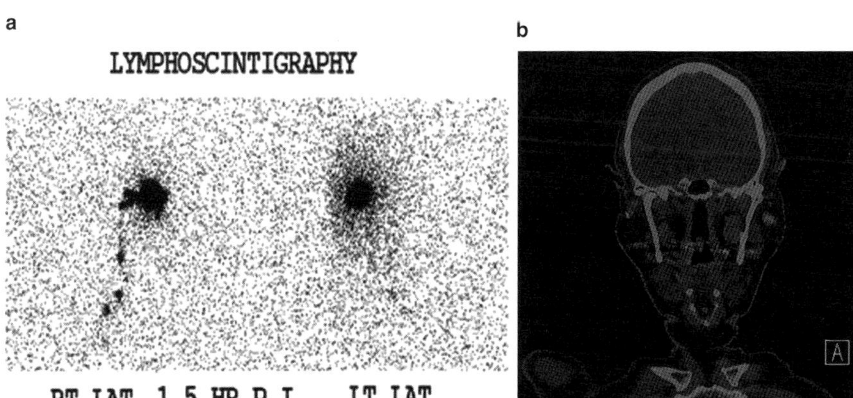

Fig. 9.6 (**a**) Preoperative lymphoscintigraphy shows drainage to a parotid node. (**b**) SPECT/CT scan provides a higher resolution and anatomic detail for the draining node(s). Note the enhancing node in the left parotid area

surgery, technetium-labeled sulfur colloid is injected into the dermal or subconjunctival space around the tumor. The tumor is then excised prior to SLN biopsy. Intraoperatively, a handheld gamma probe is used to localize the nodes that were identified during preoperative lymphoscintigraphy.

9.3.4 Nonsurgical Treatment

In certain tumors, chemotherapy, administered either topically or systemically, is an option. Imiquimod is an immune response modifier that upregulates cell-mediated immunity. Topical imiquimod 5% is approved by the US Food and Drug Administration for the treatment of superficial BCC [30] and has been successfully used for the treatment of eyelid BCC [31]. It has also been used in the treatment of SCC in situ [32] and melanoma in situ (Fig. 9.7) [33]. Topical 5-fluorouracil has been used in the treatment of actinic keratoses. Interferon has also been used for actinic keratoses. The use of intralesional interferon-2a has been reported in lentigo maligna of the eyelid [34]. Mitomycin C is used topically in the treatment of sebaceous gland carcinoma [35]. Tazarotene is a topical retinoid that has been used successfully in the treatment of BCC. In a study of the use of tazarotene for treatment of 154 BCC lesions, 71% of tumors regressed by at least 50%, while 31% of tumors were healed without recurrence at 3 years [36]. Epidermal growth factor receptor inhibitors, including erlotinib and gefitinib, have been used in the treatment of SCCs elsewhere in the body. Trials of these agents in nonmelanoma skin cancers are ongoing.

In the treatment of eyelid tumors, radiation therapy can be used as adjuvant or primary treatment. It has a role in achieving local control of disease, both for cure and for palliation. For extensive tumors that are not amenable to surgical excision,

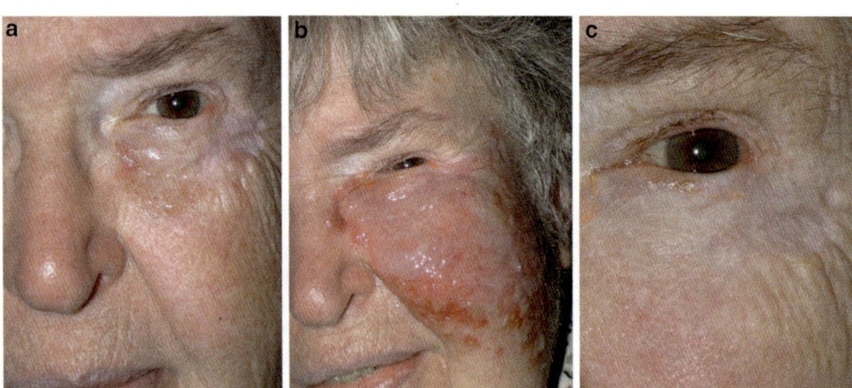

Fig. 9.7 (**a**) Recurrent lentigo maligna of the left lower eyelid and the cheek area. (**b**) Erythema and local reaction caused by topical imiquimod. (**c**) The final appearance after 6 months

radiation therapy is an option. Radiation therapy has been used as a primary treatment modality for a variety of eyelid malignancies, including Kaposi sarcoma [37], angiosarcoma [16], Merkel cell tumor, SCC, and BCC. As mentioned above, globe-preserving surgery along with postoperative radiation therapy can, in some cases, prevent the need for an orbital exenteration.

A number of other local treatment modalities have been used to treat eyelid malignancies. Photodynamic therapy has been reported in the treatment of eyelid BCC and SCC. Cryotherapy can be used to treat BCC, sebaceous carcinoma, and SCC.

In some cases, observation is the most appropriate course of management. As with any medical condition, the patient's age, social situation, and personal preferences are important factors to consider.

9.3.5 Follow-up

All patients with eyelid cancers require long-term follow-up, even after definitive treatment. The length of follow-up depends on the type of tumor. For BCC excised with negative margins, 5 years of follow-up is usually sufficient. Patients with more serious cancers, such as melanoma or sebaceous gland carcinoma, may require a longer follow-up period.

References

1. Cook BE Jr, Bartley GB. Epidemiologic characteristics and clinical course of patients with malignant eyelid tumors in an incidence cohort in Olmsted County, Minnesota. Ophthalmology 1999;106:746–50.
2. Snow SN, Sahl W, Lo JS, et al. Metastatic basal cell carcinoma. Report of five cases. Cancer 1994;73:328–35.
3. Limawararut V, Leibovitch I, Sullivan T, et al. Periocular squamous cell carcinoma. Clin Exp Ophthalmol 2007;35:174–85.
4. Faustina M, Diba R, Ahmadi MA, et al. Patterns of regional and distant metastasis in patients with eyelid and periocular squamous cell carcinoma. Ophthalmology 2004;111:1930–2.
5. Esmaeli B, Wang B, Deavers M, et al. Prognostic factors for survival in malignant melanoma of the eyelid skin. Ophthal Plast Reconstr Surg 2000;16:250–7.
6. Shields JA, Demirci H, Marr BP, et al. Sebaceous carcinoma of the eyelids: personal experience with 60 cases. Ophthalmology 2004;111:2151–7.
7. Song A, Carter KD, Syed NA, et al. Sebaceous cell carcinoma of the ocular adnexa: clinical presentations, histopathology, and outcomes. Ophthal Plast Reconstr Surg 2008;24:194–200.
8. Durairaj VD, Hink EM, Kahook MY, et al. Mucinous eccrine adenocarcinoma of the periocular region. Ophthal Plast Reconstr Surg 2006;22:30–5.
9. Mehta S, Thiagalingam S, Zembowicz A, et al. Endocrine mucin-producing sweat gland carcinoma of the eyelid. Ophthal Plast Reconstr Surg 2008;24:164–5.
10. Aurora AL, Luxenberg MN. Case report of adenocarcinoma of glands of Moll. Am J Ophthalmol 1970;70:984–90.
11. Seregard S. Apocrine adenocarcinoma arising in Moll gland cystadenoma. Ophthalmology 1993;100:1716–9.

12. Barker-Griffith AE, Streeten BW, Charles NC. Moll gland neoplasms of the eyelid: a clinical and pathological spectrum in 5 cases. Arch Ophthalmol 2006;124:1645–9.
13. Marback EF, Costa AL, Nossa LM, et al. Eyelid skin adenoid cystic carcinoma: a clinicopathological study of one case simulating sebaceous gland carcinoma. Br J Ophthalmol 2003;87:118–9.
14. Jakobiec FA. Ocular adnexal lymphoid tumors: progress in need of clarification. Am J Ophthalmol 2008;145:941–50.
15. Margo CE, Mulla ZD. Malignant tumors of the eyelid: a population-based study of non-basal cell and non-squamous cell malignant neoplasms. Arch Ophthalmol 1998;116:195–8.
16. Conway RM, Hammer T, Viestenz A, et al. Cutaneous angiosarcoma of the eyelids. Br J Ophthalmol 2003;87:514–5.
17. Eng TY, Boersma MG, Fuller CD, et al. A comprehensive review of the treatment of Merkel cell carcinoma. Am J Clin Oncol 2007;30:624–36.
18. Missotten GS, de Wolff-Rouendaal D, de Keizer RJ. Merkel cell carcinoma of the eyelid review of the literature and report of patients with Merkel cell carcinoma showing spontaneous regression. Ophthalmology 2008;115:195–201.
19. Feng H, Shuda M, Chang Y, et al. Clonal integration of a polyomavirus in human Merkel cell carcinoma. Science 2008;319:1096–100.
20. Ainbinder DJ, Esmaeli B, Groo SC, et al. Introduction of the 7th edition eyelid carcinoma classification system from the American Joint Committee on Cancer–International Union Against Cancer staging manual. Arch Pathol Lab Med 2009;133(8):1256–61.
21. Nemet AY, Deckel Y, Martin PA, et al. Management of periocular basal and squamous cell carcinoma: a series of 485 cases. Am J Ophthalmol 2006;142:293–7.
22. Malhotra R, Huilgol SC, Huynh NT, et al. The Australian Mohs database, part II: periocular basal cell carcinoma outcome at 5-year follow-up. Ophthalmology 2004;111:631–6.
23. Günalp I, Gündüz K, Dürük K. Orbital exenteration: a review of 429 cases. Int Ophthalmol 1995–1996;19:177–84.
24. Tyers AG. Orbital exenteration for invasive skin tumours. Eye 2006;20:1165–70.
25. deSousa JL, Leibovitch I, Malhotra R, et al. Techniques and outcomes of total upper and lower eyelid reconstruction. Arch Ophthalmol 2007;125:1601–9.
26. Esmaeli B. Sentinel node biopsy as a tool for accurate staging of eyelid and conjunctival malignancies. Curr Opin Ophthalmol 2002;13:317–23.
27. Nijhawan N, Ross MI, Diba R, et al. Experience with sentinel lymph node biopsy for eyelid and conjunctival malignancies at a cancer center. Ophthal Plast Reconstr Surg 2004;20:291–5.
28. Ho VH, Ross MI, Prieto VG, et al. Sentinel lymph node biopsy for sebaceous cell carcinoma and melanoma of the ocular adnexa. Arch Otolaryngol Head Neck Surg 2007;133:820–6.
29. Savar A, Ross MI, Prieto VG, Ivan D, Kim SK, Esmaeli B. Sentinel lymph node biopsy for ocular adnexal melanoma: experience in 30 patients. Ophthalmology 2009;116(11):2217–23.
30. Geisse J, Caro I, Lindholm J, et al. Imiquimod 5% cream for the treatment of superficial basal cell carcinoma: results from two phase III, randomized, vehicle-controlled studies. J Am Acad Dermatol 2004;50:722–33.
31. Choontanom R, Thanos S, Busse H, et al. Treatment of basal cell carcinoma of the eyelids with 5% topical imiquimod: a 3-year follow-up study. Graefes Arch Clin Exp Ophthalmol 2007;245:1217–20.
32. Brannan PA, Anderson HK, Kersten RC, et al. Bowen disease of the eyelid successfully treated with imiquimod. Ophthal Plast Reconstr Surg 2005;21:321–2.
33. Murchison AP, Washington CV, Soloman AR, et al. Ocular effects of imiquimod with treatment of eyelid melanoma in situ. Dermatol Surg 2007;33:1136–8.
34. Carucci JA, Leffell DJ. Intralesional interferon alfa for treatment of recurrent lentigo maligna of the eyelid in a patient with primary acquired melanosis. Arch Dermatol 2000;136:1415–6.
35. Shields CL, Naseripour M, Shields JA, et al. Topical mitomycin-C for pagetoid invasion of the conjunctiva by eyelid sebaceous gland carcinoma. Ophthalmology 2002;109:2129–33.

36. Bianchi L, Orlandi A, Campione E, et al. Topical treatment of basal cell carcinoma with tazarotene: a clinicopathological study on a large series of cases. Br J Dermatol 2004;151:148–56.
37. Shields JA, De Potter P, Shields CL, et al. Kaposi's sarcoma of the eyelids: response to radiotherapy. Arch Ophthalmol 1992;110:1689.

Chapter 10
Management of Conjunctival Neoplasms

Stella K. Kim, Dan S. Gombos, and Bita Esmaeli

Abstract Melanocytic neoplasms of the conjunctiva include nevus, primary acquired melanosis (PAM) without atypia, PAM with atypia, and conjunctival melanoma. The most common nonmelanocytic tumors of the conjunctiva are squamous cell neoplasms. Surgical excision is the cornerstone of therapy for conjunctival tumors. Proper specimen handling is critical to ensure that lesion orientation is clear to the ocular pathologist. Adjuvant therapy for conjunctival tumors can include cryotherapy and/or topical chemotherapy with mitomycin C, 5-fluorouracil, or interferon, or adjuvant radiation therapy. Tumor thickness and ulceration are important prognostic factors for local control and survival for conjunctival melanomas. Sentinel lymph node biopsy is an important recent consideration for conjunctival melanomas that are thicker than 2 mm or those that have histologic evidence of ulceration.

10.1 Introduction

Neoplasms of the conjunctiva can be subdivided into melanocytic and nonmelanocytic subtypes. Melanocytic neoplasms include nevus, primary acquired melanosis (PAM) without atypia, PAM with atypia (which some equate as the ophthalmic equivalent of cutaneous melanoma in situ), and conjunctival melanoma. The spectrum of nonmelanocytic conjunctival lesions is broad and includes epithelial, vascular, fibrous, xanthomatous, choriostomatous, myxomatous, malignant epithelial, and lipomatous varieties. In this chapter, we will discuss melanocytic lesions, including nevus, PAM, and melanoma, and squamous cell neoplasms, including both conjunctival intraepithelial neoplasia (CIN) and invasive squamous cell carcinoma.

S.K. Kim (✉)
Section of Ophthalmology, Department of Head and Neck Surgery, The University of Texas M.D. Anderson Cancer Center, Houston, TX, USA
e-mail: skim@mdanderson.org

B. Esmaeli (ed.), *Ophthalmic Oncology*, M.D. Anderson Solid Tumor Oncology Series 6, DOI 10.1007/978-1-4419-0374-7_10,

10.2 Squamous Cell Neoplasms of the Conjunctiva

Squamous cell neoplasms are the most common nonmelanocytic tumors of the conjunctiva. Generally, squamous cell tumors are subdivided into cases of CIN and frank carcinomas with invasion beyond the conjunctival basement membrane. There are a series of reports implicating the human papillomavirus as a risk factor for squamous cell carcinoma of the conjunctiva [1]. Immunosuppression (due to infectious causes or pharmacologically induced) may also play a role in tumor development and is thought to increase the risk of regional and distant metastatic disease [2].

10.2.1 Conjunctival Intraepithelial Neoplasia

CIN can be thought of as a spectrum of disease ranging from mild to severe dysplasia. If a tumor has replaced the full thickness of the epithelial layer, it is referred to as a carcinoma in situ (CIS). CIN lesions are generally located at the limbus on the bulbar conjunctiva and have a flesh-like elevation (Fig. 10.1). Leukoplakia (a white plaque) may be seen on the surface of the lesion. CIN is not thought to carry a risk of metastasis and is generally treated with surgical excision and cryotherapy (see Section 10.2.3.1).

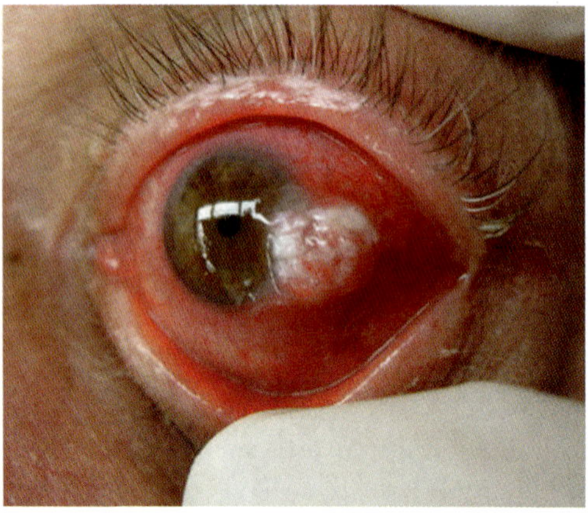

Fig. 10.1 A large perilimbal leukoplakic lesion, highly suggestive of squamous neoplasia

10.2.2 Invasive Squamous Cell Carcinoma

Squamous cell tumors with invasion beyond the conjunctival basement membrane are classified as carcinomas and have the potential for intraocular, orbital, and regional lymph node metastasis [3]. Tumors with a mucoepidermoid component noted on histopathology are generally more aggressive [4]. Clinically, squamous cell carcinomas tend to be larger than CIN lesions and require more extensive surgical and adjuvant treatment. Squamous cell carcinomas also require increased surveillance for local and distant spread. Baseline neuroimaging of the head and neck region, including the regional lymph nodes in the parotid and cervical areas, is essential and may be done with computed tomography or magnetic resonance imaging. Ultrasound of the regional lymph nodes with possible fine needle aspiration is beneficial when done by experienced echographers.

10.2.3 Management

10.2.3.1 Local Excision and Cryotherapy

As is the case for other conjunctival tumors, surgical excision is the cornerstone of therapy for squamous cell tumors of the conjunctiva. Most surgeons employ a "no-touch" technique, in which the tumor is not manipulated with instruments, and use two sets of instruments, one for excision and the other for wound closure, to avoid contaminating the surgical field with "dirty" instruments.

Smaller and more localized lesions are treated with primary excisional biopsy performed using an operating microscope. Limbal lesions that extend onto the cornea are first treated with absolute alcohol, which is tumoricidal and helps loosen the adjacent corneal epithelium. The absolute alcohol is applied with a cotton applicator, and the loosened corneal epithelium is scrolled toward the limbus and the main tumor bed. The conjunctival portion is excised with a 2-mm margin of normal tissue and resected with a layer of underlying episclera using a beaver blade. Before the specimen is submitted for pathologic evaluation, it is essential that the surgeon labels the margins to orient the ocular pathologist. Placement of the specimen on nonadherent dressing or filter paper helps prevent the tissue from scrolling up.

Once the tumor has been excised in its entirety, a new set of surgical instruments is utilized for closure. Cryotherapy is generally administered to both the underlying bulbar conjunctival margins and the scleral bed. A double freeze–thaw cycle is indicated. The wound is generally reapproximated with absorbable sutures, although some surgeons prefer closure via secondary intention, which leaves the sclera bare. Large defects can also be covered with an amniotic membrane graft [5, 6].

10.2.3.2 Treatment of More Advanced Disease

In more advanced cases, local excision may not be possible or sufficient. Diffuse surface involvement or local recurrence can be treated with adjuvant topical chemotherapy with mitomycin C, 5-fluorouracil, or interferon [7–10]. Radiotherapy can be administered focally (with ocular plaque radiotherapy) or to the entire orbit with external-beam radiotherapy.

Intraocular extension can occur, with invasion into the anterior chamber and uvea [3]. Depending on the extent of invasion, a modified enucleation with en bloc excision of the globe and the overlying conjunctiva can be considered. However, cases of diffuse conjunctival involvement (Fig. 10.2), multiple recurrent tumors, or extensive

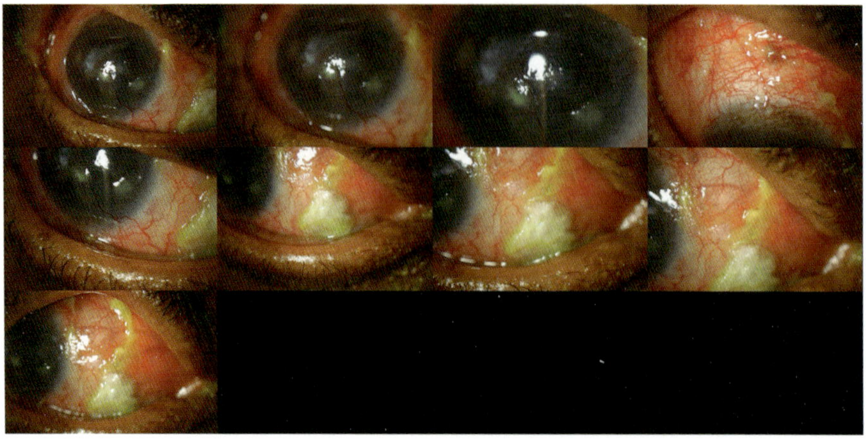

Fig. 10.2 Slit lamp photograph shows diffuse involvement of ocular surface with recurrent squamous cell carcinoma previously treated with multiple surgeries and brachytherapy. This patient underwent an orbital exenteration

orbital infiltration necessitate an orbital exenteration with or without a lid-sparing technique. If a lid-sparing technique is used, the eyelid skin can be used to line the orbital cavity [11, 12].

In high-risk patients—for example, in patients with detectable lymphadenopathy on clinical examination or imaging studies – a parotidectomy and neck dissection may be appropriate. The overall risk of lymph node metastasis from conjunctival squamous cell carcinoma is estimated to be less than 10% [13].

10.2.4 Surveillance

Patients should have follow-up visits at 3- to 6-month intervals depending on the extent of disease. Neuroimaging should be performed at the frequency of once a year, if indicated, and only for larger tumors with deep orbital or periorbital soft tissue extension and should include the head and neck region and adjacent lymph nodes.

10.3 Melanocytic Neoplasms

Melanocytic lesions of the conjunctiva behave similarly to melanocytic lesions of the skin because both types of lesions are derived from neural crest cells. Melanocytic lesions of the conjunctiva behave differently from iris and choroid lesions, which are derived from the neuroectoderm. Because conjunctival and skin melanocytic lesions have the same embryologic origin and because in clinical practice the patterns of metastasis for conjunctival melanomas are similar to cutaneous melanoma, it is reasonable to apply principles of staging, diagnosis, pathologic evaluation, and clinical course for cutaneous melanocytic lesions to conjunctival melanocytic lesions with appropriate modifications based on the clinical experience with conjunctival tumors.

10.3.1 Nevus

Nevi are the most common conjunctival melanocytic lesions in infancy and childhood (Fig. 10.3), occurring most commonly around the time of puberty [14, 15]. Nevi are benign, but 15–30% of melanomas are derived from pre-existing nevi [16, 17]. On the other hand, the rate of conversion from a pre-existing nevus to a melanoma is reported to be less than 1% over 7 years, according to a large retrospective series of over 400 patients [18]. In children, pigmented lesions are most often benign, though there are reports of melanoma in patients younger than 20 years of age [19]. Therefore, the decision whether to observe or excise a nevus must be made carefully and take into account a variety of factors, including the rate of change in the lesion, its location, the age of the patient, and associated clinical signs such as vessels or cysts; a cystic proliferation within a melanocytic lesion of conjunctiva is more characteristic of a nevus than a melanoma [14, 20].

Observation of nevi involves serial examinations and careful photodocumentation. Change in color and size may be observed [14, 20]. Benign nevi are rarely

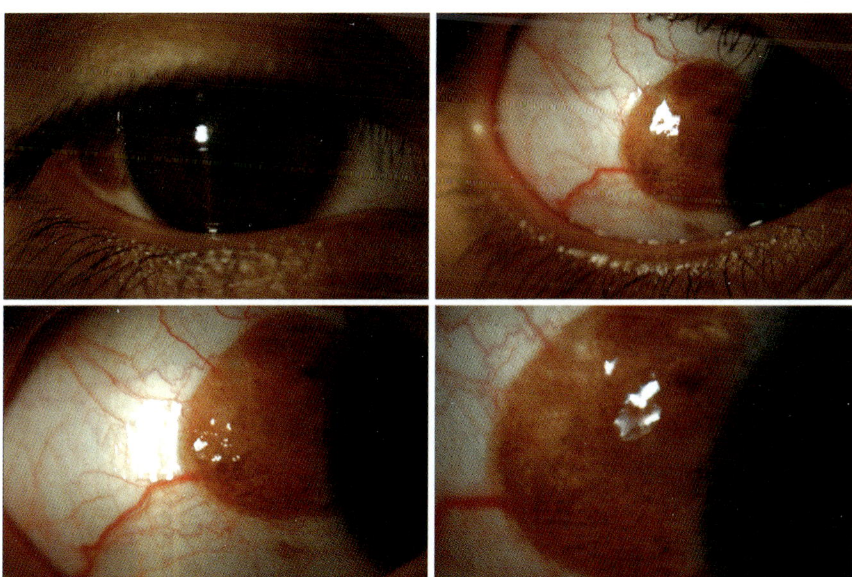

Fig. 10.3 Large conjunctival nevus in a 9-year-old boy. This lesion was surgically excised because of a history of recent enlargement

observed in the forniceal and palpebral conjunctiva; thus, biopsy of such lesions regardless of the patient's age has been advocated [14].

When a nevus is removed, careful attention to proper surgical technique is essential. It is important to avoid crush artifact by using conjunctival forceps, to excise the entire lesion with 2-mm margins when possible, to change instruments between excision and wound repair, and to handle the specimen in such a way so as to ensure that its orientation is clear to the ocular pathologist. As is true for all melanocytic lesions of the conjunctiva, frozen section evaluation of the specimen during surgery should be avoided as frozen section evaluation is not reliable for diagnosis and margin evaluation for melanomas.

Typically, if the probable diagnosis at the time of surgery is nevus, cryotherapy should be deferred. Adjuvant cryotherapy can be performed later if the diagnosis changes with the final pathology evaluation.

10.3.2 Primary Acquired Melanosis

PAM typically occurs in middle-aged Caucasians, presenting as a unilateral pigmented lesion at the limbus, on the bulbar conjunctiva, or elsewhere, including on the forniceal, caruncle, or tarsal conjunctiva [21–24]. In the ophthalmic literature, PAM is classified as PAM with atypia or PAM without atypia. Some clinicians feel that PAM with severe atypia is the ophthalmic equivalent of cutaneous melanoma in situ, and conceptualizing PAM with severe atypia as in situ disease may help patients and ophthalmic practitioners understand the severity of the diagnosis. In cases of PAM with atypia, it is helpful to have the degree of atypia (mild to severe) noted on the pathology report because the degree of atypia may be a predictor of the risk of progression to invasive melanoma [24]. In a recent large retrospective review of over 300 patients with PAM, no patients with PAM without atypia or PAM with mild atypia had progression to invasive melanoma, whereas 13% of patients with PAM with severe atypia had progression to invasive melanoma [24].

PAM with atypia and PAM without atypia typically cannot be differentiated on the basis of a clinical examination. Given the differences in the risk of progression and prognosis, some have advocated biopsy of all PAM lesions in high-risk individuals; others, though, have pointed out that one-third of middle-aged Caucasians have a unilateral pigmented lesion and have recommended against routine biopsies [25–27].

At the time of evaluation, the upper eyelids should be everted and evaluated to rule out pigmentary abnormalities, and the preauricular and cervical lymph nodes should be palpated.

The recommended treatment for PAM is complete excisional biopsy and adjuvant cryotherapy. It is important to avoid crush artifact by using conjunctival forceps, to excise the entire lesion with 2-mm margins when possible, to change instruments between excision and wound repair, and to handle the specimen in such a way so as to ensure that its orientation is clear to the ocular pathologist. It is important to excise PAM lesions and document their size and the degree of atypia because the prognosis of patients with PAM that progresses to invasive melanoma is dependent on the size of the original lesion [24]. Cryotherapy is administered to the resection margins. For large defects, amniotic membrane may be useful in reconstructing the ocular surface [28]. For diffuse lesions, conjunctival map biopsy may be needed.

As previously indicated, fresh frozen section histopathologic evaluation is not recommended for melanocytic lesions. All specimens should be subjected to permanent section histopathologic evaluation with attention to the margins. Repeat excision to clear the margins is necessary in cases of PAM with severe atypia (melanoma in situ) at the surgical margins.

If the probable diagnosis at the time of surgery is PAM rather than invasive melanoma, decisions regarding further patient workup and adjuvant treatment can be made after the final pathology evaluation. In addition to cryotherapy, adjuvant therapy may include application of topical mitomycin C or interferon alpha [29–32].

10.3.3 Conjunctival Melanoma

In the ophthalmic literature, a distinction is made between PAM with atypia and melanoma. Conjunctival melanoma is rare, accounting for fewer than 2% of ocular melanomas and fewer than 1% of malignant tumors of the eye [33]. It is typically seen in patients 40–70 years of age and most commonly occurs in the intrapalpebral region near the limbus (Fig. 10.4) but may occur anywhere on the bulbar and palpebral conjunctiva as well as in the caruncle (Fig. 10.5) [34–36]. Factors associated with a worse prognosis include greater tumor thickness (depth), a non-limbal location, higher rate of mitosis, multifocality, and intralymphatic or intravascular spread [34–36]. In addition, ulceration was recently found by our group to be an important predictor of local recurrence and lymph node metastasis[37]. Studies of conjunctival melanoma describe 5-year survival rates between 74 and 93% and 10-year survival rates between 41 and 87% [34, 35, 38].

After a thorough ocular examination, including everted eyelid evaluation, gonioscopy, and regional lymph node palpation, a workup for systemic disease should be performed, including routine blood work; imaging studies of the lymph nodes, orbital structures, and brain; and possibly computed tomography of the chest, abdomen, and pelvis for melanomas that are thicker than 2 mm. If the workup for systemic disease is negative, then surgery for definitive local control can be carefully planned.

Complete wide local excision followed by application of cryotherapy to the resection margins and the surgical bed, first described by Jakobiec et al. [39] in 1980, remains the primary surgical approach for making the diagnosis and achieving local control. A margin of at least 2 mm outside of the lesion is achieved using the no-touch technique, in which the melanoma is not manipulated with instruments. Lesions that extend onto the cornea are first treated with absolute alcohol, which is tumoricidal and helps loosen the adjacent corneal epithelium. Epitheliectomy of

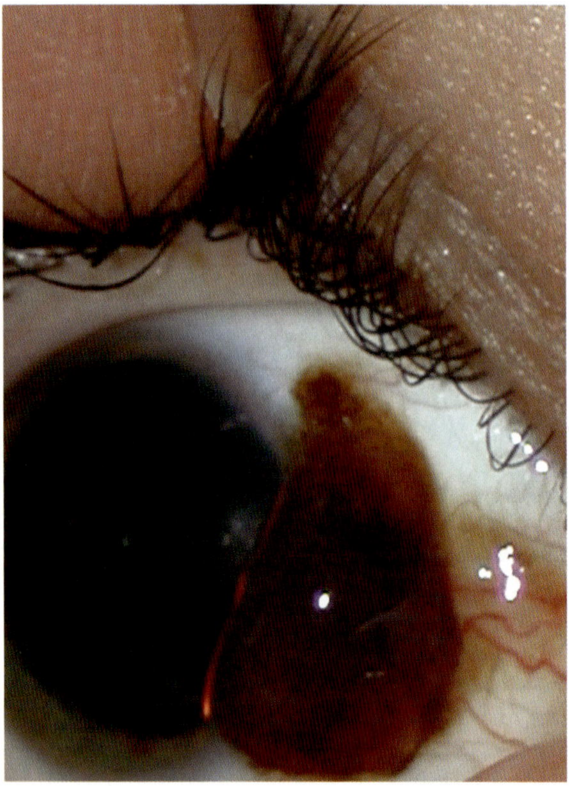

Fig. 10.4 Slit lamp photograph shows conjunctival melanoma at the limbus

corneal disease with absolute alcohol is performed. Excision is followed by double freeze–thaw cryotherapy of the conjunctival margins and the scleral bed. Proper handling of the surgical specimen is crucial to permit the pathologist to determine the true tumor thickness and to evaluate the margins [40]. Flattening of the surgical specimen and orientating the margins of interest for the pathologist are critical. A second set of clean instruments should be used for repair of the ocular surface to avoid contaminating the field with "dirty" instruments. Depending on the size of the defect, the conjunctival defect may be closed with primary closure or with amniotic membrane grafts. For widely disseminated disease on the surface of the eye, orbital exenteration with or without external-beam radiotherapy may be needed to achieve local control (Fig. 10.6). In some cases, judicious use of external-beam radiotherapy may obviate orbital exenteration [41].

If metastatic disease is found prior to surgical resection of conjunctival melanoma, the goal of surgery is to establish the definitive diagnosis as well as attempt to achieve local control by excisional biopsy and cryotherapy. However, because the patient will be treated with systemic modalities for metastatic disease, exenteration to achieve local control in such a setting is unwarranted.

For patients without evidence of metastatic disease on the initial workup, sentinel lymph node biopsy (SLNB) may be done in order to identify microscopic

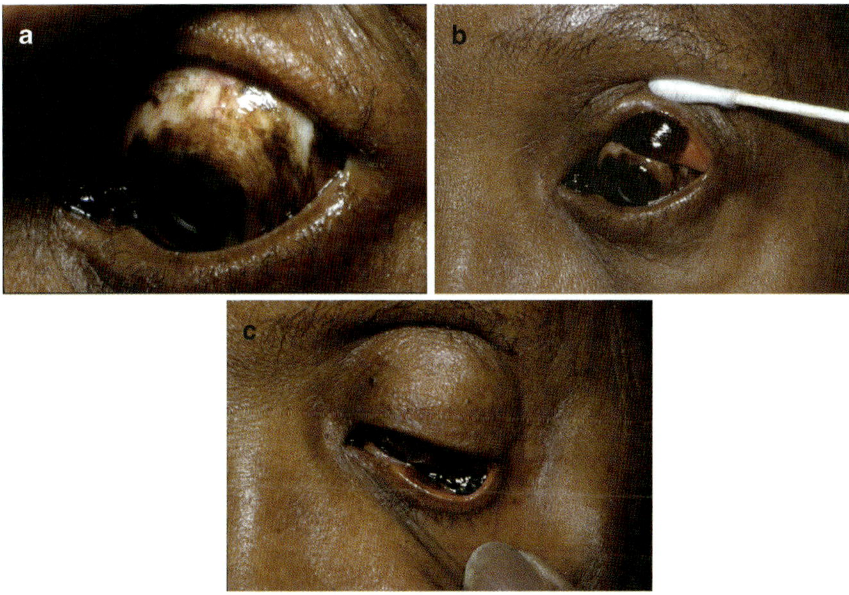

Fig. 10.5 (**a**) Bulbar conjunctival melanoma with extension onto the upper (**b**) and the lower (**c**) palpebral conjunctiva

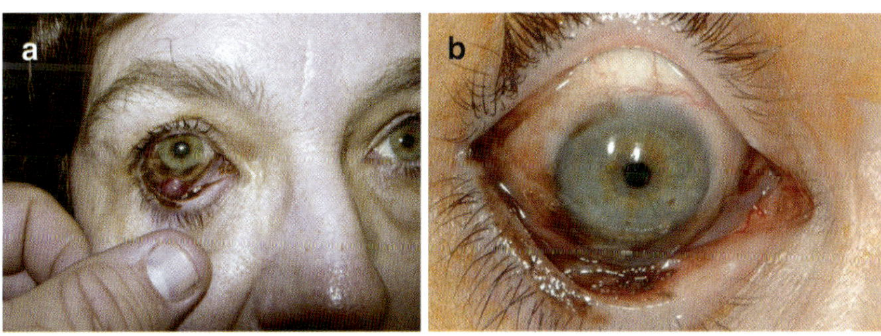

Fig. 10.6 Invasive melanoma of conjunctiva with diffuse involvement of lower eyelid margin, including an amelanotic nodule at the lid margin (**a**), as well as extensive involvement of the bulbar conjunctiva, caruncle, and parts of the upper palpebral conjunctiva (**b**). This patient had an orbital exenteration

disease in the primary ("sentinel") and secondary draining nodes [37, 42–44]. SLNB is widely accepted for evaluating whether there is microscopic lymphatic spread of cutaneous melanoma and other cancers, such as breast cancer. Our group has explored SLNB for conjunctival and eyelid melanomas in the last decade. The status of the regional lymph nodes is a crucial prognostic indicator, and SLNB can identify lymph node metastatic disease that otherwise would have gone undetected [37, 45]. At M. D. Anderson Cancer Center, a prospective trial is ongoing to evaluate the role of SLNB in patients with conjunctival melanomas with clinically and radiographically negative regional nodes [37, 46, 47]. A recent analysis of the data from this trial showed that of 30 patients with ocular adnexal (conjunctival or eyelid) melanomas who underwent SLNB, 5 patients had a positive SLN (microscopic SLN metastasis) [37]. The analysis included 14 patients with bulbar conjunctival melanoma, 8 patients with palpebral conjunctival melanoma, 4 patients with melanoma involving both the bulbar and the palpebral conjunctiva, and 4 patients with eyelid skin melanoma. At least one SLN was identified in all patients. The median number of SLNs removed was 2. The most common basin sampled was the intraparotid, followed by submandibular (level I), preauricular, and superior cervical (level II). Among the 25 patients with negative SLNB finding, there were two false-negative events, although there were no false-negative events among patients treated during the last 4.5 years of the study. The mean Breslow thickness was 2.57 mm (range, 0.62–12 mm) among patients with negative SLNB findings and 4.86 mm (range, 2.0–7.2 mm) among patients with positive SLNB findings ($p = 0.055$). Ulceration was present in 11 patients (39%)—4 (80%) of 5 patients with positive SLNB findings and 7 (28%) of 25 with negative SLNB findings, including both patients with false-negative results. We concluded that SLNB is effective for identifying nodal micrometastasis in patients with ocular adnexal melanoma and provides important prognostic information and that the false-negative event rate in our series improved in the last 4 years, most likely due to a better technique and better patient selection for SLNB [37]. On the basis of this study, SLNB may be most appropriate in patients with conjunctival melanomas greater than 2 mm thick or when ulceration is present.

References

1. Scott IU, Karp CL, Nuovo GJ. Human papillomavirus 16 and 18 expression in conjunctival intraepithelial neoplasia. Ophthalmology 2002;109(3):542–7.
2. Shelil AE, Shields CL, Shields JA, et al. Aggressive conjunctival squamous cell carcinoma in a patient following liver transplantation. Arch Ophthalmol 2003;121(2):280–2.
3. Shields JA, Shields CL, Gunduz K, et al. The 1998 Pan American lecture. Intraocular invasion of conjunctival squamous cell carcinoma in five patients. Ophthal Plast Reconstr Surg 1999;15(3):153–60.
4. Brownstein S. Mucoepidermoid carcinoma of the conjunctiva with intraocular invasion. Ophthalmology 1981;88(12):1226–30.
5. Shields JA, Shields CL, De Potter P. Surgical management of conjunctival tumors. The 1994 Lynn B. McMahan lecture. Arch Ophthalmol 1997;115(6):808–15.
6. Eichler MD, Fraunfelder FT. Cryotherapy for conjunctival lymphoid tumors. Am J Ophthalmol 1994;118(4):463–7.
7. Karp CL, Moore JK, Rosa RH Jr. Treatment of conjunctival and corneal intraepithelial neoplasia with topical interferon alpha-2b. Ophthalmology 2001;108(6):1093–8.
8. Midena E, Angeli CD, Valenti M, et al. Treatment of conjunctival squamous cell carcinoma with topical 5-fluorouracil. Br J Ophthalmol 2000;84(3):268–72.
9. Shields CL, Naseripour M, Shields JA, et al. Topical mitomycin-C for pagetoid invasion of the conjunctiva by eyelid sebaceous gland carcinoma. Ophthalmology 2002;109(11):2129–33.

10. Yeatts RP, Engelbrecht NE, Curry CD, et al. 5-Fluorouracil for the treatment of intraepithelial neoplasia of the conjunctiva and cornea. Ophthalmology 2000;107(12):2190–5.
11. Shields JA, Shields CL, Suvarnamani C, et al. Orbital exenteration with eyelid sparing: indications, technique, and results. Ophthalmic Surg 1991;22(5):292–7.
12. Shields JA, Shields CL, Demirci H, et al. Experience with eyelid-sparing orbital exenteration: the 2000 Tullos O. Coston lecture. Ophthal Plast Reconstr Surg 2001;17(5):355–61.
13. Esmaeli B, Eicher S, Popp J, et al. Sentinel lymph node biopsy for conjunctival melanoma. Ophthal Plast Reconstr Surg 2001;17(6):436–42.
14. Folberg R, Jakobiec FA, Bernardino VB, et al. Benign conjunctival melanocytic lesions. Clinicopathologic features. Ophthalmology 1989;96(4):436–61.
15. Jakobiec FA, Folberg R, Iwamoto T. Clinicopathologic characteristics of premalignant and malignant melanocytic lesions of the conjunctiva. Ophthalmology 1989;96(2):147–66.
16. Jay B. Naevi and melanomata of the conjunctiva. Br J Ophthalmol 1965;49:169–204.
17. Liesegang TJ, Campbell RJ. Mayo Clinic experience with conjunctival melanomas. Arch Ophthalmol 1980;98(8):1385–9.
18. Shields CL, Fasiuddin AF, Mashayekhi A, et al. Conjunctival nevi: clinical features and natural course in 410 consecutive patients. Arch Ophthalmol 2004;122(2):167–75.
19. McDonnell JM, Carpenter JD, Jacobs P, et al. Conjunctival melanocytic lesions in children. Ophthalmology 1989;96(7):986–93.
20. Brancato R, Campana G, Mincione G. Histopathogenetic considerations on the so-called cystic nevi of the conjunctiva [in Italian]. Arch De Vecchi Anat Patol 1969;54(3): 739–46.
21. Folberg R, McLean IW, Zimmerman LE. Conjunctival melanosis and melanoma. Ophthalmology 1984;91(6):673–8.
22. Jakobiec FA. The ultrastructure of conjunctival melanocytic tumors. Trans Am Ophthalmol Soc 1984;82:599–752.
23. Folberg R, McLean IW. Primary acquired melanosis and melanoma of the conjunctiva: terminology, classification, and biologic behavior. Hum Pathol 1986;17(7):652–4.
24. Shields JA, Shields CL, Mashayekhi A, et al. Primary acquired melanosis of the conjunctiva: experience with 311 eyes. Trans Am Ophthalmol Soc 2007;105:61–71.
25. Jakobiec FA, Rini FJ, Fraunfelder FT, et al. Cryotherapy for conjunctival primary acquired melanosis and malignant melanoma. Experience with 62 cases. Ophthalmology 1988;95(8):1058–70.
26. Jakobiec FA, Brownstein S, Wilkinson RD, et al. Adjuvant cryotherapy for focal nodular melanoma of the conjunctiva. Arch Ophthalmol 1982;100(1):115–8.
27. Gloor P, Alexandrakis G. Clinical characterization of primary acquired melanosis. Invest Ophthalmol Vis Sci 1995;36(8):1721–9.
28. Paridaens D, Beekhuis H, van Den Bosch W, et al. Amniotic membrane transplantation in the management of conjunctival malignant melanoma and primary acquired melanosis with atypia. Br J Ophthalmol 2001;85(6):658–61.
29. Finger PT, Czechonska G, Liarikos S. Topical mitomycin C chemotherapy for conjunctival melanoma and PAM with atypia. Br J Ophthalmol 1998;82(5):476–9.
30. Kurli M, Finger PT. Topical mitomycin chemotherapy for conjunctival malignant melanoma and primary acquired melanosis with atypia: 12 years' experience. Graefes Arch Clin Exp Ophthalmol 2005;243(11):1108–14.
31. Finger PT, Sedeek RW, Chin KJ. Topical interferon alfa in the treatment of conjunctival melanoma and primary acquired melanosis complex. Am J Ophthalmol 2008;145(1): 124–9.
32. Chalasani R, Giblin M, Conway RM. Role of topical chemotherapy for primary acquired melanosis and malignant melanoma of the conjunctiva and cornea: review of the evidence and recommendations for treatment. Clin Exp Ophthalmol 2006;34(7):708–14.
33. Scotto J, Fraumeni JF Jr., Lee JA. Melanomas of the eye and other noncutaneous sites: epidemiologic aspects. J Natl Cancer Inst 1976;56(3):489–91.

34. Paridaens AD, Minassian DC, McCartney AC, et al. Prognostic factors in primary malignant melanoma of the conjunctiva: a clinicopathological study of 256 cases. Br J Ophthalmol 1994;78(4):252–9.
35. Shields CL, Shields JA, Gunduz K, et al. Conjunctival melanoma: risk factors for recurrence, exenteration, metastasis, and death in 150 consecutive patients. Arch Ophthalmol 2000;118(11):1497–507.
36. Jakobiec FA. Conjunctival melanoma. Arch Ophthalmol 1980;98(8):1378–84.
37. Savar A, Ross MI, Prieto VG, et al. Sentinel lymph node biopsy for ocular adnexal melanoma: experience in 30 patients. Ophthalmology 2009;116(11):2217–23.
38. Esmaeli B, Wang X, Youssef A, et al. Patterns of regional and distant metastasis in patients with conjunctival melanoma: experience at a cancer center over four decades. Ophthalmology 2001;108(11):2101–5.
39. Jakobiec FA, Brownstein S, Wilkinson RD, et al. Combined surgery and cryotherapy for diffuse malignant melanoma of the conjunctiva. Arch Ophthalmol 1980;98(8):1390–6.
40. Esmaeli B, De Martelaere S, Ozkan Y, et al. Surgical specimen handling for conjunctival melanoma: implications for tumor thickness determination and sentinel lymph node biopsy. Ophthal Plast Reconstr Surg 2006;22(3):238–9.
41. Hsu A, Frank S, Ballo MT, et al. Postoperative adjuvant external-beam radiation therapy for cancers of the eyelid and conjunctiva. Ophthal Plast Reconstr Surg 2008;24(6):444–9.
42. Esmaeli B. Sentinel lymph node mapping for patients with cutaneous and conjunctival malignant melanoma. Ophthal Plast Reconstr Surg 2000;16(3):170–2.
43. Esmaeli B. Sentinel node biopsy as a tool for accurate staging of eyelid and conjunctival malignancies. Curr Opin Ophthalmol 2002;13(5):317–23.
44. Wilson MW, Fleming JC, Fleming RM, et al. Sentinel node biopsy for orbital and ocular adnexal tumors. Ophthal Plast Reconstr Surg 2001;17(5):338–44; discussion 44–5.
45. Esmaeli B, Reifler D, Prieto VG, et al. Conjunctival melanoma with a positive sentinel lymph node. Arch Ophthalmol 2003;121(12):1779–83.
46. Nijhawan N, Ross MI, Diba R, et al. Experience with sentinel lymph node biopsy for eyelid and conjunctival malignancies at a cancer center. Ophthal Plast Reconstr Surg 2004;20(4):291–5.
47. Ho VH, Ross MI, Prieto VG, et al. Sentinel lymph node biopsy for sebaceous cell carcinoma and melanoma of the ocular adnexa. Arch Otolaryngol Head Neck Surg 2007;133(8):820–6.

Chapter 11
Surgical Specimen Handling for Conjunctival and Eyelid Tumors

Sheri L. DeMartelaere, Frank W. Scribbick, and Doina Ivan

Abstract Ophthalmologists need to be familiar with surgical specimen handling in order to provide optimal patient care. The cornerstone of proper specimen handling is communication between the ophthalmologist and the pathologist before, during, and after surgery. Conjunctival tissue presents unique surgical specimen handling challenges as the tissue has a propensity to curl up on itself, making it difficult to maintain proper tissue orientation and alignment. For pathologic evaluation of eyelid specimens, specimen orientation is the key. Proper specimen handling and discussion with the pathologist can help alleviate these difficulties.

11.1 Introduction

Proper specimen handling is a critical component of the surgical removal of periocular tumors. Specimen handling is a critical determinant of diagnostic accuracy and the completeness of excision, which in turn influence the patient's prognosis and recommendations for adjuvant treatment [1].

For several types of periocular tumors, the first excisional biopsy provides the only opportunity to assess tumor thickness. In addition, for malignant periocular tumors for which complete surgical resection is the treatment of choice, correct evaluation of the margins of resection is essential [2]. In both situations, the surgical specimen must be prepared carefully to allow the pathologist to perform an appropriate evaluation and provide the information the surgeon needs.

Every ophthalmologist needs to be familiar with the basics of specimen handling in order to provide optimal patient care.

S.L. DeMartelaere (✉)
Ophthalmology Service, Department of Surgery, Brooke Army Medical Center, Fort Sam Houston, TX, USA
e-mail: sheri.l.demartelaere@us.army.mil

B. Esmaeli (ed.), *Ophthalmic Oncology*, M.D. Anderson Solid Tumor Oncology Series 6, DOI 10.1007/978-1-4419-0374-7_11,

11.2 Communication with the Pathologist

The cornerstone of proper specimen handling is communication between the ophthalmologist and the pathologist before, during, and after surgery. Before surgery, this communication may involve simply filling out the specimen-processing form with the patient's age, clinical history, clinical diagnosis, and lesion location or may involve speaking with the pathologist to discuss the proper tissue medium so that the appropriate studies can be obtained.

Intraoperatively, the pathologist needs to know what question the surgeon is asking. If fresh tissue is submitted, is the reason that the surgeon wants to know if the margins are clear or that the surgeon wants to determine if sufficient diagnostic tissue has been submitted? Or perhaps the tissue is being sent for special studies such as flow cytometry analysis of a suspected lymphoproliferative lesion. Do special stains need to be done to look for microorganisms? If the ophthalmologist suspects that a patient has sebaceous gland carcinoma, the Oil Red O fat stain can be used to highlight sebocytes.

Tumors in the periocular region present unique challenges for the surgeon and the pathologist. Frequently, one is trying to spare critical tissue such as the canalicular system or limbal stem cells, and thus the surgical specimens are small. If specimen tissue is limited, the pathologist needs to know which clinical diagnoses are most critical to establish or rule out so that the most pertinent diagnostic studies are performed.

Open communication with the pathologist during surgery may be necessary. It is useful to have the pathologist come to the operating room for precise specimen orientation prior to specimen removal. If this is not done, the surgeon should take the specimen to the pathologist and orient the margins of interest. This type of interaction can help the pathologist determine whether to use an en face technique or serial perpendicular sectioning of the specimen to ensure that the critical margins are tumor free [3]. The surgeon needs to consider intraoperative technique to minimize manipulation of the tissue and thereby minimize crush artifact and tissue desiccation.

Postoperatively, the surgeon and the pathologist need to continue to work together. It is not uncommon for a lesion that the surgeon considers to be clinically benign to be revealed to be malignant upon histopathologic examination. For example, what appears to be a common eyelid chalazion can turn out to be a rare tumor such as an angiosarcoma, Merkel cell carcinoma, or sebaceous gland carcinoma [4]. For this reason, it is highly recommended that all chalazion specimens be submitted for histopathologic examination and reviewed by an ocular pathologist—particularly if a chalazion has recurred after incision and curettage [5]. Surgeons need to follow up on all specimen results and keep the pathologist apprised of any supportive clinical or laboratory information that might aid in the diagnosis of a difficult case. Often this ongoing communication is facilitated by a monthly tumor board conference.

The basic steps in proper surgical specimen handling are outlined in Table 11.1.

Table 11.1 Checklist for proper surgical specimen handling

Routine specimens
Preoperative
Complete pathology request form
Patient age, sex, history of present illness, previous biopsy
Location of lesion
Clinical diagnosis
Intraoperative
Generally, use 10% neutral buffered formalin (at least five times the volume of biopsy specimen) as fixative
Place each specimen in separate formalin-filled container
Label container(s) with patient-identifying information and biopsy location
Include sketch of biopsy location to facilitate orientation by pathologist
Postoperative
Follow-up to find out diagnosis (seemingly benign lesions may turn out to be malignant and seemingly negative margins may turn out to be positive)
Communicate with pathologist about controversial findings
Fresh specimens
Preoperative
Explain to pathologist why fresh tissue is being submitted
Complete pathology request form
Patient age, sex, history of present illness, previous biopsy
Location of lesion
Clinical diagnosis
Reason for submitting fresh specimen [margin evaluation, diagnosis, determination of adequacy of tissue specimen, special studies (e.g., flow cytometry when a lymphoproliferative lesion is suspected)]
Assure whether correct fixative is available
Intraoperative
Lay out specimen on sketch labeled for orientation
Place suture or ink specimen to assist pathologist with orientation
Hand-deliver tissue to pathologist as quickly as possible
Ink margins with pathologist
Await results and submit more fresh tissue if indicated
Postoperative
Follow-up to find out diagnosis
Communicate with pathologist about controversial findings

11.3 Conjunctival Specimens

Conjunctival tissue presents unique specimen handling challenges. First and most important of these challenges is the tissue's propensity to curl up on itself, making it difficult to maintain proper tissue orientation and alignment. Second, the surgeon often wishes to preserve as much normal tissue as possible, and thus margins of normal tissue surrounding a conjunctival tumor are frequently measured in millimeters. These two factors together can result in small specimens with curled-up edges that make it difficult for the pathologist to orient the specimen, assess the margins, and provide the surgeon with meaningful data.

Proper specimen handling can help alleviate these difficulties. Intraoperatively, conjunctival specimens can be flattened out on a piece of nonadherent dressing such as Telfa. It is important not to place conjunctival specimens on sponges, which expand in fixative and distort the specimen. For orientation, surgical sutures are preferred to methylene blue or toluidine blue ink, which tend to spread out into the tissue. Ideally, the surgical site is sketched on the nonadherent dressing, and then the specimen is laid out in the correct orientation on the sketch (Fig. 11.1). This visual guide, a simple supplement to the specimen-processing paperwork, is very effective for specimen orientation.

Laying out the specimen also aids the pathologist in sectioning the specimen perpendicularly and avoiding tangential cuts. This is critical for assessing tumor invasion and tumor thickness [6]. In the specimen shown in Fig. 11.2, tangential cutting made it impossible to determine whether there had been invasion below the basement membrane and thus impossible to differentiate between invasive squamous cell carcinoma and in situ disease. In the specimen shown in Fig. 11.3, tangential sectioning of a melanoma made it impossible to appropriately assess the tumor thickness. In melanoma, tumor thickness is the most important prognostic factor, and its correct assessment is critical for patient care, as sentinel lymph node biopsy may be recommended for tumors with thickness greater than a certain Breslow-equivalent thickness (Fig. 11.4) [7].

After the specimen is received in the pathology department, it is of paramount importance that processing occurs rapidly to minimize tissue drying. The decision whether to use en face technique or serial perpendicular sectioning depends on the size of the specimen and the particulars of the case as discussed with the surgeon, emphasizing the importance of communication between the surgeon and the pathologist.

Frozen section analysis is not recommended for melanocytic conjunctival lesions. As previously mentioned, the pathologist dealing with a conjunctival

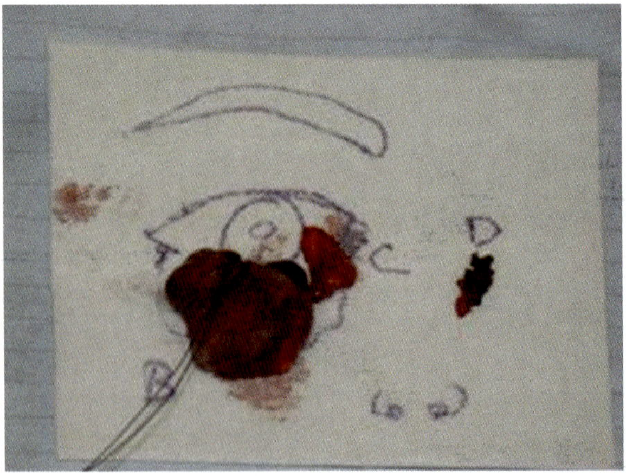

Fig. 11.1 Surgical conjunctival specimen, involving both the palpebral and the bulbar conjunctiva, placed on Telfa with a drawing of the area of resection for orientation. Photo courtesy of Dr. Bita Esmaeli

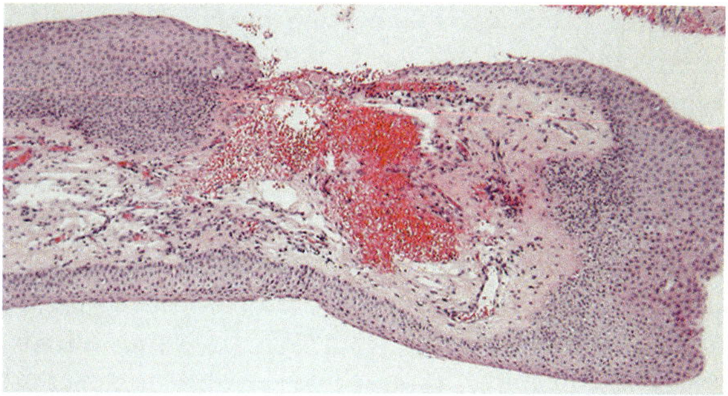

Fig. 11.2 Tangentially sectioned conjunctival biopsy specimen. It was not possible to assess whether the specimen represented carcinoma in situ or invasive squamous cell carcinoma

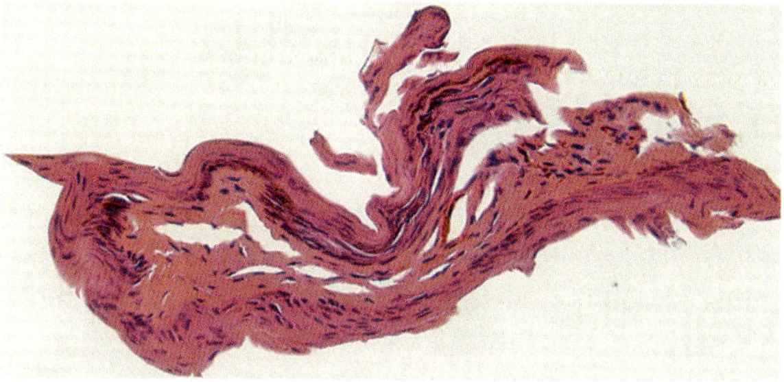

Fig. 11.3 Tangentially sectioned conjunctival biopsy specimen. It was not possible to assess whether the specimen represented primary acquired melanosis or melanoma

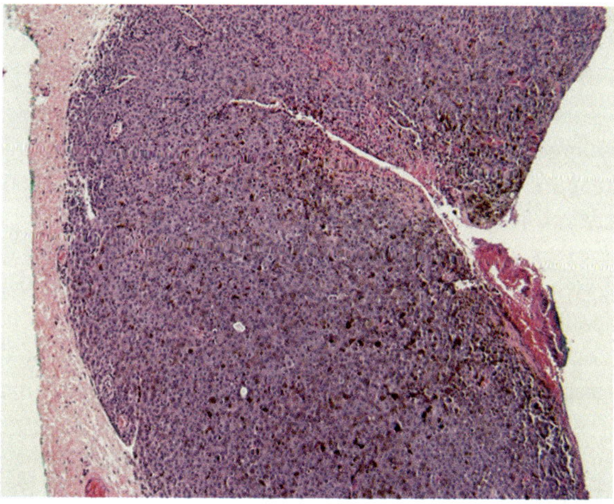

Fig. 11.4 Perpendicularly sectioned conjunctival melanoma specimen, allowing for measurement of tumor thickness

specimen is already challenged by the limited tissue and the difficulty of obliquely sectioning the tissue because of its contractile properties. An even more significant consideration is the difficulty of interpreting melanocytic cells with frozen section technique [8]. Most surgeons and pathologists would agree that permanent section technique is the gold standard for ensuring margin control for conjunctival or eyelid melanomas [9].

A few words need to be said regarding fixatives. The majority of conjunctival specimens can be sent in 10% neutral buffered formalin; however, there are a few exceptions. The possibility of pagetoid spread must be considered in cases of possible sebaceous carcinoma of the palpebral or bulbar conjunctiva. In such cases, map biopsies of the conjunctiva (representative conjunctival biopsies from each sector) should be performed and biopsy specimens sent fresh for evaluation of intraepithelial neoplasia with the use of fat stains (such as Oil Red O), if needed [10, 11]. Suspected lymphoproliferative lesions should also be sent fresh for impression cytology and flow cytometry. If electron microscopy may be diagnostically useful (for example, in cases of possible conjunctival Merkel cell carcinoma), a small fragment of the specimen should be sent in glutaraldehyde [12].

11.4 Eyelid Specimens

For pathologic evaluation of eyelid specimens, proper specimen orientation is the key. Specimens being submitted fresh for frozen section evaluation of margins need to be correctly oriented. A drawing of the eye and periocular structures is helpful for this purpose. For full-thickness lesions involving the eyelid margin, the pathologist needs to know which eye the specimen is from and whether the specimen is from the upper or the lower eyelid. With this minimum orientation, the pathologist can determine nasal, temporal, and superior or inferior margins (the eyelid margin itself is not a surgical margin).

For specimens not involving the eyelid margin yet still involving the dermis, a suture must be placed to indicate the orientation; commonly, the 12 o'clock position is tagged. However, the surgeon may choose to mark any clock hour and may choose to mark a clock hour in a segment about which there is most concern. Another method for specimen orientation is to make a drawing of the pertinent facial structures as a reference and then place the specimen in its correct orientation on the drawing (Fig. 11.5). In complex cases or when the pathologist does not frequently handle eyelid specimens, it is recommended that the surgeon hand-carry the specimen to the pathologist so that together the surgeon and the pathologist can ink the margins and discuss any questions or areas of particular concern.

If multiple specimens are being submitted, a preoperative photograph with the biopsy sites labeled is a useful tool in addition to the description of the specimen location on the specimen submission form (Fig. 11.6). Each specimen needs to be submitted in a separate container labeled with the appropriate information about patient identification and biopsy location.

Several of the recommendations for handling conjunctival specimens also apply to eyelid specimens: (1) specimens from tumors suspected of being sebaceous carcinomas or lymphoproliferative lesions need to be sent fresh, (2) frozen section margin control is not recommended for melanoma owing to the unreliability of assessment of melanocytic atypia on frozen sections, and (3) tangential cutting must be avoided in the case of melanomas because tumor thickness is the most

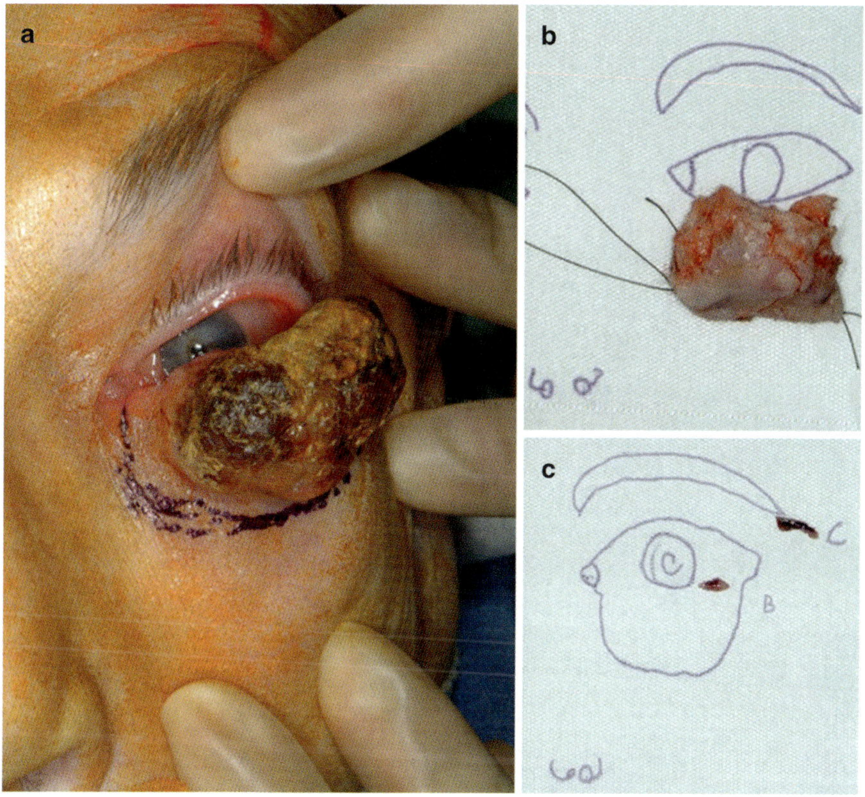

Fig. 11.5 Surgical eyelid specimen. (**a**) Preoperative surgical markings. (**b**) Primary surgical specimen A placed on sketch with sutures marking medial and lateral margins for orientation. (**c**) Additional surgical specimens B and C, removed to obtain clear margins, placed on sketch for orientation. Photos courtesy of Dr. Bita Esmaeli

important prognostic factor for melanomas. Two other factors also underscore the critical importance of proper specimen handling to enable accurate determination of melanoma tumor thickness. First, a recent study indicated that thin periocular melanomas may be excised with 5-mm margins, which are associated with less morbidity than the previously recommended 1-cm margins, which in any case are often unobtainable in the periocular region [13, 14]. Second, eyelid skin and conjunctival melanomas that are more than 1-mm thick are viewed by many authorities as being appropriate for sentinel lymph node biopsy [14, 15].

11.5 Mohs Micrographic Surgery

Mohs micrographic surgery is a technique for excising cancerous skin lesions. It utilizes microscopic margin control, enabling tumor excision with minimal sacrifice of normal surrounding tissue. This is advantageous in the eyelid, particularly in the

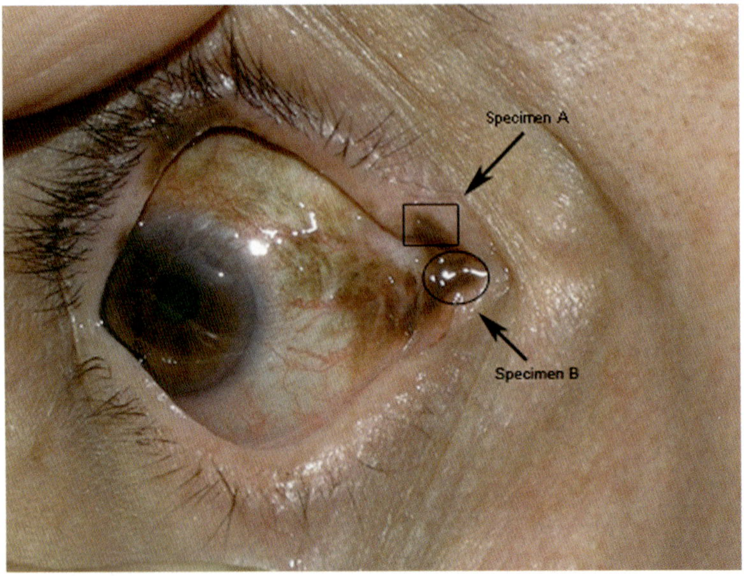

Fig. 11.6 Preoperative surgical photograph of eyelid primary acquired melanosis suggestive of melanoma. The photograph was submitted to the pathologist to aid with specimen orientation. Photo courtesy of Dr. Bita Esmaeli

medial canthal region and the lacrimal drainage system. Mohs surgery has been proven to be highly successful in the excision of basal cell carcinoma and squamous cell carcinoma [16].

In contrast, the use of Mohs surgery for melanoma, Merkel cell carcinoma, and sebaceous carcinoma is controversial [17–21]. Some investigators recommend a variant coined "slow-Mohs" or "modified Mohs technique" for such tumors [9, 18]. However, most investigators agree that for melanomas, the margins need to be assessed by permanent section technique. The tumor is excised, and the pathologist performs a 24-hour expedited assessment of the margins. Additional tissue is excised daily until the margins are clear or until both the patient and the surgeon agree to stop—for example, if the tumor has become inoperable or if other nonsurgical modalities, such as radiation therapy, or topical medications, such as imiquimod, are to be used to address microscopic residual in situ melanoma at margins.

11.6 Summary

Proper surgical specimen handling of conjunctival and eyelid tumors is not difficult, but it is a critical component of a successful surgical ablation of periocular and ocular adnexal tumors. The basic concepts of specimen orientation and effective communication between the surgeon and the pathologist will enable the ophthalmologist to provide optimal patient care.

References

1. Wang Q, Prieto V, Esmaeli B, et al. Cellular blue nevi of the eyelid: a possible diagnostic pitfall. J Am Acad Dermatol 2008;58:257–60.
2. Plowman PN. Eyelid tumours. Orbit 2007;26:207–13.
3. Wong VA, Marshall JA, Whitehead KJ, et al. Management of periocular basal cell carcinoma with modified en face frozen section controlled excision. Ophthal Plast Reconstr Surg 2002;18:430–5.
4. Peters GB III, Meyer DR, Shields JA, et al. Management and prognosis of Merkel cell carcinoma of the eyelid. Ophthalmology 2001;108:1575–9.
5. Pereira PR, Odashiro AA, Rodrigues-Reyes AA, et al. Histopathological review of sebaceous carcinoma of the eyelid. J Cutan Pathol 2005;32:496–501.
6. Esmaeli B, DeMartelaere S, Ozkan Y, et al. Surgical specimen handling for conjunctival melanoma: implications for tumor thickness determination and sentinel lymph node biopsy [letter]. Ophthal Plast Reconstr Surg 2006;22:238–9.
7. Nijhawan N, Ross MI, Diba R, et al. Experience with sentinel lymph node biopsy for eyelid and conjunctival malignancies at a cancer center. Ophthal Plast Reconstr Surg 2004;20:291–5.
8. Chévez-Barrios P. Frozen section diagnosis and indications in ophthalmic pathology. Arch Pathol Lab Med 2005;129:1626–34.
9. Chan FM, O'Donnell BA, Whitehead K, et al. Treatment and outcomes of malignant melanoma of the eyelid: a review of 29 cases in Australia. Ophthalmology 2007;114:187–92.
10. Wolfe JT III, Yeatts RP, Wick MR, et al. Sebaceous carcinoma of the eyelid: errors in clinical and pathologic diagnosis. Am J Surg Pathol 1984;8:597–606.
11. Folberg R, Whitaker DC, Tse DT, et al. Recurrent and residual sebaceous carcinoma after Mohs' excision of the primary lesion. Am J Ophthalmol 1987;103:817–23.
12. Leibovitch I, Davis G, Huilgol SC, et al. An unusual presentation of periocular Merkel cell carcinoma. J Cutan Pathol 2006;33(Suppl 2):39–41.
13. Esmaeli B, Youssef A, Naderi A, et al; for Collaborative Eyelid Skin Melanoma Group. Margins of excision for cutaneous melanoma of the eyelid skin: the Collaborative Eyelid Skin Melanoma Group Report. Ophthal Plast Reconstr Surg 2003;19:96–101.
14. Berdahl JP, Pockaj BA, Gray RJ, et al. Optimal management and challenges in treatment of upper facial melanoma. Ann Plast Surg 2006;57:616–20.
15. Esmaeli B, Wang B, Deavers M, et al. Prognostic factors for survival in malignant melanoma of the eyelid skin. Ophthal Plast Reconstr Surg 2000;16:250–7.
16. Bernardini FP. Management of malignant and benign eyelid lesions. Curr Opin Ophthalmol 2006;17:480–4.
17. Song A, Carter K, Syed N, et al. Sebaceous cell carcinoma of the ocular adnexa: clinical presentations, histopathology, and outcomes. Ophthal Plast Reconstr Surg 2008;24:194–200.
18. Boulos PR, Rubin PA. Cutaneous melanomas of the eyelid [review]. Semin Ophthalmol 2006;21:195–206.
19. O'Connor WJ, Roenigk RK, Brodland DG. Merkel cell carcinoma: comparison of Mohs micrographic surgery and wide excision in eighty-six patients. Dermatol Surg 1997;23:929–33.
20. Pathai S, Barlow R, Williams G, et al. Mohs' micrographic surgery for Merkel cell carcinomas of the eyelid. Orbit 2005;24:273–5.
21. Boyer JD, Zitelli JA, Brodland DG, et al. Local control of primary Merkel cell carcinoma: review of 45 cases treated with Mohs micrographic surgery with and without adjuvant radiation. J Am Acad Dermatol 2002;47:885–92.

Chapter 12
Neuroradiology of Ocular and Orbital Tumors

J. Matthew Debnam

Abstract This chapter on neuroradiology for ophthalmologic tumors discusses the basic utilization of computed tomography and magnetic resonance imaging in the evaluation of lesions involving the globe and orbit. The protocol for these techniques, relevant imaging anatomy, and imaging features of the more common ophthalmologic tumors are discussed. The common radiographic features of ocular lesions, such as retinoblastoma, melanoma, and uveal metastases, as well as orbital lesions, including lymphoma, rhabdomysarcoma, nerve sheath tumors, fibrous lesions, and orbital pseudotumors are discussed. Lesions of the optic nerve, including glioma and meningioma, are also covered. The final section discusses radiographic findings for lesions of the lacrimal gland, secondary spread of tumors to the orbit and periocular region, and cutaneous lesions of the periocular region, including perineural tumor spread.

12.1 Introduction: Imaging and Protocol

Advances in computed tomography (CT), magnetic resonance imaging (MRI), and positron emission tomography/computed tomography (PET/CT) have aided in the diagnosis of ocular and orbital lesions. Most orbital and some ocular lesions can be evaluated by CT imaging. CT is superior to MRI for evaluation of the bony structures around the orbit and detection of calcifications within lesions. CT is also used to exclude foreign bodies in preparation for MRI. With multidetector CT, imaging can be performed in the axial plane, and multiplanar reformatted images can be provided in any plane deemed necessary. However, because MRI provides exquisite soft tissue detail, it is the preferred imaging modality for some lesions of the orbit.

J.M. Debnam (✉)
Section of Neuroradiology, Department of Radiology, The University of Texas M.D. Anderson Cancer Center, Houston, TX, USA
e-mail: matthew.debnam@mdanderson.org

B. Esmaeli (ed.), *Ophthalmic Oncology*, M.D. Anderson Solid Tumor Oncology Series 6, DOI 10.1007/978-1-4419-0374-7_12,

The use of multiple pulse sequences provides different signal characteristics for the various types of orbital lesions, aiding in the differential diagnosis.

The MRI examination should be tailored to the patient's specific symptom. Orbital imaging protocols generally include an axial T1 precontrast sequence, a T1 postcontrast sequence in three orthogonal planes, and an axial T2 sequence. Fat suppression technique may be employed on both T1 postcontrast and T2 sequences. Some institutions obtain at least one sequence without fat suppression because magnetic susceptibility, related to the patient's makeup, dental amalgam, and braces, is increased with the fat suppression technique. For optic nerve lesions, oblique-sagittal T1 postcontrast images along the optic nerve and coronal T2 images for comparison of the optic nerve size and signal intensity may be added. A 3-mm slice section thickness with a 0.5- to 1.0-mm gap between slices may be utilized for these sequences. An axial T1 postgadolinium sequence of the brain can also be added to assess for intracranial spread of orbital tumors and metastasis. An axial T2 sequence with fat saturation of the neck can be used to assess for associated lymphadenopathy.

The standard CT examination of the brain and orbits can be completed with the patient on the CT table for only a few minutes. The average MRI examination may take up to 1 hour. Administration of iodinated contrast material for CT or gadolinium for MRI is contraindicated in patients with renal failure. When intravenous contrast cannot be administered because of renal failure, a nephrologist should be consulted, as obtaining a diagnostic radiological study of the orbits without contrast is often of little benefit.

PET/CT involves the administration of 18F-fluorodeoxyglucose (FDG), which competes with serum glucose for uptake within the body. FDG accumulates in tumors, which have a high metabolic demand. In ophthalmic imaging, this modality may be used for both staging and assessing treatment response in lesions such as ocular adnexal lymphoma [1].

12.2 Anatomy

The bony anatomy of the orbit is well visualized with CT, especially utilizing bone windows. This includes the optic canal, lateral and medial orbital walls, superior and inferior orbital fissures, lacrimal fossa and nasolacrimal duct, and infraorbital canal. Coronal CT can be used to assess the orbital roof and floor (Fig. 12.13).

The extraocular muscles run parallel to the orbital walls. The medial and lateral rectus muscles are best visualized in the axial plane, while the superior and inferior rectus muscles are best visualized in the oblique sagittal plane. The levator palpebrae superioris muscle lies in close approximation to the superior rectus muscle and can be seen as a separate entity on oblique coronal imaging. The superior oblique muscle is best evaluated in the coronal plane and the inferior oblique muscle is best evaluated in the coronal, sagittal, or parasagittal plane. The trochlea, best seen in the axial plane, is often calcified and should not be misinterpreted as a foreign body. The lacrimal gland lies in the lacrimal fossa and is adjacent to the tendinous insertion of the superior and lateral rectus muscles.

The optic nerve, which is 2–3 cm in length and 3–4 mm in width, has imaging characteristics similar to the white matter in the brain [2]. The nerve leaves the posterior aspect of the globe, and there is a slight inferolateral bowing of the midportion of the nerve. The nerve courses posteriorly, medially, and superiorly to exit the orbit through the optic canal. The optic nerves join in the suprasellar cistern to form the optic chiasm.

The ophthalmic division of the trigeminal nerve (V_1) provides sensory innervation to the eye, lacrimal gland, conjunctiva, upper eyelids, forehead, and scalp. The largest branch, the frontal nerve, enters the orbit through the superior orbital fissure (Fig. 12.8). Within the orbit, the nerve divides into the supratrochlear and supraorbital nerves, which run along the orbital roof. These nerves are difficult to see on imaging when not involved with tumor (Fig. 12.17).

Branches of the maxillary division of the trigeminal nerve (V_2) provide sensory innervation to the skin of the nose, midface, and cheek. This nerve extends through the foramen rotundum to the pterygopalatine fossa (Fig. 12.18b, c) and enters the orbit through the inferior orbit fissure. The nerve then courses through the infraorbital canal, where it is named the infraorbital nerve (Fig. 12.18a), and extends through the infraorbital foramen.

The zygomatic nerve is a branch of V_2 that arises in the pterygopalatine fossa. The nerve enters the orbit through the inferior orbital fissure, traverses the lateral wall, and exits the orbit along the lateral orbital wall. Branches of the nerve supply the skin of the temporal region and lateral cheek (zygomaticotemporal and zygomaticofacial nerves).

The intraocular structures can be appreciated to some extent on imaging studies. The lens is hyperdense on CT and the vitreous is hypodense. The sclera, choroid, and retina form a well-defined, enhancing line on CT. On MRI, the vitreous has high water content and thus is hyperintense on T2-weighted images and does not enhance. The lens has low signal intensity on T1 and T2 images. The sclera, choroid, and retina are hypointense.

12.3 Intraocular Lesions

12.3.1 Retinoblastoma

Retinoblastoma is a type of primitive neuroectodermal tumor caused by a mutation in the tumor suppressor oncogene *RB1*, located on chromosome 13q14 [3, 4]. Approximately 30% of retinoblastomas are hereditary and 85% of these are bilateral [5]. The remainder arises from spontaneous mutations and occurs unilaterally. It is important to recognize retinoblastoma in the early stages [5–8], as patients with tumors confined to the globe have a 5-year survival rate of greater than 90% whereas patients with tumors extending outside the globe have a 5-year survival rate of less than 10% [9]. Retinoblastoma and its management are discussed in great detail in Chapter 14.

As most cases of retinoblastoma are initially diagnosed by the patient's primary ophthalmologist, the role of the radiologist is to use imaging to confirm the diagnosis, evaluate for metastasis along the optic pathway, and detect other intracranial masses [10]. MRI is primarily used to evaluate the globe and brain. CT may also be used in questionable cases to identify calcification, which occurs in 90% of cases and is highly characteristic, especially in children under 3 years [11].

On CT, the tumor is smoothly marginated and hyperdense with punctate or nodular calcification (Fig. 12.1a). Associated subretinal and vitreous hemorrhage appears as nonenhancing areas of hyperdensity. Lesions in the vitreous are intermediate to slightly hyperintense on T1 sequences and hypointense on T2 sequences

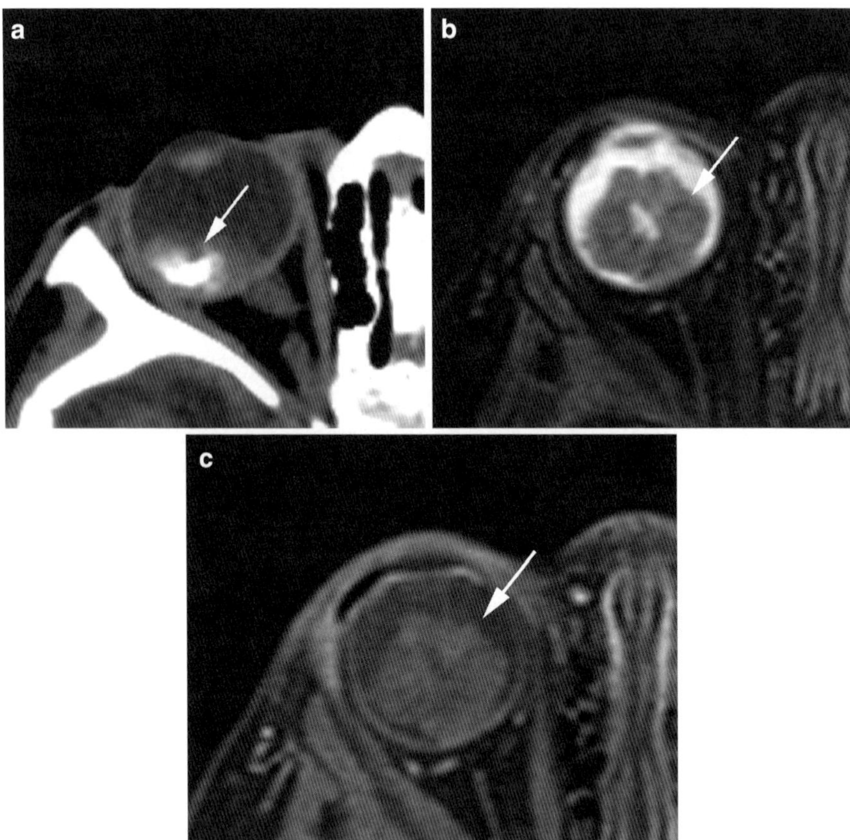

Fig. 12.1 Retinoblastoma, right globe. (**a**) Axial precontrast-enhanced CT demonstrates a calcified mass in the right globe (*arrow*). (**b**) Axial T2 image shows a T2 hypointense mass extending into the vitreous (*arrow*). (**c**) Axial T1 postcontrast image with heterogeneous enhancement of the mass (*arrow*)

(Fig. 12.1b). In children, the hypointensity on T2 sequences is relatively specific for retinoblastoma. The lesions usually have moderate to marked enhancement (Fig. 12.1c).

With optic nerve involvement, the nerve appears thickened and enhancing. Seeding of the cerebrospinal fluid may present as diffuse leptomeningeal enhancement. Bilateral retinoblastoma may be accompanied by an intracranial primitive neuroectodermal tumor along the midline of the brain; this tumor occurs most commonly in the pineal gland (pineoblastoma), suprasellar region, or parasellar region [12, 13]. These lesions are hypointense on T1 sequences and intermediate to hyperintense on T2 images, and there may be associated hydrocephalus. Response to treatment appears on MRI as a reduction in the volume of the lesion, loss of vascularity, and replacement of the tumor with calcification. Secondary tumors, such as osteosarcoma and chondrosarcoma, may develop in the radiation field.

12.3.2 Uveal Melanoma

Uveal melanoma is the most common intraocular tumor in adults. Lesions usually occur unilaterally and may be associated with retinal detachment and vitreous hemorrhage. The role of imaging studies is complimentary to echography; imaging studies can help determine the size and extent of the mass, including extraocular extension, and detect associated retinal detachment. On CT, uveal melanoma presents as a hyperdense thickening of the wall of the globe, which is enhancing. Because of the paramagnetic properties of melanin, lesions are often hyperintense on T1 images, are often hypointense on T2 images, and demonstrate moderate enhancement (Fig. 12.2). The lesions are often well defined and may extend into

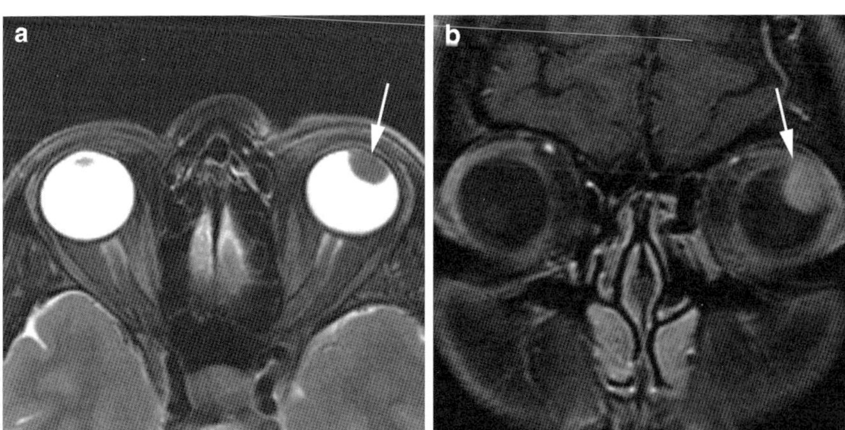

Fig. 12.2 Uveal melanoma, left globe. (**a**) Axial T2 image demonstrates a hypointense uveal lesion (*arrow*). (**b**) Coronal T1 postcontrast image demonstrates the homogeneously enhancing uveal mass (*arrow*)

the vitreous. Hemorrhage may be difficult to distinguish from mass on the T1 pre-contrast sequence as both may be T1 hyperintense, but the hemorrhagic component does not enhance.

12.3.3 Uveal Metastases

Carcinoma from primary lesions, such as those in the breast or lung, may metastasize to the orbit. Lesions generally are hypointense on T1 images, are generally hyperintense on T2 images, and demonstrate enhancement.

12.4 Orbital Lesions

12.4.1 Lymphoma

Involvement of the orbit with lymphoma may be primary or secondary to systemic disease. Orbital lymphoma is generally a low-grade marginal zone B-cell lymphoma of the mucosa-associated lymphoid tissue, accounting for 40–70% of lesions [14], and is associated with systemic disease in about 30% of patients [15]. In patients with lymphoma of the orbit, the risk of systemic involvement increases with grade. The average age at presentation is 50–70 years, but this disease can occur in children and young adults. Ocular adnexal lymphomas may involve the conjunctiva, eyelid, and orbital soft tissue, including the lacrimal gland [16]. Lymphoma is often contained by facial planes and grows by molding around adjacent structures rather than presenting as a solid mass. Lymphoma almost never indents the globe [16].

The appearance varies from diffusely infiltrative in high-grade lesions to solid tumors with defined margins in less aggressive forms. Usually, there is less bone destruction than in other disease processes. On CT, lymphoma is similar in density to muscle and demonstrates enhancement. Lymphoma is isointense to muscle on T1 images and demonstrates moderate to marked enhancement (Fig. 12.3a). Since lymphoma is hypercellular, it tends to be isointense to hypointense to muscle on T2 sequences (Fig. 12.3b), which differentiates this lesion from rhabdomyosarcoma. Central nervous system lymphoma may also show decreased diffusion (Fig. 12.3c) [17]. On PET/CT, lymphoma is seen as an FDG-avid lesion (Fig. 12.3d), and systemic disease may also be demonstrated (Fig. 12.4).

12.4.2 Orbital Rhabdomyosarcoma

Rhabdomyosarcoma arises from primitive undifferentiated mesenchymal cells in the orbit. The tumor can occur in patients at any age, but the average age at presentation is 7 years. Rhabdomyosarcoma has a predilection for the upper outer quadrant [18] of the orbit, but it may occur in the lid or conjunctiva. Lesions range from moderately well defined to ill-defined and demonstrate mild to moderate enhancement.

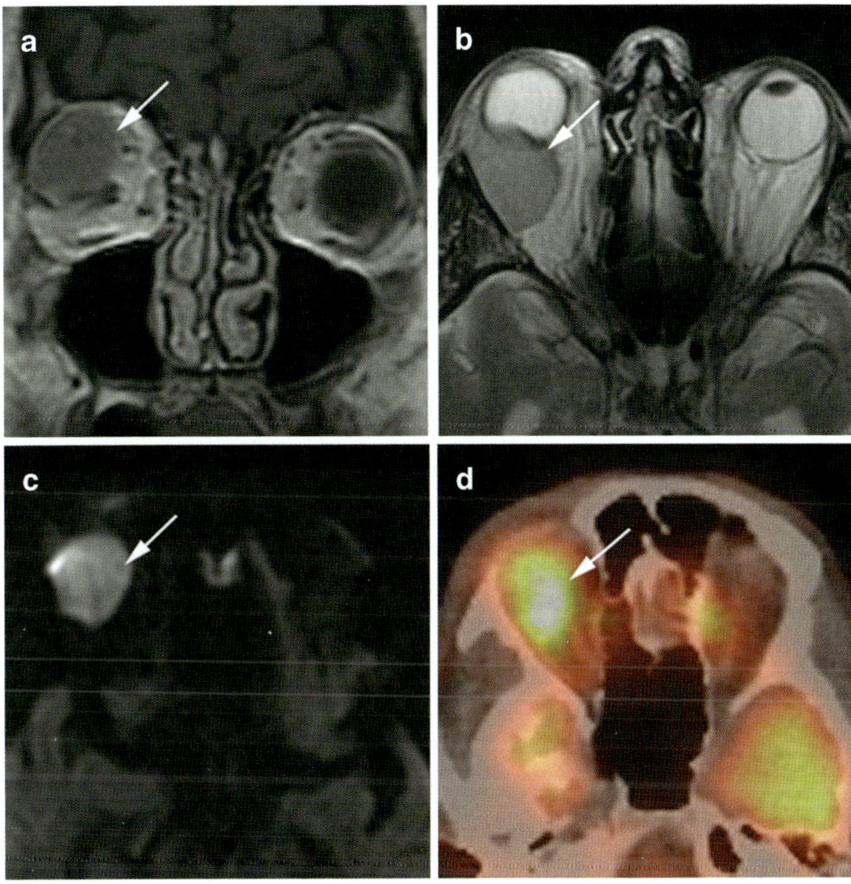

Fig. 12.3 Orbital lymphoma, right orbit. (**a**) Coronal T1 postcontrast image demonstrates an enhancing superior right orbital mass (*arrow*). (**b**) Axial T2 image shows the mass is isointense to brain parenchyma (*arrow*). (**c**) Axial diffusion-weighted sequence shows decreased diffusion within the mass (*arrow*). (**d**) PET/CT axial plane image shows an 18F-fluorodeoxyglucose avid right orbital lesion (*arrow*)

Invasion of paranasal sinuses and intracranial extension may occur [19, 20]. On CT, lesions are similar in density to soft tissue and heterogeneous in appearance, and bone destruction may be seen. On MRI, rhabdomyosarcoma is isointense to muscle on T1 images, hyperintense to muscle on T2 images, and demonstrates enhancement (Fig. 12.5). The globe is often displaced but rarely invaded [18].

12.4.3 Orbital Nerve Sheath Tumors

Neurofibroma and schwannoma most commonly arise from the peripheral nerves of the orbit [21] and therefore have a predilection for the extroconal, superior orbit [22]; they are well defined and oval or fusiform. Nerve sheath tumors present in

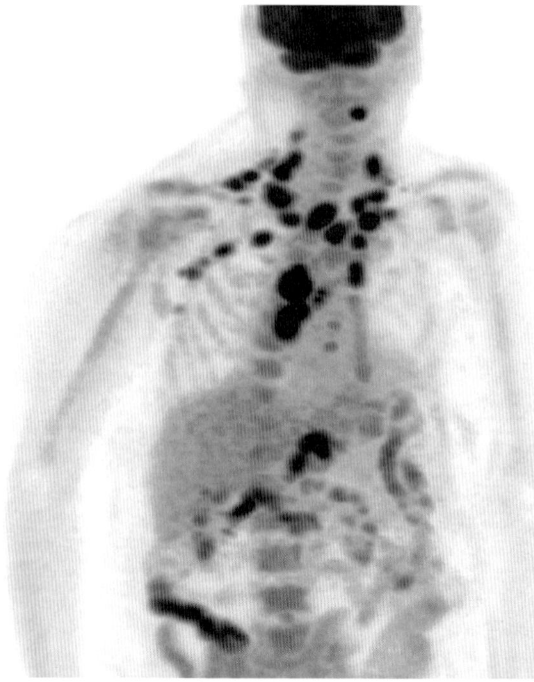

Fig. 12.4 Orbital lymphoma with systemic disease. PET/CT image shows 18F-fluorodeoxyglucose avid adenopathy within the neck, axilla, and mediastinum

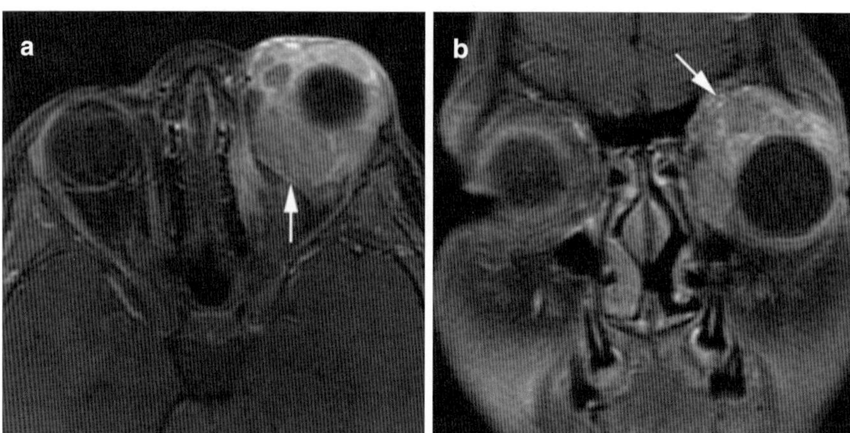

Fig. 12.5 Orbital rhabdomyosarcoma, left orbit. (**a**) Axial T1 postcontrast image demonstrates an enhancing pre- and postseptal left orbital mass (*arrow*). (**b**) Coronal T1 postcontrast image demonstrates an enhancing mass (*arrow*) with inferior displacement of the left globe. Figures courtesy of Dr. Bita Esmaeli

young to middle-aged adults are noninvasive and are associated with a painless proptosis [21]. On CT, these tumors are isodense to slightly hyperdense and demonstrate mild to marked enhancement. On MRI (Fig. 12.6) these tumors are isointense to slightly hyperintense to muscle on T1 images, hyperintense on T2 images, and also

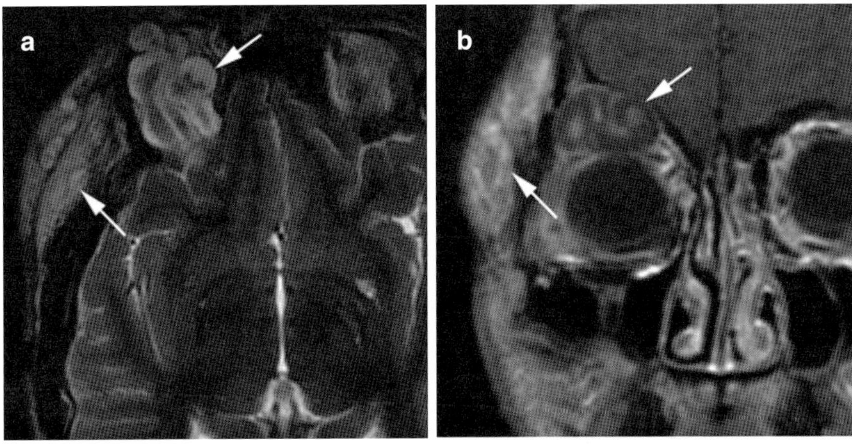

Fig. 12.6 Plexiform neurofibroma, right orbit. (**a**) Axial T2 image demonstrates the lesion within the right temporal soft tissue and superior right orbit (*arrows*). (**b**) Coronal T1 postcontrast image shows the enhancing characteristics of the lesions (*arrows*)

demonstrate moderate to marked enhancement. As lesions age, they become more hypocellular with a predominance of collagen and may not significantly enhance. Associated expansion of the orbit and bone erosion may be seen.

12.4.4 Mesenchymal Tumors of the Orbit

Mesenchymal tumors of the orbit include fibrous histiocytoma, fibroma, and fibrosarcoma. Fibrous histiocytoma probably arises from a fibroblast precursor and may be benign or malignant [23, 24]. Fibroma is usually found in young adults [25] and grows slowly. On CT, these lesions appear well circumscribed and demonstrate moderate to marked enhancement. The benign form can cause bony remodeling, and the malignant form causes bone erosion [26, 27]. On MRI, the lesion is hypointense to isointense on T1 images and demonstrates moderate enhancement. On T2 images, fibrous tumors are hypointense to hyperintense. The fibrous component is hypointense on both sequences.

Other mesenchymal tumors include chondrosarcoma, osteosarcoma, Ewing sarcoma, and synovial sarcoma. These lesions may occur within or around the orbit with secondary extension. CT demonstrates a soft tissue mass of muscle density with variable enhancement (Fig. 12.7). Associated bone destruction may occur with more aggressive lesions. On MRI, lesions are often nonspecific with T1 signal hypointensity, T2 signal isointensity to hyperintensity, and variable enhancement.

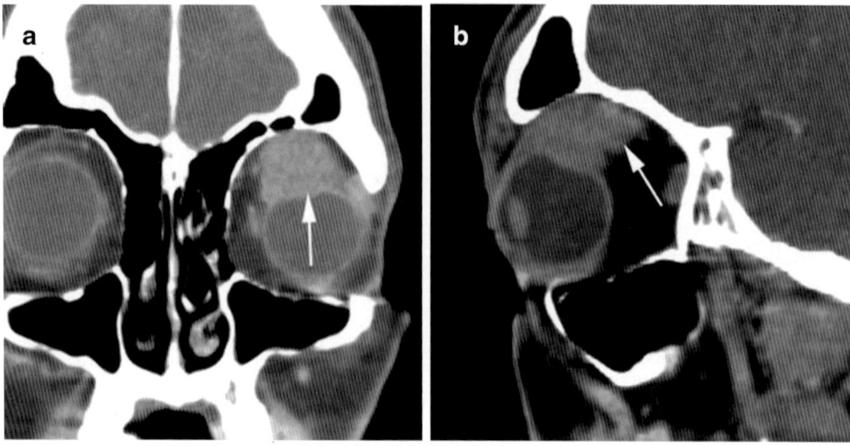

Fig. 12.7 Synovial sarcoma, left orbit. (**a**) Coronal postcontrast CT demonstrates a lesion within the superior left orbit with impression upon and inferior displacement of the globe (*arrow*). (**b**) Sagittal postcontrast CT shows the superior left orbital mass (*arrow*) indenting the globe

12.4.5 Orbital Pseudotumor

Orbital pseudotumor is an idiopathic inflammatory process usually presenting as unilateral painful ophthalmoplegia, proptosis, and lid erythema. This process may affect any intraorbital soft tissue. Pseudotumor is the most common cause of an intraorbital mass in adults, but it may occur at any age, usually in young women. Orbital pseudotumor presents as a moderately enhancing, poorly defined mass with inflammation of the orbital fat and extraocular muscles. On CT, there is increased density of the retro-orbital fat and variable enhancement (Fig. 12.8). Pseudotumors are isointense on T1 images and hypointense to isointense on T2 images with variable enhancement. The primary alternative lesion to consider in the differential diagnosis in children is primary orbital rhabdomyosarcoma. When extraocular muscle involvement occurs, pseudotumor involves the tendon insertion, in contradistinction to Graves disease, which spares the tendon.

12.4.6 Orbital Metastases

In adults, metastases to the orbit arise most commonly from primary tumors in the breast or lung. In children, orbital metastases may occur from neuroblastoma, Ewing sarcoma, and Wilms tumor. On CT, metastases from solid tumors are usually of intermediate density to muscle and demonstrate enhancement. On MRI, these

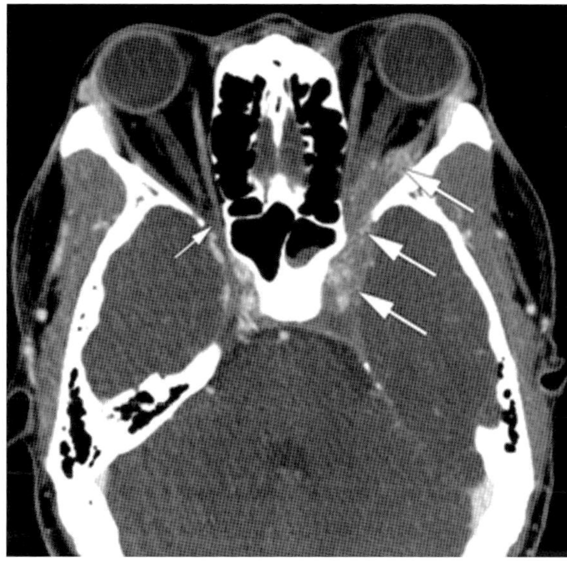

Fig. 12.8 Orbital pseudotumor, left orbit. Axial postcontrast CT demonstrates mass involving the left lateral rectus muscle and tendinous insertion with extension through the superior orbital fissure to involve the cavernous sinus (*large arrows*). Note the normal right superior orbital fissure (*small arrow*). Figure courtesy of Dr. Bita Esmaeli

generally are hypointense on T1 images, are hyperintense on T2 images, and enhance with contrast (Fig. 12.9). An exception would be a mucin-producing tumor, such as adenocarcinoma, which can be hypointense on T2 images.

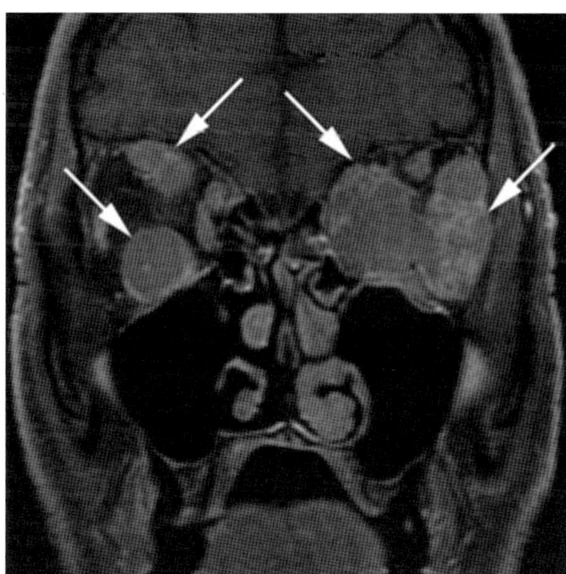

Fig. 12.9 Breast cancer metastasis, bilateral orbits. Coronal T1 postcontrast image shows bilateral enhancing mass lesions centered around the extraocular muscles (*arrows*)

12.5 Optic Nerve Tumors

12.5.1 Optic Nerve Glioma

Optic nerve glioma is the most common cause of optic nerve enlargement, and patients present with proptosis and decreased vision. Optic nerve glioma is a juvenile pilocytic astrocytoma in children [28]. The average age at presentation is 7 years, with 90% of patients presenting prior to age 20 [29]. The childhood form grows slowly with no tendency for malignant transformation and may even undergo spontaneous regression with improved vision [30]. The malignant form may extend to the hypothalamus and third ventricle.

Optic gliomas are well circumscribed with fusiform enlargement [31]. On CT, an optic glioma is isodense to the optic nerve and demonstrates mild to moderate enhancement. There may be associated enlargement of the bony optic canal. Calcification may be seen following radiation therapy. On MRI, the lesion is hypointense to isointense to muscle on T1 images, hyperintense on T2 images, and demonstrates variable enhancement with widening and kinking of the optic nerve (Fig. 12.10) [31].

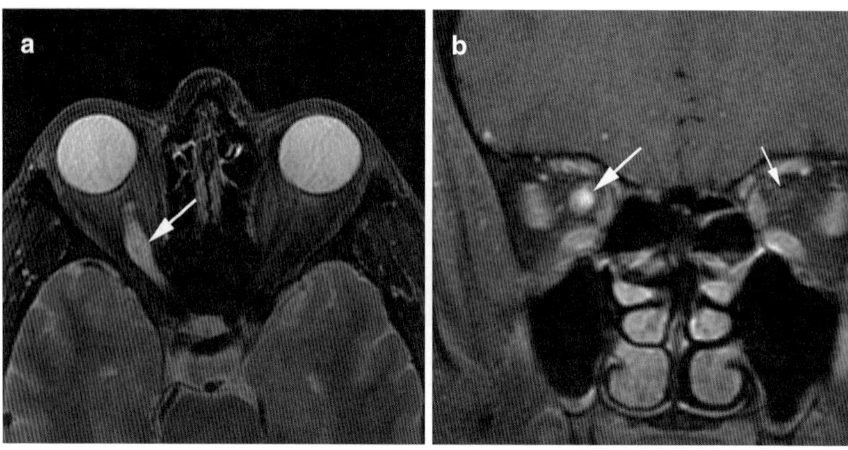

Fig. 12.10 Optic nerve glioma, right optic nerve. (**a**) Axial T2 image demonstrates a hyperintense lesion involving the right optic nerve (*arrow*). (**b**) Coronal T1 postcontrast image shows homogeneous enhancement of the optic glioma (*arrow*). Note the normal appearance of the left optic nerve (*small arrow*)

12.5.2 Optic Nerve Sheath Meningiomas

Meningiomas arise from arachnoid rests in the dural sheath of optic nerves. Patients may present with proptosis and signs of optic neuropathy [32]. These generally occur in middle-aged and elderly women, are slightly more aggressive in children, and are associated with neurofibromatosis type 2 [33]. Optic nerve sheath meningiomas demonstrate a tubular configuration or may grow eccentrically over the optic nerve. On CT, the lesion is hyperdense, with intensely enhancing linear bands seen around the nerve. Calcification is frequent and highly suggestive of meningioma. On MRI, the soft tissue mass surrounding the optic nerve is hypointense to isointense to brain on T1 and T2 images. Some lesions have cystic components. The tumor shows marked enhancement around the optic nerve, resulting in linear enhancement along the course of the optic nerve in the axial plane (the so-called railroad track or tram track sign), and a rim-like appearance around the nerve in the coronal plane (Fig. 12.11). This enhancement pattern may differentiate meningioma from optic nerve glioma. Orbital meningiomas can also occur that primarily involve the greater wing of the sphenoid (Fig. 12.12), causing proptosis and visual loss.

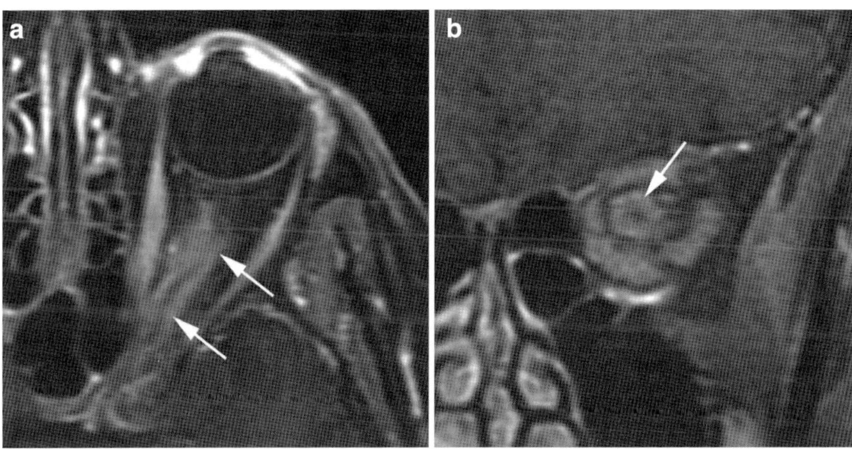

Fig. 12.11 Optic nerve meningioma, left optic nerve. (**a**) Axial T1 postcontrast image demonstrates enhancement of the mass parallel to the left optic nerve (*arrows*), the so-called tram track appearance. (**b**) Coronal T1 postcontrast image shows circumferential enhancement around the left optic nerve (*arrow*)

12.6 Lacrimal Gland Tumors

Fifty percent of lacrimal gland lesions are epithelial tumors, with the rest being lymphoma or inflammatory processes [34]. Metastasis to the lacrimal gland is rare [34]. Half of epithelial lacrimal gland tumors are pleomorphic adenoma (benign mixed), and half are malignant, with adenoid cystic carcinoma of the lacrimal gland being the most common. Benign tumors are often smooth with well-defined margins (Fig. 12.13), while malignant lesions have irregular margins, suggestive of infiltration, and may have associated perineural spread (Fig. 12.14) [35]. Benign or slow

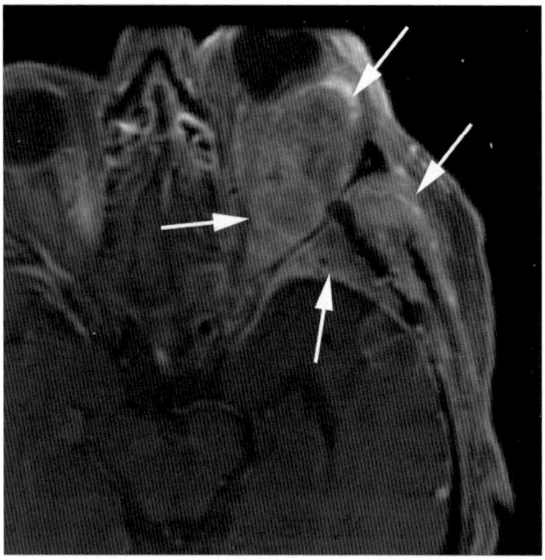

Fig. 12.12 Recurrent meningioma, left sphenoid wing. Axial T1 postcontrast image shows a mass involving the left sphenoid bone and infratemporal fossa, with intraorbital extension, compression upon the globe and proptosis (*arrows*)

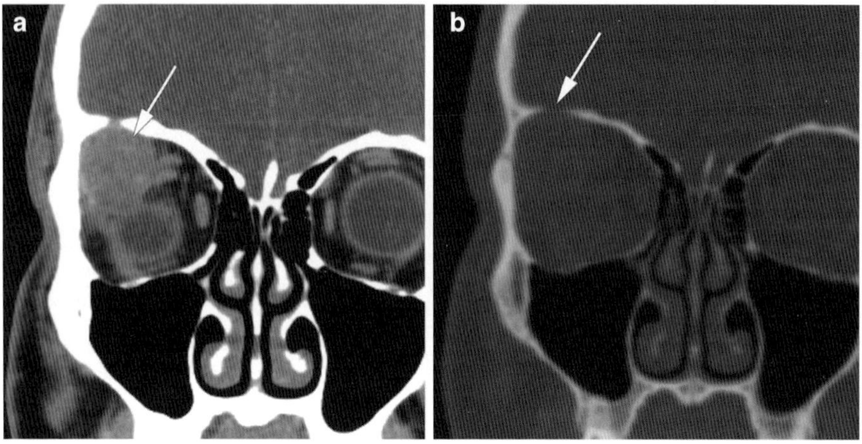

Fig. 12.13 Pleomorphic adenoma, right lacrimal gland. (**a**) Coronal postcontrast, soft tissue window, CT soft tissue window demonstrates a well-defined mass involving the superior orbit with inferior displacement of the globe and remodeling of the lacrimal gland bony fossa. (**b**) Coronal CT, bone window, demonstrates bony remodeling of the orbital roof (*arrow*)

growing lacrimal gland tumors are associated with bony remodeling of the walls of the lacrimal gland fossa whereas malignant processes are more likely to cause bony erosion. Neoplastic lesions rarely arise in the anterior aspect of the lacrimal gland and tend to grow posteriorly. Epithelial lesions may indent the globe [35] and may produce bone changes [34]. Lymphoid tumors show diffuse enlargement with a pancake-like spread and frequently have anterior and posterior extensions.

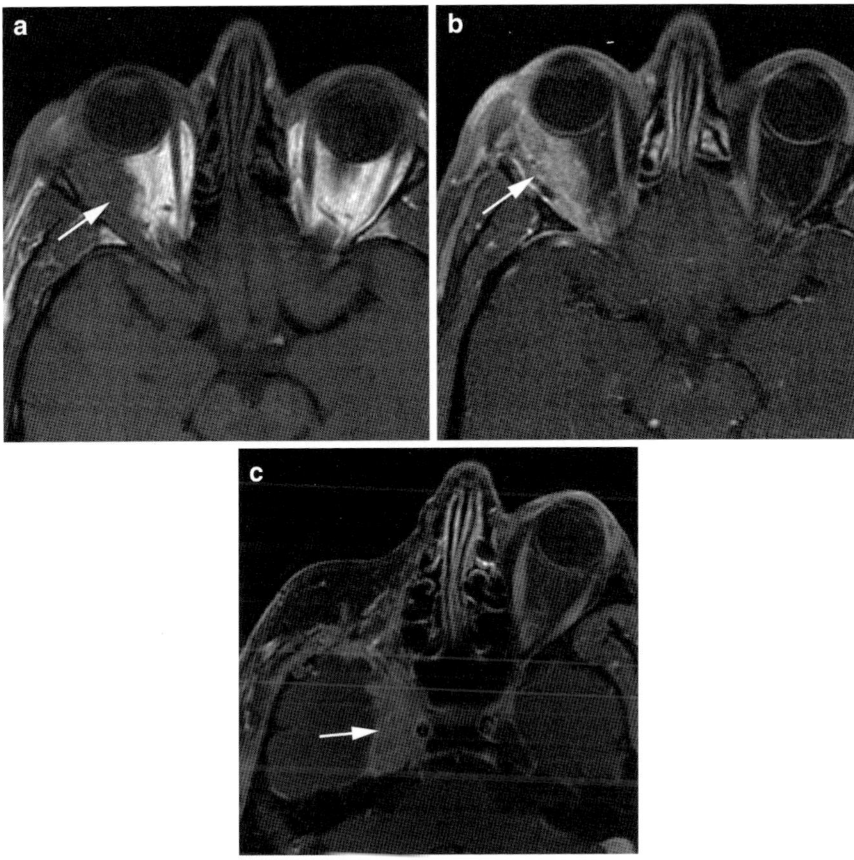

Fig. 12.14 Adenoid cystic carcinoma, right lacrimal gland. (**a**) Axial T1 precontrast-enhanced image shows a right orbital mass (*arrow*) with an ill-defined medial margin that is well visualized because of the adjacent retro-orbital fat. (**b**) Axial T1 contrast-enhanced image shows the enhancing characteristics of the mass (*arrow*). (**c**) Axial T1 contrast-enhanced study following orbital exenteration demonstrates perineural spread to involve the cavernous sinus (*arrow*)

These lesions rarely produce bone changes [34]. Inflammatory lesions cause diffuse enlargement of the gland, often with adjacent myositis. The lymphomatous and inflammatory lesions tend to involve the entire gland, whereas neoplastic lesions often show only posterior extension.

12.7 Secondary Tumor Spread to the Orbit

Tumors from adjacent soft tissue structures can extend directly into the orbit. Lesions of the sinonasal cavity can extend into the orbit through the orbital floor and lamina papyracea (Fig. 12.15). Intracranial lesions of the frontal lobes, such

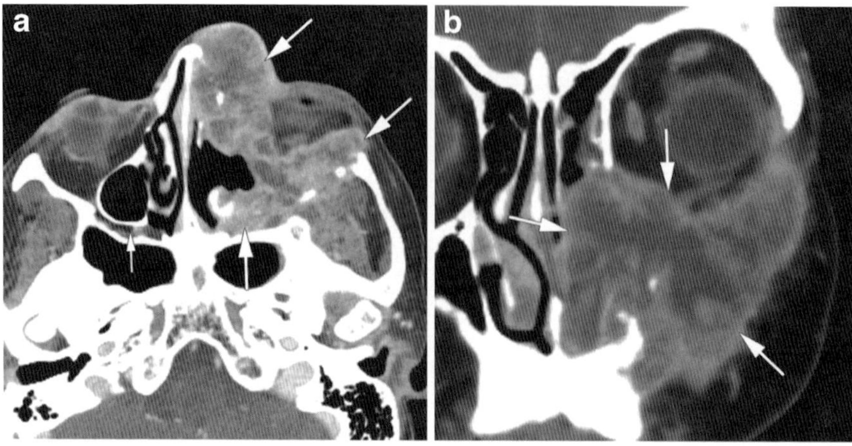

Fig. 12.15 Adenoid cystic carcinoma, left maxillary sinus. (**a**) Axial postcontrast CT image demonstrates a mass involving the left orbit, periorbital soft tissue, and pterygopalatine fossa (*large arrows*). Note the normal right pterygopalatine fossa (*small arrow*). (**b**) Coronal postcontrast CT image shows an invasive left maxillary sinus mass with destruction of the orbital floor (*arrows*)

as meningioma and glioblastoma, can grow into the orbit through the superior and posterior walls, superior orbital fissure, and optic canal. Skin cancers and lesions of subcutaneous soft tissue can grow into the preseptal space and directly invade the orbit. Lesions such as adenoid cystic carcinoma of the oral and sinonasal cavities can also extend into the pterygopalatine fossa, through the inferior orbital fissure, and then into the orbit, either by direct extension or by perineural spread.

12.8 Periorbital Skin Cancer and Perineural Spread

Tumors of the skin, including basal cell carcinoma, squamous cell carcinoma, and melanoma, can appear as an exophytic mass (Fig. 12.16) of the periorbital soft tissues or invade deep into the subcutaneous soft tissue. These lesions can also extend along the first and second divisions of the trigeminal nerve.

Skin cancers involving the forehead, upper eyelid, and scalp may spread along distal branches of the frontal nerve, a component of the ophthalmic division of the trigeminal nerve (V_1). Perineural spread may extend along these nerves in the orbital roof (Fig. 12.17), through the superior orbital fissure, and into the cavernous sinus.

Lesions of the temporal region and lateral cheek may extend in a retrograde fashion along the zygomatic nerve, a branch of the maxillary division of the trigeminal nerve (V_2). The nerve extends along the lateral orbital wall, through the inferior orbital fissure, and into the pterygopalatine fossa. Perineural tumor spread of lesions

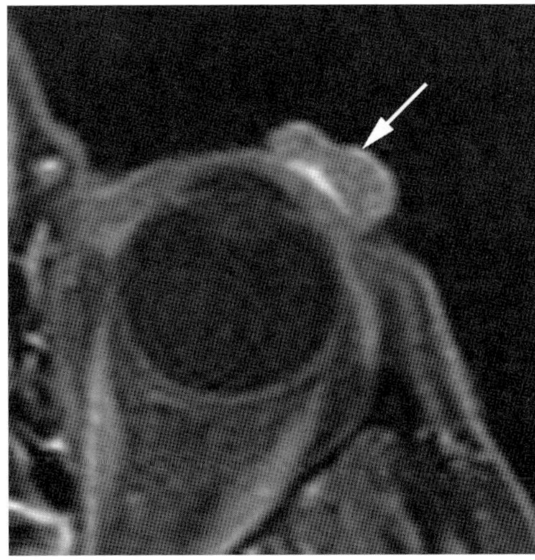

Fig. 12.16 Melanoma, left eyelid. Axial T1 postcontrast image demonstrates an exophytic lesion arising on the left eyelid (*arrow*)

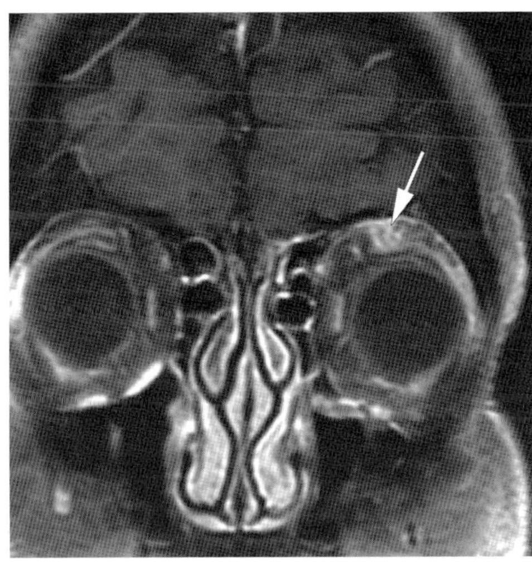

Fig. 12.17 Squamous cell carcinoma, left forehead. Coronal T1 postcontrast image demonstrates perineural spread along the first division of the left trigeminal nerve (V_1) (*arrow*)

involving the nose, midface, and cheek may occur along the infraorbital nerve. The nerve extends through the infraorbital foramen, traveling along the floor of the orbit (Fig. 12.18), through the inferior orbital fissure, and into the pterygopalatine fossa. From the pterygopalatine fossa, lesions may extend in an antegrade fashion along other branches or in a retrograde fashion through the foramen rotundum to the cavernous sinus.

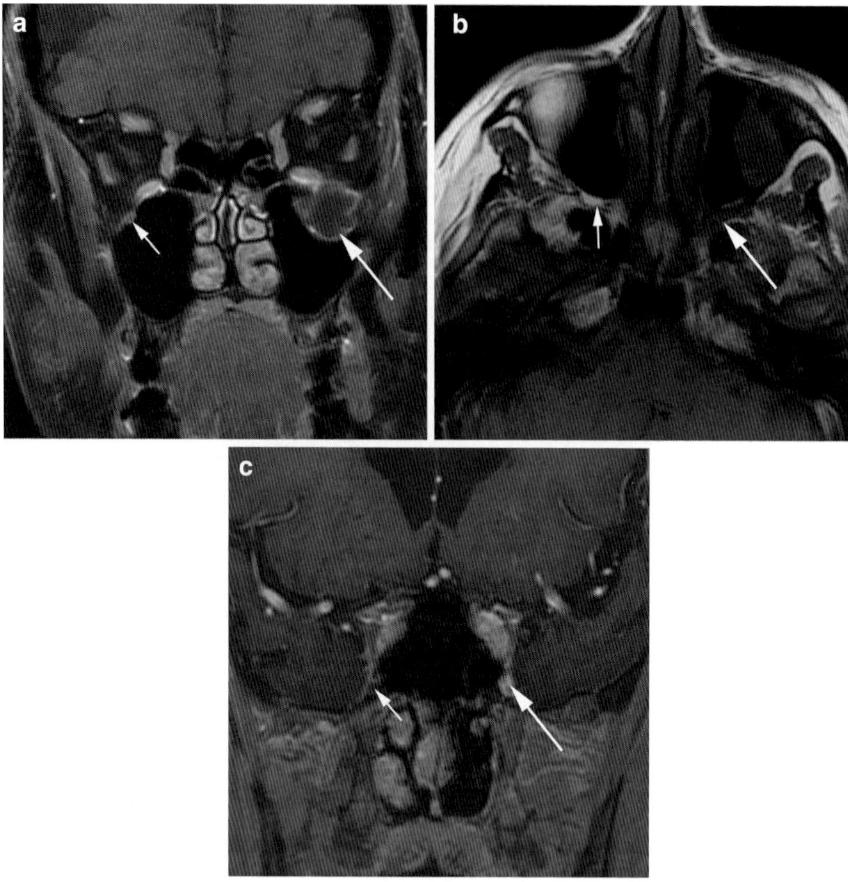

Fig. 12.18 Squamous cell carcinoma, left cheek. (**a**) Coronal T1 postcontrast image demonstrates perineural spread along the left infraorbital nerve (V_2) (*large arrow*). Note the normal right infraorbital nerve (*small arrow*). (**b**) Axial T1 precontrast-enhanced image shows a mass filling the left pterygopalatine fossa (*large arrow*). Note the normal right pterygopalatine fossa (*small arrow*). (**c**) Coronal T1 demonstrates the perineural spread to involve the left foramen rotundum (*large arrow*). Note the normal right foramen rotundum (*small arrow*)

12.9 Conclusion

Orbital and ocular tumors encompass a wide range of lesions. Both CT and MRI are used in the assessment of these tumors, including the initial evaluation of the lesion, adjacent soft tissue, and bony structures, associated perineural spread, and metastatic disease.

References

1. Gayed I, Eskandari MF, McLaughlin P, et al. Value of positron emission tomography in staging ocular adnexal lymphomas and evaluating their response to therapy. Ophthalmic Surg Lasers Imaging 2007;110:809–15.
2. Ettl A, Salomonowitz E, Koorneef L, et al. High resolution MR imaging anatomy of the orbit: correlation with comparative cryosectional anatomy. Radiol Clin North Am 1998;36:1021–45.
3. Francke U. Retinoblastoma and chromosome 13. Cytogenet Cell Genet 1976;16:131–4.
4. Knudson AG, Meadows AT, Nichols WW, et al. Chromosomal deletion and retinoblastoma. N Engl J Med 1976;295:1120–3.
5. Kaufman LM, Mafee MF, Song CD. Retinoblastoma and simulating lesion: role of CT, MR imaging, and the use of GD-DTPA contrast enhancement. Radiol Clin North Am 1998;36:1101–17.
6. Kadom N, Sze RW. Radiological reasoning: leukocoria in a child. AJR Am J Roentgenol 2008,191:40–4.
7. Devesa SS. The incidence of retinoblastoma. Am J Ophthalmol 1975;80:236–65.
8. Abramson DH, Ellsworth RM, Tretter P, et al. Treatment of bilateral groups I through III retinoblastoma with bilateral radiation. Arch Ophthalmol 1981;99:1762.
9. Wycliffe ND, Mafee MF. Magnetic resonance imaging in ocular pathology. Top Magn Reson Imaging 1999;10:384–400.
10. Apushkin MA, Shapiro MJ, Mafee MF. Retinoblastoma and simulating lesions: role of imaging. Neuroimaging Clin N Am 2005;15:49–67.
11. Mafee MF, Goldberg MF, Greenwald MJ, et al. Retinoblastoma and simulating lesions: role of CT and MR imaging. Radiol Clin North Am 1987;25:667–81.
12. Bader JL, Meadows AT, Zimmerman LE, et al. Bilateral retinoblastoma with ectopic intracranial retinoblastoma: trilateral retinoblastoma. Cancer Genet Cytogenet 1982;5:203–13.
13. Bader JL, Miller RW, Meadows AT, et al. Trilateral retinoblastoma. Lancet 1980;2:582–3.
14. Demirci H, Shields CL, Karatza EC, et al. Orbital lymphoproliferative tumors: analysis of clinical features and systemic involvement in 160 cases. Ophthalmology 2008;115:1626–31.
15. Hatef E, Roberts D, McLaughlin P, et al. Prevalence and nature of systemic involvement and stage at initial examination in patients with orbital and ocular adnexal lymphoma. Arch Ophthalmol 2007;125:1663–7.
16. Valvassori GE, Sabnis SS, Mafee RF, et al. Imaging of orbital lymphoproliferative disorders. Radiol Clin North Am 1999;37:135–50.
17. Zacharia TT, Law M, Naidich TP, et al. Central nervous system lymphoma characterization by diffusion-weighted imaging and MR spectroscopy. J Neuroimaging 2008;18:411–17.
18. Sohaib SA, Moseley I, Wright JE. Orbital rhabdomyosarcoma: the radiological characteristics. Clin Radiol 1998;53:357–62.
19. Shields JA, Shields CL. Rhabdomyosarcoma: review for the ophthalmologist. Ophthalmology 2003;48:39–57.
20. Folpe AL, McKenney JK, Bridge JA, et al. Sclerosing rhabdomyosarcoma in adults: report of four cases of hyalinizing, matrix-rich variant of rhabdomyosarcoma that may be confused with osteosarcoma, chondrosarcoma, or angiosarcoma. Am J Surg Pathol 2002;26:1175–83.
21. Albert DM, Jakobiec FA. Principles and Practice of Ophthalmology, second edition. Philadelphia, PA: WB Saunders, 2000.
22. DePotter P, Shields JA, Shields CL. MRI of the Eye and Orbit. Philadelphia, PA: JB Lippincott, 1995.
23. Font RL, Hidayat AA. Fibrous histiocytoma of the orbit: a clinicopathologic study of 150 cases. Hum Pathol 1982;13:199.
24. Ros PR, Kursunoglu S, Batle JF, et al. Malignant fibrous histiocytoma of the orbit. J Clin Neuroophthalmol 1985;5:116.

25. Dalley R. Fibrous histiocytoma and fibrous tissue tumors of the orbit. Radiol Clin North Am 1999;37:185–94.
26. Shields JA. Diagnosis and Management of Orbital Tumors. Philadelphia, PA: WB Saunders, 1989.
27. Krishnakumar S, Subramanian N, Mohan ER, et al. Solitary fibrous tumor of the orbit: a clinicopathologic study of six cases with review of the literature. Surv Ophthalmol 2003;48:544–54.
28. Eggers H, Jakobiec FA, Jones IS. Optic nerve gliomas. In: Jones IS, Jakobiec FA, editors. Diseases of the Orbit. New York, NY: Harper & Row, 1979:417–33.
29. Dutton JJ. Gliomas of the anterior visual pathways. Surv Ophthalmol 1994;384:27–52.
30. Parsa CF, Hoyt CS, Lesser RL, et al. Spontaneous regression of optic gliomas: thirteen cases documented by serial neuroimaging. Arch Ophthalmol 2001;119:516–29.
31. Weber AL, Klufas R, Pless M. Imaging evaluation of the optic nerve and visual pathway including cranial nerves affecting the visual pathway. Neuroimaging Clin N Am 1996;6: 143–77.
32. Mehra KS, Khanna S, Dube B. Primary meningiomas of the intraorbital optic nerve. Ann Ophthalmol 1979;11:758–60.
33. Dutton JJ. Optic nerve sheath meningiomas. Surv Ophthalmol 1992;37:167–83.
34. Hecht SD. Dacryocystorhinostomy. In: Hornblas A, Hanig CJ, editors. Oculoplastic, Orbital, and Reconstructive Surgery. Baltimore, MD: Williams & Wilkins, 1990:1433–40.
35. Jakobiec FA, Yeo JH, Trokel SL, et al. Combined clinical and computed tomographic diagnosis or primary lacrimal fossa lesions. Am J Ophthalmol 1982;94:785–807.

Chapter 13
Radiation Therapy for Orbital and Adnexal Tumors

Steven J. Frank and Anita Mahajan

Abstract Radiation therapy is used in the multimodality treatment of many orbital and adnexal tumors to enhance local control and possibly, in some patients, overall survival. In this chapter we will review the indications, modern techniques, potential toxic effects, and expectations of tumor control for a variety of orbital and adnexal tumors. Typically, treatments are delivered in fractions of 1.8–2.0 Gy per day, with the total number of fractions depending on the inherent radiosensitivity of the lesion. Radiotherapy technique and field design depends on the required dose, the tumor type, and the surrounding normal structures such as the lens, which is at risk of a cataract after a dose as low as 2 Gy. Excellent functional outcomes are evident for patients with optic nerve meningiomas with 5-year local control rates greater than 90% after local radiation therapy alone. In patients with orbital rhabdomyosarcoma, chemotherapy with radiation therapy results in excellent 5-year survival rates. Recently, we have been evaluating the role of oculoplastic procedures followed by adjuvant radiation therapy in lieu of orbital exenteration for patients with locally advanced ocular adnexal cancers.

13.1 Indications

Radiation therapy is used in the multimodality treatment of many orbital and adnexal tumors. Benign orbital and adnexal tumors and conditions that are successfully treated with radiation therapy alone include hemangioma, meningioma, orbital pseudotumor, and Graves ophthalmopathy. Malignant orbital and adnexal tumors that may require the use of radiation therapy include lymphoma, sarcoma, carcinoma, and metastatic disease. Radiation therapy may be used as the sole treatment modality or in combination with surgery and/or chemotherapy. For all of the

S.J. Frank (✉)
Department of Radiation Oncology, The University of Texas M.D. Anderson Cancer Center, Houston, TX, USA
e-mail: sjfrank@mdanderson.org

B. Esmaeli (ed.), *Ophthalmic Oncology*, M.D. Anderson Solid Tumor Oncology Series 6, DOI 10.1007/978-1-4419-0374-7_13,

indications described above, the role of radiation therapy is to enhance local control and possibly, in some patients, overall survival.

13.2 Radiation Therapy Terminology

Radiation therapy is prescribed in the unit of Gray (Gy), which measures the energy absorbed in a material (J/kg). Typically, orbital and adnexal radiation treatments are delivered in fractions of 1.8–2.0 Gy per day. The total number of fractions varies according to the inherent radiosensitivity of the lesion; for example, Graves disease may be treated in 10 fractions with a total dose of 20 Gy, whereas a sarcoma may require up to 30 fractions with a total dose of 60 Gy. Another factor that determines final treatment dose is the normal tissue in the irradiated volume and the associated morbidity risk (see Section 13.7).

Three-dimensional (3D) radiation therapy planning allows careful optimization of a plan to improve the tumor control probability while minimizing the normal tissue complication rate. The tumor volumes and normal tissue are identified on a planning computed tomography scan that is usually obtained in the radiation therapy department. These images can be fused with other diagnostic scans, including magnetic resonance imaging scans, positron emission tomography scans, or angiograms, to better visualize the regions of interest. Once all of the areas of concern and the tumor are delineated, a plan is generated on one of many available treatment planning systems. The treatment plan is then assessed through evaluation of the isodose curves and dose–volume histograms. These histograms are graphical representations of the volume of each region of interest receiving a particular dose. This analysis provides the radiation oncologist an objective method of appraising a heterogeneous dose distribution. Typically, normal tissue receives a nonuniform dose; however, an effort is made to maintain a uniform dose distribution within the tumor volumes.

13.3 Radiation Therapy Techniques

A variety of different radiation therapy techniques and modalities are available for treatment of the orbit and adnexal areas. All of the current treatment techniques use 3D algorithms that calculate dose in all planes and display dose in the axial, coronal, and sagittal views.

The basic form of radiation therapy based on 3D planning is called 3D conformal radiation therapy (3DCRT). With 3DCRT, conformal fields from different angles are optimized to meet the individual patient's needs. Any radiation therapy modality—i.e., photons, electrons, or protons—can be used for 3DCRT.

Stereotactic radiosurgery and fractionated stereotactic radiation therapy are techniques that use stereotactic positioning accomplished with an external fiducial system to immobilize and position patients, allowing submillimeter precision for radiation therapy treatments. With stereotactic radiosurgery, a large single fraction of radiation is given; with fractionated stereotactic radiation therapy, multiple fractions of radiation are given, and the patient is positioned before delivery of each fraction by using a noninvasive stereotactic frame.

Intensity-modulated radiation therapy (IMRT) is typically delivered with photon beams; a few centers now deliver it with proton beams ("intensity-modulated proton therapy"). Intensity modulation can also be implemented with the stereotactic approach, which may allow an increase in precision of delivery and conformality. IMRT plans use multiple beams optimized for the tumor location and patient. For each beam, the multileaf collimation varies during the dose delivery to modulate the dose from that beam to "paint" the dose and allow improved conformality and reduction in normal tissue doses.

Electron and proton radiation therapy differ from photon radiation therapy (X-ray or Cobalt) in that they lack an exit dose. Electron radiation therapy is an excellent modality for treating shallow, superficial tumors while sparing the underlying tissues. A lead eye shield is necessary when ocular adnexal lesions are treated with KV photons, and a tungsten eye shield is necessary when adnexal lesions are treated with electrons because of the risk of acute and late side effects from definitive or adjuvant radiation therapy.

Proton radiation therapy is becoming more available worldwide and allows treatment of larger, deeper tumors without an exit dose, thereby reducing the volume of normal tissue receiving low to moderate doses and potentially reducing acute and late toxic effects [1]. Proton radiation therapy may be a useful technology for young patients with curable tumors.

Radiation therapy implants (brachytherapy) are not typically used for orbital or adnexal tumors; the experience with brachytherapy for orbital tumors is limited to a few case reports of brachytherapy for lacrimal gland tumors and recurrent conjunctival tumors. We currently do not use brachytherapy at our center for lesions involving the orbit or ocular adnexal structures.

13.4 Radiation Therapy for Squamous Cell Carcinoma of the Eyelid

For patients presenting with squamous cell carcinoma of the eyelid, radiation therapy can be used in both the definitive and adjuvant settings. Recently, we have reviewed our institutional experience from 1950 to 2005 with 42 tumors in 39 patients [2]. Thirty-two of the tumors were treated with primary radiation therapy to a dose of 66–70 Gy, and 10 tumors were treated with adjuvant radiation therapy to 60 Gy. With a median follow-up of 76 months, the local disease-free, regional disease-free, and overall disease-free survival rates at 5 years in the entire group were 88, 95, and 90%, respectively. There was no significant difference between the patients treated with radiotherapy alone versus those treated after surgery. While there were no grade 3 or 4 complications, patients did experience grade 1 and 2 complications, including epiphora, symptomatic cataract, neovascular glaucoma, dry eye syndrome, and keratitis.

We recommend primary radiation therapy for patients refusing surgery and patients who are poor surgical candidates because of medical comorbidities or large lesions, removal of which would result for poor function and cosmesis. Adjuvant radiation therapy is recommended for patients with residual disease, positive or close margins, perineural invasion, lymph node-positive disease, lymphovascular invasion, or deep muscle invasion. Our institutional experience has revealed no difference in 5-year regional lymph node control in those patients who received radiation therapy to the regional nodes in comparison to those who did not—100 versus 93%, respectively. Prophylactic nodal irradiation is, therefore, not recommended.

13.5 Adjuvant Radiation Therapy for Ocular Adnexal Tumors

Recently, we have begun to investigate the role of adjuvant radiation therapy following oculoplastic procedures in lieu of orbital exenteration for some patients with locally advanced or aggressive ocular adnexal tumors. A review of our orbit-sparing approach from 2000 to 2006 with 20 consecutive patients presenting with primary eyelid or conjunctival tumors was recently published [3]. Pathologic subtype varied within this cohort of patients and included melanoma (three patients), Merkel cell carcinoma (three patients), squamous cell carcinoma (three patients), sebaceous gland carcinoma (three patients), basal cell carcinoma (one patient), mucinous eccrine adenocarcinoma (one patient), adenoid cystic carcinoma (one patient), and myxoid sarcoma (one patient). Most patients in this study (12 patients) presented with lower eyelid lesions; nine patients had tumors involving more than one site. In the majority of cases, oculoplastic surgery consisted of placement of local flaps or direct closure of the eyelid; also used were tarsoconjunctival flaps and grafts, full-thickness skin grafts, amniotic membrane grafts, and lacrimal stenting. The indications for adjuvant radiation therapy were high-grade disease, recurrent tumor, positive or close margins, perineural invasion, and advanced-stage disease. Radiation therapy for melanoma was 30 Gy delivered in 6-Gy fractions over 2.5 weeks. Radiation therapy for other tumors was 60 Gy delivered in 2-Gy fractions over 6 weeks.

With a median follow-up of 21 months, there were no local or regional relapses, and no salvage surgery was required. Fifteen patients had 20/40 vision or better, and the majority maintained their visual acuity after radiation therapy. Complications following surgery and adjuvant radiation therapy were dry eye syndrome (13 patients), keratinization of the conjunctivae (3 patients), blepharitis (1 patient), trichiasis (1 patient), optic neuropathy (1 patient), and exposure keratopathy (1 patient). We have observed that in patients with ocular adnexal cancers, local control rates after oculoplastic procedures and external-beam radiation therapy are acceptable; however, for an orbit-sparing approach to be considered, meticulous radiation techniques are a prerequisite, and realistic expectations regarding risk of ocular toxicity need to be discussed with the patient.

13.6 Radiation Therapy for Optic Nerve Meningiomas and Orbital Rhabdomyosarcomas

Optic nerve meningiomas are typically diagnosed on the basis of their characteristic radiographic appearance. A pathologic diagnosis is not mandatory if an orbital biopsy would entail risk to visual function. With definitive radiation therapy with doses ranging from 50.4 to 54 Gy in 28–30 fractions, the 5-year overall control rate is 90% [4, 5]. Potential morbidities include retinal injury, cataract, further visual compromise, and neuroendocrine compromise. Vision may improve or stabilize after radiation therapy. Typically, 3DCRT, fractionated stereotactic radiation therapy, or IMRT is used. Proton radiation therapy may be used if late toxic effects are of concern. Stereotactic radiosurgery is usually not recommended because of the unacceptable risk to vision.

The treatment strategy for orbital rhabdomyosarcoma usually involves a biopsy and surgical debulking of tumor followed by chemotherapy with radiation therapy. The recommended dose is 45 Gy given in 25 fractions. Particular concerns in individuals with this tumor, who tend to be young, are potential adverse effects of radiation on orbital bone growth and vision and the risk of secondary malignancies. These morbidities may be reduced with the use of highly conformal techniques such as IMRT or proton radiation therapy [6, 7]. The 5-year overall survival rate is excellent, and efforts to minimize late toxic effects are paramount. For further discussion of orbital rhabdomyosarcoma, please see Chapter 4.

13.7 Toxic Effects of Radiation Therapy

Toxic effects of radiation therapy are divided into two categories: acute toxic effects, which occur during or shortly after treatment, and late toxic effects, which can occur months or years after treatment. The probability and nature of toxic effects depends on the area of treatment, the volume of the organ being treated, and dose that it receives. For the orbit and the ocular adnexal structures, the anatomic structures at risk are the eyelid, lacrimal gland, nasolacrimal duct, intraocular structures, optic nerve(s), optic chiasm, bone (in young patients), brain, and neuroendocrine structures.

Acute toxic effects that are not unusual are eyelid erythema and swelling, eyebrow and eyelash alopecia, and conjunctival irritation with mild dry eye. The lacrimal gland secretes the aqueous layer of tear film; keratoconjunctivitis sicca (also known as dry eye syndrome) occurs when the gland receives doses in excess of 30 Gy [8]. The eyelashes protect the eye; a dose of 20 Gy will lead to eyelid alopecia, which in turn causes irritation of the conjunctivae and cornea. Subsequent regrowth may be associated with trichiasis and eyelid entropion. Additionally, meibomian gland dysfunction as a result of irradiation results in dry eye symptoms [9, 10].

Late toxic effects of radiation therapy are important because they can permanently affect visual function or cosmetic outcome. The cornea serves as the "clear window" for the eye and refracts light. Doses up to 30 Gy are well tolerated by the cornea; however, doses exceeding 50 Gy can result in keratitis, stromal edema, ulceration, and resultant vision loss [11]. The lens transmits and refracts light and is considered the most radiosensitive organ in the body. Doses exceeding 2 Gy in a single fraction can result in cataract formation; the time of onset and severity of the cataract can vary with lens exposure [11]. The retina contains the neuroreceptors for the eye and produces the image-forming signals. Doses greater than 45 Gy can result in retinopathy, including retinal hemorrhages, microaneurysms, hard exudates, cotton-wool spots, telangiectases, and retinal neovascularization [12]. The optic nerve transmits signals from the retina to the brain; optic neuropathy can occur if greater than 1 cm of the nerve receives 60 Gy or greater [11, 13]. The optic nerves cross at the optic chiasm, where doses exceeding 54 Gy in 2-Gy fractions can result in bilateral blindness [11]. The sclera maintains the globe shape and is, fortunately, extremely radioresistant, tolerating doses up to 200 Gy. The tolerance of the sclera has allowed orbit-sparing approaches and improved outcomes for patients presenting with intraocular melanoma. Doses to the sclera exceeding 200 Gy result in atrophy of the globe [13].

The nasolacrimal duct allows tears to drain into the nasal cavity. When the duct receives a dose of 60 Gy or more, stenosis of the duct can occur, leading to epiphora, which may necessitate silicone intubation or dacryocystorhinostomy with Pyrex glass tube placement to relieve epiphora [14].

In the pediatric population, orbital bone hypoplasia and facial asymmetry are of concern in areas receiving more than 20 Gy. Secondary malignancies are of particular concern in younger patients who are expected to have an extended survival. Proton radiation therapy may reduce the risk of secondary malignancies because of the low dose of radiation that is "sprayed" out with the photon techniques because of the exit dose [15].

13.8 Summary

In summary, radiation therapy is an integral component in the management of orbital and adnexal tumors. Various technologies are used in this treatment, and the optimal treatment technique should be chosen for each patient's needs.

References

1. Miralbell R, Cella L, Weber D, et al. Optimizing radiotherapy of orbital and paraorbital tumors: intensity-modulated X-ray beams vs. intensity-modulated proton beams. Int J Radiat Oncol Biol Phys 2000;47(4):1111–9.

2. Petsuksiri J, Frank SJ, Garden AS, et al. Outcomes after radiotherapy for squamous cell carcinoma of the eyelid. Cancer 2008;112(1):111–8.
3. Hsu A, Frank S, Ballo MT, et al. Postoperative adjuvant external-beam radiation therapy for cancers of the eyelid and conjunctiva. Ophthal Plast Reconstr Surg 2008;24(6):444–9.
4. Melian E, Jay WM. Primary radiotherapy for optic nerve sheath meningioma. Semin Ophthalmol 2004;19(3–4):130–40.
5. Eddleman CS, Liu JK. Optic nerve sheath meningioma: current diagnosis and treatment. Neurosurg Focus 2007;23(5):E4.
6. Timmermann B, Schuck A, Niggli F, et al. "Spot-scanning" proton therapy for rhabdomyosarcomas of early childhood. First experiences at PSI. Strahlenther Onkol 2006;182(11):653–9.
7. Yock T, Schneider R, Friedmann A, et al. Proton radiotherapy for orbital rhabdomyosarcoma: clinical outcome and a dosimetric comparison with photons. Int J Radiat Oncol Biol Phys 2005;63(4):1161–8.
8. Parsons JT, Bova FJ, Fitzgerald CR, et al. Severe dry-eye syndrome following external beam irradiation. Int J Radiat Oncol Biol Phys 1994;30:775–80.
9. Brady LW, Shields J, Augusburger J, et al. Complications from radiation therapy to the eye. Front Radiat Ther Oncol 1989;23:238–50.
10. Hungerford J. Current management of choroidal malignant melanoma. Br J Hosp Med 1985;34:287–93.
11. Jiang GL, Tucker SL, Guttenberger R, et al. Radiation-induced injury to the visual pathway. Radiother Oncol 1994;30:17–25.
12. Parsons JT, Bova FJ, Fitzgerald CR, et al. Radiation retinopathy after external-beam irradiation: analysis of time–dose factors. Int J Radiat Oncol Biol Phys 1994;30(4):765–73.
13. Parsons JT, Bova FJ, Fitzgerald CR, et al. Radiation optic neuropathy after megavoltage external-beam irradiation: analysis of time–dose factors. Int J Radiat Oncol Biol Phys 1994;30(4):755–63.
14. Diba R, Saadati H, Esmaeli B. Outcomes of dacryocystorhinostomy in patients with head and neck tumors. Head Neck 2005;27:72–75.
15. Miralbell R, Lomax A, Cella L, et al. Potential reduction of the incidence of radiation-induced second cancers by using proton beams in the treatment of pediatric tumors. Int J Radiat Oncol Biol Phys 2002;54(3):824–9.

Part II
Intraocular Tumors

Section Editor: Dan S. Gombos

Chapter 14
Multidisciplinary Management of Retinoblastoma: Diagnosis, Treatment, and Future Direction

Maurizio L. Ghisoli, Peter E. Zage, Cindy Herzog, Patty Chevez-Barrios, Murali Chintagumpala, Richard L. Hurwitz, Anita Mahajan, and Dan S. Gombos

Abstract Retinoblastoma is a relatively uncommon tumor of childhood that arises from the retina and accounts for about 3% of the cancers occurring in children younger than 15 years. The treatment of retinoblastoma is complex and requires a multidisciplinary team that includes pediatric oncologists, ophthalmologists, ocular pathologists, geneticists, and radiation oncologists, all of whom have expertise in retinoblastoma management. This chapter includes a brief discussion of the presentation, classification, and pathologic features of the disease. Available treatment options are also discussed, including enucleation, chemoreduction, systemic or local chemotherapy, focal therapy with cryotherapy, laser photocoagulation, or plaque brachytherapy, and external-beam radiation therapy.

14.1 Historical Perspective

Retinoblastoma is a relatively uncommon tumor of childhood that arises from the retina and accounts for about 3% of the cancers occurring in children younger than 15 years. The estimated annual incidence in the United States is approximately 10–14 cases per 1 million children between birth and 4 years. Although retinoblastoma may occur at any age, it most often occurs in young children, usually before 2 years, and 95% of cases are diagnosed before 5 years. Retinoblastoma occurs in heritable (40%) and nonheritable (60%) forms. It is usually confined to the eye and, as a result, has a cure rate in the United States approaching 98–99%. The present challenge for those who treat retinoblastoma is to help the patient avoid loss of an eye, blindness, and other late effects of treatment, including secondary nonocular tumors.

The treatment of retinoblastoma is complex and requires a multidisciplinary team that includes pediatric oncologists, geneticists, ocular pathologist, ophthalmologists,

---

M.L. Ghisoli (✉)
Department of Hematology and Oncology, Medical City Children's Hospital, Texas Oncology, Dallas, TX, USA
e-mail: maurizio.ghisoli@usoncology.com

B. Esmaeli (ed.), *Ophthalmic Oncology*, M.D. Anderson Solid Tumor Oncology Series 6, DOI 10.1007/978-1-4419-0374-7_14,

and radiation oncologists, all of whom have expertise in retinoblastoma management. Treatment options for the involved eye include enucleation, external-beam radiation therapy (EBRT), systemic or local chemotherapy, and focal therapy with laser photocoagulation, cryotherapy, or plaque brachytherapy.

Within the last 20 years, there have been significant changes in the treatment strategies employed for retinoblastoma. Historically, chemotherapy was reserved for use in patients with extraocular or metastatic disease or as adjuvant chemotherapy after enucleation. However, the realization that patients who underwent EBRT have an increased risk of developing secondary malignancies has led to the increased use of primary chemotherapy. Chemoreduction (i.e., chemotherapy followed by focal consolidation) has now become the standard approach to eye-sparing treatment.

14.2 Presentation and Workup

In the United States and developed countries, the most common presenting symptom of retinoblastoma is leukocoria or a white pupillary reflex (Fig. 14.1). Less common symptoms include strabismus, redness, pain, and periocular cellulitis. Patients with a family history of retinoblastoma are likely to be diagnosed earlier and may be asymptomatic at presentation. Assessment requires an examination under anesthesia by an experienced ocular oncologist who can confirm the diagnosis based on clinical features. Most retinoblastoma foci have a typical chalky white appearance with associated calcification. As these tumors are generally not biopsied because of the risk of extraocular spread, diagnosis is made by ophthalmoscopy combined with noninvasive testing, such as ocular echography, fluorescein angiography, or neuroimaging.

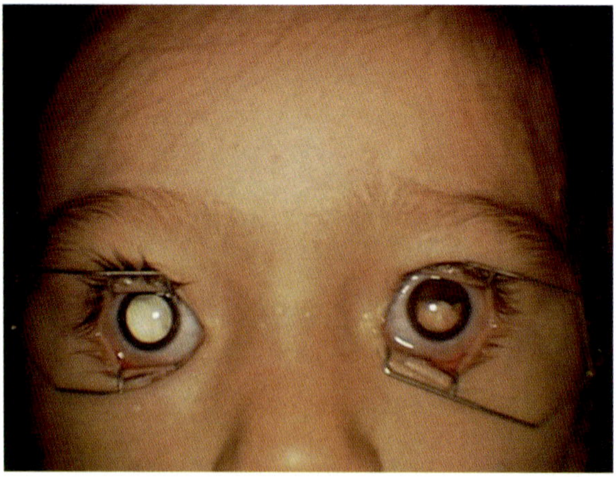

Fig. 14.1 Bilateral leukocoria in a patient with retinoblastoma

The majority of retinoblastoma foci harbor calcium, which can be easily confirmed on ultrasonography and/or computed tomography. Increasingly, however, many specialty centers prefer magnetic resonance imaging over computed tomography because of magnetic resonance imaging's superiority in visualizing the orbital portion of the optic nerve and pineal region. Ret Cam (Clarity Medical Systems, Pleasanton, CA) imaging allows digital photographs to be taken of the ocular fundus and has become the standard of care in baseline and follow-up intraocular tumor imaging. Historically, lumbar puncture and bone marrow biopsies were performed routinely in all patients. Today, this is limited to those at increased risk for developing extraocular disease.

14.3 Classification

Since the 1960s, the most common classification system used to describe intraocular retinoblastoma has been the Reese–Ellsworth (R–E) system, developed by Algernon Reese and Robert Ellsworth [1]. This system was initially designed to predict prognosis in patients treated with EBRT and, therefore, is a classification (or grouping) system rather than a true staging system. The R–E system has been used consistently to compare outcomes of different treatment modalities and classifies eye tumors into five groups (Table 14.1).

Because current treatment strategies more commonly consist of primary chemotherapy combined with focal treatment, a new classification system was developed by Dr. Linn Murphree [2]. The international classification for intraocular retinoblastoma (also called the ABC system) [2] incorporates the natural history of the disease and better predicts outcomes of current treatments, including systemic

Table 14.1 The Reese Ellsworth classification system for intraocular retinoblastoma. From reference 1. Reprinted with permission

Group	Features	Prognosis
I	A) Solitary tumor; <4 disc diameter; at or behind the equator B) Multiple tumors; none >4 disc diameter; all at or behind the equator	Very favorable
II	A) Solitary tumor; 4–10 disc diameter; at or behind the equator B) Multiple tumors; 4–10 disc diameter; behind the equator	Favorable
III	A) Any lesion anterior to the equator B) Solitary tumors; >10 disc diameter; behind the equator	Uncertain
IV	A) Multiple tumors; some >10 disc diameter B) Any lesion extending anterior to the ora serrata	Unfavorable
V	A) Massive tumors involving over half the retina B) Vitreous seeding	Very unfavorable

chemotherapy [3]. It consists of five groups (A–E), with specific criteria for determination of tumor volume and dissemination to the subretinal and vitreous portions of the globe (Table 14.2). It is the preferred classification for ongoing Children's Oncology Group (COG) trials (see Section 14.8).

Table 14.2 International classification for intraocular retinoblastoma, ABC system

Group	Reference	Features
A	Small tumor	Retinoblastoma ≤3 mm Tumor not adjacent to fovea or optic nerve
B	Larger tumor Macula Juxtapapillary Subretinal fluid	Retinoblastoma >3 mm Macular retinoblastoma ≤3 mm from fovea, any size Juxtapapillary retinoblastoma ≤1.5 mm from disc, any size
C	Focal seeds (fine)	Retinoblastoma with subretinal and/or vitreous seeds ≤3 mm from tumor
D	Diffuse seeds (greasy)	Retinoblastoma with subretinal and/or vitreous seeds >3 mm from tumor
E	Extensive retinoblastoma	Retinoblastoma occupying >50% of globe Neovascular glaucoma Opaque media from hemorrhage in anterior chamber, vitreous, or subretinal space Invasion of postlamina optic nerve, choroid (>2 mm), sclera, orbit, or anterior chamber

14.4 Genetics

Retinoblastoma tumors are characterized as having biallelic inactivation of the *retinoblastoma* gene on chromosome 13q14 [4]. The protein encoded by the *retinoblastoma* gene (pRB) prevents activation of the genes necessary for DNA replication and cell division [5]. Absent or deficient pRB allows cells to replicate continuously. In about 40% of patients, the mutation that occurs in the first allele is a germline mutation; 30% of these cases are de novo, and 10% are inherited from a parent. In the remaining 60% of patients, the mutation in the first allele occurs in a retinal precursor cell. The second allele then also mutates in the retina [4, 6]. The presence of multiple tumors in both eyes of young patients (less than 1 year old) who have the germline mutation contrasts with single retinal tumors observed in older patients, which can be explained by this "two-hit" theory [4–7].

Patients with hereditary retinoblastoma are at increased risk for second nonocular tumors [8, 9]. Thus, detection of the *retinoblastoma* gene mutation in both the leukocytes and tumor cells of a patient with unilateral retinoblastoma confirms the presence of a germline mutation. This information is especially useful in those patients with unilateral retinoblastoma who have no family history of the disease but are at risk for developing additional retinoblastoma foci and need frequent follow-up eye examinations, enabling early diagnosis of new tumors; this information is also valuable when it comes to counseling the family of the patient. DNA analysis can reduce health-care costs by eliminating follow-up evaluations of patients who do not have the germline mutation and their close relatives [10], and it enhances genetic counseling of family members of patients who have the germline mutation and are thus at increased risk of developing retinoblastoma [11]. Fresh tumor samples are necessary to perform the complete genetic testing; thus, adequate planning is necessary when enucleating eyes with unilateral retinoblastoma.

14.5 Pathologic Features

The tumor is composed of small cells with basophilic nuclei, scanty cytoplasm, and numerous mitoses and apoptotic cells. Tumor cells alternate with geographic areas of necrotic tumor cells and deposits of calcium (Fig. 14.2a). The tumor arises from the retina and invades the vitreous, occasionally forming free-floating spheres of tumor seeds. In some tumors, the tumor cells form rosette structures

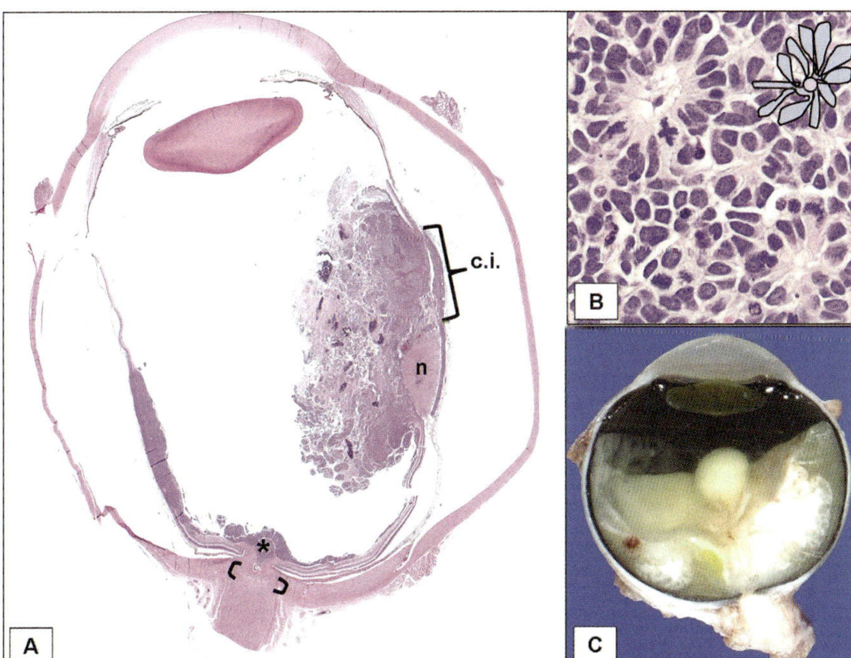

Fig. 14.2 (**a**) Histopathologic slide of retinoblastoma demonstrating choroidal invasion (c.i.). Careful assessment must be made in the region of the optic nerve (*star*) as to whether there is laminar or posterior laminar optic nerve invasion (*brackets*). (**b**) High magnification view demonstrating Homer Wright rosette. (**c**) Gross photo of eye demonstrating combined endophytic and exophytic growth pattern

that resemble photoreceptors. Flexner–Wintersteiner rosettes are characteristic of retinoblastoma, and Homer Wright rosettes may be seen in other nonocular tumors (Fig. 14.2b). Tumors may also form fleurette clusters, which are highly differentiated structures closely resembling photoreceptors [12]. The tumor growth pattern may be primarily endophytic growth into the vitreous, primarily exophytic growth into the subretinal space, or combined growth (which is the most common pattern) (Fig. 14.2c). Multivariate statistical analysis has suggested correlation between certain histopathologic findings and prognostic risk factors [13–15]. Histopathologic risk factors include invasion of the tumor into the postlamina cribrosa portion of the optic nerve or beyond the cut margin of the nerve.

The most frequent route of spread of retinoblastoma is through the optic nerve into the brain [12, 13]. The extent of tumor invasion in the optic nerve correlates with prognosis. Superficial invasion of the optic disc is associated with a mortality rate of 10%. The presence of tumor up to the lamina cribrosa is associated with a mortality rate of 29%. Invasion of tumor posterior to the lamina cribrosa is associated with a mortality rate of 42%, and tumor at the transected surgical margin is associated with a mortality rate of 80% [14, 15]. Choroidal invasion when the tumor is massive (3 mm or more) may increase the risk of metastasis, especially when such invasion is associated with scleral invasion and extraocular extension. Given the importance of architecture features in determining prognosis, when eyes with retinoblastoma are subjected to pathologic examination or to sampling of fresh tissue for genetic studies, it is important to avoid disturbing the architecture of the eye so that the necessary data for evaluation of risk factors for metastasis remain available.

14.6 Treatment Options

14.6.1 General Considerations

The treatment required depends on both the extent of the disease within the eye and whether the disease has spread beyond the eye, either to the brain or elsewhere. For those with bilateral disease, therapy should be designed to treat the more severely affected eye. The goals of therapy are to cure the patient, eradicate the disease, preserve as much vision as possible, and minimize the late sequelae from treatment.

14.6.2 Enucleation

Enucleation remains the treatment of choice for significantly advanced retinoblastoma and for retinoblastoma with no potential for visual salvage. It is curative in the majority of cases. Enucleation involves the removal of the intact globe, with care taken to not perforate or penetrate the globe and to limit the risk of tumor cell spread within the orbital cavity. The optic nerve should then be cut in such a way as to obtain as long a section as possible and minimize the risk of tumor cells distal to the cut margin. Because unilateral disease is often diagnosed late, when the stage is advanced and the potential for vision preservation is poor, enucleation is generally the preferred treatment modality, although in select cases more conservative therapy may be considered.

14.6.3 Chemoreduction

During the past decade, chemoreduction (systemic chemotherapy to reduce tumor volume before focal consolidation) has become the preferred modality for ocular salvage. Multiagent chemotherapy is generally used, and the standard regimen currently consists of combinations of carboplatin and vincristine, with or without etoposide. Systemic chemotherapy may also decrease the risk of development of trilateral retinoblastoma and may be effective against small undetected lesions.

The results of a number of trials have been published using systemic chemotherapy for patients whose intraocular tumors are too large to be treated with focal therapy alone, in situations where local therapy would limit vision and offer little improvement over enucleation. All centers reporting to date have demonstrated that globe and vision salvage is achievable in many cases, especially for tumors that are classified as R–E group IV or lower. Advanced retinoblastoma tumors with diffuse vitreous seeding (group D and higher) have proven extremely difficult to treat, however. Several strategies have been used in an attempt to overcome this problem.

The lack of high eye salvage rates in advanced cases has led to the development of newer adjuvant therapies, including subtenon (subconjunctival) carboplatin (see Section 14.6.4) and use of higher doses of carboplatin or etoposide. There is no absolute agreement between different institutions regarding the best combination of chemotherapy agents and the number of treatment cycles. In comparisons of different studies, similar outcome is seen between two-drug combinations (carboplatin combined with either etoposide or vincristine) and three-drug combinations (vincristine, etoposide or teniposide, and carboplatin or cisplatin, with or without the addition of cyclosporine) (Table 14.3).

Friedman et al. [16] treated 75 eyes with 6 cycles of chemotherapy consisting of carboplatin, etoposide, and vincristine, with a median follow-up of 13 months. Almost half of the treated eyes (30) were group V. The response in R–E groups I and II was excellent, with avoidance of EBRT or enucleation in all of them. For groups IV and V, the success rate was lower, with 33% of 6 eyes and 53% of 30 eyes, respectively, requiring EBRT and/or enucleation. In a prospective study with a medium follow-up of 21 months, Brichard et al. [17] treated 24 eyes (21 were group V), with 2 to 6 cycles of chemotherapy. Chemotherapy was combined with

Table 14.3 Comparison of outcomes of recent retinoblastoma treatment trials

Study (reference)	R–E groups	# eyes	Therapy	Globe salvage w/o EBRT	Enucleations	EBRT	f/u duration[a]
Zage et al. [21]	I–IV	23	CE + focal	19/23 (83%)	4/23	0/23	Mean 59 months
	V	25		6/25 (24%)	18/25	7/25	
Schiavetti et al. [20]	I–IV	41	CE + focal	28/41 (68%)	10/41	6/41	Mean 53 months
	V	17		1/17 (6%)	11/17	4/17	
Chantada et al. [23]	I–III	24	CV + focal	10/24 (42%)	1/24	14/24	Mean 48 months
	IV/V	54	CEV + focal	10/54 (19%)	27/54	25/54	
Gunduz et al. [46]	I–IV	69	CEV + focal	n/a	9/69	15/69	Mean 26 months
	I–III	34		25/34 (74%)			
	IV/V	71		28/71 (40%)	30/71	18/71	
	V	36		n/a	23/36	11/36	
Rodriguez-Galindo et al. [19]	I–IV	27	CV	15/27 (56%)	7/27	10/27	Med 32 months
	V	16		5/16 (32%)	6/16	9/16	
Lee et al. [52]	I–IV	21	CEV + focal	17/21 (81%)	4/21	0/21	Mean 44 months
	V	6		0/6 (0%)	0/6	0/6	
Hadjistilianou et al. [24]	I–IV	13	CE + focal	9/13 (69%)	4/13	0/13	Mean 21 months
	V	3		2/3 (67%)	1/3	0/3	

Table 14.3 (continued)

Study (reference)	R–E groups	# eyes	Therapy	Globe salvage w/o EBRT	Enucleations	EBRT	f/u duration[a]
Brichard et al. [17]	I–III	12	CEV + focal	12/12 (100%)	0/12	0/12	Mean 21 months
	V	21		8/21 (38%)	11/21	0/21	
Shields et al. [25][b]	I–IV	83	CEV + focal	78/83 (94%)[c]	5/83	8/83	Med 28 months
	V	75		43/75 (57%)[c]	32/75	32/75	
Beck et al. [26]	I–IV	19	CE + focal	18/19 (95%)	0/19	1/19	Med 31 months
	V	14		2/14 (14%)	5/14	7/14	
Friedman et al. [16][b]	I–IV	45	CEV + focal	96%[d]	n/a	n/a	Med 13 months
	V	30		39%[d]	n/a	n/a	
Levy et al. [27]	I–IV	18	CE + focal	8/18 (44%)	0/18	10/18	Mean 18 months
	V	20		0/20 (0%)	11/20	13/20	

Abbreviations: R–E, Reese–Ellsworth; EBRT, external-beam radiation therapy; f/u, follow-up; C, carboplatin; E, etoposide; V, vincristine; n/a, data not available

[a]Values expressed as mean or median (med)

[b]Some patients were included in both of these studies

[c]Globe salvage both with and without the use of EBRT

[d]Estimated from Kaplan–Meier calculations

thermotherapy plus cryotherapy in 16 eyes and thermotherapy plus cryotherapy plus radioactive iodine 125 plaque radiation therapy in 4 eyes; this strategy made EBRT unnecessary in 60% of the eyes. Enucleation remained the treatment of choice in 70% of the group V eyes. One of the more recent studies with a large number of treated eyes (145, with 74 eyes in group V) was done by Antoneli et al. [18] in 2006. These authors used two to six cycles of vincristine, carboplatin, and etoposide plus focal therapy with cryotherapy, laser photocoagulation, and thermotherapy or plaque radiation therapy during and/or after the chemotherapy. In the group of patients with R–E stages I, II, and III disease, the success rate (ocular salvage) for unilateral and bilateral tumors was 50 and 79% ($P = 0.179$), respectively. In contrast, in the group with R–E stages IV and V disease, children with bilateral tumors responded significantly better (40.7%) than children with unilateral tumors (0%) ($P = 0.012$) [18].

These studies indicate that for patients with R–E eye groups I, II, or III, systemic chemotherapy in combination with local ophthalmic therapies can avoid the need for enucleation or EBRT. More aggressive therapy is required for R–E eye groups IV and V.

The efficacy of two-drug chemotherapy regimens has been investigated in recent studies [19–21]. Schiavetti et al. [20] achieved an overall complete response rate of 88% after four to eight courses of carboplatin plus etoposide in conjunction with focal therapy (either laser photocoagulation or cryotherapy). The response rate was 100, 94, and 100% for R–E groups I, II, and III, respectively, and 83 and 70% for groups IV and V, respectively. However, the relapse rate was found to be 57% after a mean of 7 months (range, 2–36 months) and was 100% for group V eyes. St. Jude's researchers reported better outcomes, with 43 eyes in 25 patients treated with 8 courses of vincristine and carboplatin. Focal treatment was given in 39 of the eyes, only after documentation of progression. EBRT was required in 18 eyes (44.2%), and 13 eyes (30.2%) were enucleated. With this treatment, the ocular salvage rate was 83.3% for R–E group I, II, and III eyes and 52.6% for group IV and V eyes. More recently, Zage et al. [21] at Children's Memorial Hospital in Chicago, treated 48 eyes in 29 patients with a combination of carboplatin and etoposide and early local therapy. The reported response rate was 85.4%; the vision salvage rate was 82.6% without EBRT for eye groups A and B but only 20% for R–E group V eyes. The evidence suggests that a regimen with only two chemotherapy agents (i.e., carboplatin combined with either etoposide or vincristine) and a total of six to eight cycles is a suitable approach for low-stage tumors, but for R–E groups IV and V a more aggressive regimen is still required.

The presence of extraocular disease, particularly invasion of the central nervous system, has prompted the use of drugs like carboplatin that have better central nervous system penetration [22]. Regimens of chemotherapy that use carboplatin, etoposide, and vincristine have been used to treat patients with extraocular disease. There are emerging data suggesting that the use of systemic chemotherapy may decrease the risk of development of trilateral retinoblastoma. Local tumor recurrence is not uncommon in the first few years after treatment and can often be successfully treated with focal therapy [23]. Among patients with heritable disease, younger patients and those with a positive family history are more likely to develop additional tumors.

14.6.4 Subtenon (Subconjunctival) Chemotherapy

Carboplatin can be administered by the treating ophthalmologist into the subconjunctival space. This modality is undergoing testing in clinical trials (see Section 14.8) and is generally used in conjunction with systemic chemotherapy and local ophthalmic therapies for patients with retinoblastoma with vitreous seeding. This approach offers some promise in this group of patients.

14.6.5 Unilateral Disease

Because unilateral disease is usually extensive, often with no expectation that useful vision can be preserved, surgery (enucleation) is usually undertaken. However, recent studies in patients with unilateral disease have used chemotherapy in an attempt to preserve vision in the affected eye [2, 24, 25]. One study [26] revealed that children with retinoblastoma who present with obvious external findings of leukocoria, strabismus, or red eye detectable by their family or pediatrician most often require enucleation. Children who manifest no obvious external findings can often avoid enucleation [26].

When there is potential for preservation of vision, treatment with globe-sparing modalities (radiation therapy, photocoagulation, cryotherapy, thermotherapy, chemoreduction, and brachytherapy) should be considered. In select children with unilateral disease, chemoreduction reduced the need for enucleation or EBRT within 5 years of treatment to 68%. R–E group correlated with successful chemoreduction: 11% of children classified as having R–E group II or III disease, 60% of children having R–E group IV disease, and 100% of children having R–E group V disease required enucleation or EBRT within 5 years of treatment [27].

Because a proportion of children who present with unilateral retinoblastoma will eventually develop contralateral disease, it is important that children with unilateral retinoblastoma receive periodic examinations of the unaffected eye. Asynchronous bilateral disease occurs most frequently in families with affected parents.

Careful examination of the enucleated specimen by an experienced pathologist is necessary to determine whether features indicating high risk for metastatic disease are present. These include anterior chamber seeding, choroidal involvement, tumor beyond the lamina cribrosa, intraocular hemorrhage, and scleral and extrascleral extensions [12, 14]. Systemic adjuvant therapy has been suggested to prevent the development of metastatic disease in patients with certain high-risk features detected on pathologic review after enucleation. Clinical trials are currently ongoing to determine precisely what features indicate the highest risk for metastatic spread (see Section 14.8).

14.6.6 Bilateral Disease

The management of bilateral disease depends on the extent of the disease in each eye. Systemic therapy should be chosen based on the eye with more extensive disease.

Usually the disease is more advanced in one eye, with less involvement in the other. The standard of care in the past has been to enucleate the more involved eye; however, if there is potential for preservation of vision, chemoreduction with close follow-up for response and focal treatment (e.g., cryotherapy or laser therapy) is indicated.

A number of large centers in Europe and North America have published results of trials using systemic chemotherapy for patients whose intraocular tumors are not initially amenable to local management [2, 18, 20, 22, 23, 25–40]. Examples of such tumors are those that are too large to be treated with cryotherapy, laser photocoagulation, or plaque radiation therapy (brachytherapy). Another example is the newborn with a tumor over the optic nerve head. All of these situations share the likelihood that local therapy would limit vision and would not be curative. Most centers have limited this approach to patients with bilateral disease, reasoning that for patients with unilateral disease, the morbidity of enucleation is modest.

In all cases, the goal of chemotherapy is the reduction (hence the term *chemoreduction*) of tumor volume, making possible the use of focal therapy (cryotherapy, laser photocoagulation, thermotherapy, plaque radiation therapy).

The backbone of the chemoreduction protocols has generally been carboplatin, etoposide, and vincristine. Studies from the Children's Hospital of Philadelphia and Wills Eye Hospital reported complete success in the avoidance of enucleation or EBRT in R–E group I, II, and III eyes when patients were treated for six cycles. However, local control was often transient in patients with vitreous seeding or very large tumors (R–E group V). Several strategies have been used in an attempt to overcome this problem. Researchers reported the use of nine courses of carboplatin, etoposide, and vincristine with the addition of high-dose cyclosporine A as a modulator of the p-glycoprotein for eight R–E group V eyes with an 88% (seven of eight eyes) success rate (no need for EBRT or enucleation). However, researchers using this regimen in 10 R–E group V eyes reported only a 20% (2 of 10 eyes) success rate.

Using the international classification system for intraocular retinoblastoma applied to these data retrospectively, approximately 30% of group C and 70% of group D eyes failed systemic chemotherapy alone (i.e., chemotherapy was not enough) and achieved responses in pilot studies [30].

This has led to newer adjuvant therapies, including subtenon (subconjunctival) carboplatin, in pilot studies that also use higher doses of carboplatin or etoposide [41–44] (see Section 14.8).

Currently unresolved issues include long-term tumor control and the long-term consequences of chemotherapy. Most of these patients treated by chemotherapy are exposed to etoposide, which has been associated with secondary leukemia in patients without predisposition to cancer; however, the risk of secondary leukemia after etoposide treatment is modest compared to the risk of secondary tumors following EBRT in patients with heritable retinoblastoma. In a retrospective database and literature review, ocular and pediatric oncologists at referral centers in Europe and the Americas and the retinoblastoma databases at the National Institutes of Health and the Ophthalmic Oncology Service at Memorial Sloan-Kettering Cancer Center conducted a study of secondary acute myeloid leukemia among patients treated for retinoblastoma [45]. Fifteen patients were identified; 12 patients (79%) had received chemotherapy with a topoisomerase II inhibitor (etoposide or teniposide). Ten children died of their leukemia [45].

Whether patients with heritable retinoblastoma have greater susceptibility to chemotherapy-induced second tumors is unknown. Some patients will experience disease progression, and the risk of exposure to both chemotherapy and irradiation in this population has not been determined.

14.7 Focal Therapies

The need for supplemental focal therapy for the control and eradication of retinoblastoma has been demonstrated in several studies [28–30, 46]. Wilson et al. [30] utilized up to eight cycles of chemotherapy with carboplatin and vincristine, initially without focal therapy. A total of 36 eyes were treated (4 patients with unilateral and 16 with bilateral disease). Eighteen eyes had R–E group I, II, or III tumors, and 16 eyes had R–E group IV or V tumors. Only three eyes were treated successfully with chemotherapy alone; in 92% of eyes, disease progressed after completion of the treatment, and at the end of treatment, 42% of the eyes required EBRT.

14.7.1 Cryotherapy

Cryotherapy is used mainly with small peripheral tumors. It induces damage to the tumor vasculature through rapid freezing, with subsequent thrombosis and necrosis of the tissue. Usually patients are treated one to two sessions per month, and a triple freeze–thaw technique is used. A tumor control rate of up to 90% has been reported for small tumors (<3 mm) with minimal complications [31, 32]. Cryotherapy also can be used to treat small recurrences in tumors previously treated with other modalities.

14.7.2 Laser Photocoagulation

Focal laser therapy is occasionally used alone with small tumors. Photocoagulation is used for posteriorly located tumors that are smaller than four DD, distinct from the optic nerve head and macula, and without the involvement of large nutrient vessels or choroid involvement. Photocoagulation requires multiple (at least two to three) sessions. Thermotherapy delivered via infrared radiation (see Section 14.7.4) is an alternative to laser photocoagulation [34].

14.7.3 Brachytherapy

Brachytherapy with radioactive plaques can be used for either focal unilateral presentations or recurrent disease following previous EBRT. The goal is to deliver up to 4000–4500 cGy transsclerally for a total of 2–4 days. The tumor must be no more than 16 mm wide and 8 mm thick. Shields et al. [33] reported in a series of 208 eyes that brachytherapy achieved tumor control in 79% of cases at 5 years and proved to be especially useful in tumors for which treatment with chemoreduction, laser photocoagulation, thermotherapy, or cryotherapy failed (see Section 14.7.5).

14.7.4 Thermotherapy

Thermotherapy involves the application of a source of heat (usually via infrared 810 nm laser) directly to the tumor to achieve temperatures up to 60°C. As with other types of focal therapy, thermotherapy is used for small retinoblastoma tumors (less than 3 mm in diameter), and the success rate is reported to be up to 92% [34]. In many centers it is the preferred modality over traditional photocoagulation.

14.7.5 Radiation Therapy

Retinoblastoma is a radiosensitive tumor with control rates exceeding 90% with EBRT alone. Because of the potential late consequences of radiation therapy, however, the role of this modality has changed to a salvage role following failed chemoreduction. Technological advances for EBRT, including megavoltage photon and electron beams, three-dimensional treatment planning, intensity-modulated radiation therapy, and proton beam radiation, have allowed improved treatment conformality, which should, in theory, lead to a reduction of unwanted sequelae.

EBRT planning strategies should maximize conformality of high doses to the areas at risk and minimize the dose to surrounding uninvolved structures. In patients treated with EBRT, the radiation oncologist should explicitly understand the extent of tumor involvement, which requires direct communication with the evaluating ophthalmologist. This knowledge allows delineation of the gross tumor volume and definition of the clinical target volume to encompass the areas at risk of microscopic disease. The clinical target volume could extend from the ora serrata to the anterior 1 cm of the optic nerve, thereby including the vitreous body. Alternatively, in patients with discrete limited disease, the clinical target volume may not include the entire retina or vitreous body, allowing lens-sparing techniques to be used. The planning target volume, which includes an extra margin of uncertainty, is patient and machine dependent. Optimal immobilization allows minimum planning target volume and increases the possibility of lens sparing. Techniques have been described to immobilize the eye so that the beam orientation can be optimized for treatment delivery.

Proton beam radiation therapy, electron beam therapy, and intensity-modulated radiation therapy are EBRT modalities that have been used to reduce the dose of radiation to the brain, orbital and facial bones, and contralateral eye and lens. Dosimetric studies have been reported; however, long-term benefits and reduction of possible secondary malignancies have not been established yet. Proton radiation therapy is particularly interesting in these vulnerable patients because of the reduction of the integral dose to the patient's head. The fractionation schemes remain the same as those used for other forms of EBRT, with a typical dose of 40–45 Gy delivered over 20–25 treatments over 4–5 weeks.

Brachytherapy is another effective radiation therapy delivery system. A plaque is sutured on the sclera directly over the tumor using either ruthenium 106 (Ru-106) plaque or a plaque with radioactive seeds (iodine 125 [I-125]). Ru-106 is a beta-emitting isotope that is well suited for patients with retinoblastoma; however, availability is a problem in the United States. I-125 is a gamma-emitting isotope that can be customized to the size and shape of the tumor. Brachytherapy is ideally used in patients who have small, accessible, discrete single tumors.

14.8 Multi-institutional Clinical Trials

For many decades, pediatric oncologists in North America were involved in multi-institutional clinical trials through the establishment of cooperative groups like the Pediatric Oncology Group, Children's Cancer Group, National Wilms Tumor Study Group, and Intergroup Rhabdomyosarcoma Study Group. In 2001, these groups were brought together to form the COG. The formation of COG gave fresh impetus to the study of retinoblastoma as a disease and the establishment of clinical trials to develop a uniform approach to the management of retinoblastoma in children in order to improve outcomes.

A retinoblastoma committee was formed within the COG, which included ophthalmologists, oncologists, pathologists, statisticians, radiation oncologists, epidemiologists, and researchers interested in the study of the biology of the tumor. The goal of this committee is to investigate all aspects of the disease. For the first time, there is an opportunity to enroll most of the approximately 300 patients diagnosed each year with retinoblastoma in North America in clinical trials. The new international retinoblastoma classification and staging systems for intraocular and extraocular disease are used in the staging and assignment of patients to specific protocols.

A study of patients with unilateral disease was the first protocol to open; the study's main objective was estimating the incidence of "high-risk" histopathologic features following enucleation. There is consensus about the definitions of high-risk features that predict recurrence in patients who undergo enucleation for unilateral advanced disease. Involvement of the choroid by the tumor and extension of the tumor into the optic nerve posterior to the lamina cribrosa are features that are generally considered to be predictive of recurrence. However, this is not widely accepted, as the previous studies were mostly retrospective and had different definitions of choroid and optic nerve involvement. In an effort to prospectively evaluate all enucleated eyes from patients with unilateral disease for specific histopathologic features, a committee of three pathologists was formed as part of this study to develop a consensus pathology report based on definite criteria for choroidal involvement and other features. In addition, patients who meet the criteria for choroidal involvement and postlamina optic nerve involvement receive chemotherapy consisting of three agents as per the protocol. This protocol is currently accruing.

With the wide acceptance of the ABC international classification system for intraocular retinoblastoma [2], the role of chemotherapy can be more definitively evaluated in multi-institutional studies. Extensive intraocular disease that corresponds to group B disease requires chemotherapy in addition to local therapies to salvage the vision and eye. Chemotherapy regimens include carboplatin, vincristine, and etoposide. However, data from a single institution suggest that carboplatin and vincristine without the use of etoposide can be effective in this stage of the disease. This would decrease toxicity as well as the number of visits to the hospital. Therefore, a study was initiated by the COG to evaluate the efficacy of two drugs—carboplatin and vincristine—in conjunction with local treatments to salvage eyes with group B intraocular disease. This study also evaluates the response to the initial course of chemotherapy that is not accompanied by local therapies.

A third COG study addresses group C and D intraocular disease and evaluates the efficacy of high-dose carboplatin given over 2 days along with etoposide and vincristine in saving the globe from enucleation. This study is based on pilot data from Children's Hospital Los Angeles who received high doses of carboplatin along with subtenon carboplatin. The recommended number of subtenon injections is 3. When six injections were given, there was evidence of orbital retraction and cosmetic defects. With this regimen, clinicians from the Children's Hospital Los Angeles were able to save 2 of 3 group C eyes and 11 of 19 group D eyes without EBRT or enucleation. This study is open only to a limited number of institutions. The goal of this study is to salvage the globes and the residual vision of patients with group C or D disease.

The fourth COG study that is currently accruing patients addresses patients with extraocular disease. This involves patients with orbital disease, extracranial metastatic disease, and central nervous system disease. Staging for this protocol is based on the international staging system for extraocular disease. High-dose chemotherapy and stem cell rescue are part of the treatment for patients with extensive disease beyond the orbit. Radiation therapy is also part of the treatment, and the dose and the volume irradiated depend on response to systemic chemotherapy. This study is actively recruiting patients from institutions from countries all over the world and is an international collaboration.

14.9 Animal Models of Retinoblastoma

Retinoblastoma is uniquely a disease of human children. Rb1 mutations do not result in the development of retinal tumors in other animals. This has been hypothesized to be due to redundancy in the expression of retinoblastoma gene family members during fetal eye development in animals other than humans. Two approaches have been used to create animal models of retinoblastoma: the xenografting of human tissue in animals and the development of transgenic mice.

Establishing xenografts of human retinoblastoma cell lines necessitates the use of immune-compromised animals to prevent rejection. Such xenografts have been successfully established in the eyes of mice, rats, and rabbits, using either transgenic immune-compromised animals or drug-induced immune suppression. Because the animals receive intravitreous injections of tumor cells, these models mimic retinoblastoma with vitreous seeds rather than disease originating from primary retinal tumors. A murine model that exhibits extensive optic nerve and choroidal invasive disease that can result in central nervous system metastasis has been described [47]. These models have been successfully used to model gene transfer and oncolytic virus strategies to treat human disease [48, 49].

Another approach to animal models of retinoblastoma has been the development of murine transgenic models. The oncogenic viral protein SV40 T-antigen binds to and sequesters all retinoblastoma family members and p53. Introduction of the gene encoding this SV40 protein driven by appropriate promoters into embryonic mice has resulted in primary retinal tumors that are similar to retinoblastoma in appearance and, to varying degrees, biology. Another approach has been to knock out varying combinations of *retinoblastoma* gene family members in mice. Again, retinal tumors develop in these animals. Transgenic models have been used to study intraocular tumor response to chemotherapy and tumor biology.

While both types of animal models have proven useful to study preclinical response to potential novel therapeutic interventions, both have drawbacks. Xenograft models use immune-deficient animals, and therefore the host immune response to the therapies cannot be monitored. Transgenic tumors are not the result of the same genetic mutations as human tumors, and nonhuman cells do not respond to therapeutic modalities in the same way as do human cells. Therefore, the animal tumors might respond differently than the human counterparts, especially to therapies using delivery systems derived from viral vectors. These caveats must be kept in mind when interpreting therapeutic results of preclinical trials.

14.10 Gene Transfer Technology for Treatment of Retinoblastoma

Adenoviral vectors have been shown to transfer transgenes to human retinoblastoma both in vitro and in vivo [48, 50]. While the introduction of the normal *Rb1* gene can reduce the proliferation of retinoblastoma, the transfer of the herpes simplex thymidine kinase gene using adenoviral vectors into retinoblastoma tumors and then treating the animal with the anti-herpes drug ganciclovir (suicide gene therapy) is superior [48]. The cytotoxic phosphorylated ganciclovir can be transported to adjacent tumor cells and result in the killing of cells that have not been transduced by the viral vector. This is termed a "bystander effect" and can greatly amplify the therapeutic potential of therapeutic gene transfer.

The successful validation of this preclinical strategy in xenograft models of retinoblastoma led to the development of a phase I trial to test the use of intravitreous adenoviral vector delivery of the herpes simplex thymidine kinase gene followed by ganciclovir for bilateral retinoblastoma complicated by vitreous seeds in children in whom all standard therapies for the disease had failed and who were facing a second enucleation. Nine children were treated and all had a complete clinical response of their vitreous seeds to this potential therapy. However, recurrent retinal disease and local toxic effects resulted in the subsequent enucleation of these eyes. Toxic reactions consisted of a transient inflammatory response that could be controlled with anti-inflammatory therapy. The inflammation appeared to be more severe in children with more extensive tumor seeding. Importantly, the intraocular injections did not result in the spread of the tumor through the needle track, suggesting that other therapies could be delivered by intraocular injection [51].

Use of an oncolytic picornavirus for the treatment of metastatic retinoblastoma has also been studied in a murine xenograft model of retinoblastoma [49]. In contrast to gene transfer using a viral vector, for which the virus is made replication incompetent, this oncolytic virus is a naturally occurring replication-competent virus. All of the treated animals had at least a partial response and most of the animals had a complete extraocular response to a single intravenous injection of this virus. None of the treated animals developed central nervous system metastases. Intravenous delivery of the virus did not control intraocular disease. A phase I trial to determine the toxicity of this virus in adults is ongoing, and a phase I trial to treat neuroendocrine tumors in children is under development.

14.11 Future Development

As translational research progresses from the laboratory to the clinic, it is likely that new approaches to retinoblastoma will be focused on localizing drug delivery directly to the eye, thereby avoiding systemic toxicity associated with current modalities. Intra-arterial chemotherapy and transscleral depot reservoirs are two such approaches that hold promise for the future.

References

1. Reese AB, Ellsworth RM. The evaluation and current concept of retinoblastoma therapy. Trans Am Acad Ophthalmol Otolaryngol 1963;67:164–72.
2. Murphree AL. Intraocular retinoblastoma: the case for a new group classification. Ophthalmol Clin North Am 2005;18(1):41–53, viii.

3. Shields CL, Mashayekhi A, Au AK, et al. The International Classification of Retinoblastoma predicts chemoreduction success. Ophthalmology 2006;113(12):2276–80.
4. Dryja TP, Cavenee W, White R, et al. Homozygosity of chromosome 13 in retinoblastoma. N Engl J Med 1984;310:550–3.
5. Classon M, Harlow E. The retinoblastoma tumour suppressor in development and cancer. Nat Rev Cancer 2002;2:910–7.
6. Hagstrom SA, Dryja TP. Mitotic recombination map of 13cen-13q14 derived from an investigation of loss of heterozygosity in retinoblastomas. Proc Natl Acad Sci U S A 1999;96:2952–7.
7. Sherr CJ. Cancer cell cycles. Science 1996;274:1672–7.
8. Wong FL, Boice JD Jr, Abramson DH, et al. Cancer incidence after retinoblastoma: radiation dose and sarcoma risk. JAMA 1997;278:1262–7.
9. Rubenfeld M, Abramson DH, Ellsworth RM, et al. Unilateral vs. bilateral retinoblastoma: correlations between age at diagnosis and stage of ocular disease. Ophthalmology 1986;93:1016–9.
10. Noorani HZ, Khan HN, Gallie BL, et al. Cost comparison of molecular versus conventional screening of relatives at risk for retinoblastoma. Am J Hum Genet 1996;59:301–7.
11. Cohen JG, Dryja TP, Nicholls KB, et al. RB1 genetic testing as a clinical service: a follow-up study. Med Pediatr Oncol 2001;37:372–8.
12. McLean IW, Burnier M, Zimmerman L, et al. Tumors of the retina. In: McLean IW, Burnier MN, Zimmerman LE, Fa J, editors. Atlas of Tumor Pathology. Tumors of the Eye and Ocular Adnexa. Washington, DC: Armed Forces Institute of Pathology, 1994: 100–35.
13. Hurwitz RL, Chévez-Barrios P, Chintagumpala M, et al. Retinoblastoma. In: Pizzo PA, Poplack D, editors. Principles and Practice of Pediatric Oncology, 6th edition. Philadelphia, PA: Lippincott-Raven, 2002:825–46.
14. Chévez-Barrios P, Eagle RC, Marbach P. Histological features and risks for metastatic spread of retinoblastoma. In: Singh AD, Damato B, Pe'er J, Murphree AL, Perry JD, editors. Clinical Ocular Oncology, first edition. London: Elsevier Saunders, 2007:468–76.
15. Karcioglu ZA, al Mesfer SA, Abboud E, et al. Workup for metastatic retinoblastoma. A review of 261 patients. Ophthalmology 1997,104:307 12.
16. Friedman DL, Himelstein B, Shields CL, et al. Chemoreduction and local ophthalmic therapy for intraocular retinoblastoma. J Clin Oncol 2000;18(1):12–7.
17. Brichard B, De Bruycker JJ, De Potter P, et al. Combined chemotherapy and local treatment in the management of intraocular retinoblastoma. Med Pediatr Oncol 2002;38(6): 411–5.
18. Antoneli CB, Ribeiro KC, Steinhorst F, et al. Treatment of retinoblastoma patients with chemoreduction plus local therapy: experience of the AC Camargo Hospital, Brazil. J Pediatr Hematol Oncol 2006;28(6):342–5.
19. Rodriguez-Galindo C, Wilson MW, Haik BG, et al. Treatment of intraocular retinoblastoma with vincristine and carboplatin. J Clin Oncol 2003;21(10):2019–25.
20. Schiavetti A, Hadjistillianou T, Clerico A, et al. Conservative therapy in intraocular retinoblastoma: response/recurrence rate. J Pediatr Hematol Oncol 2005;27(1):3–6.
21. Zage PE, Reitman AJ, Seshadri R, et al. Outcomes of a two-drug chemotherapy regimen for intraocular retinoblastoma. Pediatr Blood Cancer 2008;50(3):567–72.
22. Williams PC, Hemer WD, Roman-Goldstein S, et al. Toxicity and efficacy of carboplatin and etoposide in conjunction with disruption of the blood-brain tumor barrier in the treatment of intracranial neoplasms. Neurosurgery 1995;37(1):17–27; discussion 27–8.
23. Chantada GL, Fandino AC, Raslawski EC, et al. Experience with chemoreduction and focal therapy for intraocular retinoblastoma in a developing country. Pediatr Blood Cancer 2005;44(5):455–60.
24. Hadjistilianou T, Mastrangelo D, De Francesco S, et al. Brief report: conservative treatment in unilateral retinoblastoma: a preliminary report. Med Pediatr Oncol 2002;38(6):439–41.

25. Shields CL, Shelil A, Cater J, et al. Development of new retinoblastomas after 6 cycles of chemoreduction for retinoblastoma in 162 eyes of 106 consecutive patients. Arch Ophthalmol 2003;121(11):1571–6.
26. Beck MN, Balmer A, Dessing C, et al. First-line chemotherapy with local treatment can prevent external-beam irradiation and enucleation in low-stage intraocular retinoblastoma. J Clin Oncol 2000;18(15):2881–7.
27. Levy C, Doz F, Quintana E, et al. Role of chemotherapy alone or in combination with hyperthermia in the primary treatment of intraocular retinoblastoma: preliminary results. Br J Ophthalmol 1998;82(10):1154–8.
28. Hungerford JL, Toma NM, Plowman PN, et al. External beam radiotherapy for retinoblastoma: I. Whole eye technique. Br J Ophthalmol 1995;79(2):109–11.
29. Shields CL, Shields JA, DePotter P, et al. The effect of chemoreduction on retinoblastoma-induced retinal detachment. J Pediatr Ophthalmol Strabismus 1997;34(3):165–9.
30. Wilson MW, Rodriguez-Galindo C, Haik BG, et al. Multiagent chemotherapy as neoadjuvant treatment for multifocal intraocular retinoblastoma. Ophthalmology 2001;108(11):2106–14; discussion 2114–5.
31. Abramson DH, Ellsworth RM, Rozakis GW. Cryotherapy for retinoblastoma. Arch Ophthalmol 1982;100(8):1253–6.
32. Shields JA, Shields CL, Donoso LA, et al. Current treatment of retinoblastoma. Trans Pa Acad Ophthalmol Otolaryngol 1989;41:818–22.
33. Shields CL, Shields JA, Cater J, et al. Plaque radiotherapy for retinoblastoma: long-term tumor control and treatment complications in 208 tumors. Ophthalmology 2001;108(11):2116–21.
34. Abramson DH, Schefler AC. Transpupillary thermotherapy as initial treatment for small intraocular retinoblastoma: technique and predictors of success. Ophthalmology 2004;111(5):984–91.
35. Lee SY, Kim DK, Cho JH, et al. Inhibitory effect of bevacizumab on the angiogenesis and growth of retinoblastoma. Arch Ophthalmol 2008;126(7):953–8.
36. Dalgard CL, Van Quill KR, O'Brien JM. Evaluation of the in vitro and in vivo antitumor activity of histone deacetylase inhibitors for the therapy of retinoblastoma. Clin Cancer Res 2008;14(10):3113–23.
37. Laurie NA, Donovan SL, Shih CS, et al. Inactivation of the p53 pathway in retinoblastoma. Nature 2006;444:61–6.
38. Wadhwa L, Hurwitz MY, Chevez-Barrios P, et al. Treatment of invasive retinoblastoma in a murine model using an oncolytic picornavirus. Cancer Res 2007;67(22):10653–6.
39. Kleinerman RA, Tucker MA, Tarone RE, et al. Risk of new cancers after radiotherapy in long-term survivors of retinoblastoma: an extended follow-up. J Clin Oncol 2005;23(10): 2272–9.
40. Dunkel IJ, Aledo A, Kernan NA, et al. Successful treatment of metastatic retinoblastoma. Cancer 2000;89(10):2117–21.
41. Kremens B, Wieland R, Reinhard H, et al. High-dose chemotherapy with autologous stem cell rescue in children with retinoblastoma. Bone Marrow Transplant 2003;31(4):281–4.
42. Lee SH, Yoo KH, Sung KW, et al. Tandem high-dose chemotherapy and autologous stem cell rescue in children with bilateral advanced retinoblastoma. Bone Marrow Transplant 2008;42(6):385–91.
43. Matsubara H, Makimoto A, Higa T, et al. A multidisciplinary treatment strategy that includes high-dose chemotherapy for metastatic retinoblastoma without CNS involvement. Bone Marrow Transplant 2005;35(8):763–6.
44. Namouni F, Doz F, Tanguy ML, et al. High-dose chemotherapy with carboplatin, etoposide, and cyclophosphamide followed by a hematopoietic stem cell rescue in patients with high-risk retinoblastoma: a SFOP and SFGM study. Eur J Cancer 1997;33(14):2368–75.
45. Gombos DS, Hungerford JH, Abramson DH, et al. Secondary acute myelogenous leukemia in patients with retinoblastoma: is chemotherapy a factor? Ophthalmology 2007;114(7): 1378–83.

46. Gunduz K, Shields CL, Shields JA, et al. The outcome of chemoreduction treatment in patients with Reese-Ellsworth group V retinoblastoma. Arch Ophthalmol 1998;116(12):1613–7.
47. Chevez-Barrios P, Hurwitz MY, Louie K, et al. Metastatic and nonmetastatic models of retinoblastoma. Am J Pathol 2000;157:1405–12.
48. Hurwitz MY, Marcus KT, Chevez-Barrios P, et al. Suicide gene therapy for treatment of retinoblastoma in a murine model. Hum Gene Ther 1999;10: 441–8.
49. Wadhwa L, Hurwitz MY, Chevez-Barrios P, et al. Treatment of invasive retinoblastoma in a murine model using an oncolytic picornavirus. Cancer Res 2007;67:10653–6.
50. Mallam JN, Hurwitz MY, Mahoney T, et al. Efficient gene transfer into retinal cells using adenoviral vectors: dependence on receptor expression. Invest Ophthalmol Vis Sci 2004;45:1680–7.
51. Chevez-Barrios P, Chintagumpala M, Mieler W, et al. Response of retinoblastoma with vitreous tumor seeding to adenovirus-mediated delivery of thymidine kinase followed by ganciclovir. J Clin Oncol 2005;23:7927–35.
52. Lee V, Hungerford JL, Bunce C, et al. Globe conserving treatment of the only eye in bilateral retinoblastoma. Br J Ophthalmol 2003;87(11):1374–80.

Chapter 15
Management of Uveal Melanoma

Michelle Ludwig, Adam S. Garden, Michelle D. Williams, and Dan S. Gombos

Abstract About 3% of all melanomas are of ocular origin; of these, 85% are uveal. Uveal melanomas are rare, with standardized incidence rates ranging from approximately 2 to 8 cases per 1 million people in the United States and Europe. The typical presentation of uveal melanoma depends on the site of origin: choroid, iris, or ciliary body. About 80–90% of all uveal melanomas develop in the posterior choroid. Uveal melanoma is typically a clinical rather than a pathologic diagnosis. Currently, several options are available for the management of uveal melanoma, including observation, transpupillary thermotherapy, brachytherapy, stereotactic radiotherapy, proton radiotherapy, and tumor resection.

15.1 Epidemiology

About 3% of all melanomas are of ocular origin; of these, 85% are uveal, and the majority are choroidal. Uveal melanomas are rare, with standardized incidence rates ranging from approximately 2 to 8 cases per 1 million people in the United States and Europe. Mean age at diagnosis is approximately 60 years, with the incidence rate increasing to age 70. Risk factors for development of uveal melanoma include history of choroidal nevi, ipsilateral nevus of Ota, and atypical mole syndrome. Weak correlations have suggested sunlight exposure as a possible causative agent. Welders and metal workers have also been reported as having a slightly higher incidence of uveal melanoma, possibly due to ultraviolet light exposure [1].

M. Ludwig (✉)
Department of Radiation Oncology, The University of Texas M.D. Anderson Cancer Center, Houston, TX, USA
e-mail: mludwig@mdanderson.org

B. Esmaeli (ed.), *Ophthalmic Oncology*, M.D. Anderson Solid Tumor Oncology Series 6, DOI 10.1007/978-1-4419-0374-7_15,

15.2 Clinical Features

The typical presentation of uveal melanoma depends on the site of origin: choroid, iris, or ciliary body. About 80–90% of all uveal melanomas develop in the posterior choroid. Patients with these tumors generally present with complaints of blurred vision or floaters. Occasionally, pain, inflammation, or double vision is noted. Metamorphopsia (distortion of vision) and photopsias (flashing lights) are not uncommon symptoms and may be associated with an exudative retinal detachment [2, 3].

Iris melanomas are generally smaller at diagnosis than those of the choroid. Iris melanomas can grow in a circumscribed or diffuse pattern. The circumscribed type can vary in color and invade the anterior chamber, ciliary body, or posterior chamber. Diffuse iris melanomas can infiltrate the iris stroma, causing pupillary distortion.

Ciliary body melanoma can develop as a circumscribed or annular type. The circumscribed type is often brown and can invade the anterior chamber, causing elevated intraocular pressure. In contrast, the annular type grows around the ciliary body in a ring-type fashion. Ciliary body melanoma may be initially misdiagnosed as open-angle glaucoma because of the difficulty in visualizing a distinct mass [3, 4].

As the uvea has no intrinsic lymphatic drainage, metastasis occurs by hematogenous dissemination. Ciliary body melanomas can invade anteriorly toward the sclerocorneal limbus. Posteriorly located tumors can spread via the vortex veins or ciliary arteries, or they can have frank invasion past the sclera. Large peripapillary tumors can invade the optic nerve and adjacent meninges. The liver is the primary site of distant metastasis, followed by the skin and lung; brain metastasis rarely occurs [3].

15.3 Diagnosis

Uveal melanoma is typically a clinical rather than a pathologic diagnosis. A 20–40% misdiagnosis rate has been reported in historical series following enucleation. Yet with recent advances, this has been reduced to less than 1%. As is the case with any malignancy, a thorough systematic history should be obtained.

An external ocular examination should be performed to evaluate for dilated episcleral vessels or pigmented nodules suggestive of extraocular extension. Slit-lamp evaluation can reveal bulging of the iris, a distinct iris or ciliary body mass, cataract, or subluxation of lens. Indirect ophthalmoscopy can demonstrate details regarding tumor color, size, and configuration. Features such as drusen, subretinal fluid, retinal pigment epithelial changes, and orange pigment are important prognostic indicators that should be documented [5].

Gonioscopy should be performed for all tumors in the anterior segment. Fluorescein angiography can demonstrate pinpoint hyperfluorescence or a distinct "second" choroidal vasculature [6]. Echography should be performed in all cases and is the single most important noninvasive test. Typical ultrasonographic features of choroidal melanomas on B-scan echography include an internal acoustic quiet zone, choroidal excavation, and orbital shadowing (Fig. 15.1a). A-scan echography demonstrates low internal reflectivity with an angle kappa (Fig. 15.1b) [7, 8]. In rare cases in which these noninvasive techniques do not establish the diagnosis, tissue biopsy can be performed via an ab externo or ab interno approach.

Baseline testing should include liver function tests and chest and liver imaging (generally a computed tomography of the chest and abdomen with contrast) to rule out distant metastasis. Magnetic resonance imaging of the brain and orbit can be helpful in identifying intraocular features consistent with melanoma (Fig. 15.2).

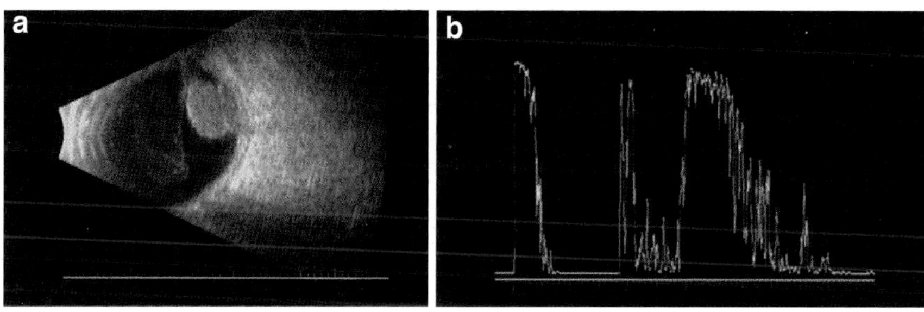

Fig. 15.1 Ultrasonography demonstrates the features of a mass consistent with left-sided ciliochoroidal melanoma. (**a**) The first scan is a B-scan sonogram with a collar-button appearance. (**b**) The second scan is an A-scan sonogram with low internal reflectivity

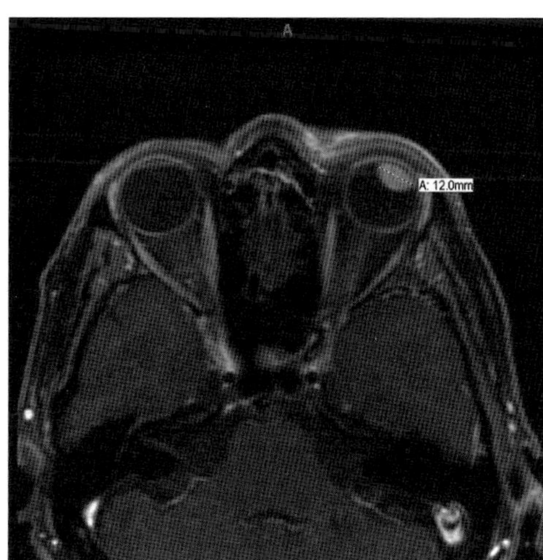

Fig. 15.2 Magnetic resonance imaging showing an intraocular melanoma, left eye

15.4 Staging and Prognostic Factors

Currently, the staging process is less than ideal for uveal melanoma. Accurate use of the American Joint Committee on Cancer TNM staging system requires pathologic diagnosis, which is often not obtained in uveal melanoma cases since most are treated with brachytherapy. No widely accepted staging system is used for most iris melanomas.

In patients with uveal melanoma, prognostic factors for patient survival differ from prognostic factors for eye and vision preservation. The most important feature predicting mortality in uveal melanoma is largest basal diameter. Other factors correlating with increased morbidity include extrascleral extension, diffuse presentation, older age, male gender, rapid growth, and recurrence after treatment. Pathologic features in enucleated specimens indicative of poor prognosis include a large number of mitotic figures per high-power field or high Ki-67; a high number of tumor-infiltrating lymphocytes; and periodic acid Schiff identification of vasculogenic mimicry patterns. Fine-needle biopsy for tissue prognostication is currently undergoing scientific testing in a number of centers. Fluorescence in situ hybridization studies have suggested molecular abnormalities associated with chromosomes 1, 3, 6, and 8. Monosomy 3 strongly correlates with metastatic disease. Gene expression profiling using microarray analysis suggests that uveal melanomas can be divided into two groups. "Class 1" tumors (low grade) are thought to have a much lower risk of distant metastasis than "class 2" tumors (high grade) [9–13].

15.5 Background Studies

Historically, enucleation was considered the only acceptable method of managing uveal melanomas. In the late 1970s, this practice was brought into question by suggestions that enucleation might expedite metastasis by promoting intraoperative seeding of tumor cells (Zimmerman's hypothesis) [14]. To evaluate this hypothesis, the Collaborative Ocular Melanoma Study (COMS) was organized in 1986. This was a multicenter effort with 43 participating centers in the United States and Canada. The COMS investigators conducted several studies, including two randomized trials and an observational study; in addition to reports on these studies, several technical papers have been published on the basis of the COMS results [15–17].

The observational study evaluated risk factors for growth of small melanomas (less than 3.0 mm in apical height) [18]. A total of 204 patients were enrolled and 188 were observed. On multivariate analysis, tumor characteristics associated with greater likelihood of growth included the presence of orange pigment, tumor thickness of at least 2 mm, and largest basal diameter of at least 12 mm [19].

One of the randomized clinical trials was conducted for medium-sized choroidal melanomas (2.5–10 mm in apical height and no more than 16 mm in largest basal diameter); patients were randomized to receive either enucleation or iodine-125 plaque brachytherapy [20]. Patients with tumors touching the optic disc or primarily in the ciliary body were excluded. A total of 1317 patients were randomized, and 12-year follow-up data showed no difference in melanoma-related morbidity between the two treatment arms. Visual loss secondary to brachytherapy correlated with tumor thickness, tumor proximity to the foveal avascular zone, and a history of diabetes. Visual loss was significant, with 43% of patients progressing to an acuity of 20/200 (legal blindness) within 3 years. The contralateral eye, however, was not affected by treatment. Patients with recurrence after brachytherapy were treated with enucleation for salvage; about 10% of patients who underwent enucleation had recurrence at 5 years [21]. A quality-of-life study was performed on 209 of the 1317 patients and found that visual acuity in patients who received brachytherapy was greater than that in patients who underwent enucleation until about 3–5 years after treatment [22].

In the second randomized trial, a total of 1003 patients with large tumors (greater than 10 mm in apical height or 16 mm in largest basal diameter) were randomized to enucleation with or without presurgical radiotherapy consisting of 20 Gy in five fractions [23]. This study was designed to address concerns regarding the possibility of tumor seeding during enucleation and the potential benefit of pre-enucleation radiotherapy. On 10-year follow-up, no difference was noticed in melanoma-related mortality, and neither harm nor benefit was ascribed to pre-enucleation radiotherapy [23].

In both of the randomized COMS trials—for medium and large choroidal melanoma—annual screening after treatment included liver function tests and chest radiography. The use of liver function tests to identify distant metastasis had a sensitivity of 15% and specificity of 92%; thus, the COMS authors recommended annual liver imaging. Liver echography and computed tomography are the most common methods of liver imaging, but some centers advocate the use of routine positron emission tomography scans.

15.6 Overview of Management

Currently, several options for the management of uveal melanoma are available, including observation, transpupillary thermotherapy, brachytherapy, stereotactic radiotherapy, charged-particle radiotherapy, and tumor resection. A choice between these modalities depends on tumor size, location, and growth pattern and the condition of the patient. The goal of vision and organ preservation should be balanced with that of tumor control. Asymptomatic tumors that are less than 10 mm in basal diameter and less than 2.5 mm in thickness may be reasonable candidates for observation. Medium-sized uveal melanomas generally receive brachytherapy but may be amenable to charged-particle radiotherapy or resection. Larger tumors are often treated by enucleation [14, 19].

15.7 Brachytherapy

The concept of treating uveal melanoma with brachytherapy began in the 1930s when Sir Foster Moore inserted radon 222 seeds directly into a choroidal melanoma. This technique was later changed to use of episcleral cobalt 60 and then to ruthenium 106 and iodine 125 eye plaques. Iodine 125 was used in the COMS protocol and is a practical isotope because low-energy photon radiation allows for shielding with 1 mm of lead, reducing dose to hospital personnel. Iodine 125's half-life of 59 days allows for re-use of the seeds [24]. The plaque is shielded with gold, and the iodine 125 seeds are set in a template. These plaques can be customized to fit specific tumor locations, e.g., a notch can be placed to fit around the optic nerve. Plaques are available in various sizes ranging from 12 to 22 mm in diameter with multiple suture holes (Fig. 15.3) [24].

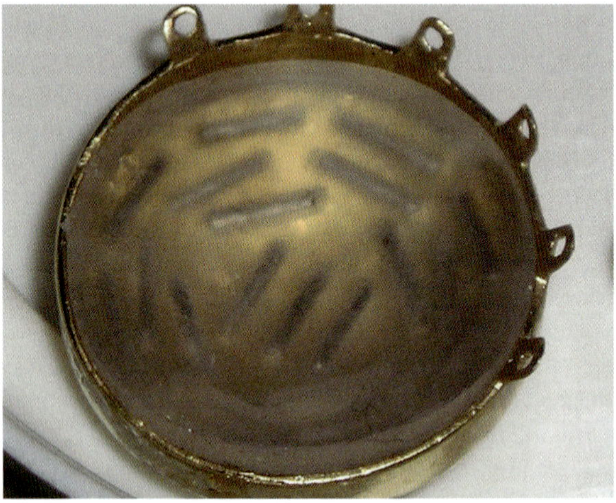

Fig. 15.3 An 18-mm iodine 125 plaque with 21 seeds

Ruthenium 106 is used at some institutions in Europe and has been used at our institution, but it is no longer commercially available in the United States. It is a beta emitter with a steeper dose gradient than iodine 125, allowing for lower dose delivery to surrounding structures. The half-life of ruthenium 106 is about 1 year, allowing for re-use of the plaque. This source is generally used for tumors with apical height of less than 5 mm. These plaques are thinner than the COMS iodine 125 plaques, making surgical placement easier and more comfortable for the patient.

Treatment planning begins with indirect ophthalmoscopy and ocular ultrasonography to delineate the location and exact dimensions of the tumor. The plaque size is chosen to give a 2–3 mm margin around the tumor base. As per the COMS protocol, dosing is based on the apical height measured from the scleral surface. A total dose of 85 Gy is prescribed to the apex of the tumor if the tumor apical height is greater than 5 mm; a total dose of 85 mm is prescribed to 5-mm height if the apical height is 5 mm or less. Because of the sharp dose gradient of the brachytherapy system, the apex is the prescription point and the area of minimum tumor dose. As such, much of the tumor actually receives more than the prescribed dose. Total dose rates should fall between 42.5 and 106 cGy/h. The use of a three-dimensional treatment planning system allows for decreased dose to be delivered to critical structures while ensuring dose delivery to the tumor by collimation of individual seeds [24].

Placement of the plaque is done in the operating room. The ophthalmologist transilluminates the globe and outlines the tumor shadow on the sclera. A dummy plaque is then placed over the marking, and loose sutures are placed in the suture holes. With the radiation oncologist present, the dummy plaque is removed, replaced by the radioactive plaque, and fastened in place with the sutures. A lead shield is placed over the affected eye as a safety precaution. The plaque is left in place for a number days, after which the patient is taken back to the operating room for removal of the plaque (Fig. 15.4).

This treatment is well tolerated in the short term. Late effects include dry eye, retinopathy, glaucoma, maculopathy, and scleral necrosis, depending on the proximity of the tumor and the radiation dose to adjacent structures. A significant percentage of patients develop radiation retinopathy. In a large review, poor long-term visual acuity was found to be associated with tumor location less than 5 mm from the fovea, age greater than 60 years, and use of cobalt 60 plaques [25].

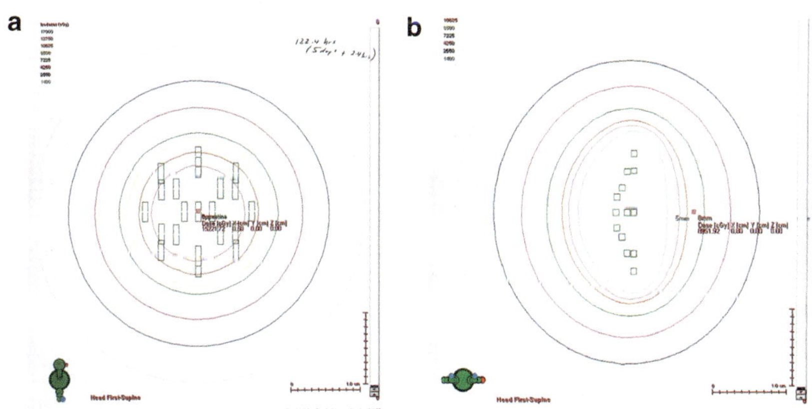

Fig. 15.4 Dose distribution of iodine 125; 85 Gy prescribed to apical height of 8.3 mm

15.8 Charged-Particle Radiotherapy

Proton radiotherapy offers the potential to deliver a homogenous and conformal dose to tumors, particularly those located close to critical structures such as the macula or optic disc. The physical properties of protons are such that stopping power is great, allowing for a high-dose deposition in the desired location with no exit dose. Restrictions related to tumor size or location are less than those with brachytherapy. The use of charged particles in treatment of uveal melanoma began in 1975, and about 20 institutions around the world have employed this approach [24].

Treatment planning is similar to the typical evaluation for uveal melanoma, with the addition of surgical tumor localization. Patients undergo intraoperative transillumination, and the base of the tumor is marked by suturing radio-opaque tantalum rings to the sclera around the tumor. Tumor and eye dimensions are entered into the treatment planning computer, and an aperture is designed for the proton beam that approximates the shape of the tumor with a 3-mm lateral margin. Doses to critical structures are calculated in the treatment plan made by the computer but assessed by the MD. During treatment, patients are immobilized, and the eye is aligned on a flashing light; the eye is monitored for movement. Lid retraction is used to reduce treatment of the eyelid. The standard dose is 60–70 cobalt Gy equivalents in four to five fractions [24].

Several extensive series of uveal melanoma patients treated with proton radiotherapy have been published. Neovascular glaucoma was the most common cause of subsequent enucleation and was more prominent in patients with larger tumor volumes [25]. Other complications included radiation maculopathy and papillopathy, which was greater among patients with tumors close to the optic disc. Vision loss was associated with dose to the macula of greater than 35 cobalt Gy equivalents, larger apical height, and a history of diabetes. Local tumor control is excellent with protons. Comparison of complication and survival rates between proton and plaque treatment is difficult since many patients are referred to proton centers because of larger tumor size or tumor location close to the optic disc or macula [26–30].

15.9 Surgical Techniques

15.9.1 Uveal Resection

Depending on the size and location of the tumor, uveal resection can be a good treatment option for globe salvage. Small iris and ciliary body tumors (less than 4 clock hours) can be safely resected by iridectomy or iridocyclectomy techniques. Some surgeons advocate hypotensive anesthesia to reduce the risk of expulsive hemorrhage. The main complications are iris coloboma and lens instability from ciliary body excision. Visually, this can lead to photophobia and polyopia. Transscleral resection of choroidal tumors was popularized in the late 1970s and 1980s; however, given the high percentage of scleral invasion in many uveal melanomas, there is concern about inadequate resection with such procedures [31]. As a result, some centers routinely treat patients with adjuvant plaque brachytherapy at the time of resection [31, 32]. This approach (uveal resection) also exposes the patient to the possibility of expulsive hemorrhage and the risk of orbital tumor seeding.

15.9.2 Enucleation

Primary enucleation is typically used with large uveal melanomas that involve greater than one-half of the globe. Integrated implants, such as hydroxyapatite and Medpor, are generally implanted and provide excellent cosmesis with good ocular motility. When local extraocular extension is present, a modified enucleation can be performed with excision of the overlying tissue removed en bloc with the globe. Exenteration is rarely indicated but can provide good local control in cases of diffuse orbital involvement.

15.9.3 Transpupillary Thermotherapy

Transpupillary thermotherapy involves a low-energy diode laser that heats the tumor and surrounding choroid to 45–60°C. The laser is generally administered in multiple sessions. As a primary treatment modality, this technique is recognized as being associated with a risk of local recurrence, especially for thicker tumors and tumors that overhang the optic nerve. Transpupillary thermotherapy is increasingly used as an adjuvant modality following plaque brachytherapy (also referred to as "sandwich" therapy, which is brachytherapy followed by thermotherapy). Significant visual field loss can occur in the area treated; other complications include extrascleral extension, hemorrhage, and vascular occlusion [33].

15.9.4 Pathologic Assessment

An enucleation specimen is the most common tissue specimen obtained for pathologic evaluation. The intact globe is received fresh from the operating room when tissue is harvested for research purposes and/or tissue banking. Initial pathologic assessment of the specimen includes three-dimensional measurements of the globe and the length of the attached optic nerve. Also, the iris is examined for any deformity or gross involvement by the tumor. Each external component of the eye and anterior chamber is evaluated, and any abnormalities are documented. Samples of the vortex veins, located in the posterior portion of each quadrant, should be obtained for histologic examination. The entire extraocular portion of each vein is removed, and its location is noted (Fig. 15.5). A compound microscope may be used for gross assessment of ocular specimens, as needed.

Transillumination is used to locate the intraocular mass. When a light is held directly proximal to the pupil or sclera, light is transmitted into the vitreous, which glows through the sclera when the normal ocular structures are in place. A shadow, when noted, is marked on the sclera with a colored pencil, and its location is noted relative to its distance from the limbus, optic nerve, and region involved (i.e., 11:00 to 2:00) (Fig. 15.6). The basal dimensions of the tumor are also noted. Although the

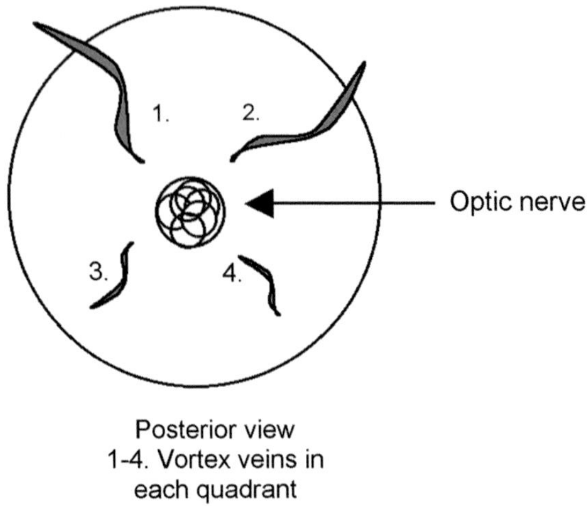

Fig. 15.5 Histologic sampling of the extraocular portions of the vortex veins, which exit the globe posteriorly in each quadrant, is recommended

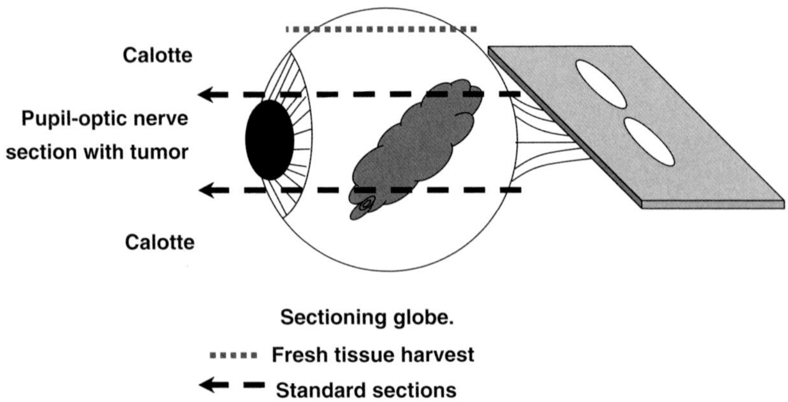

Fig. 15.6 Once the tumor base is located using transillumination, the globe is oriented with the tumor in the plane of the optic nerve and pupil and transected directly above the optic nerve to the edge of the pupil, as shown

shadow may correspond directly to the mass, retinal detachment can also cause a shadow that may obscure the exact size and location of the tumor.

Optimal sectioning of the tumor, following fixation in 10% buffered formalin, is generally achieved when the pupil and optic nerve are seen in cross section along with the tumor (Fig. 15.6) [34]. Horizontal, vertical, or oblique sectioning of the globe can be used to obtain this orientation.

If fresh tissue is to be harvested prior to fixation, a window or flap is opened adjacent to the tumor in the same plane from which the main tissue sections will be taken (Fig. 15.6). Normal retina and choroid are removed from the scleral flap. The tumor is then incised, using a sterile scalpel blade parallel to the window, and removed with forceps. No more than one-third of any tumor should be harvested to ensure the integrity of the specimen for histologic diagnosis. Also, tissue harvesting should be avoided when the tumor is small or flat or when it is poorly visualized.

15.9.5 Histologic Examination

Histologic parameters include the initial determination that the lesion is a melanoma [35]. Among the primary intraocular tumors, uveal melanoma is the most common [36]. Uveal melanomas arise most commonly in the choroidal space and less frequently in the ciliary body and iris [35]. Large choroidal melanomas may involve adjacent structures, and any such involvement is noted in the pathologic report. Both the largest tumor dimension and tumor cell types (epithelioid, spindle, or mixed), which are important predictors of outcome, are documented [37, 38]. The growth pattern of a thin, diffuse, spreading melanoma should be documented, and additional hematoxylin and eosin-stained levels of the tumor should be examined, as this growth pattern portends a higher risk of extraocular extension and high risk of metastatic potential (25% at 5 years) despite its flatness [38, 39]. Multiple hematoxylin and eosin-stained levels are examined to check for invasion of the sclera directly or around nerves and vessels and exclude extraocular tumor extension, which would warrant additional therapy. Likewise, involvement of the optic nerve, optic nerve margin, or meninges must be assessed [40].

Unlike retinoblastomas, uveal melanomas generally do not spread via the optic nerve; however, they are more likely than retinoblastomas to invade the vortex veins [38]. Thus, both the vortex veins as they course through the sclera and the extraocular portions of the vortex veins are sampled and assessed [34].

Additional intratumoral factors—including complex vascular loops (which are optimally visualized for evaluation by a periodic acid Schiff stain) and mitotic figures (number of mitoses per 10 high-power fields)—may provide additional prognostic information [40, 41]. The final pathologic report includes both the findings on gross assessment and the pathologic parameters of the uveal melanoma, which facilitates determination of mortality risk for patients with this disease.

15.10 Conclusion

The past two decades have seen significant advances in the ocular treatment of uveal melanomas. Large prospective randomized trials, such as the COMS, have demonstrated the efficacy and benefits of globe-salvaging approaches, such as plaque brachytherapy. Charged-particle radiotherapy has also become an accepted standard of care, particularly for tumors adjacent to critical ocular structures such as the disc and macula. Unfortunately, these advances in treatment of the primary tumor have not been accompanied by advances in treatment for distant metastatic disease, for which limited effective therapy exists. The next decade is likely to see further research in gene expression and identification of specific tumors with high metastatic potential. Those tumors should be targeted with adjuvant therapies to treat and prevent extraocular recurrence and reduce patient morbidity.

References

1. Singh AD, Damato B, Howard P, et al. Uveal melanoma: genetic aspects. Ophthalmol Clin North Am 2005;18(1):85–97, viii.
2. McLean IW, Saraiva VS, Burnier MN Jr. Pathological and prognostic features of uveal melanomas. Can J Ophthalmol 2004;39(4):343–50.
3. Woll E, Bedikian A, Legha SS. Uveal melanoma: natural history and treatment options for metastatic disease. Melanoma Res 1999;9(6):575–81.
4. McLean IW, Keefe KS, Burnier MN. Uveal melanoma. Comparison of the prognostic value of fibrovascular loops, mean of the ten largest nucleoli, cell type, and tumor size. Ophthalmology 1997;104(5):777–80.
5. Damato BE. An approach to the management of patients with uveal melanoma. Eye 1993;7(Pt 3):388–97.
6. Damato B. Detection of uveal melanoma by optometrists in the United Kingdom. Ophthalmic Physiol Opt 2001;21(4):268–71.
7. Liu T, Lizzi FL, Silverman RH, et al. Ultrasonic tissue characterization using 2-D spectrum analysis and its application in ocular tumor diagnosis. Med Phys 2004;31(5):1032–9.
8. Bakri SJ, Sculley L, Singh AD. Imaging techniques for uveal melanoma. Int Ophthalmol Clin 2006;46(1):1–13.
9. Onken MD, Worley LA, Person E, et al. Loss of heterozygosity of chromosome 3 detected with single nucleotide polymorphisms is superior to monosomy 3 for predicting metastasis in uveal melanoma. Clin Cancer Res 2007;13(10):2923–7.
10. Onken MD, Worley LA, Davila RM, et al. Prognostic testing in uveal melanoma by transcriptome profiling of fine-needle biopsy specimens. J Mol Diagn 2006;8(5):567–73.
11. Onken MD, Worley LA, Ehlers JP, et al. Gene expression profiling in uveal melanoma reveals two molecular classes and predicts metastatic death. Cancer Res 2004;64(20):7205–9.
12. Damato B, Eleuteri A, Fisher AC, et al. Artificial neural networks estimating survival probability after treatment of choroidal melanoma. Ophthalmology 2008;115(9):1598–607.
13. Damato B, Duke C, Coupland SE, et al. Cytogenetics of uveal melanoma: a 7-year clinical experience. Ophthalmology 2007;114(10):1925–31.
14. Singh AD, Damato BE, Pe'er J. Clinical Ophthalmic Oncology. Philadelphia, PA: Saunders Elsevier, 2007.
15. Astrahan MA, Luxton G, Jozsef G, et al. An interactive treatment planning system for ophthalmic plaque radiotherapy. Int J Radiat Oncol Biol Phys 1990;18(3):679–87.
16. Chiu-Tsao ST, Anderson LL, O'Brien K, et al. Dosimetry for 125I seed (model 6711) in eye plaques. Med Phys 1993;20(2 Pt 1):383–9.
17. de la Zerda A, Chiu-Tsao ST, Lin J, et al. 125I eye plaque dose distribution including penumbra characteristics. Med Phys 1996;23(3):407–18.
18. The Collaborative Ocular Melanoma Study Group. Factors predictive of growth and treatment of small choroidal melanoma. COMS report no. 5. Arch Ophthalmol 1997;115(12):1537–44.
19. The Collaborative Ocular Melanoma Study Group. Mortality in patients with small choroidal melanoma. COMS report no. 4. Arch Ophthalmol 1997;115(7):886–93.
20. Jampol LM, Moy CS, Murray TG, et al. The COMS randomized trial of iodine 125 brachytherapy for choroidal melanoma: IV. Local treatment failure and enucleation in the first 5 years after brachytherapy. COMS report no. 19. Ophthalmology 2002;109(12):2197–206.
21. Diener-West M, Earle JD, Fine SL, et al. The COMS randomized trial of iodine 125 brachytherapy for choroidal melanoma, III: initial mortality findings. COMS report no. 18. Arch Ophthalmol 2001;119(7):969–82.
22. Melia M, Moy CS, Reynolds SM, et al. Quality of life after iodine 125 brachytherapy vs

enucleation for choroidal melanoma: 5-year results from the Collaborative Ocular Melanoma Study: COMS QOLS report no. 3. Arch Ophthalmol 2006;124(2):226–38.
23. Hawkins BS. The Collaborative Ocular Melanoma Study (COMS) randomized trial of pre-enucleation radiation of large choroidal melanoma: IV. Ten-year mortality findings and prognostic factors. COMS report number 24. Am J Ophthalmol 2004;138(6):936–51.
24. Brady L. Radiotherapy of Intraocular and Orbital Tumors, second revised edition. New York, NY: Springer, 2003.
25. Shields CL, Shields JA, Cater J, et al. Plaque radiotherapy for uveal melanoma: long-term visual outcome in 1106 consecutive patients. Arch Ophthalmol 2000;118(9):1219–28.
26. Damato B, Kacperek A, Chopra M, et al. Proton beam radiotherapy of iris melanoma. Int J Radiat Oncol Biol Phys 2005;63(1):109–15.
27. Kodjikian L, Roy P, Rouberol F, et al. Survival after proton-beam irradiation of uveal melanomas. Am J Ophthalmol 2004;137(6):1002–10.
28. Dendale R, Lumbroso-Le Rouic L, Noel G, et al. Proton beam radiotherapy for uveal melanoma: results of Curie Institut-Orsay proton therapy center (ICPO). Int J Radiat Oncol Biol Phys 2006;65(3):780–7.
29. Gragoudas ES, Lane AM, Regan S, et al. A randomized controlled trial of varying radiation doses in the treatment of choroidal melanoma. Arch Ophthalmol 2000;118(6):773–8.
30. Egan KM, Gragoudas ES, Seddon JM, et al. The risk of enucleation after proton beam irradiation of uveal melanoma. Ophthalmology 1989;96(9):1377–82; discussion 1382–3.
31. The Collaborative Ocular Melanoma Study Group. Histopathologic characteristics of uveal melanomas in eyes enucleated from the Collaborative Ocular Melanoma Study. COMS report no. 6. Am J Ophthalmol 1998;125(6):745–66.
32. Damato B. Treatment of primary intraocular melanoma. Expert Rev Anticancer Ther 2006;6(4):493–506.
33. Damato B, Jones AG. Uveal melanoma: resection techniques. Ophthalmol Clin North Am 2005;18(1):119–28, ix.
34. Folberg R, Verdick R, Weingeist TA, et al. The gross examination of eyes removed for choroidal and ciliary body melanomas. Ophthalmology 1986;93(12):1643–7.
35. The Collaborative Ocular Melanoma Study Group. Histopathologic characteristics of uveal melanomas in eyes enucleated from the Collaborative Ocular Melanoma Study. COMS report no. 6. Am J Ophthalmol 1998;125(6):745–66.
36. Shields CL, Shields JA, Gross NE, et al. Survey of 520 eyes with uveal metastases. Ophthalmology 1997;104(8):1265–76.
37. Gamel JW, Greenberg RA, McLean IW, et al. A clinically useful method for combining gross and microscopic measurements to select high-risk patients after enucleation for ciliochoroidal melanoma. Cancer 1986;57(7):1341–4.
38. Singh AD, Shields CL, Shields JA. Prognostic factors in uveal melanoma. Melanoma Res 2001;11(3):255–63.
39. Shields CL, Shields JA, De Potter P, et al. Diffuse choroidal melanoma. Clinical features predictive of metastasis. Arch Ophthalmol 1996;114(8):956–63.
40. Folberg R, Salomao D, Grossniklaus HE, et al. Recommendations for the reporting of tissues removed as part of the surgical treatment of common malignancies of the eye and its adnexa. The Association of Directors of Anatomic and Surgical Pathology. Hum Pathol 2003;34(2):114–8.
41. McLean IW, Saraiva VS, Burnier MN Jr. Pathological and prognostic features of uveal melanomas. Can J Ophthalmol 2004;39(4):343–50.

Chapter 16
Uveal Metastases from Solid Tumors

Gerardo D. Camoriano and Dan S. Gombos

Abstract Because the uveal tract is a highly vascular structure with a low-flow microenvironment, it is well suited for seeding of circulating cancer cells. Numerous studies have shown that uveal metastases are the most common intraocular malignancies in adults. The most common primary cancers metastasizing to the uvea are breast and lung cancers. The most common symptom of uveal metastasis is blurred vision; however, patients may also present with vision loss, intraocular pain, scotoma, floaters, photopsias, and metamorphopsia. Treatment modalities include observation, external-beam radiation therapy, chemotherapy, plaque brachytherapy, transpupillary thermotherapy, and enucleation. For many patients, uveal metastasis is associated with advanced systemic disease, which portends a poor prognosis; however, early diagnosis and treatment of uveal metastasis can result in good visual outcomes and high rates of ocular salvage.

16.1 Introduction

Cancer is the second most common cause of death in the United States, contributing to nearly one in four deaths. As the incidence rate of cancer increases, it is likely that an ophthalmologist in general practice will encounter a patient with ocular metastasis.

Numerous studies in the past 10 years have shown that uveal metastases are the most common intraocular malignancies in adults. Given that the uveal tract is a highly vascular structure with a low-flow microenvironment, it is not surprising that the uveal tract is well suited for seeding of circulating cancer cells. Cases of ocular metastases outnumber cases of primary uveal melanoma by a ratio of approximately 2:1 [1–3]. Within the uvea, the most common site of involvement is the choroid,

G.D. Camoriano (✉)
Department of Ophthalmology and Visual Sciences, The University of Texas Medical Branch, Galveston, TX, USA
e-mail: gdcamori@utmb.edu

B. Esmaeli (ed.), *Ophthalmic Oncology*, M.D. Anderson Solid Tumor Oncology Series 6, DOI 10.1007/978-1-4419-0374-7_16,

which has a comparatively large surface area and distribution of blood flow. In some cases, metastatic disease goes clinically unrecognized during the patient's lifetime and is only identified when the eye is examined at autopsy. In most patients, however, uveal metastasis presents with painless blurred vision, which, in the context of a previous history of systemic malignancy, mandates an urgent ocular assessment. Hence, the ophthalmologist may be the first physician to discover the recurrence of a previously treated cancer or detect a previously unknown primary cancer in a patient without any history of cancer.

16.2 Patient Characteristics

Uveal metastases have been reported in patients in every decade of life. Women (70–85% of cases) are more commonly affected than men. Lung and breast adenocarcinomas account for the majority of uveal metastases, with estimates ranging from 71 to 92% of cases. Incidences of uveal metastatic tumors parallel those of the corresponding primary tumors. In men with uveal metastases, the most common primary cancer site is the lung (40–60% of cases), while in women with uveal metastases, the most common primary cancer site is the breast (70–80% of cases), followed by the lung (10% of cases) [4–6]. It should be noted that uveal metastases related to primary breast cancer have also been reported in men and that lung cancer-associated uveal metastases are expected to become more common in women as the incidence of primary lung cancer in women continues to increase. Other adenocarcinomas that metastasize to the eye include gastrointestinal, prostate, kidney, and thyroid adenocarcinomas [7]. Germinal tumors from the ovaries and testes and cutaneous melanoma have also been shown to metastasize to the uvea. Although rare, metastasis from neuroendocrine tumors, particularly carcinoid tumors, has also been known to occur [8].

16.3 Symptoms

Symptoms of ocular metastases depend on the location of the tumor. Tumors affecting the posterior pole often present earlier, and visual complaints are common, particularly when the macula is involved. The most common initial symptom is blurred vision, which may result from exudative retinal detachment or subretinal fluid or from a hyperopic shift secondary to mass effect. Similarly, iris or ciliary body metastases may result in displacement of the lens diaphragm, causing new refractive errors. Alternatively, vision loss may be caused by an iritis or iridocyclitis-like inflammation due to tumor seeding in the anterior chamber. Extensive seeding in the anterior segment may also result in the formation of a pseudohypopyon. Visual acuity can range from 20/20 to no light perception; visual acuity is commonly severely affected at presentation [4, 5].

Intraocular pain is not common but may be present in up to 16% of patients who have ocular metastases. This is generally a dull, boring, and constant pain; however, it may be sharp and intermittent. Secondary angle closure from tumor debris, neovascular glaucoma from anterior segment ischemia, and perineural invasion of the ciliary nerves may also lead to intraocular pain. Other symptoms of ocular metastases include scotoma (6–31% of patients), floaters (5–21% of patients), photopsias (13% of patients), and metamorphopsia (3–5% of patients).

16.4 Clinical Features

All patients with a history of cancer should have a thorough annual ophthalmic examination. The iris should be carefully inspected with a slit lamp for the presence of nodules. Most iris metastases occur in the inferior quadrant (42% of cases), and iris metastases are more likely to affect the midzone than the pupillary margin or iris root. Ciliary body metastases are usually sessile or dome shaped. They are often difficult to visualize directly but should be suspected when there is segmental distortion of the pupil or lens diaphragm. If not apparent on slit lamp or ophthalmoscopy, ciliary body metastases can often be seen with gonioscopy or high-frequency ultrasound biomicroscopy. Ciliary body metastases, like their iris counterparts, often occur in the inferior quadrant (48% of cases). Other clinical signs associated with iris or ciliary body metastases include conjunctival hyperemia, glaucoma, corectopia, iridocyclitis, pseudohypopyon, and hyphema.

A dilated fundus examination should be performed to identify choroidal lesions, since the choroid is the most common site for metastasis to the uvea. Choroidal lesions are most commonly seen in the near periphery (52–83% of cases), followed by the macula (up to 40% of cases) and mid and far periphery (together accounting for 8–17% of cases). Radially, the lateral quadrant (35% of cases) is affected slightly more often than the superior (22% of cases), inferior (17% of cases), nasal (14% of cases), and central (macula) quadrants (12% of cases). Choroidal tumors are usually cream-colored or pale yellow and placoid or slightly dome shaped, with oval or irregular margins. They may be associated with subretinal fluid and shallow exudative retinal detachments.

Uveal metastases of bronchial carcinoids, renal cell carcinoma, and thyroid cancer may be orange, and cutaneous melanomas are brown. Overlying lipofuscin deposits may confer a leopard skin appearance. Careful examination reveals the presence of multifocal disease in 29–35% of cases and bilateral eye involvement in up to 50% of patients.

16.5 Diagnosis

In the diagnosis of uveal metastases, the importance of obtaining a patient's complete medical history cannot be overemphasized. Particular attention should be given to the patient's chief complaint and past medical history, which often narrows the differential diagnosis.

Ancillary techniques, such as gonioscopy and high-frequency ultrasound biomicroscopy, may be necessary to evaluate lesions involving the iris root or ciliary body. Traditional A- and B-scan ocular echographic images are helpful in assessing most choroidal lesions. A-scan ultrasonography often shows moderate- to high-amplitude internal reflectivity. The thickness and largest basal diameter of metastatic foci can be determined by B-scan ultrasonography, which usually shows moderate-to-high acoustic solidity. Ultrasonography may be particularly helpful when a view of the fundus is compromised by a dense cataract or other optical media opacity, such as vitreous hemorrhage.

Other imaging modalities that may help establish the diagnosis of uveal metastasis include fluorescein angiography and ocular coherence tomography. Fluorescein angiography of choroidal lesions may reveal early blockage of the choroidal circulation, which is associated with hypofluorescence in the arterial and early venous phases and leakage in the later phases. In contrast to the double circulation pattern sometimes seen with primary uveal melanoma, no large intralesional blood vessels are normally seen in choroidal metastases. Ocular coherence tomography provides a cross-sectional image of the retina, retinal pigment epithelium, and choriocapillaris, which may further aid in mapping these lesions and demonstrating subretinal fluid.

Magnetic resonance imaging should be considered, especially when central nervous system (CNS) involvement is suspected [9]. Magnetic resonance imaging may also help differentiate metastatic lesions from primary choroidal melanoma, as the latter often exhibits high signal intensity on T1-weighted images. Computed tomography or magnetic resonance imaging of the CNS is indicated in all patients with newly diagnosed metastases and should be part of any staging workup to rule out CNS metastasis.

The differential diagnosis of uveal metastasis includes amelanotic nevus, amelanotic melanoma, granulomatous iritis, lymphoma, leukemia, leiomyoma, choroidal osteoma, choroidal hemangioma, and eccentric disciform degeneration. If, after a complete workup, the diagnosis of uveal metastasis remains elusive because of an atypical presentation or failure to identify the primary tumor, a biopsy may be considered. However, the benefits of pathologic verification of the lesion and prediction of the primary tumor site must be carefully weighed against the risk of complications related to the procedure itself or the possibility of tumor spread by seeding. Biopsy techniques include ab externo and ab interno approaches, including pars plana fine-needle aspiration biopsy. Of these techniques, fine-needle aspiration biopsy is the least invasive and has a reported sensitivity of up to 84% after cytological analysis. The main risks associated with this procedure are dissemination of tumor cells along the needle tract or into the bloodstream and ocular complications leading to visual loss and blindness (endophthalmitis, vitreous hemorrhage, rhegmatogenous retinal detachment, or suprachoroidal hemorrhage).

16.6 Treatment

Once the diagnosis of uveal metastasis is made, close collaboration with an oncologist is essential to provide the best care for the patient. This is particularly important in cases in which the ophthalmologist initially makes the diagnosis in a patient with no history of cancer. In this setting, an oncology consultation should take place promptly to determine the location of the primary tumor and to dictate systemic treatment. Several treatment modalities have been investigated and are presented in the following sections. These therapies aim at selectively targeting the metastatic foci while minimizing collateral damage and optimizing visual outcomes.

16.6.1 Observation

Not all uveal metastases are considered sight threatening or require specific ocular therapy. Ophthalmologists may choose to follow lesions that remain stable in size, are asymptomatic, or are not threatening the macula or the optic nerve. Often these lesions are diagnosed in patients who have undergone prior systemic treatment, such as chemotherapy, and are detected on routine ophthalmic examination. In such cases, local treatment is not likely to result in any appreciable benefit.

16.6.2 External-Beam Radiation Therapy

External-beam radiation therapy is an excellent treatment modality for most uveal metastatic lesions. It is well suited for the patient with bilateral multifocal disease and should be considered when the macula is threatened or involved in one or both eyes. Treatment is usually tailored, in part, to the type of primary lesion and its relative radiosensitivity. When CNS lesions are identified at the same time as uveal metastasis, whole brain radiation therapy inclusive of both globes may be indicated. Close coordination with the treating radiotherapist is essential to review the size and ocular location of the tumor foci. In select cases (with posterior tumors), a lens-sparing approach can be used, decreasing ocular side effects such as dry eye and cataract formation. In most cases, radiation therapy is well tolerated and has minimal side effects, such as lash loss and dry eye, which can be addressed with the use of supplemental artificial tears. Cataracts, if clinically significant, can be removed in the usual fashion; however, given that most patients with uveal metastasis have a short life expectancy (see Section 16.7), cataracts often do not become a clinically significant complication [4, 10].

16.6.3 Chemotherapy

In some cases, systemic chemotherapy can be used to treat ocular metastatic lesions. Generally, newly diagnosed patients with systemic disease that includes ocular involvement are candidates for systemic chemotherapy. If systemic chemotherapy is considered, the oncologist and ophthalmologist should review the relative ocular and CNS penetration of the chemotherapeutic regimen selected. Patients should be monitored closely with each cycle of treatment since initial regression may be followed by late recurrence. Adjuvant radiation therapy or laser hyperthermia therapy may be necessary. In many cases, there is good correlation between ocular and systemic response. We have observed that uveal metastases from newly diagnosed breast cancers are most responsive to systemic chemotherapy.

16.6.4 Plaque Brachytherapy

Brachytherapy is an excellent modality for select patients with choroidal metastasis. Patients with a single isolated tumor focus and no CNS disease are good candidates for this approach. Iodine 125 and ruthenium plaques are the most common sources used. Charged-particle radiation therapy has also been described. Careful presurgical measurements are critical to ensure that the basal and apical dimensions of the metastatic tumor are considered in radiation and dosimetric planning. Treatment dose is dependent on the relative radiosensitivity of the primary lesion [10–12].

16.6.5 Transpupillary Thermotherapy

For most patients, transpupillary thermotherapy (laser hyperthermia) is not a first-line modality in the treatment of uveal metastases. However, in treating recurrent disease, transpupillary thermotherapy can be a helpful adjunct in the management of select lesions. Smaller pigmented tumors tend to respond best to this type of therapy. The treatment is administered in an outpatient setting and requires local retrobulbar anesthesia. Before treatment is begun, a review of the patient's blood counts should be performed to ensure that retrobulbar injection can be performed safely with minimal risk of orbital hemorrhage. Most centers administer multiple treatment cycles at intervals over a 1–3 month period. We have found transpupillary thermotherapy to be helpful in cases in which there was a relative contraindication to ocular radiation therapy in the form of either prior radiation therapy or concurrent chemotherapy; however, transpupillary thermotherapy is associated with a higher risk of scotoma than other modalities.

16.6.6 Enucleation

In severe and advanced cases of uveal metastases that involve poor visual prognosis and ocular pain, enucleation may be considered. In such cases, the surgeon should carefully assess the patient's systemic disease and life expectancy as well as whether the patient's pain or glaucoma can be controlled using alternative methods. Enucleation can provide local tumor control in patients with otherwise nonresponsive lesions.

16.7 Prognosis

For many patients, the development of uveal metastasis is associated with significant and diffuse neoplasia, particularly of the CNS. Some ocular metastases, particularly breast cancer metastases, can have a very good response to local treatment, resulting in an excellent prognosis for visual and ocular preservation. However, the association of uveal metastasis with advanced systemic disease often portends poor survival and high morbidity. Life expectancy in patients with advanced systemic disease varies greatly depending on the primary neoplasm—breast cancer and carcinoid tumors are associated with longer survival, while cutaneous melanoma and lung carcinoma are associated with a dismal prognosis.

16.8 Conclusions

As the incidence of cancer continues to increase in the United States, a greater numbers of patients are expected to present with ocular metastases. Early treatment of uveal metastases can result in good visual outcomes and high rates of ocular salvage. Many cases of uveal metastasis respond to radiation therapy or systemic chemotherapy. It is critical in all patients when radiation therapy or systemic chemotherapy is being considered to pursue a systemic workup, as uveal metastases are often associated with CNS metastasis. In many patients, findings from the systemic workup reveal diffuse disease, which generally indicates a poor overall morbidity. However, in some cases, particularly distant spread of breast cancer, long-term survival, and excellent quality of life have been observed.

References

1. Ferry AP, Font RL. Carcinoma metastatic to the eye and orbit III. A clinicopathologic study of 28 cases metastatic to the orbit. Cancer 1976;38(3):1326–35.
2. Ferry AP, Font RL. Carcinoma metastatic to the eye and orbit II. A clinicopathological study of 26 patients with carcinoma metastatic to the anterior segment of the eye. Arch Ophthalmol 1975;93(7):472–82.
3. Ferry AP, Font RL. Carcinoma metastatic to the eye and orbit. I. A clinicopathologic study of 227 cases. Arch Ophthalmol 1974;92(4):276–86.
4. Shields CL, Shields JA, Gross NE, Schwartz GP, Lally SE. Survey of 520 eyes with uveal metastases. Ophthalmology 1997;104(8):1265–76.
5. Amichetti M, Caffo O, Minatel E, et al. Ocular metastases from breast carcinoma: a multicentric retrospective study. Oncol Rep 2000;7(4):761–5.
6. Demirci H, Shields CL, Chao AN, Shields JA. Uveal metastasis from breast cancer in 264 patients. Am J Ophthalmol 2003;136(2):264–71.
7. Kurli M, Finger PT. The kidney, cancer, and the eye: current concepts. Surv Ophthalmol 2005;50(6):507–18.
8. Harbour JW, De Potter P, Shields CL, Shields JA. Uveal metastasis from carcinoid tumor. Clinical observations in nine cases. Ophthalmology 1994;101(6):1084–90.
9. Chang EL, Lo S. Diagnosis and management of central nervous system metastases from breast cancer. Oncologist 2003;8(5):398–410.

10. Kanthan GL, Jayamohan J, Yip D, Conway RM. Management of metastatic carcinoma of the uveal tract: an evidence-based analysis. Clin Exp Ophthalmol 2007;35(6):553–65.
11. Shields CL, Shields JA, De Potter P, et al. Plaque radiotherapy for the management of uveal metastasis. Arch Ophthalmol 1997;115(2):203–9.
12. Shields CL. Plaque radiotherapy for the management of uveal metastasis. Curr Opin Ophthalmol 1998;9(3):31–7.

Chapter 17
Vascular Tumors of the Posterior Pole

Dan S. Gombos

Abstract Vascular tumors of the posterior pole represent a significant percentage of lesions managed by ocular oncologists. The spectrum of disorders includes retinal vascular tumors, choroidal lesions, and various neuro-oculo-cutaneous syndromes. Management of the ocular lesions varies, depending on the size and location of the lesion and its associated ocular damage. Small, asymptomatic peripheral lesions can be observed. Larger and symptomatic lesions can be treated successfully with radiation therapy, either through an external approach or with a radioactive plaque. Some can be treated with laser photocoagulation or photodynamic therapy. While vascular tumors of the retina are benign, they often can be associated with various syndromes that harbor neoplastic potential, and it is important to identify those lesions that may be associated with neoplastic risk.

17.1 Introduction

Vascular tumors of the posterior pole represent a significant percentage of lesions managed by ocular oncologists. The spectrum of disorders includes retinal vascular tumors, choroidal lesions, and various neuro-oculo-cutaneous syndromes (i.e., phakomatoses). This chapter will focus on the most common vascular tumors encountered at a tertiary cancer center. It is by no means an exhaustive review of all vascular lesions encountered in the posterior pole.

17.2 Retinal Capillary Hemangioma and von Hippel–Lindau Disease

Retinal capillary hemangiomas, also known as hemangioblastomas, are acquired circumscribed vascular tumors of the retina. Retinal capillary hemangiomas often have

D.S. Gombos (✉)
Section of Ophthalmology, Department of Head and Neck Surgery, The University of Texas M.D. Anderson Cancer Center, Houston, TX, USA
e-mail: dgombos@mdanderson.org

B. Esmaeli (ed.), *Ophthalmic Oncology*, M.D. Anderson Solid Tumor Oncology Series 6, DOI 10.1007/978-1-4419-0374-7_17,

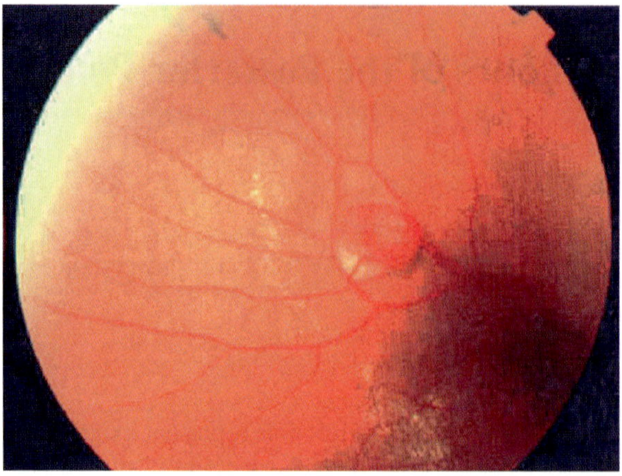

Fig. 17.1 Fundus photograph of an untreated retinal hemangioma in a patient with von Hippel–Lindau syndrome. Note the adjacent subretinal exudation

an orange-red appearance with associated prominent feeder vessels, vascular dilatation, and tortuosity (Fig. 17.1). Associated retinal and subretinal exudations are not uncommon in larger or more active lesions. Small lesions may be asymptomatic, while actively growing tumors are often associated with blurry vision or photopsias (flashing lights). While most lesions have a characteristic appearance that is diagnostic on ophthalmoscopy, fluorescein angiography can be helpful in identifying feeder vessels and active areas of leakage.

Ocular oncologists must be aware of the association between retinal capillary hemangiomas and von Hippel–Lindau disease. While many retinal capillary hemangiomas are idiopathic and occur spontaneously, a significant percentage are associated with von Hippel–Lindau disease, a disorder that occurs in 1 in 32,000 to 1 in 40,000 live births per year and presents in an autosomal dominant fashion. Pathogenesis is associated with the lack of production of the protein associated with the von Hippel–Lindau disease gene, which leads to excessive production of vascular endothelial growth factor. This excessive production leads to various vascular tumors of the brain, spine, and retina as well as renal cell carcinomas, pheochromocytomas, and neuroendocrine tumors of the pancreas. Genetic testing is available to screen asymptomatic family members. Those who possess the gene defect should undergo annual ocular screening, including dilated funduscopic assessment, with more frequent exams during pubescent years [1].

Management of ocular lesions depends on the size and location of the lesion and its associated ocular damage. Small, asymptomatic peripheral lesions can be observed, particularly if they are not associated with exudation and remain smaller than 0.5–1 mm. Tumors that are actively leaking can be treated with laser photocoagulation. Generally, this approach requires multiple treatments applied to the tumor and feeding artery. Argon photocoagulation is often used, but recent reports have also described the role of infrared 810-nm diode laser therapy (thermotherapy).

Thermotherapy tends to be most effective with tumors that are 1.5 mm or smaller. For larger lesions and lesions in the peripheral transscleral region, cryotherapy can be effective.

As retinal capillary hemangiomas increase in size, they become more resistant to focal modalities, such as laser and cryotherapy. Lesions larger than 4 mm can be treated successfully with radiation therapy, either through an external approach or with a radioactive plaque. Vitreoretinal procedures are generally required for large hemangiomas that have a complex detachment of significant size and elevation. Increasingly, clinicians have also utilized anti-vascular endothelial growth factor compounds, such as bevacizumab and ranibizumab, to treat lesions that have demonstrated resistance to more traditional modalities [2, 3].

Because of the risk of systemic neoplasia and central nervous system vascular tumors, patients with von Hippel–Lindau disease benefit from a multidisciplinary approach, including consultation with medical oncologists, urologists, neurosurgeons, and endocrinologists who are experienced in treating patients with this disorder.

17.3 Circumscribed Choroidal Hemangioma

Circumscribed choroidal hemangiomas are acquired vascular tumors of the choroid. They generally develop in the second to fourth decade of life and have a classic orange pigmentation on ophthalmoscopy. Because of their location and amelanotic features, circumscribed choroidal hemangiomas are often misdiagnosed as metastatic tumors of the choroid.

Circumscribed choroidal hemangiomas are often asymptomatic, but they can present with metamorphopsia and photopsias when associated with subretinal fluid. They demonstrate early hyperfluorescence on fluorescein angiography, but indocyanine green angiography is particularly helpful in making a diagnosis [4]. Indocyanine green angiography demonstrates an intrinsic choroidal vascular pattern that occurs shortly after injection. As the study progresses, there is a significant reduction in the dye's intensity. On A-scan ocular echography, these lesions typically demonstrate high internal reflectivity.

17.4 Management of Posterior Choroidal Hemangiomas

Patients with asymptomatic choroidal lesions do not require treatment and can be monitored. It is best to provide these patients with an Amsler grid and instruct them to monitor their vision closely. Historically, radiation therapy was the treatment of choice for these lesions. Low-dose external-beam radiation therapy can be highly effective in reducing the associated subretinal fluid and tumor thickness. Some patients, however, continue to experience metamorphopsia with limited visual improvement. A number of experts prefer to treat choroidal lesions with plaque brachytherapy, which provides not only resolution of exudation and reduction of tumor thickness but improved vision. Since the introduction of photodynamic therapy, a number of investigators have commented on the role of this modality in treating these vascular tumors. Photodynamic therapy can result in dramatic reduction and near resolution of some hemangiomas. Increasingly, a number of centers employ this modality as the treatment of choice, using protocols similar to those described for managing choroidal neovascular membranes. Multiple treatments may be required before response and improvement of vision occur [5–9].

17.5 Acquired Vasoproliferative Tumors of the Retina

Acquired vasoproliferative tumors of the retina are known by various names in the medical literature. *Acquired retinal hemangioma* is a term preferred by some oncologists. These lesions may be asymptomatic, but patients often present to the ocular oncologist with decreased vision and photopsias. Acquired vasoproliferative tumors of the retina have a yellowish vascular appearance and are often identified in the peripheral retina. One of the important distinguishing features of these lesions is the presence of associated subretinal exudation and exudative retinal detachment. In some cases, these lesions are misdiagnosed as atypical amelanotic melanomas. A-scan ocular echography can be helpful in distinguishing between these conditions, as most melanomas have lower internal reflectivity than vascular tumors.

With regard to management, patients with asymptomatic lesions can be observed. However, patients with significant exudation or subretinal fluid are generally treated. Most tumors are quite responsive to cryotherapy, which can be applied with a triple freeze–thaw transscleral technique. Large tumors may be resistant to this approach and may require alternative treatment, such as plaque radiation. Following treatment, tumor response can be dramatic—there can be significant reduction in size and resolution of exudation [10–12].

17.6 Conclusions

While vascular tumors of the retina are benign, they often can be associated with various syndromes that harbor neoplastic potential. It is important to identify those lesions that may be associated with neoplastic risk. Most vascular tumors, if asymptomatic, can be observed. Larger lesions are generally responsive to some form of focal therapy, such as cryotherapy or laser photocoagulation. Resistant cases are often amenable to radiation therapy. Increasingly, anti-vascular endothelial growth factor compounds, such as bevacizumab and ranibizumab, show additional promise in treating these intraocular vascular tumors.

References

1. Wong WT, Chew EY. Ocular von Hippel–Lindau disease: clinical update and emerging treatments. Curr Opin Ophthalmol 2008;19(3):213–7.
2. Dahr SS, Cusick M, Rodriguez-Coleman H, et al. Intravitreal anti-vascular endothelial growth factor therapy with pegaptanib for advanced von Hippel–Lindau disease of the retina. Retina 2007;27(2):150–8.
3. Aiello LP, George DJ, Cahill MT, et al. Rapid and durable recovery of visual function in a patient with von Hippel–Lindau syndrome after systemic therapy with vascular endothelial growth factor receptor inhibitor su5416. Ophthalmology 2002;109(9):1745–51.
4. Horgan N, O'Keefe M, McLoone E, et al. Fundus fluorescein angiographic characterization of diffuse choroidal hemangiomas. J Pediatr Ophthalmol Strabismus 2008;45(1):26–30.
5. Ritland JS, Eide N, Tausjø J. External beam irradiation therapy for choroidal haemangiomas. Visual and anatomical results after a dose of 20 to 25 Gy. Acta Ophthalmol Scand 2001;79(2):184–6.
6. Chao AN, Shields CL, Shields JA, et al. Plaque radiotherapy for choroidal hemangioma with total retinal detachment and iris neovascularization. Retina 2001;21(6):682–4.
7. Boixadera A, Arumí JG, Martínez-Castillo V, et al. Prospective clinical trial evaluating the efficacy of photodynamic therapy for symptomatic circumscribed choroidal hemangioma. Ophthalmology 2009;116(1):100–105.
8. Vicuna-Kojchen J, Banin E, Averbukh E, et al. Application of the standard photodynamic treatment protocol for symptomatic circumscribed choroidal hemangioma. Ophthalmologica 2006;220(6):351–5.
9. Shields JA. Photodynamic therapy for choroidal hemangioma. Graefes Arch Clin Exp Ophthalmol 2006;244(9):1071–2.
10. Irvine F, O'Donnell N, Kemp E, et al. Retinal vasoproliferative tumors: surgical management and histological findings. Arch Ophthalmol 2000;118(4):563–9.
11. Tripathi A. Retinal vasoproliferative tumors: a conservative approach. Arch Ophthalmol 2001;119(1):145–6.
12. Singh AD, Rundle PA, Rennie I. Retinal vascular tumors. Ophthalmol Clin North Am 2005,18(1):167–76.

Part III
Oculoplastic and Periocular Reconstructive Surgery in Cancer Patients

Section Editor: Bita Esmaeli

Chapter 18
Reconstructive Surgery for Eyelid Defects

Roman Shinder and Bita Esmaeli

Abstract With a depleting ozone layer and increasing ultraviolet radiation exposure, the incidence of eyelid cancers is on the rise, and we can expect a growing need for eyelid reconstruction. Several reconstructive techniques may be appropriate for a particular eyelid defect. The choice of procedure by the surgeon depends on the patient's age, the degree of eyelid laxity and quality of eyelid skin, the location and size of the defect, and the surgeon's preference. Regardless of the surgical procedure chosen, the goals of the procedure should be restoration of both the anatomy and the dynamic function of the eyelid, creation of a stable eyelid margin, acceptable vertical eyelid height, adequate eyelid closure, smooth posterior epithelial surface, and maximum cosmesis and symmetry.

18.1 Introduction

With a depleting ozone layer and increasing ultraviolet radiation exposure, the incidence of eyelid cancers is on the rise, and we can expect a growing need for eyelid reconstruction. The following chapter details eyelid reconstruction following tumor resection.

18.2 General Principles

Regardless of the surgical procedure chosen, the goals of the procedure should be restoration of both the anatomy and the dynamic function of the eyelid, creation of a stable eyelid margin, acceptable vertical eyelid height, adequate eyelid closure, smooth posterior epithelial surface, and maximum cosmesis and symmetry. The

R. Shinder (✉)
Section of Ophthalmology, Department of Head and Neck Surgery, The University of Texas M.D. Anderson Cancer Center, Houston, TX, USA
e-mail: romanshinder@hotmail.com

B. Esmaeli (ed.), *Ophthalmic Oncology*, M.D. Anderson Solid Tumor Oncology Series 6, DOI 10.1007/978-1-4419-0374-7_18,

reconstructive technique chosen for eyelid defects largely depends on the extent of full-thickness horizontal lid resection. The surgeon may be surprised at the final size of a lid defect following tumor excision if frozen-section histopathologic examination proves the tumor to be more extensive than clinically estimated. Therefore, the patient should be counseled about the potential extent of the eyelid defect based on the anatomic location and type of cancer.

For the purposes of repair, the eyelids can be thought of as being made of an anterior and a posterior lamella. The anterior lamella consists of the skin and orbicularis muscle, while the posterior lamella is made up of the tarsus and conjunctiva. It is important to reconstruct both the anterior and posterior lamellae. Reconstruction of either the anterior or the posterior lamella may be accomplished with a graft, but grafts should not be used to reconstruct both lamellae since one of the layers must act as a pedicle flap and provide the blood supply. A graft placed upon another graft has a high probability of failure. Horizontal tension should be maximized at the expense of vertical tension to avoid postoperative eyelid malposition. In so doing, the surgeon must evaluate for horizontal lid laxity.

Medial and lateral canthal fixation should always be optimized, and an attempt should be made to match like tissue to like tissue in each lamella. Before any graft is sized, the anatomical defect should be narrowed as much as possible. The surgeon should avoid, whenever feasible, creating a defect that cannot be closed. When presented with alternatives, choosing the simplest technique is often wise. Finally, for complex and large defects encompassing more than the immediate periorbital soft tissues, it may be necessary to engage specialists from other disciplines, such as facial plastic surgery, to collaborate with the oculoplastic surgeon in surgical planning and reconstruction.

18.3 Eyelid Defects Not Involving the Eyelid Margin

Partial-thickness eyelid defects not involving the eyelid margin frequently result from Mohs surgery for skin cancers. Defects that do not involve the eyelid margin can be repaired by direct closure as long as the procedure does not distort the eyelid margin. Undermining of superficial tissues may sometimes be necessary to avoid undue wound tension. Tension of wound closure should be directed horizontally to avoid lower eyelid ectropion, eyelid retraction, and lagophthalmos. Avoiding vertical tension requires the placement of vertically oriented incision lines.

When undermining does not allow direct approximation, advancement or transposition procedures utilizing local skin flaps may be undertaken. The most commonly used flaps are advancement flaps, including sliding and rotation flaps, and transposition flaps, including z-plasty and rhomboid flaps [1]. The simplest skin-and-muscle flap is a sliding flap. It requires wide undermining to allow it to "slide" into the defect. The second simplest flap is the advancement flap, which requires wide undermining followed by relaxing incisions to allow the flap to "advance" into the defect. The resultant excess tissue adjacent to the flap can be trimmed by removing Burrow's triangles of skin on either side of the flap [2]. Semicircular and rotation flaps are types of advancement flaps that are rotated into the defect. Z-plasty and rhomboid flaps are transposition flaps, entailing transfer of the flap from a non-adjacent area into the defect by lifting the flap over normal tissue [3]. Transposition flaps are often helpful in the repair of larger defects. These different flaps are often used in combination to work around facial contours. Flaps typically provide the best tissue match and cosmetic result but necessitate planning to limit secondary deformities. Although skin graft procedures are usually less challenging to perform, a skin graft may not be an appropriate choice for a deep defect or if postoperative adjuvant radiation therapy is planned.

Upper eyelid defects involving the anterior lamella are best repaired with full-thickness skin grafts from the contralateral upper lid. Preauricular or retroauricular grafts may also be utilized, but their greater thickness may hinder upper lid mobility and cosmesis. Lower eyelid defects not involving the margin and without significant soft tissue depth can be repaired using a skin graft from the upper eyelid or the preauricular or retroauricular skin. When tissue is not available from the upper lid or periauricular locations, full-thickness grafts may be harvested from the supraclavicular fossa or the inner upper arm. It should be remembered that skin grafts will shrink, somewhat, and produce some traction on the eyelid in the direction of the graft [2]. Surgeons must be vigilant not to place hair-bearing skin grafts near the eyelid margin as this may lead to future corneal irritation.

Split-thickness grafts should be avoided in periocular reconstructions as the cosmetic result is inferior to full-thickness grafts. They are only recommended in the surgical care of severe facial burns when adequate full-thickness skin is unavailable.

18.4 Small Defects Involving the Lower Eyelid Margin

Small defects that involve the lower eyelid margin can be repaired by direct closure assuming that the surrounding tissue is sufficiently lax so that undue tension is not placed on the wound. Primary closure is typically carried out when less than 33% of the lid margin is involved (Fig. 18.1). If a larger defect is present, adjacent tissue advancement or grafting of distant tissue may be needed. During primary closure, an additional 3–5 mm of medial mobilization may be obtained from the remaining lateral lid margin by severing the inferior limb of the lateral canthal tendon via a canthotomy and a cantholysis. During closure, the lid margin should be repaired with interrupted 6-0 silk sutures, which are left long and incorporated into subsequent skin sutures to ensure that they do not rub against the cornea. Three margin sutures should be placed—through the tarsus, the lash line, and the gray line. The tarsus should be repaired with 5-0 absorbable polyglactin suture.

Possible complications resulting from direct closure include a notch at the eyelid margin and wound dehiscence. A notch at the eyelid margin can be prevented by ensuring precise approximation of the tarsal margin and placing additional silk sutures at the eyelid margin [2]. Occasionally, wound dehiscence may occur. This

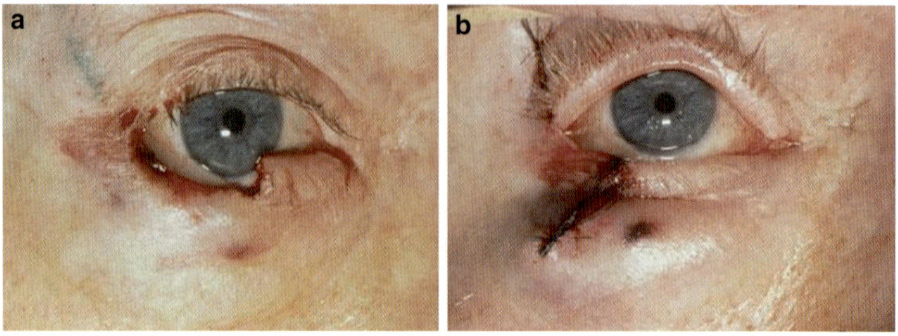

Fig. 18.1 Small right lower eyelid margin defect closed directly (pentagonal wedge). (**a**) Defect. (**b**) Intraoperative appearance after closure

tends to happen when there is excess tension on the wound or when the tissues are chronically inflamed. If the wound is too tight, thought should be given to performing a cantholysis to relieve the tension. Additionally, well-placed tarsal sutures at the lid margin and tarsal base help prevent dehiscence.

18.5 Moderate Defects Involving the Lower Eyelid Margin

Moderate defects are defined as those involving 33–50% of the margin. They are repaired by advancement of the lateral portion of the eyelid using semicircular advancement or rotation flaps. The most common repair technique utilizes a modified superior Tenzel semicircular rotation flap in conjunction with an inferior cantholysis. The flap should not extend as far as the brow superiorly, nor should it extend beyond the lateral orbital rim laterally [2]. Complications resulting from the use of the semicircular flap are usually caused by poor placement of the flap at the lateral canthus. The deep tissue of the flap must be securely fixed to the periorbita on the inner aspect of the lateral orbital rim [2], since ectropion is likely to result from poor fixation. Also, the semicircular rotation flap may result in a rounded lateral canthus, making secondary revisions necessary.

Tarsoconjunctival flaps are very useful for larger lower eyelid defects. These flaps are taken from the undersurface of the upper eyelid and may be transplanted into the lower lid defect to reconstruct the posterior lamella. Please see the next section for more details.

18.6 Large Defects Involving the Lower Eyelid Margin

Lower eyelid defects that involve greater than 50% of the lid margin—require adjacent tissue advancement for repair (Fig. 18.2a). One such approach involves the use of a modified tarsoconjunctival flap (Hughes flap) taken from the undersurface of

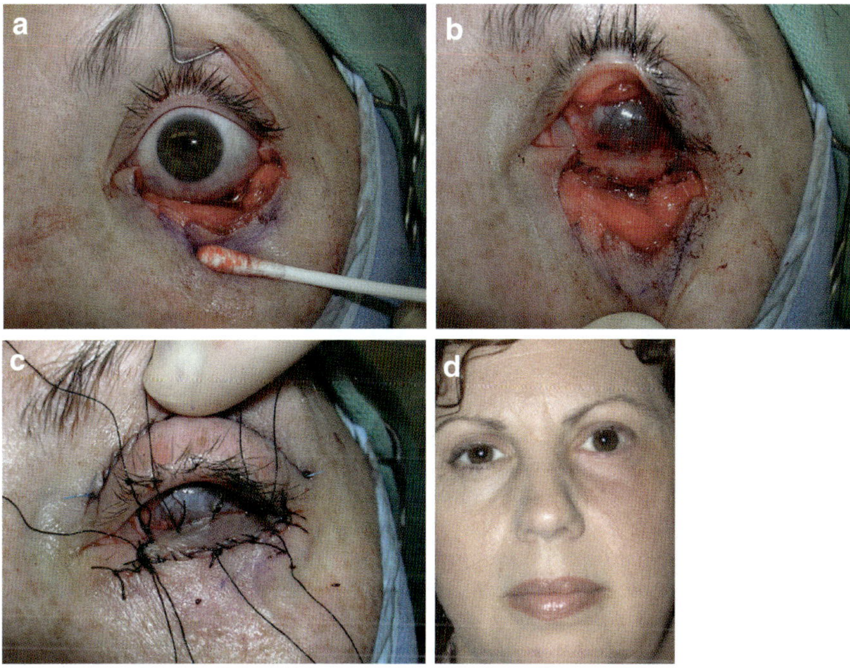

Fig. 18.2 Large left lower eyelid defect closed with a Hughes flap. (**a**) Defect. (**b**) Intraoperative appearance after tarsoconjunctival flap harvested from upper eyelid has been sutured to lower eyelid. (**c**) Intraoperative appearance after full-thickness skin graft harvested from upper eyelid has been sutured over tarsoconjunctival flap of lower eyelid. (**d**) Postoperative appearance 6 months after repair and administration of postoperative adjuvant radiation therapy

the upper eyelid. The flap is advanced from the upper lid into the posterior lamellar defect of the lower lid (Fig. 18.2b) [4]. Care should be taken when tarsal grafts are harvested to preserve the marginal 3–4 mm tarsal height in the upper eyelid to prevent donor-lid margin distortion. The tarsoconjunctival flap can be covered with various types of skin flaps or a full-thickness skin graft; the latter is our preferred choice for anterior lamella reconstruction over the tarsoconjunctival flap [5, 6]. The skin graft can be harvested from the upper eyelid using a blepharoplasty-type incision, usually from the same side, or it can be harvested from the retroauricular area (Fig. 18.2c). The modified Hughes procedure thus results in a bridge of conjunctiva from the upper lid across the visual axis for approximately 6 weeks. The vascularized pedicle of conjunctiva is subsequently released in a staged, second procedure once vascularization of the lower lid flap is achieved (Fig. 18.2d). The timing of the second stage of the modified Hughes procedure (when the pedicle of the flap is severed) depends on many factors. From the standpoint of vascular supply, studies have shown that a Hughes flap with good blood supply can be separated as early as 2 weeks after the first stage. However, there is a higher likelihood of lower eyelid ectropion after early separation of the flap. When postoperative adjuvant radiation therapy is planned for cutaneous cancers of the lower eyelid, it is necessary to separate the Hughes flap within 4–6 weeks after the first stage to allow for shielding of the globe and to allow radiation therapy to begin in a timely fashion (within 4–6 weeks after ablative surgery).

Because it is an eyelid-sharing technique and may result in complications, the modified Hughes procedure should be avoided in certain patient groups whenever possible. Children under age 7 should not undergo this procedure as it may precipitate occlusion amblyopia. This procedure should also be avoided in the seeing eye of a monocular patient. Several complications may result following a modified Hughes procedure. For instance, the patient may develop an eyelid malposition. If the lower eyelid margin skin rotates inward, the patient is likely to develop keratitis, either from the keratinized skin surface or from the fine lanugo hairs arising from the skin [2]. The risk of this complication can be reduced during the second stage of the procedure when the surgeon transects the advancement flap. Specifically, care should be taken to angle the incision to create a longer posterior lamella with more conjunctiva than skin [2]. The conjunctiva can then be advanced over the lid margin, leaving it nonkeratinized. Another complication that may occur following the modified Hughes procedure is upper lid retraction. To reduce this risk, the Müller muscle should be dissected away from conjunctiva and not be advanced with the tarsoconjunctival flap during the first stage of the procedure [2]. During the second stage of the procedure, the conjunctiva of the upper lid is left unsutured; it may even be recessed if retraction is a concern [2]. Sloughing of the skin graft may also occur following the Hughes procedure, but this is an uncommon occurrence. If blood or fluid collect beneath the donor graft, poor donor–host apposition will occur, resulting in graft failure. Drainage holes in the skin graft will prevent any fluid accumulation under the graft [2]. A bolster suture that is placed over the graft will keep it firmly apposed to the underlying vascular bed [2]. Necrosis of the tarsoconjunctival flap is another rare complication and results from a poorly vascularized flap.

Alternative procedures include full-thickness pedicled flaps [7, 8] and a free tarsoconjunctival graft from the contralateral upper lid with an overlying vascularized bipedicled skin-and-muscle flap [9]. Another useful technique is the tarsal transposition flap, as described by Hewes et al. [10]. The advantage of these procedures is that only one surgical stage is needed and visual axis occlusion is avoided, but in our experience the outcomes are not as predictable as those of a modified Hughes procedure for large defects of the lower eyelid.

A large rotating cheek flap (Mustardé flap) works well for repair of a large anterior lamellar defect, but for posterior lamellar replacement, it must be coupled with a tarsal substitute, such as a free tarsoconjunctival autograft, hard palate mucosa, nasal septum cartilage and mucosa, full-thickness buccal mucous membrane, Hughes flap, free periosteal graft, or homologous tarsus [11–17]. The Mustardé cheek rotation flap often results in a rounded lateral canthus and is associated with a high risk of lower eyelid ectropion; thus, secondary revisions are often needed.

18.7 Small Defects Involving the Upper Eyelid Margin

Upper eyelid defects involving less than 33% of the lid margin can be repaired by primary closure. Mirroring what is possible with the lower lid, the superior crus of the lateral canthal tendon can be lysed to obtain an additional 3–5 mm of medial mobilization of the remaining lateral lid margin.

18.8 Moderate Defects Involving the Upper Eyelid Margin

Upper eyelid defects involving 33–50% of the lid margin are repaired by advancement of the lateral portion of the lid. A lateral canthotomy and superior cantholysis are performed, and a reverse Tenzel semicircular skin flap is created inferior to the lateral brow and canthus to allow additional mobilization of the lid [18–20].

Tarsal sharing procedures, which consist of an adjacent sliding tarsoconjunctival flap from the remaining part of the upper lid covered by either a skin–orbicularis advancement flap or a full-thickness skin graft, have also been described for repair of the upper lid.

18.9 Large Defects Involving the Upper Eyelid Margin

Upper eyelid defects involving greater than 50% of the lid margin are most commonly repaired utilizing a Cutler–Beard procedure (Fig. 18.3a). This technique involves advancing a composite full-thickness lower eyelid flap into the upper eyelid defect by passing it posterior to the remaining lower lid margin (Fig. 18.3b) [21] Lysis of the flap is the second stage of the procedure and typically is performed 6–8 weeks after the first stage (Fig. 18.3c) [2].

This procedure, however, results in a relatively thick and immobile upper eyelid. Upper eyelid stability is enhanced by placing a spacer graft, such as donor sclera or AlloDerm, in the upper eyelid [2]. To decrease postoperative keratitis, it is also helpful to lyse the flap in such a way that the conjunctival surface is longer than the skin surface. The conjunctiva can then be draped forward over the lid margin and sutured to the skin anteriorly [2]. Other potential complications of a Cutler–Beard procedure include blepharoptosis, lagophthalmos, and even lid retraction [2]. Upper eyelid retraction can be avoided by waiting a minimum of 6 weeks before performing the second-stage procedure and by transecting the flap approximately 2 mm below the level of the upper lid [2]. Necrosis of the bridge in the lower lid may result if the vascular supply is compromised. In creating the bridge during the first-stage procedure, the marginal arterial arcade should be avoided by making the incision 4 mm below the lid margin [2].

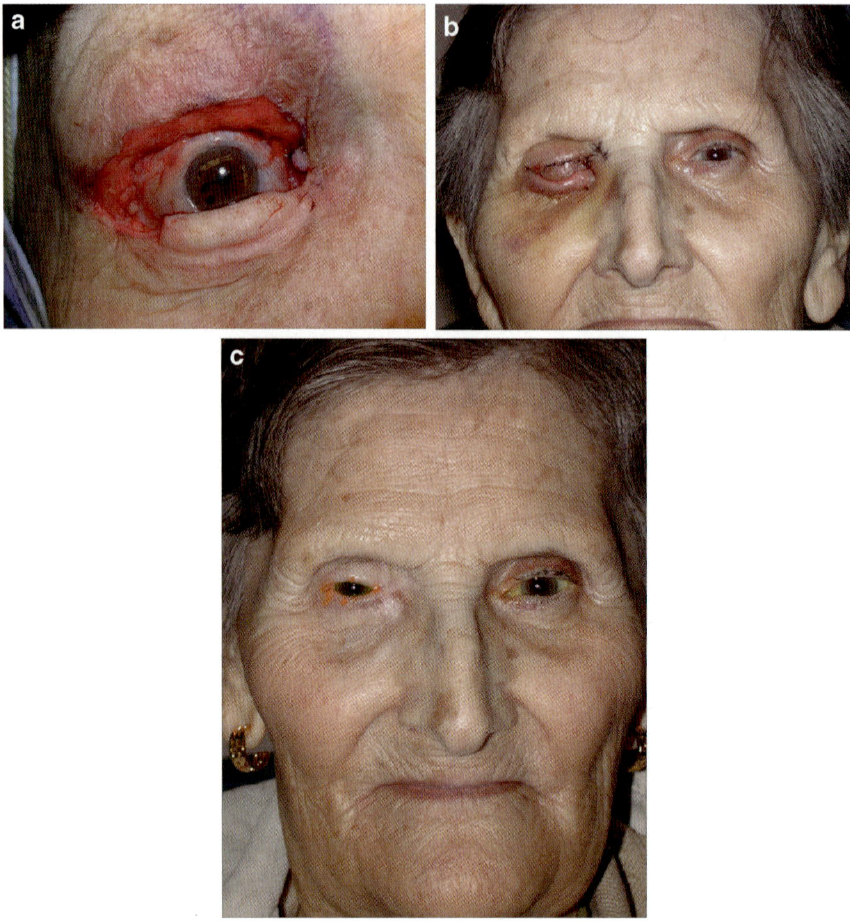

Fig. 18.3 Large right upper eyelid defect closed with a Cutler–Beard flap. (**a**) Defect. (**b**) Postoperative appearance following first stage of procedure showing the full-thickness lower eyelid flap sutured into the upper eyelid defect, coursing posterior to the intact lower eyelid margin. (**c**) Postoperative appearance of reconstructed right upper eyelid 6 months after repair

A potential alternative to a Cutler–Beard procedure for large upper lid defects is placement of a free tarsoconjunctival graft from the contralateral upper lid and coverage of this graft with a skin–muscle flap if the amount of redundant upper lid skin is adequate. However, for deep defects of the upper eyelid with loss of tissue extending into the conjunctival fornix and anterior orbit, a free tarsoconjunctival graft is not adequate, and a Cutler–Beard flap would be more appropriate.

A lower eyelid switch flap or median forehead flap has also been described for use in repairing large upper lid defects. If the upper lid defect is wide but shallow, involving only the lid margin, a tarsoconjunctival flap from the area just superior to the defect can be advanced inferiorly to replace the posterior lamella [2]. This flap must be well dissected toward the fornix. The levator aponeurosis is dissected away from the anterior face of the tarsus to prevent upper lid retraction during the postoperative period [2]. It may then be covered by either a full-thickness skin graft or a skin–orbicularis flap.

18.10 Lateral Canthal Defects

A key element of reconstruction in the lateral canthus is maintenance of the lower eyelid position and avoidance of lower eyelid ectropion. This is usually achieved by a lower eyelid tightening procedure that involves attaching the lower eyelid to the lateral orbital rim [2]. If the periorbita is of poor quality or absent, drill holes can be placed in the lateral orbital rim near Whitnall's tubercle (the lateral orbital tubercle) [2]. In most individuals, the vertical position of the lateral canthus is approximately 2 mm higher than the vertical position of the medial canthus. Following extensive lower lid surgery, the lateral canthus tends to retract inferiorly. Thus, the lateral canthus should be positioned superiorly enough that the lower lid and canthus maintain good anatomic orientation.

Laterally based transposition flaps or upper lid tarsus and conjunctiva can be utilized for large lower lid defects that extend to the lateral canthus [22]. Free skin grafts can be used to cover these flaps. Semicircular advancement skin flaps may also be used for defects extending to the lateral canthus. Occasionally, strips of periosteum and temporalis fascia still attached at the lateral orbital rim can be used to attach the remaining lateral lid margins to the lateral orbital rim [22, 23].

18.11 Medial Canthal Defects

Large medial canthal defects require good fixation of the residual upper and lower eyelid to the medial canthal tendon insertion area (Fig. 18.4a). The fixation suture should be posterior enough and with solid attachment to the bone to achieve good apposition of the eyelid against the globe. Fixation may be carried out with heavy permanent suture, wire, or titanium miniplates [24]. In the majority of cases, the lid can be fixated by suturing its medial aspect to the deep tissues in the region of the posterior lacrimal crest, where the posterior limb of the medial canthal tendon normally inserts [2]. Various local flaps and grafts can be used to cover soft tissue defects in the medial canthal area. Full-thickness skin grafts are ideal for shallow defects of the medial canthus. For deeper defects, various forms of transposition flaps are more appropriate. A very useful flap for this location is a glabellar flap (Fig. 18.4b) [25–27]. Flaps can withstand postoperative adjuvant radiation therapy, if it is needed [27].

Loss of the lacrimal drainage apparatus, including the canaliculi, is common after removal of medial canthal cancers. We typically do primary repair of canaliculi with silicone stenting only for defects that involve up to 5 mm of canalicular loss;

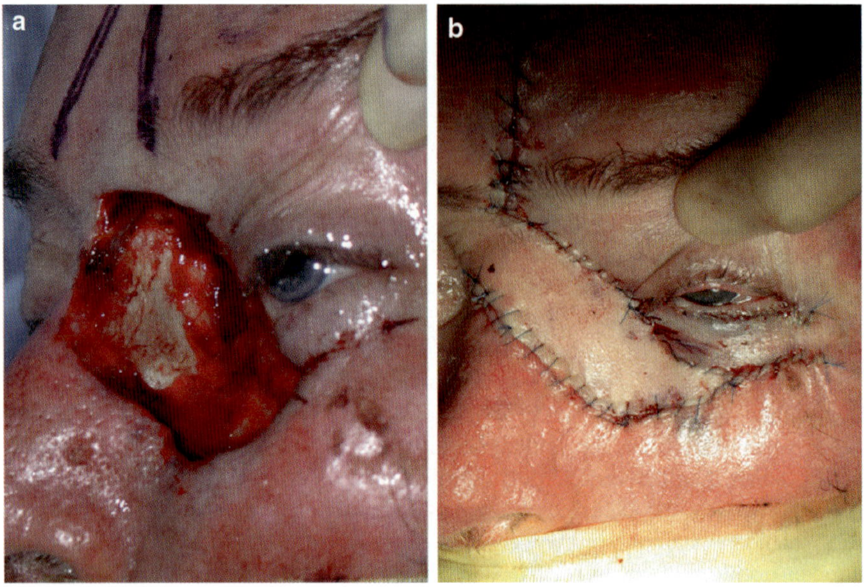

Fig. 18.4 Large left medial canthal defect closed with a combination of a glabellar flap and other local flaps. (**a**) Defect. (**b**) Intraoperative appearance after flap placement

otherwise, we prefer to perform lacrimal bypass surgery, including placement of a Pyrex glass tube ("Jones tube"), after the soft tissue reconstruction in the medial canthal angle has stabilized and only if the patient has symptomatic epiphora.

Spontaneous granulation ("laissez faire" granulation) of anterior lamellar defects has been used with varying success because of cicatrix formation [28]. This is best used when the defect straddles the medial canthal tendon with approximately equal areas above and below the tendon [2]. In such cases, tissue shrinkage that occurs postoperatively should be symmetrical, minimizing the risk of displacement of the canthus or of lower lid ectropion. Of note, healing with a laissez faire strategy takes much longer than healing with grafts and flaps and requires daily care to avoid infection and prominent scars.

References

1. Patrinely JR, Marines HM, Anderson RL. Skin flaps in periorbital reconstruction. Surv Ophthalmol 1987;31:249–61.
2. Arthurs BP. Tumor excision and eyelid reconstruction. In: Della Rocca RC, Bedrosian EH, Arthurs BP, editors. Ophthalmic Plastic Surgery Decision Making and Techniques. New York, NY: McGraw-Hill, 2002:117–35.
3. Harvey J. Modified "double Z-plasty" in the closure of medial canthal defects. Ophthalmic Surg 1987;18:120–2.
4. Hughes WL, editor. Reconstructive Surgery of the Eyelids, second edition. St. Louis, MO: Mosby, 1954.

5. Smith B, Lisman R. Preparation of split thickness auricular cartilage for use in ophthalmic plastic surgery. Ophthalmic Surg 1982;13:1018–21.
6. Baylis HI, Rosen N, Neuhaus RW. Obtaining auricular cartilage for reconstructive surgery. Am J Ophthalmol 1982;93:709–12.
7. Anderson RL, Weinstein GS. Full thickness bipedicle flap for total lower eyelid reconstruction. Arch Ophthalmol 1987;105:570–6.
8. Anderson RL, Jordan DR, Beard C. Full-thickness unipedicle flap for lower eyelid reconstruction. Arch Ophthalmol 1988;106:122–5.
9. Leone CR, Van Gemert JV. Lower lid reconstruction using tarsoconjunctival grafts and bipedicle skin–muscle flap. Arch Ophthalmol 1989;107:758–60.
10. Hewes EH, Sullivan JH, Beard C. Lower eyelid reconstruction by tarsal transposition. Am J Ophthalmol 1976;81:512–4.
11. Kanski JJ, editor. Clinical Ophthalmology: A Systematic Approach, fifth edition. London: Butterworth Heinemann, 2003:25–6.
12. Putterman AM. Viable composite grafting in eyelid reconstruction. Am J Ophthalmol 1978;85:237–41.
13. Cohen MS, Shorr N. Eyelid reconstruction with hard palate mucosa grafts. Ophthal Plast Reconstr Surg 1992;8:183–95.
14. Siegel RJ. Palatal grafts for eyelid reconstruction. Plast Reconstr Surg 1985;76:411–4.
15. Brown BZ. The use of homologous tarsus as a donor graft in lid surgery. Ophthal Plast Reconstr Surg 1985;1:91–5.
16. Hurwitz JJ, Corin SM, Tucker SM. The use of free periosteal grafts in extensive lower lid reconstruction. Ophthalmic Surg 1989;20:415–9.
17. Jordan DR, Tse DT, Anderson RL, et al. Irradiated homologous tarsal plate banking: a new alternative in eyelid reconstruction: part II. Human data. Ophthal Plast Reconstr Surg 1990;6:168–76.
18. Tenzel RR. Reconstruction of the central one-half of an eyelid. Arch Ophthalmol 1975;93:125–6.
19. Tenzel RR, Stewart WB. Eyelid reconstruction by the semicircle flap technique. Ophthalmology 1978;85:1164–9.
20. Levine MR, Buckman G. Semicircular flap revisited. Arch Ophthalmol 1986;104:915.
21. Cutler NL, Beard C. A method for partial and total upper eyelid reconstruction. Am J Ophthalmol 1955;39:1.
22. Leone CR. Lateral canthal reconstruction. Ophthalmology 1987;94:238–41.
23. Holt JE, Holt GR, Van Kirk M. Use of temporalis fascia in eyelid reconstruction. Ophthalmology 1984;91:89–93.
24. Howard GR, Nerad JA, Kersten RC. Medial canthoplasty with microplate fixation. Arch Ophthalmol 1992;110:1793–7.
25. Dortzbach RK, Hawes MJ. Midline forehead flap in reconstructive procedures of the eyelids and exenterated socket. Ophthalmic Surg 1981;12:257–68.
26. Teske SA, Kersten RC, Devoto MH, et al. The modified rhomboid transposition flap in periocular reconstruction. Ophthal Plast Reconstr Surg 1998;14:360–6.
27. Spinelli HM, Jelks GW. Periocular reconstruction: a systematic approach. Plast Reconstr Surg 1993;91:1017–24.
28. Lowry JC, Bartley GB, Garrity JA. The role of second-intention healing in periocular reconstruction. Ophthal Plast Reconstr Surg 1997;13:174–88.

Chapter 19
Nasolacrimal Duct Obstruction and Lacrimal Surgery in Cancer Patients

Aaron Savar and Bita Esmaeli

Abstract Nasolacrimal duct obstruction is often seen in patients with cancer. Iatrogenic causes such as surgery, radiation therapy, and chemotherapy are among the most common causes. Primary lacrimal drainage tumors are less common causes. The evaluation of patients with suspected nasolacrimal duct obstruction should include a thorough history and a comprehensive ophthalmic examination, including probing and irrigation of the lacrimal drainage apparatus and a Schirmer's test. Imaging studies may also be necessary. Treatment depends on the degree and location of the obstruction and may consist of probing and irrigation alone; balloon dilation; intubation of the drainage system with silicone stents; or dacryocystorhinostomy, usually with placement of silicone stents to maintain duct patency during healing.

19.1 Introduction

Obstruction of the nasolacrimal drainage apparatus can occur in cancer patients for a variety of reasons. Patients typically present with epiphora, which can be extremely bothersome. Indeed, it can be one of the most troubling symptoms experienced by patients as it can interfere with vision and appearance.

19.2 Anatomy

Tears drain from the ocular surface to the nose via the lacrimal drainage apparatus (Fig. 19.1). Tears enter the superior and inferior puncta and pass into the lacrimal canaliculi, which join to form the common canaliculus. The valve of Rosenmüller

A. Savar (✉)
Section of Ophthalmology, Department of Head and Neck Surgery, The University of Texas M.D. Anderson Cancer Center, Houston, TX, USA
e-mail: asavar@gmail.com

B. Esmaeli (ed.), *Ophthalmic Oncology*, M.D. Anderson Solid Tumor Oncology Series 6, DOI 10.1007/978-1-4419-0374-7_19,

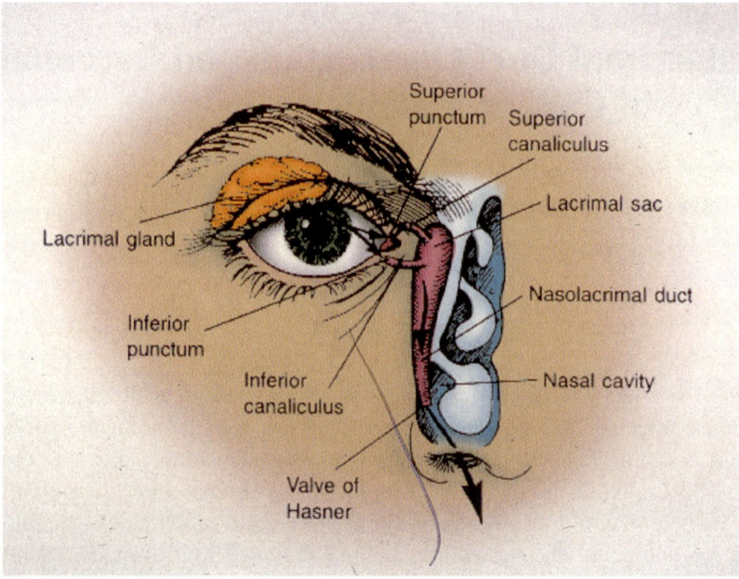

Fig. 19.1 Anatomic components of the lacrimal drainage apparatus

separates the common canaliculus from the nasolacrimal sac. Once in the sac, tears pass inferiorly into the nasolacrimal duct, cross the valve of Hasner, and enter the nose under the inferior turbinate.

19.3 Causes of Obstruction

Causes of nasolacrimal duct obstruction in cancer patients include primary obstruction from a malignancy and secondary obstruction as a result of therapies, such as surgical manipulation, radiation therapy, and chemotherapy [1–3].

Lacrimal drainage system neoplasms are uncommon. A study of 202 lacrimal sac specimens obtained at the time of dacryocystorhinostomy (DCR) from patients thought to have primary acquired nasolacrimal duct obstruction showed no evidence of neoplasia in any of the specimens [4]. On rare occasions, however, nasolacrimal duct obstruction can occur secondary to neoplasia. Epiphora is the most common presentation of tumors of the lacrimal drainage system [5]. In a series of 115 patients with lacrimal sac tumors, 53% presented with epiphora, 37% had dacryocystitis, and 36% had a lacrimal sac mass [6]. Epithelial tumors—including transitional, squamous cell, mucoepidermoid, and basaloid carcinomas—are the most common type of lacrimal drainage system malignancy (Fig. 19.2) [5]. Other, less common malignancies include lymphomas and leukemias [7], melanoma [5], and metastases from primary tumors at other sites [8].

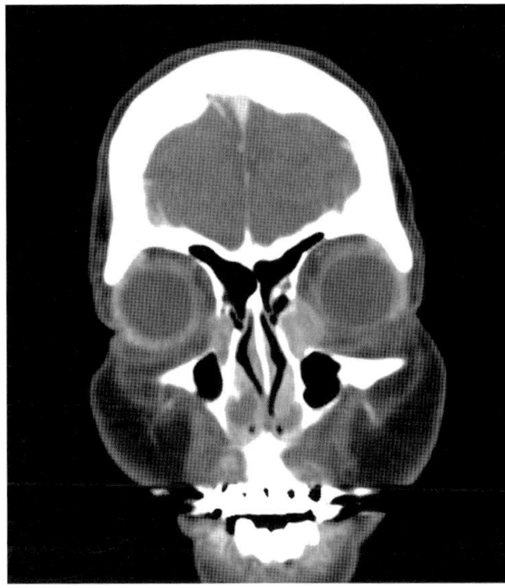

Fig. 19.2 Computed tomography scan in a patient with a primary squamous cell carcinoma of the left lacrimal sac

Secondary causes of nasolacrimal duct obstruction are commonly seen in patients with head and neck cancer. Resection of midface tumors may require removal of portions of the nasolacrimal drainage system or nearby tissues. Treatment with external-beam radiation therapy can damage the mucosa of the nasolacrimal drainage system, as can chemotherapy. In many patients with head and neck cancer, the cause of obstruction is a combination of damage from surgery, radiation therapy, and chemotherapy [9].

Treatment of thyroid carcinoma with radioactive iodine (I-131) is also known to cause nasolacrimal duct obstruction [10, 11]. Iodine is taken up in the thyroid gland by the sodium iodide symporter. This transport protein is also present in the basolateral surface of the epithelium of the lacrimal sac and nasolacrimal duct [12]. Treatment with I-131 can result in fibrosis of these tissues, causing nasolacrimal duct obstruction. Kloos et al. [10] looked at a large cohort of 390 patients who had received I-131 treatment and found 10 with nasolacrimal duct obstruction.

A number of chemotherapy drugs have been shown to cause nasolacrimal stenosis and obstruction, including 5-fluorouracil, docetaxel, mitomycin C, and S-1.

5-Fluorouracil is a pyrimidine analog used in the treatment of a variety of malignancies. Systemic 5-fluorouracil was first reported to cause lacrimal outflow obstruction by Haidak et al. [13]. The mechanism of this effect is thought to be due to chronic inflammation leading to stenosis of the lacrimal drainage system caused by 5-fluorouracil secreted in the tears [14, 15]. While tearing may be seen in 27% of patients treated with systemic 5-fluorouracil, punctal–canalicular stenosis is seen only in 6% [15].

Docetaxel is an antimitotic chemotherapy drug used in the treatment of metastatic carcinomas, frequently breast and prostate cancer. Secreted in tears, docetaxel has been shown to cause nasolacrimal duct obstruction in a dose-dependent manner [16]. Histopathologic analysis of tissue from the lacrimal drainage system and nasal mucosa of patients with nasolacrimal duct obstructions due to docetaxel has shown fibrosis and chronic inflammation [17]. The risk of obstruction is greatest in patients receiving weekly doses and is much less frequent in patients receiving doses every third week (Fig. 19.3a) [18]. A high index of suspicion for this complication is important, and all patients receiving weekly doses of docetaxel should have a baseline ophthalmic examination and monthly follow-up examinations. If epiphora develops, prophylactic silicone intubation is recommended (Fig. 19.3b). In patients who develop epiphora while receiving doses of docetaxel every third week, frequent probing and irrigation and a taper of topical steroids is sufficient to address epiphora in the majority of patients [19]. In advanced cases and in patients who are evaluated after many months of treatment with weekly doses of docetaxel, a DCR and placement of a Pyrex glass tube ("Jones tube") (Fig. 19.3c) may be the only way to alleviate epiphora [20].

Paclitaxel has also been reported to cause nasolacrimal duct obstruction, though only in a single case report of a patient who had also received radiation therapy [21]. We have evaluated many patients complaining of epiphora associated with the use of paclitaxel but to date have not observed anatomic closure of the puncta and canaliculi in association with paclitaxel's use.

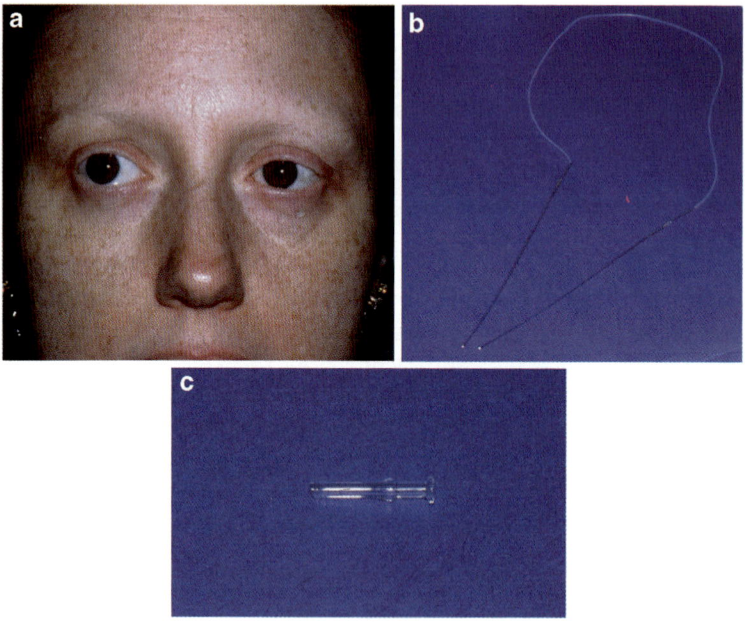

Fig. 19.3 (**a**) Obvious epiphora in a patient treated with weekly doses of docetaxel for several months. (**b**) A silicone tube can be used as a stent for bicanalicular intubation. (**c**) A Pyrex glass tube ("Jones tube")

Punctal stenosis has been reported with the topical use of mitomycin C [22]. The puncta and canaliculi are the most commonly affected sites [23].

S-1 is an antineoplastic prodrug of 5-fluorouracil used in the treatment of gastrointestinal carcinomas. It has been reported to cause punctal, canalicular, and nasolacrimal duct obstruction [24].

Idiopathic acquired nasolacrimal duct obstruction is a diagnosis of exclusion in cancer patients, but this type of nasolacrimal duct obstruction would be expected to be at least as common in cancer patients as in noncancer patients.

19.4 Evaluation

Evaluation of cancer patients with suspected nasolacrimal duct obstruction requires taking a thorough history with attention to symptoms and signs of epiphora, medical problems, cancer history, medications used (including previous chemotherapy), radiation therapy, and surgeries in the orbital area. A comprehensive ophthalmic examination is necessary and should include particular attention to the appearance and position of the puncta and a careful search for masses in the nose or the periorbital area. Probing and irrigation of the lacrimal drainage apparatus should be performed, and it should be noted whether there is any resistance in the canalicular system, how far a probe is able to be passed, and whether fluid refluxes out of or passes into the nasopharynx. A Schirmer's test should be performed to provide an objective measurement of tear production. This can also help identify dry eye syndrome, a common cause of "pseudoepiphora."

Although not typically used in most patients, tear testing can be performed to further evaluate flow through the tear drainage system. Tear testing can include the dye disappearance test, Jones I test, and Jones II test.

In certain cases, imaging may be necessary to further assess the lacrimal drainage system. Available modalities include fluoroscopy, dacryoscintigraphy, computed tomography, ultrasonography, and magnetic resonance imaging.

19.5 Treatment

In the case of mild, early obstruction associated with chemotherapy, probing and irrigation alone may provide relief. Balloon dilation, though not used in our practice, is another noninvasive option; however, it must be repeated, and its efficacy in the treatment of chemotherapy-induced lacrimal obstruction is unclear.

In many cases, if the nasolacrimal duct obstruction is identified early, before it is complete, intubation of the drainage system with silicone stents can prevent progression to complete obstruction and the need for more invasive surgical procedures. Use of stents should be based on findings on probing and irrigation of the system; stents should not be placed solely because of exposure in the absence of signs and symptoms of obstruction.

For anatomic blockage of the nasolacrimal duct, DCR is the standard treatment. This procedure creates an artificial connection between the lacrimal sac and the middle meatus of the nose, bypassing the nasolacrimal duct. Silicone stents are placed at the time of surgery to maintain patency during healing. The outcome of DCR in head and neck cancer patients was evaluated by Diba et al. [9], who found a failure rate of 17% in these patients. This increased rate is likely due to the multifactorial nature of nasolacrimal duct obstruction in head and neck cancer patients, many of whom are exposed to chemotherapy, high-dose radiation therapy with its sequelae of nasal mucosal chronic long-term inflammation and fibrosis, and previous surgery including complex reconstruction with free flaps in the area. In patients with a history of irradiation of the area, surgery should be delayed for at least 12 months if possible as the risk of recurrent obstruction is higher. Additionally, in patients who have received radiation to the lacrimal drainage system, stents should be left in place for an extended period of time, usually at least 6 months.

DCR can be performed via an open external approach or via an endoscopic approach. Debate exists over which method is preferable. Similar results have been reported with the two methods in various studies of idiopathic acquired nasolacrimal duct obstruction, but most studies report a higher failure rate with the endoscopic approach. Although the underlying mechanism of obstruction in cancer patients is different from that of idiopathic acquired nasolacrimal duct obstruction, DCR by either method is reasonable for cancer patients. In our practice, external DCR is preferred because the anatomy is often markedly abnormal due to prior surgery or other therapies.

If the canaliculi are significantly obstructed, conjunctivodacryocystorhinostomy with Pyrex glass tube ("Jones tube") placement is usually necessary. Complications are more common in patients requiring Jones tube placement than in patients undergoing standard DCR. In a study of 49 patients who had Jones tube placement, extrusion, obstruction, and malposition were the most common complications, seen in 49%, 47%, and 33% of treated patients, respectively. Other complications included discomfort, infection, and diplopia. Despite this, 70% of patients reported being satisfied after the procedure [25].

References

1. Bartley GB. Acquired lacrimal drainage obstruction: an etiologic classification system, case reports, and a review of the literature. Part 1. Ophthal Plast Reconstr Surg 1992;8:237–42.
2. Bartley GB. Acquired lacrimal drainage obstruction: an etiologic classification system, case reports, and a review of the literature. Part 2. Ophthal Plast Reconstr Surg 1992;8:243–9.
3. Bartley GB. Acquired lacrimal drainage obstruction: an etiologic classification system, case reports, and a review of the literature. Part 3. Ophthal Plast Reconstr Surg 1993;9:11–26.
4. Lee-Wing MW, Ashenhurst ME. Clinicopathologic analysis of 166 patients with primary acquired nasolacrimal duct obstruction. Ophthalmology 2001;108:2038–40.
5. Valenzuela AA, McNab AA, Selva D, et al. Clinical features and management of tumors affecting the lacrimal drainage apparatus. Ophthal Plast Reconstr Surg 2006;22:96–101.
6. Stefanyszyn MA, Hidayat AA, Pe'er JJ, et al. Lacrimal sac tumors. Ophthal Plast Reconstr Surg 1994;10:169–84.

7. Yip CC, Bartley GB, Habermann TM, et al. Involvement of the lacrimal drainage system by leukemia or lymphoma. Ophthal Plast Reconstr Surg 2002;18:242–6.
8. Wladis EJ, Frempong T, Gausas R. Nasolacrimal metastasis from hepatocellular carcinoma masquerading as dacryocystitis. Ophthal Plast Reconstr Surg 2007;23:333–5.
9. Diba R, Saadati H, Esmaeli B. Outcomes of dacryocystorhinostomy in patients with head and neck tumors. Head Neck 2005;27:72–5.
10. Kloos RT, Duvuuri V, Jhiang SM, et al. Nasolacrimal drainage system obstruction from radioactive iodine therapy for thyroid carcinoma. J Clin Endocrinol Metab 2002;87:5817–20.
11. Shepler TR, Sherman SI, Faustina MM, et al. Nasolacrimal duct obstruction associated with radioactive iodine therapy for thyroid carcinoma. Ophthal Plast Reconstr Surg 2003;19: 479–81.
12. Morgenstern KE, Vadysirisack DD, Zhang Z, et al. Expression of sodium iodide symporter in the lacrimal drainage system: implication for the mechanism underlying nasolacrimal duct obstruction in I(131)-treated patients. Ophthal Plast Reconstr Surg 2005;21:337–44.
13. Haidak DJ, Hurwitz BS, Yeung KY. Tear-duct fibrosis (dacryostenosis) due to 5-fluorouracil. Ann Intern Med 1978;88:657.
14. Caravella LP Jr, Burns JA, Zangmeister M. Punctal–canalicular stenosis related to systemic fluorouracil therapy. Arch Ophthalmol 1981;99:284–6.
15. Eiseman AS, Flanagan JC, Brooks AB, et al. Ocular surface, ocular adnexal, and lacrimal complications associated with the use of systemic 5-fluorouracil. Ophthal Plast Reconstr Surg 2003;19(3):216–24.
16. Esmaeli B, Ahmadi MA, Rivera E, et al. Docetaxel secretion in tears: association with lacrimal drainage obstruction. Arch Ophthalmol 2002;120:1180–2.
17. Esmaeli B, Burnstine MA, Ahmadi MA, et al. Docetaxel-induced histologic changes in the lacrimal sac and the nasal mucosa. Ophthal Plast Reconstr Surg 2003;19:305–8.
18. Esmaeli B, Amin S, Valero V, et al. Prospective study of incidence and severity of epiphora and canalicular stenosis in patients with metastatic breast cancer receiving docetaxel. J Clin Oncol 2006;24:3619–22.
19. Esmaeli B, Hidaji L, Adinin RB, et al. Blockage of the lacrimal drainage apparatus as a side effect of docetaxel therapy. Cancer 2003;98:504–7.
20. Ahmadi MA, Esmaeli B. Surgical treatment of canalicular stenosis in patients receiving weekly docetaxel. Arch Ophthalmol 2001;119:1802–4.
21. McCartney E, Valluri S, Rushing D, et al. Upper and lower system nasolacrimal duct stenosis secondary to paclitaxel. Ophthal Plast Reconstr Surg 2007;23:170–1.
22. Billing K, Karagiannis A, Selva D. Punctal–canalicular stenosis associated with mitomycin-C for corneal epithelial dysplasia. Am J Ophthalmol 2003;136(4):746–7.
23. Kopp ED, Seregard S. Epiphora as a side effect of topical mitomycin C. Br J Ophthalmol 2004;88(11):1422–4.
24. Esmaeli B, Golio D, Lubecki L, et al. Canalicular and nasolacrimal duct blockage: an ocular side effect associated with the antineoplastic drug S-1. Am J Ophthalmol 2005;140:325–7.
25. Lim C, Martin P, Benger R, et al. Lacrimal canalicular bypass surgery with the Lester Jones tube. Am J Ophthalmol 2004;137:101–8.

Chapter 20
Eyelid Malposition: Unique Scenarios in Cancer Patients

Aaron Savar and Bita Esmaeli

Abstract Eyelid malposition in cancer patients encompasses a variety of conditions, including ectropion, entropion, ptosis, eyelid retraction, and eyelid malposition due to periorbital edema. Ectropion is by far the most commonly encountered form of eyelid malposition in cancer patients. In some situations, the eyelid abnormality is the presenting sign of an underlying malignancy, but most often, it is the result of therapeutic interventions for cancer.

20.1 Introduction

A variety of forms of eyelid malposition can be seen in cancer patients. Eyelid malposition in cancer patients can result from direct effects on the lids by a nearby tumor; scarring or nerve damage from surgery; or radiation therapy or chemotherapy.

20.2 Ectropion

Ectropion is the most common form of eyelid malposition seen in cancer patients.

20.2.1 Ectropion Due to Facial Nerve Paralysis

Paralytic ectropion is common in patients with facial nerve paralysis, which is often seen after parotid tumor resection. It can also be seen with a variety of other conditions, including infiltration of the facial nerve by tumor and central nervous system

A. Savar (✉)
Section of Ophthalmology, Department of Head and Neck Surgery, The University of Texas M.D. Anderson Cancer Center, Houston, TX, USA
e-mail: asavar@gmail.com

B. Esmaeli (ed.), *Ophthalmic Oncology*, M.D. Anderson Solid Tumor Oncology Series 6, DOI 10.1007/978-1-4419-0374-7_20,

lesions involving the facial nerve nucleus. Patients with facial nerve paralysis typically present with multiple eyelid abnormalities due to loss of tone of the orbicularis oculi muscle, including upper eyelid retraction and paralytic ectropion of the lower eyelid. This combination of eyelid abnormalities can predispose patients to exposure keratopathy and necessitates multifaceted surgical repair. In addition, loss of frontalis muscle tone can result in brow ptosis, which can further exacerbate these problems.

Initial treatment of patients with facial nerve paralysis consists of frequent lubrication with artificial tears and ointment. Tape tarsorrhaphies can be performed at night to avoid excessive exposure.

Surgical options for patients with facial nerve paralysis include implantation of an upper eyelid gold weight, lower eyelid horizontal tightening procedures, lateral tarsorrhaphy, cerclage, palpebral springs, or a combination of these. In our experience, placement of a gold weight, lateral tarsal strip procedure, and lateral tarsorrhaphy performed together yield good results. A direct brow lift can be added if necessary. More information about these techniques is available in Chapter 24. In patients who are not good operative candidates, external weights are available to assist in eyelid closure.

Review of a series of 72 patients from our institution with facial nerve palsy found good results with periocular reconstruction. All 72 patients underwent placement of a gold weight, 71 underwent lateral tarsorrhaphy, 53 underwent lateral tarsal strip procedure, and 21 underwent direct brow lift. Complications included gold weight extrusion in two patients and mild ptosis in four patients [1].

20.2.2 Cicatricial Ectropion

Another common type of ectropion in cancer patients is cicatricial ectropion. This type of ectropion can occur after combined treatment with surgery and postoperative external-beam radiation therapy for various head and neck cancers (Fig. 20.1) or with either of these modalities used alone. Chemotherapeutic agents can also

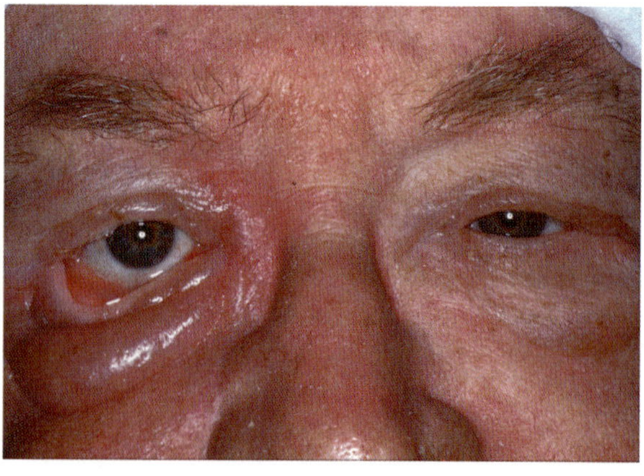

Fig. 20.1 Cicatricial ectropion of the lower eyelid in a patient with maxillary sinus carcinoma treated with maxillectomy and postoperative radiation therapy

cause cicatricial ectropion. Erlotinib and cetuximab, both inhibitors of the epidermal growth factor receptor, have been reported to cause cicatricial ectropion [2, 3], as has systemic fluorouracil [4, 5].

Periorbital tumors can present with ectropion. In a large series of patients with cutaneous T-cell lymphoma, 17 (0.8%) of 2155 patients had ectropion attributable to their disease. The majority of the cases of ectropion were cicatricial in nature [6]. Basal cell carcinoma has also been reported to present with ectropion [7].

In symptomatic cases of cicatricial ectropion, surgical repair is indicated. This most commonly consists of placement of a large full-thickness skin graft—usually harvested from the upper eyelid skin using a blepharoplasty incision—combined with an eyelid-shortening procedure such as the lateral tarsal strip procedure and a medial or a lateral tarsorrhaphy (Fig. 20.2). In our experience,

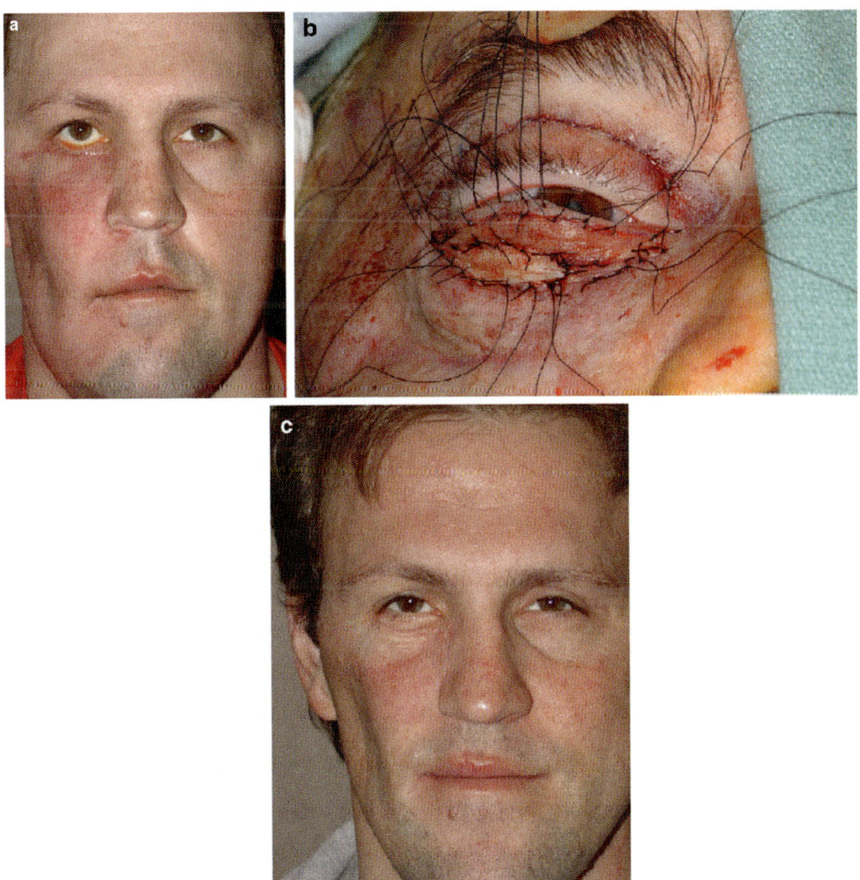

Fig. 20.2 Cicatricial ectropion of the lower eyelid in a patient with a history of maxillary sinus sarcoma. (**a**) Preoperative appearance. (**b**) Intraoperative photo: a full-thickness skin graft is placed and scar tissue released. (**c**) Improved position and function of the lower eyelid after surgical correction of cicatricial ectropion

full-thickness skin grafts are quite viable and effective in the periocular region even when the area has previously been treated with high-dose radiation therapy.

20.3 Entropion

Entropion is much less common than ectropion in cancer patients. As in the general population, the most common form of entropion in cancer patients is caused by lower eyelid laxity and disinsertion of the lower eyelid retractors. Cancer patients can also have cicatricial entropion as a complication of eyelid reconstruction in the periocular region or as a result of conjunctival scarring after surgery or radiation therapy. An eyelid-shortening procedure such as the lateral tarsal strip procedure is the typical corrective procedure.

20.4 Ptosis

The most common cause of ptosis in cancer patients is surgery. Postsurgical ptosis can be due to extensive resection of the upper eyelid or damage to the levator complex during surgery (Fig. 20.3).

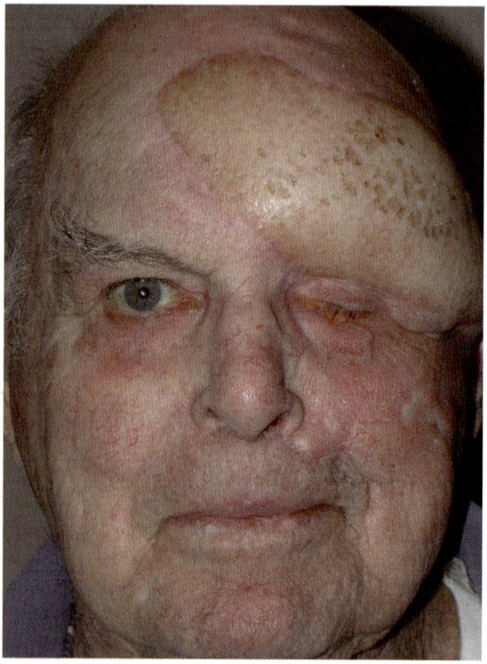

Fig. 20.3 Iatrogenic ptosis of the upper eyelid due to damage to the levator complex during resection of a squamous cell carcinoma of the forehead and brow area. There is also a component of mechanical ptosis due to the free flap in the forehead

Malignancies can cause a neurogenic ptosis in the form of Horner's syndrome. Tumors in the lateral medulla can affect the first-order neuron. Apical lung cancers, Pancoast tumors, and head and neck cancers necessitating extensive neck dissection can cause a second-order Horner's syndrome. In children, malignancy can produce an acquired Horner's syndrome. In a study of 56 pediatric patients with Horner's syndrome, 23% of the cases were due to neoplasm, most commonly neuroblastoma [8]. Loss of sympathetic stimulation of Mueller's muscle typically results in 1–2 mm of ptosis. Patients also have the other classic findings in Horner's syndrome, including elevation of the lower eyelid, miosis, anhidrosis, conjunctival injection, and a drop in intraocular pressure. If the ptosis is causing visual compromise or is cosmetically unacceptable, repair using the posterior müllerectomy technique or a Fasanella–Servat procedure (tarsoconjunctival müllerectomy) would be adequate.

Compressive neoplasms, particularly skull base tumors, can be a cause of third-nerve palsy and resultant upper eyelid ptosis. Patients with this type of ptosis would be expected to have other oculomotor disturbances as well as a dilated pupil.

Lambert–Eaton myasthenic syndrome is a cause of ptosis in some cancer patients. It is a paraneoplastic syndrome, seen most commonly in small cell lung cancer, that can cause ptosis as well as proximal muscle weakness and autonomic dysfunction. In some cases, these symptoms precede the diagnosis of the underlying malignancy. The syndrome is caused by immunoglobulins directed against presynaptic calcium channels.

Plexiform neurofibromas can cause mechanical ptosis. These lesions typically present with an S-shaped deformity of the upper eyelid (please see Chapter 2).

20.5 Eyelid Retraction

In cases of massive proptosis due to large orbital tumors, the eyelid may not adequately cover the surface of the globe (Fig. 20.4). In this situation, there are often severe symptoms of exposure. Depending on the tumor type, treatment with chemotherapy, local radiation therapy, or surgical resection may allow the globe to return to the normal position in the orbit.

20.6 Periorbital Edema Secondary to Imatinib Mesylate

Imatinib mesylate (Gleevec) is a tyrosine kinase receptor inhibitor used in the treatment of certain cases of chronic myelogenous leukemia and gastrointestinal stromal tumor. In a phase I study, imatinib mesylate was noted to cause periorbital edema in 30% of patients [9]. In some cases, the edema is so severe that visual compromise develops and surgical debulking is necessary (Fig. 20.5) [10]. It has been shown that the cells in the periocular dermis express tyrosine kinase

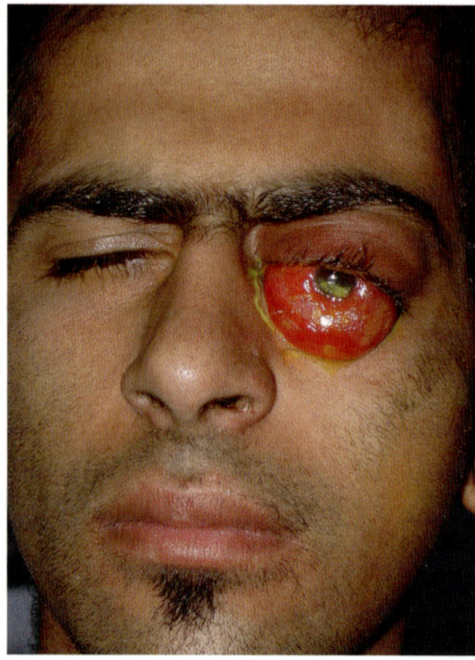

Fig. 20.4 Metastatic Ewing sarcoma causing massive proptosis, upper and lower eyelid retraction, and exposure keratopathy. From Savar A, Trent J, Al-Zubidi N, et al. Efficacy of adjuvant and neoadjuvant therapies for adult orbital sarcomas. Ophthal Plast Reconstr Surg 2010;26(3):185–189. Reprinted with permission

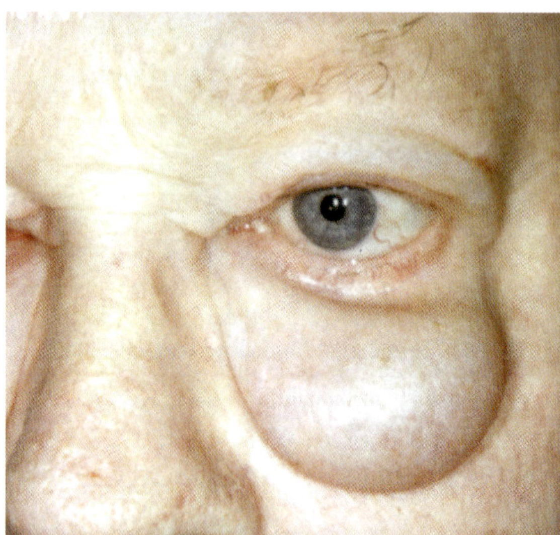

Fig. 20.5 Severe periorbital edema and lower eyelid festoons caused by imatinib mesylate in a patient with chronic myelogenous leukemia. From Esmaeli B, Diba R, Ahmadi MA, et al. Periorbital oedema and apiphora as ocular side effects of imatinib mesylate (Gleevec) [letter]. Eye 2004;18:760–762

receptors targeted by imatinib, including the platelet-derived growth factor receptor. This receptor is known to be involved in the regulation of tissue fluid, which may explain the propensity for edema formation in this area with imatinib treatment [10, 11].

References

1. Golio D, De Martelaere S, Anderson J, et al. Outcomes of periocular reconstruction for facial nerve paralysis in cancer patients. Plast Reconstr Surg 2007;119:1233–7.
2. Methvin AB, Gausas RE. Newly recognized ocular side effects of erlotinib. Ophthal Plast Reconstr Surg 2007;23:63–5.
3. Garibaldi DC, Adler RA. Cicatricial ectropion associated with treatment of metastatic colorectal cancer with cetuximab. Ophthal Plast Reconstr Surg 2007;23:62–3.
4. Straus DJ, Mausolf FA, Ellerby RA, et al. Cicatricial ectropion secondary to 5-fluorouracil therapy. Med Pediatr Oncol 1977;3:15–9.
5. Hurwitz BS. Cicatricial ectropion: a complication of systemic fluorouracil. Arch Ophthalmol 1993;111:1608–9.
6. Cook BE Jr, Bartley GB, Pittelkow MR. Ophthalmic abnormalities in patients with cutaneous T-cell lymphoma. Ophthalmology 1999;106:1339–44.
7. Beyer TL, Dryden RM. Basal cell carcinoma masquerading as ectropion. Arch Ophthalmol 1988;106:170–1.
8. Mahoney NR, Liu GT, Menacker SJ, et al. Pediatric Horner syndrome: etiologies and roles of imaging and urine studies to detect neuroblastoma and other responsible mass lesions. Am J Ophthalmol 2006;142:651–9.
9. van Oosterom AT, Judson I, Verweij J, et al. European Organisation for Research and Treatment of Cancer Soft Tissue and Bone Sarcoma Group. Safety and efficacy of imatinib (STI571) in metastatic gastrointestinal stromal tumours: a phase I study. Lancet 2001;358:1421–3.
10. Esmaeli B, Prieto VG, Butler CE, et al. Severe periorbital edema secondary to STI571 (Gleevec). Cancer 2002;95:881–7.
11. Larson JS, Bergstrom LK, Cameron JD, et al. Severe periorbital edema secondary to imatinib mesylate for chronic myelogenous leukemia. Arch Ophthalmol 2007;125:985–6.

Chapter 21
Craniofacial Surgery in the Orbit and Periorbital Region

Dominick Golio

Abstract Orbital reconstruction after ablative cancer surgery is one of the most challenging procedures in facial reconstruction. Thorough knowledge of the anatomy of the orbit and its contents is critical for successful orbital reconstruction. The principal objectives of orbital reconstruction are (1) to provide support to the orbital contents to avoid displacement of the globe and diplopia; (2) to prevent ascending infections by obliterating any communication between the orbit and the nose, mouth, nasopharynx, and anterior skull base; (3) to reconstruct the palatal surface to enhance articulation and deglutition; (4) to reconstruct the lacrimal apparatus; and (5) to provide enough tissue volume to achieve facial symmetry and a good aesthetic result. Following maxillectomy with orbital exenteration, postoperative high-dose adjuvant radiation therapy is often required; therefore, reconstruction usually requires grafting of free tissue flaps from distant donor sites. Reconstruction in patients who have undergone maxillectomy with preservation of the orbital contents but resection of the floor of the orbit can be particularly challenging. The primary goal of reconstruction after orbital exenteration is to either line or fill the orbit with durable tissue that excludes the nasal cavity and paranasal sinuses and, when there is a cranial defect, protects the brain.

21.1 Introduction

Orbital reconstruction after ablative cancer surgery is one of the most challenging procedures in facial reconstruction. Significant advances in the field of craniofacial surgery have improved the functional and aesthetic outcomes of orbital reconstruction.

D. Golio (✉)
Departments of Surgery and Ophthalmology, State University of New York, Downstate Medical Center, Brooklyn, NY, USA
e-mail: dominickgoliomd@pol.net

B. Esmaeli (ed.), *Ophthalmic Oncology*, M.D. Anderson Solid Tumor Oncology Series 6, DOI 10.1007/978-1-4419-0374-7_21,

The unique and complex anatomy of the orbit means that small errors can produce suboptimal functional and cosmetic results. Thus, thorough knowledge of the anatomy of the orbit and its contents is critical for successful orbital reconstruction. The operative plan must be constructed on the basis of an accurate physical examination of the soft tissues, facial skeleton, and visual sensory system, combined with high-resolution computed tomographic scans in the axial and coronal planes with three-dimensional reconstruction. The addition of medical modeling adds the benefit of hands-on models on which to base the reconstructive plan. The overall success of the reconstructive procedure depends on adequate repositioning or reconstruction of the bony orbit and correction of any soft tissue defects. In the oncologic setting, extensive tumor resection may necessitate adequate soft tissue coverage of large defects.

21.2 Anatomic Considerations

Familiarity with the correct anatomic relationships of the orbit is essential in maintaining proper form and function.

In adults, the lateral orbital walls are approximately 90° from each other and angle 45° from anterior to posterior. The medial orbital walls are nearly straight anteroposterior, angling only slightly medially anteriorly. The divergent axis of each orbit is 23° (Fig. 21.1).

The orbit is widest 1 cm behind the orbital rim, which corresponds to the equator of the globe. The depth of the orbit is approximately 45 mm, but there is substantial variation between individuals and slight interindividual variation between the left and right orbits.

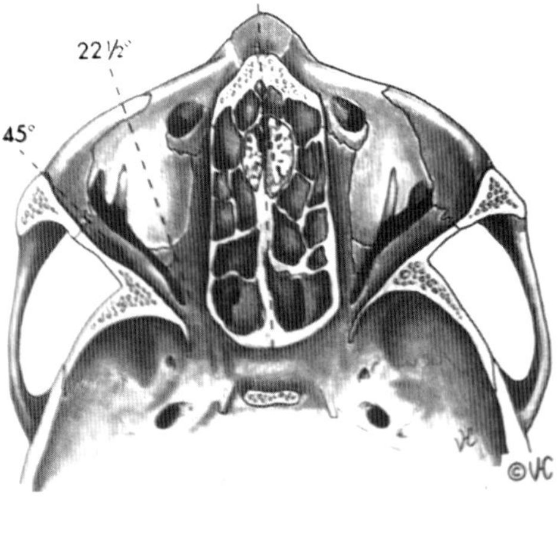

Fig. 21.1 Horizontal section through orbits. From Lemke BN, Lucarelli MJ. Anatomy of the ocular adnexa, orbit, and related facial structures. In: Nesi FA, Lisman RD, Levine MR, eds. Smith's Ophthalmic Plastic and Reconstructive Surgery. St. Louis, MO: Mosby-Year Book; 1998; p.4. Reprinted with permission

21.2.1 Orbital Margin

The orbital margin is a discontinuous spiral. It is roughly rectangular with a horizontal dimension of 40 mm and a vertical dimension of 32 mm. The zygomatic bone forms most of the lateral margin and the lateral half of the inferior rim. This is the facial buttress and provides significant protection to the globe. The zygomatic bone is also an important aesthetic component, providing elevation and projection to the midface. Any reconstruction should focus on returning as much symmetry as possible to the face.

The frontal bone encompasses the superior orbital margin and extends laterally and medially to form portions of the lateral and medial borders. In most skulls, the supraorbital neurovascular bundle rising to the forehead forms the medial superior notch. In some patients, the frontal bone actually forms a foramen.

The maxillary bone, rising to meet the maxillary process of the frontal bone, forms the medial orbital margin inferiorly. The lacrimal sac complicates the medial rim by indenting the maxillary bone and forming anterior (maxillary bone) and posterior (lacrimal bone) crests.

The infraorbital neurovascular bundle exits the maxilla via a foramen approximately 1 cm below the inferior orbital rim.

21.2.2 Nasal and Paranasal Sinuses

The orbital roof, floor, and medial wall are intimately related to the nasal cavity. These bones are pneumatized by paranasal sinuses arising from and maintaining communication with the nasal cavity.

The maxillary sinus is the largest paranasal sinus (15 mL) and is the first to develop. The roof of the maxillary sinus is the orbital floor. Medially, the orbital floor is thin and prone to fracture. It thickens laterally near the infraorbital canal. The roof of the sinus (orbital floor) declines from the medial wall to the lateral wall at an angle of 30°. The pterygopalatine fossa lies posteriorly with the internal maxillary artery intimately related to the posterior sinus wall. The nasal cavity lies medially except where the nasolacrimal canal and then inferior turbinate intervene.

The ethmoidal sinuses are the most exuberantly growing sinuses and may pneumatize the frontal, sphenoid, palatine, and lacrimal bones. Normally, 3–15 air cells expand from each lateral border of the cribriform plate. The air cell masses convolute medially to form the middle, superior, and supreme (if present) turbinates. The anterior and middle air cells drain into the middle meatus. The posterior air cells drain into the superior meatus.

The frontal sinus evaginates from the frontal recess superior to the nasal hiatus semilunaris. Pits are present at birth, but the infundibulum is not well developed or radiographically evident until approximately 6 years of age. The frontal sinus then expands until early adulthood, with greater expansion occurring in males. The frontonasal duct drains into the anterior middle meatus.

The sphenoid sinus evaginates from the most posterior portion of the nasal roof. Growth of this sinus continues until adulthood. There is usually a midline septum that divides the two portions of the sinus.

21.2.3 The Lacrimal System

The bony passage of the lacrimal system consists of the lacrimal sac fossa above, continuing inferiorly as the nasolacrimal canal to end under the inferior turbinate bone in the nose.

The lacrimal sac fossa is bounded in front by the anterior lacrimal crest of the maxillary bone frontal process and behind by the posterior lacrimal crest of the lacrimal bone.

21.2.4 Maxilla

The maxillary bone provides structure and support to the overlying structures, is critical to the functions of mastication, speech, and deglutition, and contributes significantly to facial projection and appearance. The maxilla has been described as a hexahedron (a geometric structure with six walls) (Fig. 21.2). The roof of the maxilla supports the globe. The medial wall is part of the lacrimal system. The floor of the maxilla forms the anterior portion of the hard palate and alveolar ridge. Several walls contribute to the paranasal sinuses, and the maxillary antrum is contained within the central portion of the maxilla. In addition, a majority of the muscles of facial expression and mastication insert on the maxilla. These muscles, together with the overlying skin and intraoral mucosa, constitute the lower eyelid, the cheek, the

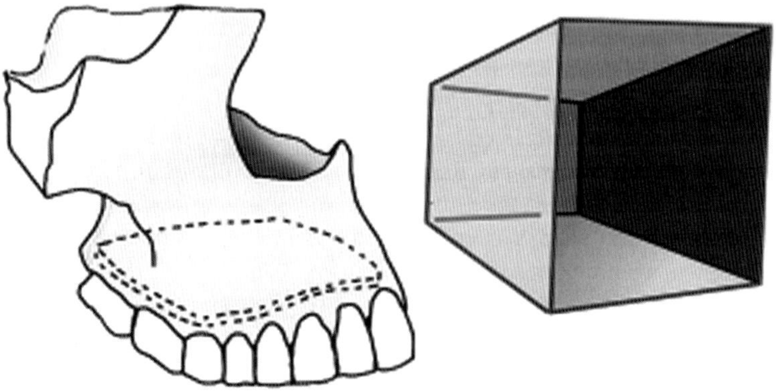

Fig. 21.2 View of maxilla demonstrating its hexahedron shape. The roof of the maxilla is the floor of the orbit. The floor of the maxilla is the hard palate. The vertical buttresses consist of the anterior, posterior, medial and lateral walls. The antrum of the maxilla in inside. From Cordeiro PG, Santamaria E. A classification system and algorithm for reconstruction of maxillectomy and midfacial defects. Plast Reconstr Surg 2000;80:2331–46. Reprinted with permission

upper lip, and the oral commissure. The two horizontal and three vertical buttresses of the maxilla are responsible for the projection of the midface and vertical facial height.

21.3 Repair of Orbital Defects

Orbital defects range from defects resulting from limited or subtotal maxillectomy to defects resulting from total maxillectomy with orbital exenteration. A varying number of adjacent structures are often excised in combination with the maxilla.

The principal objectives of orbital reconstruction are (1) to provide support to the orbital contents to avoid displacement of the globe and diplopia; (2) to prevent ascending infections by obliterating any communication between the orbit and the nose, the mouth, the nasopharynx, and the anterior skull base; (3) to reconstruct the palatal surface to enhance articulation and deglutition; (4) to reconstruct the lacrimal apparatus; and (5) to provide enough tissue volume to achieve facial symmetry and a good aesthetic result [1].

21.3.1 Overview of Approaches

The various approaches available for repair of orbital defects can be divided into two main categories: repair after maxillectomy with orbital exenteration and repair after maxillectomy without orbital exenteration. Reconstruction after total maxillectomy with preservation of the orbital contents is technically more challenging than reconstruction after maxillectomy combined with orbital exenteration.

21.3.1.1 Maxillectomy with Orbital Exenteration

Maxillectomy with orbital exenteration is a disfiguring and complex surgical procedure that is required when there is extensive invasion of cancer in the maxillary sinus with significant involvement of the orbital soft tissues. Given the frequent need for postoperative high-dose adjuvant radiation therapy, reconstruction usually requires grafting of free tissue flaps from distant donor sites, such as transverse rectus abdominis myocutaneous flaps and anterolateral thigh free flaps. The size of the defect dictates from where sufficient soft tissue can be harvested and transferred. It is possible to choose flaps that may allow for a concave orbital cavity so that the patient can use an orbital prosthesis if desired. In a recent study from M.D. Anderson Cancer Center, it was found that a radial forearm flap or a temporoparietal muscle flap may be the best choices in terms of potentially allowing for an orbital prosthesis. In some patients, especially those with complete obliteration of the orbital contents on the affected side, the choice of a free flap is limited to more bulky tissues, such as anterolateral thigh or abdominal flaps.

21.3.1.2 Maxillectomy Without Orbital Exenteration

Reconstruction in patients who have undergone maxillectomy with preservation of the orbital contents but resection of the floor of the orbit can be particularly challenging. The orbital floor has to be reconstructed, and often the orbit and maxillary sinus area have to be irradiated after reconstruction, which limits the use of synthetic material to rebuild the orbital floor. In such cases, the best option may be autologous vascularized tissue flaps with bone grafts supplemented with titanium or other similar material to provide support. In many cases, despite all efforts, there may be ocular morbidity associated with removal of the orbital floor—e.g., there may be entrapment of the inferior soft tissues of the orbit, including the inferior rectus muscle.

Multiple approaches to reconstruction of the radical maxillectomy defect with preservation of the orbit have been described. These include prosthesis attached to the palate alone [2], soft tissue pedicled flaps [3], free flaps with secondary bone grafting [4, 5], vascularized osteocutaneous free flaps [5–9], and nonvascularized bone grafts in conjunction with a soft tissue free flap or pedicled muscle flap [1]. Cordeiro and Santamaria [10] describe a systematic approach for reconstruction of the complex maxillectomy and midfacial defect.

21.3.2 Types of Maxillary Defects and Strategies for Their Repair

21.3.2.1 Type I Defect

Type I defects result from limited maxillectomy, which includes resection of one or two walls of the maxilla, excluding the palate and occasionally the orbital rim. In most patients, the anterior wall is partially removed with either the medial wall

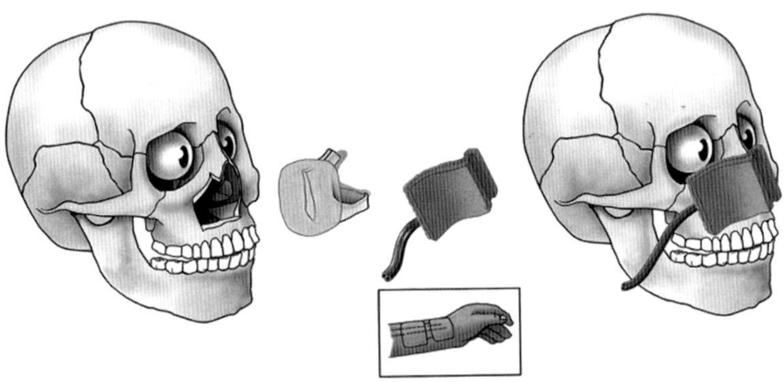

Fig. 21.3 Type I defect (limited maxillectomy). There is resection of anterior and medial walls of the maxilla (*left*). The resected area has skin, soft tissue, and bone creating a large surface area/low volume defect (*center, left*). The radial forearm fasciocutaneous flap provides multiple large surface areas with minimal volume (*center, right*). (*Right*) The radial forearm flap is shown in place with a skin island to resurface the anterior cheek and nasal lining. From Cordeiro PG, Santamaria E. A classification system and algorithm for reconstruction of maxillectomy and midfacial defects. Plast Reconstr Surg 2000;80:2331–46. Reprinted with permission

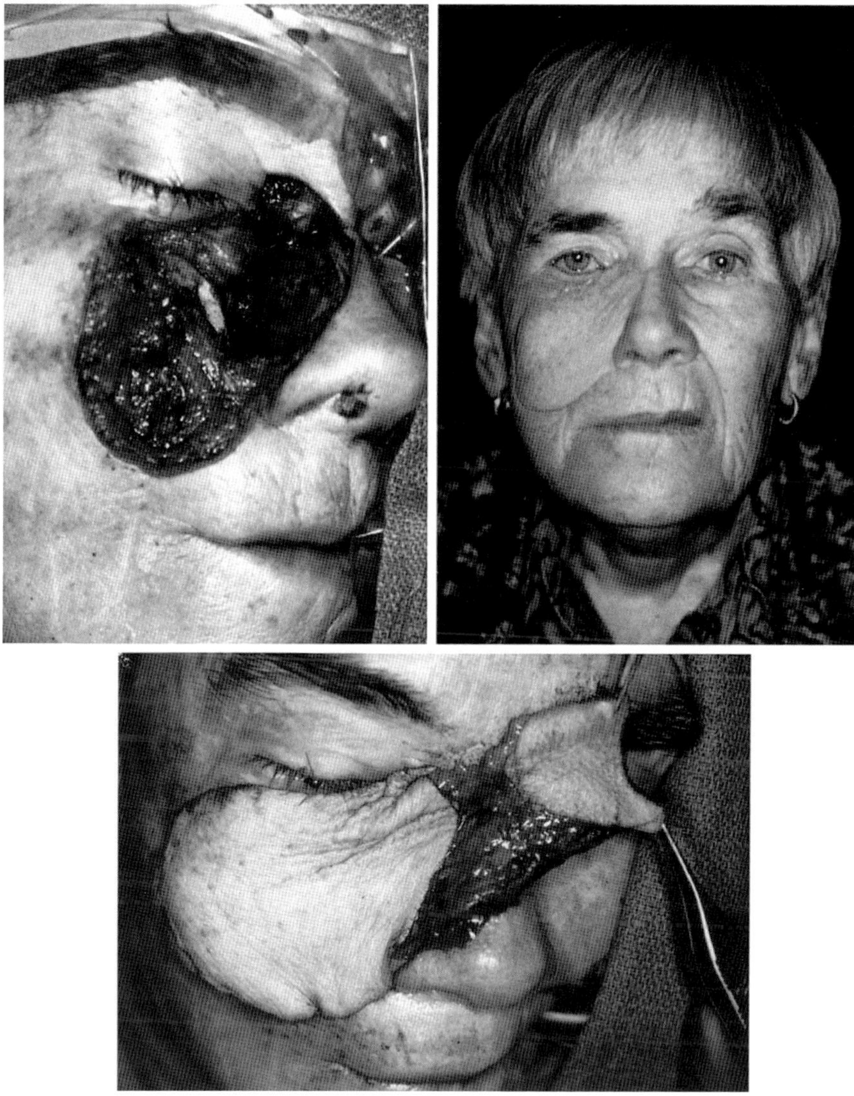

Fig. 21.4 Type I defect (*above, left*) after partial resection of orbital floor, external skin, and medial and anterior walls of the maxilla in a 68-year-old woman with a recurrent desmoplastic melanoma of the right cheek. (*Above, right*) Post operative photograph demonstrating excellent facial contour and cosmesis. (*Below*) Two skin island radial forearm flap demonstrating large surface area and minimal volume. From Cordeiro PG, Santamaria E. A classification system and algorithm for reconstruction of maxillectomy and midfacial defects. Plast Reconstr Surg 2000;80:2331–46. Reprinted with permission

or the orbital floor (Figs. 21.3 and 21.4). These defects have small volume and large surface area requirements. If critical segments of bone are missing, such as the orbital rim or the anterior floor of the orbit, nonvascularized bone grafts can be used. The radial forearm flap provides good external skin coverage and minimal bulk with multiple skin islands that can be deepithelialized to improve contour, wrap around bone grafts, or supply nasal lining.

21.3.2.2 Type II Defects

Type II defects result from subtotal maxillectomy, which includes resection of the maxillary arch, palate, and anterior and lateral walls (lower five walls) with preservation of the orbital floor (Fig. 21.5). These defects usually have medium volume and large surface area requirements. The radial forearm flap, when folded over, provides ample skin to reline the palatal mucosal surface as well as the nasal floor. Another alternative is the "osteocutaneous sandwich flap" [16], which supplies a vascularized bony strut to support the upper lip and maintain anterior projection. The bone of this flap is also adequate for osteointegration. This "sandwich" provides a moderate amount of bulk and is usually sufficient for the volume requirements of reconstruction. The osteocutaneous sandwich flap is also an excellent solution for reconstruction after bilateral subtotal maxillectomy.

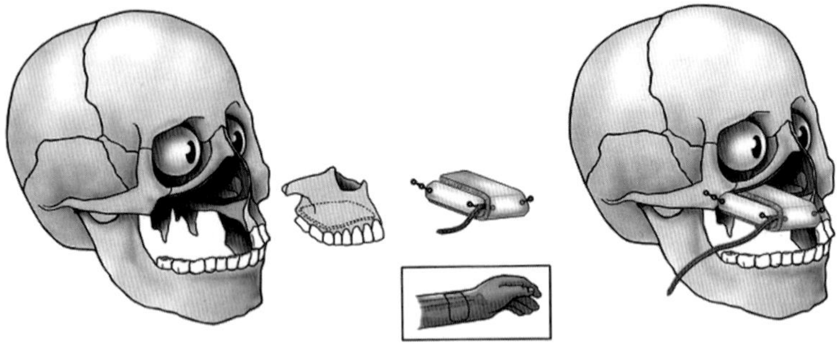

Fig. 21.5 Type II defects (subtotal maxillectomy). (*Left*) There is resection of five walls of the maxilla sparing the roof (orbital floor). The resected specimen palate/nasal floor lining and bone. (*Center, left*) The radial forearm "sandwich flap" provides moderate volume and large skin surface area with vascularized bone. (*Center, right*) The radial forearm "sandwich flap" in place (*right*) showing a vascularized bone strut to reconstruct the maxillary arch defect in between two skin islands that replace palatal and nasal lining. From Cordeiro PG, Santamaria E. A classification system and algorithm for reconstruction of maxillectomy and midfacial defects. Plast Reconstr Surg 2000;80:2331–46. Reprinted with permission

21.3.2.3 Type III Defects

Type III defects result from total maxillectomy, which includes resection of all six walls of the maxilla, the floor of the orbit, and often the orbital contents [11]. When the orbital soft tissues are not involved with extension of cancer from the maxillary sinus, the orbital contents can often be preserved [12, 13]. This type of defect can be subdivided into type IIIa, in which the orbital contents are preserved (Fig. 21.6), and type IIIb, in which the orbital contents are exenterated (Fig. 21.7).

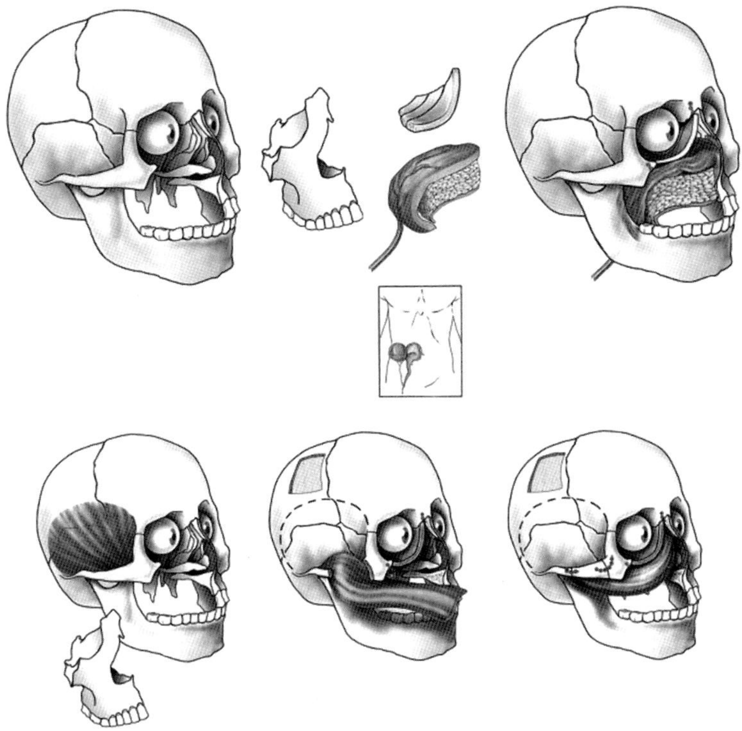

Fig. 21.6 Type IIIa defects. There is preservation of the orbit, but all six walls of the maxilla have been resected (*above, left*). The resected specimen demonstrates the orbital floor (roof of maxilla), vertical maxillary buttress, and palate creating a medium surface area/medium volume defect (*center, left*). Cranial or rib bone graft is used to reconstruct the floor of the orbit and is covered with a single island rectus abdominis myocutaneous free flap (*center, right*). The free flap is inset with the skin island used to close the roof of the palate, soft tissue to fill in the midfacial defect, and muscle to cover the bone graft. (*Below*) The patients that are not free-flap candidates can benefit from split calvarial bone grafts covered with temporalis muscle, transposed anteriorly. The zygomatic arch should be osteotomized temporarily to increase the excursion of the temporalis muscle. From Cordeiro PG, Santamaria E. A classification system and algorithm for reconstruction of maxillectomy and midfacial defects. Plast Reconstr Surg 2000;80:2331–46. Reprinted with permission

Type IIIa defects are medium to large volume and surface area defects. The two functional requirements that need to be addressed are support of the orbital contents and reconstruction of the palate. Without exception, the orbital floor must be reconstructed. If this is not done, the orbital contents will sink into the cheek, creating orbital dystopia and diplopia. The orbital floor can be addressed with nonvascularized bone grafts. The bone graft must be sandwiched between a healthy flap below (rectus abdominis or temporalis) and the orbital contents above. The rectus abdominis flap, according to Cordeiro and Santamaria, provides the muscle coverage for bone grafts and also adequate subcutaneous fat that can be contoured for soft tissue fill (usually on a delayed basis) [10]. The temporalis flap covers bone effectively

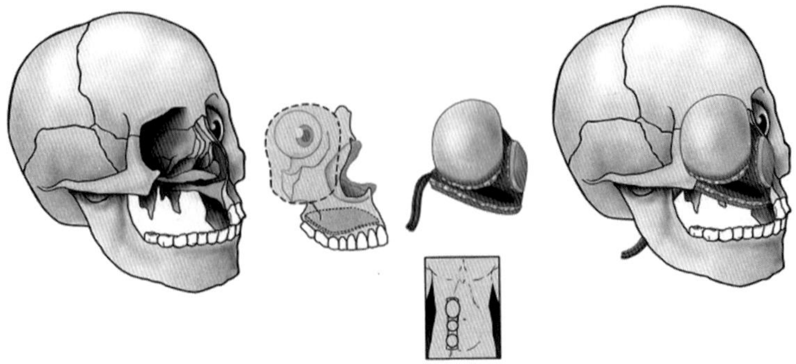

Fig. 21.7 Type IIIb defects: total maxillectomy and orbital exenteration. The resected specimen contains external eyelid, cheek skin, orbital contents including entire maxilla and palate. (*Center, left*) This creates a large surface area/large volume defect. A three-skin-island rectus abdominis myocutaneous free flap is shown (*inset*). This flap provides multiple large surface areas with large volume of soft tissue and muscle to fill the defect (*center, right*). From Cordeiro PG, Santamaria E. A classification system and algorithm for reconstruction of maxillectomy and midfacial defects. Plast Reconstr Surg 2000;80:2331–46. Reprinted with permission

but does not close the palate. This causes a need for an obturator. Reconstruction with a temporalis flap is usually indicated in patients who are older or are not good candidates for a free tissue transfer. In type IIIa resections, if the malar eminence is preserved, there is usually good anterior projection of the upper midface, which obviates the need for anterior maxillary wall reconstruction.

Type IIIb defects are extensive and have large volume and surface area requirements (Figs. 21.7 and 21.8). Of significant importance is that the anterior cranial base, in the area of the sphenoid, is often exposed, meaning that coverage of the brain becomes essential.

21.3.2.4 Type IV Defects

Type IV defects result from orbitomaxillectomy, which involves resection of the upper five walls of the maxilla and the orbital contents and preservation of the palate (Fig. 21.9). Type IV defects are generally large volume and surface area defects. Because the palate is intact, the reconstructive objectives are primarily soft tissue fill and external skin resurfacing, if required. The rectus abdominis flap allows effective accomplishment of all these objectives. Conceptually, these are simple reconstructive procedures; technically, however, they are challenging and best left in the hands of an experienced microvascular free-flap surgeon.

The algorithm of Cordeiro and Santamaria is principally based on the extent of resection of the maxillary bone, which is the key building block of the structure of the midface. First, the bony defect must be addressed; then the associated soft tissue, skin, palate, and cheek-lining deficits must be assessed; and finally the palate, oral commissure, nasal airway, and eyelids need to be addressed individually. The most common walls needing reconstruction to maintain the functional and aesthetic unit

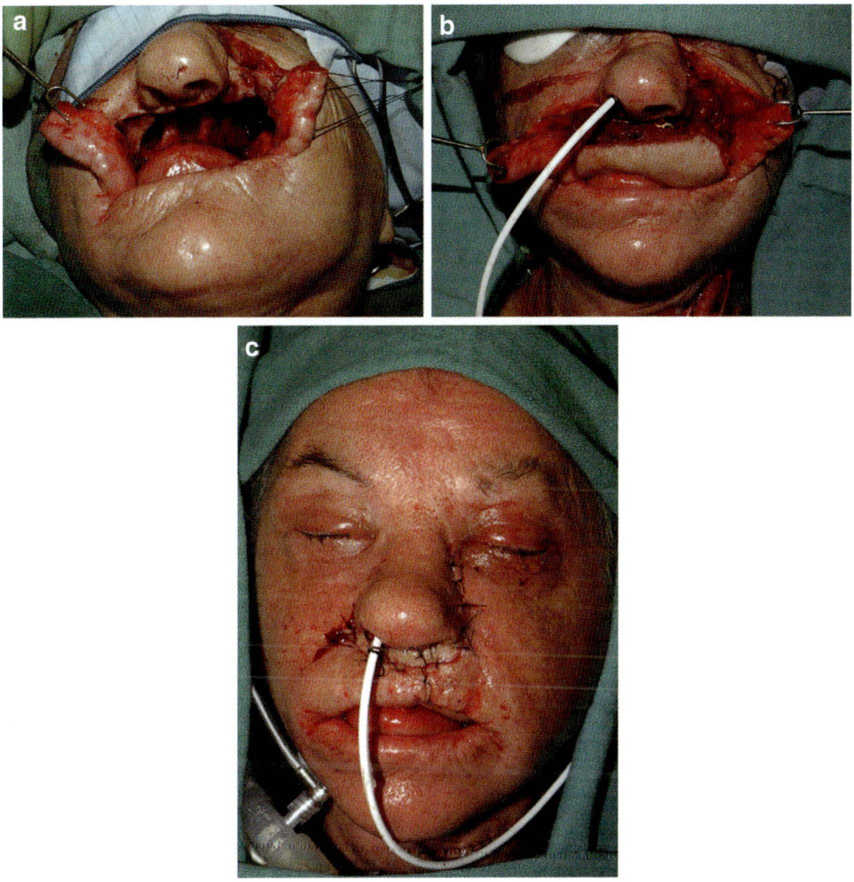

Fig. 21.8 A 75-year-old woman with recurrent maxillary sinus SCCA. She had had a prior partial maxillectomy and underwent a complete bilateral maxillectomy. She was reconstructed with a fibula osteocutaneous free flap. The orbital floors were spared

are the anterior (cheek), superior (orbital floor), and inferior (palate). Bone replacement is essential so that the orbital floor can maintain the position of the globe [1, 9, 14]. Bone replacement is also useful in the maxillary arch to provide anterior projection of the midface and bone stock for osteointegrated implants [15–17]. For reconstruction of the orbital floor, bone grafts can be effectively used in conjunction with soft tissue flaps (free or pedicled) because this area requires minimal supportive strength. Vascularized bone is indicated in the maxillary arch if osteointegration is required and when high-dose postoperative radiation therapy is planned. Free flaps are usually required when skin islands are necessary for intraoral, cheek, palatal, nasal lining, or external resurfacing. The space between the restored anterior, superior, and inferior walls of the maxilla can usually be filled with soft tissue, and the nasal lining may or may not be restored.

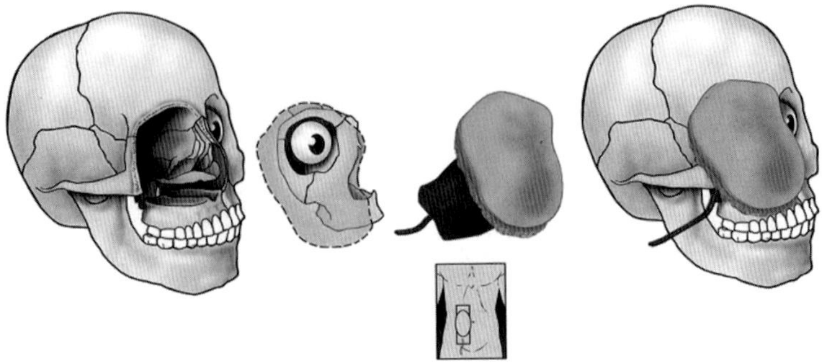

Fig. 21.9 Type IV defects (orbitomaxillectomy). There is resection of the five upper walls of the maxilla, including the orbital contents, but sparing the palate (*left*). The resected specimen consists of the orbital contents, eyelid, cheek skin, and bone creating a large surface area/large volume defect (*center, left*). Note design (*inset*) of single skin island rectus abdominis myocutaneous free flap. This flap provides a large surface area with significant volume to reconstruct the defect (*center, right*). Rectus abdominis free flap in place, demonstrating the skin island used to resurface the external skin defect and subcutaneous fat with muscle used to fill in the soft tissue defect (*right*). From Cordeiro PG, Santamaria E. A classification system and algorithm for reconstruction of maxillectomy and midfacial defects. Plast Reconstr Surg 2000;80:2331–46. Reprinted with permission

21.3.3 Reconstruction After Orbital Exenteration

Orbital exenteration involves removal of the contents of the orbit, including the globe, the extraocular muscles, and the periorbital soft tissues. It is most commonly performed for orbital and periorbital malignancies, including squamous cell carcinoma, basal cell carcinoma, sebaceous gland carcinoma, conjunctival and uveal melanoma, sarcoma, and adenoid cystic carcinoma of the lacrimal gland [18]. Invasive cancers may necessitate extended resections, resulting in communication of the orbit with the cranial vault, nasal cavity, and paranasal sinuses.

The primary goal of reconstruction after orbital exenteration is to either line or fill the orbit with durable tissue that excludes the nasal cavity and paranasal sinuses and, when there is a cranial defect, protects the brain. The tissues used for the reconstruction may need to be able to tolerate radiation therapy, and when the patient desires, the orbit should be able to accommodate a prosthesis. Numerous reconstructive methods that attempt to fulfill these goals have been described in case reports and small case series [19–23].

Recently, Hanasono et al. [24] at M.D. Anderson suggested an algorithm (Fig. 21.10) for surgical reconstruction and prosthetic rehabilitation after orbital exenteration. Based on their experience, numerous reconstructive options are available to successfully line the socket. The determining factor in the choice of reconstructive method is whether the patient underwent preoperative irradiation or is anticipated to undergo postoperative irradiation [24].

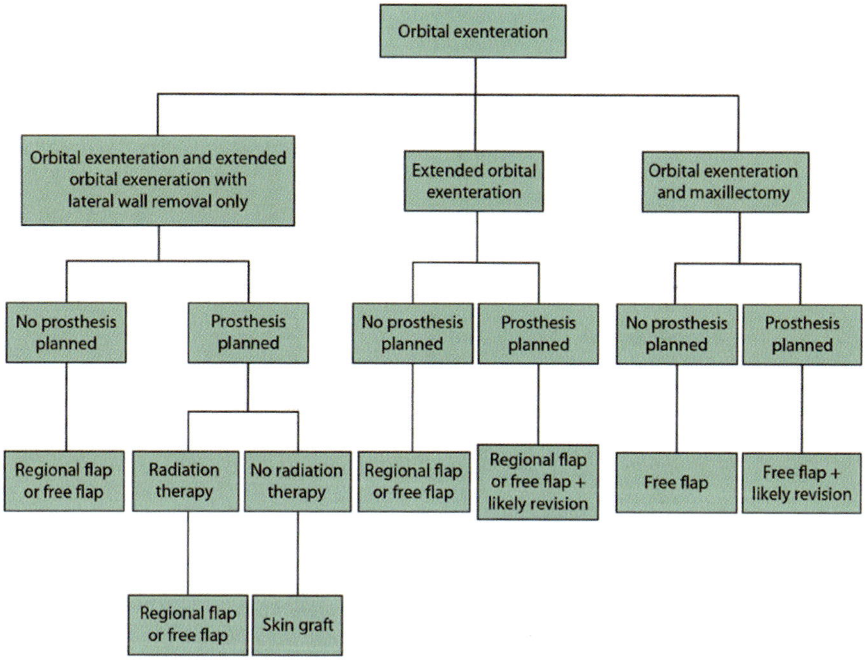

Fig. 21.10 Algorithm for reconstruction after orbital exenteration. From Hanasono MM, Lee JC, Yang JS, et al. Plast Reconstr Surg 2009;123:98. Reprinted with permission

Split-thickness or full-thickness skin grafts are used for reconstruction when an open cavity is desired; when there is no need to isolate the orbital cavity from the sinonasal, oral, or intracranial cavities; and when radiation therapy is not given preoperatively or postoperatively. Preoperative or postoperative radiation therapy is a contraindication to skin grafting because of the risk of poor graft take or subsequent graft loss [24].

Regional flaps and microvascular free flaps are used for reconstruction when orbital exenteration is combined with removal of orbital walls or if a patient received preoperative radiation therapy or is expected to receive postoperative radiation therapy. These flaps are used to provide soft tissue coverage of the bony walls of the orbit, isolate the orbit from the paranasal sinuses, or protect the intracranial contents in cases of exposure.

Aside from radiation therapy, the other major factor influencing the choice of reconstructive option is whether the cavity will be left open or closed. An open-cavity reconstruction of the orbital socket is preferred when use of an orbital prosthesis is planned postoperatively. The open cavity allows for a more secure fit of the prosthesis and usually requires less extensive reconstructive surgery. The free flaps of choice to allow for an open cavity are radial forearm fasciocutaneous flaps, temporoparietal muscle flaps, and any myocutaneous flaps in which flap design can keep soft tissue bulk to a minimum.

A potential drawback of using skin grafts to line the orbital cavity is that they may result in downward displacement of the brow and cheek due to soft tissue contracture [21]. This may be less of a concern with full-thickness skin grafts as they contract less than split-thickness grafts.

Closed-cavity reconstructions tend to contract less and do not undergo the same amount of atrophy as skin grafts [21] but tend to be less amenable to a prosthesis. Prostheses over closed cavities may protrude excessively such that the affected side is not symmetric with the contralateral face. According to Hanasono et al. [24], closed cavities required surgical revisions before being able to accommodate a prosthesis successfully. These revisions consisted of flap debulking by direct tissue excision, usually combined with suction-assisted lipectomy.

21.4 Conclusion

Orbital reconstruction in cancer patients can be approached by many different avenues. The most important factors determining the reconstructive approach are the size of the defect, the periorbital structures exposed, and whether the area was irradiated preoperatively or will be irradiated postoperatively. There are several different new algorithms that provide a strong foundation for surgical planning. These, in addition to free-flap techniques, will continue to expand the options available to the orbital reconstructive surgeon.

References

1. Cordeiro PG, Santamaria E, Kraus DH, et al. Reconstruction of total maxillectomy defects with preservation of the orbital contents. Plast Reconstr Surg 1998;102(6):1874–84.
2. Ali A, Fardy MJ, Patton DW. To reconstruct or to obturate? Results of a UK survey of oral and maxillofacial surgeons. Br J Oral Maxillofac Surg 1995;33:207–10.
3. Shestak KC. Soft tissue reconstruction of craniofacial defects. Clin Plast Surg 1994;21: 107–11.
4. Wells MD, Luce EA. Reconstruction of mid-facial defects after surgical resection of malignancies. Clin Plast Surg 1995;22:79–89.
5. Coleman JJ III. Osseous reconstruction of the midface and orbits. Clin Plast Surg 1994;21:113–24.
6. Nakayama B, Matsuura H, Hasegawa Y, et al. New reconstruction for total maxillectomy defect with a fibula osteocutaneous free flap. Br J Plast Surg 1994;47:247–9.
7. McLoughlin PM, Gilhooly M, Phillips JG. Reconstruction of the infraorbital margin with a composite microvascular free flap. Br J Oral Maxillofac Surg 1993;31:227–9.
8. Schusterman MA, Reece GP, Miller MJ. Osseous free flaps for orbit and midface reconstruction. Am J Surg 1993;166:341–5.
9. Swartz WM, Banis JC, Newton ED, et al. The osteocutaneous scapular flap for mandibular and maxillary reconstruction. Plast Reconstr Surg 1986;77:530–45.
10. Cordeiro PG, Santamaria E. A classification system and algorithm for reconstruction of maxillectomy and midfacial defects. Plast Reconstr Surg 2000;80:2331–46.
11. Spiro RH, Strong EW, Shah JP. Maxillectomy and its classification. Head Neck 1997;19: 309–14.

12. Larson DL, Christ JE, Jesse RH. Preservation of the orbital contents in cancer of the maxillary sinus. Arch Otolaryngol 1982;108:370–2.
13. Stern S, Goepfert H, Clayman G, et al. Orbital preservation in maxillectomy. Otolaryngol Head Neck Surg 1993;109:111–5.
14. Schusterman MA. Discussion of reconstruction of total maxillectomy defects with preservation of the orbital contents (discussion). Plast Reconstr Surg 1998;102:1885.
15. Yamamoto Y, Minakawa H, Kawashima K, et al. Role of buttress reconstruction in zygomaticomaxillary skeletal defects. Plast Reconstr Surg 1998;101:943–50.
16. Cordeiro PG, Bacilious N, Schantz S, et al. The radial forearm osteocutaneous "sandwich" free flap for reconstruction of the bilateral subtotal maxillectomy defect. Ann Plast Surg 1998;40:397–402.
17. Kyutoku S, Tsuji H, Inoue T, et al. Experience with the rectus abdominis myocutaneous flap with vascularized hard tissue for immediate orbitofacial reconstruction. Plast Reconstr Surg 1999;103:395–402.
18. Rapıdis AD, Liarikos S. Malignant orbital and orbitomaxillary tumors: surgical considerations. Orbit 1998;17:77–88.
19. Reese A. Exenteration of the orbit with transplantation of the temporalis muscle. Am J Ophthalmol 1958;45:386–90.
20. Goldberg RA, Kim JW, Shorr N. Orbital exenteration: results of an individualized approach. Ophthal Plast Reconstr Surg 2003;19:229–36.
21. Chepeha DB, Wang SJ, Marentette LJ, et al. Restoration of the orbital aesthetic subunit in complex midface defects. Laryngoscope 2004;114:1706–13.
22. Pryor SG, Moore EJ, Kasperbauer JL. Orbital exenteration reconstruction with rectus abdominis microvascular free flap. Laryngoscope 2005;115:1912–6.
23. Taylan G, Yildirim S, Aköz T. Reconstruction of large orbital exenteration defects after resection of periorbital tumors of advanced stage. J Reconstr Microsurg 2006;22:583–9.
24. Hanasono MM, Lee JC, Yang JS, et al. An algorithmic approach to reconstructive surgery and prosthetic rehabilitation after orbital exenteration. Plast Reconstr Surg 2009;123:98–105.

Chapter 22
Enucleation, Evisceration, Orbital Implants, and Management of the Irradiated Socket

Miguel Gonzalez-Candial and Aaron Savar

Abstract Removal of an eye is somctimes necessary in the management of ocular malignancies. The most common intraocular malignancies necessitating enucleation are uveal melanoma in adults and retinoblastoma in children. In patients with retinoblastoma, the segment of optic nerve removed during enucleation must be long enough to ensure that the entire tumor has been removed. A number of different types of orbital implants are available, each with advantages and disadvantages. Radiation can cause atrophy and contraction of orbital tissues; thus, management of the socket in patients who have undergone radiation therapy is challenging. There is considerable debate over the benefits of enucleation versus evisceration. Evisceration is not appropriate in patients with intraocular tumors as it may leave tumor behind. Before evisceration is performed for an indication not related to cancer, the eye should be carefully examined to rule out the presence of intraocular tumor.

22.1 Introduction

The management of ocular malignancies sometimes necessitates the removal of an eye. The most common intraocular malignancies leading to enucleation are uveal melanoma in adults and retinoblastoma in children. Enucleation is also occasionally required in the management of ophthalmic complications resulting from the treatment of other cancers. Management of anophthalmic sockets in cancer patients presents unique challenges, especially in patients who have previously undergone radiation treatment. Evisceration may be appropriate in some cancer patients without intraocular malignancy.

M. Gonzalez-Candial (✉)
Department of Orbital and Ophthalmic Plastic Surgery, Universitat Autonoma de Barcelona, I.M.O. Barcelona, Barcelona, Spain
e-mail: mgcandial@mac.com

B. Esmaeli (ed.), *Ophthalmic Oncology*, M.D. Anderson Solid Tumor Oncology Series 6, DOI 10.1007/978-1-4419-0374-7_22,

22.2 Surgical Technique

The surgical technique used for enucleation for treatment of malignancy is essentially the same as the surgical technique used for enucleation for other indications. This procedure is well described and can be performed with or without suturing the extraocular muscles to the implant [1]. There are, however, certain special considerations when enucleation is performed for treatment of an intraocular tumor.

22.2.1 Confirmation of Correct Eye

Identification of the correct eye must be confirmed and reconfirmed before enucleation. Often an eye being removed because it is blind and painful is abnormal in appearance; in contrast, an eye with an intraocular tumor may have a completely normal appearing anterior segment. This underscores the importance of confirming the correct eye prior to proceeding with enucleation. The eye to be removed should be confirmed with the patient, and the information provided by the patient should be checked against the patient's chart and confirmed by the operating surgeon. It is also a good policy to dilate the eye to be operated on and confirm the presence of the tumor as an extra safety measure prior to enucleation.

22.2.2 Resection of Optic Nerve in Patients with Retinoblastoma

In patients with retinoblastoma, as in patients with many other malignancies, complete resection of the tumor portends a better prognosis. Because retinoblastoma can spread via the optic nerve, it is of the utmost importance to obtain a sufficiently long piece of optic nerve during enucleation to ensure that the entire tumor has been removed. Survival is worse when the tumor has spread to the optic nerve than when the tumor is confined to the globe. The prognosis is worst if the cut end of the nerve is involved [2]. It has been recommended that as much optic nerve as safely possible be removed, 15 mm or more according to some authors [3].

To obtain a sufficiently long segment of optic nerve, several techniques can be added to the standard enucleation procedure. A medial approach when scissors are used can allow for removal of a longer section of nerve [4]. Sutures can be passed through the muscle insertions or the muscle stumps can be grasped with clamps to elevate the globe out of the orbit. This stretches the optic nerve so that it is more easily cut and also makes it easier to pass scissors further posteriorly. Havre [5] described a technique in which an incision is made into the posterior tendon's fascia behind the globe to facilitate acquisition of a longer piece of optic nerve.

Another method to obtain a longer segment of optic nerve involves the use of a snare [6]. Schiedler and associates [7] retrospectively compared the use of a snare to the use of scissors during enucleation for retinoblastoma. They found that significantly longer segments of optic nerve were resected with the snare than with scissors (mean of 13.35 mm versus 11.05 mm). They also noted improved hemostasis with the use of the snare, but more crush artifact.

22.2.3 *Maintenance of Globe Integrity*

While efforts are made to avoid penetration of the globe during any enucleation, there is no situation in which maintenance of globe integrity is more important than it is in the case of an intraocular cancer. It is crucial that the integrity of the globe be maintained to avoid spillage of tumor into the orbit. After the globe is removed, it should be examined to ensure that it is intact and to determine whether there is gross extrascleral extension.

22.3 Choice of Implant

After enucleation, placement of an implant is necessary to maintain orbital volume to allow for motility and for retention of a prosthesis. A variety of orbital implants are available, each with possible advantages and disadvantages. Implants can be solid or porous, synthetic or natural, and wrapped or unwrapped; cost varies according to the implant features.

Solid orbital implants used today include implants made from silicone and implants made from acrylic. Porous orbital implants have become available over the past 20 years and include implants made of hydroxyapatite, which is harvested from coral, and implants made of porous polyethylene, a synthetic polymer.

Porous implants allow for fibrovascular ingrowth, which allows integration of the implant into the orbit and is thought to decrease the rate of implant extrusion and infection [8, 9]. However, studies have shown lower rates of exposure with solid implants than with porous implants [10, 11]. Solid implants are also considerably less expensive than porous implants [1]. A prospective randomized trial comparing motility between hydroxyapatite (porous) and acrylic (solid) orbital implants showed no difference between the two implant types [12]. Lyle and associates [13] compared porous to solid implants in patients who underwent enucleation for treatment of retinoblastoma and found no significant difference in orbital volume between the side with the implant and the uninvolved side for either type of implant.

Despite the benefits of and length of experience with solid implants, porous implants remain very popular. Porous implants do have certain advantages. They allow for the placement of a motility coupling peg, which can potentially improve motility. In addition, extraocular muscles can be attached directly to porous polyethylene implants, which may shorten operative time compared to operative time with other orbital implants. Sadiq and associates [14] retrospectively compared 26 patients with hydroxyapatite implants to 26 patients with porous polyethylene implants and found no significant differences between the two groups in terms of postoperative complications; however, they did note improved motility of the porous polyethylene implants.

Implants can be wrapped or unwrapped [1, 15]. A variety of different materials have been used for wrapping implants, including polyglactin mesh, donor sclera, and bovine pericardium. Wrapping the implant provides a surface for attachment of the extraocular muscles and may also provide an extra barrier to extrusion (Fig. 22.1). Polymer-coated hydroxyapatite implants are also available [16]. This absorbable coating makes wrapping of the implant unnecessary. Before the extraocular muscles can be attached to the polymer coating, a high-temperature disposable cautery device must be used to fashion openings in the coating to allow the muscles to contact the hydroxyapatite and sutures to be attached to it (Fig. 22.2).

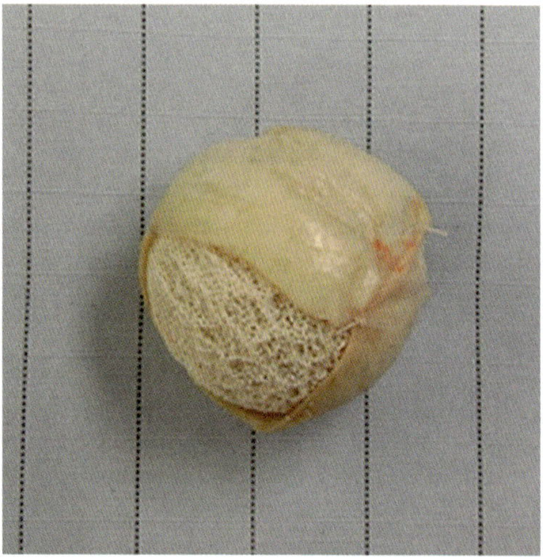

Fig. 22.1 Photograph of a hydroxyapatite orbital implant wrapped in donor sclera. The posterior aspect of the implant is left exposed to allow for fibrovascular ingrowth

All of the implants discussed above maintain a fixed orbital volume. This is appropriate in an adult. In a child, however, in order for the orbit to grow normally, the implant size must gradually increase. This can be accomplished with successive implant exchanges. Another option is the placement of a dermis-fat graft [17]. This graft has the potential to grow with the child. Heher and associates [18] reported 16 cases of unilateral pediatric dermis-fat grafts for varying indications. They noted maintenance of or improvement in orbital symmetry in all patients. Atrophy with associated volume loss can be a concern with dermis-fat grafts; however, in this series, it was not seen in any of the children 4 years of age or younger. Six of the eight patients 4 years of age or younger required surgical debulking of their graft. Mitchell and associates [19] reported a series of eight pediatric enucleations followed by dermis-fat grafting; good orbital symmetry was achieved in all cases.

Clearly, there are numerous options for implants after enucleation. The choice of implant needs to be tailored to the patient. On the ocular oncology service at The University of Texas M.D. Anderson Cancer Center, the implant most frequently

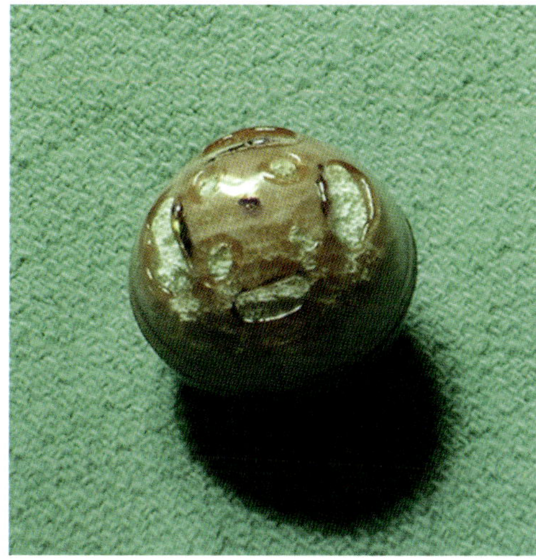

Fig. 22.2 Photograph of a polymer-coated hydroxyapatite orbital implant. Openings have been created in the anterior surface to attach the extraocular muscles

placed after primary enucleation in children or adults is a hydroxyapatite implant, either polymer coated or wrapped in donor sclera.

22.4 Management of the Anophthalmic Socket After Enucleation and Radiation Therapy

Radiation therapy is sometimes necessary after enucleation for malignancy. Managing an anophthalmic socket in a patient who has undergone radiation therapy can be difficult.

22.4.1 Patients with Retinoblastoma

Management of the anophthalmic socket is especially difficult in patients who have undergone irradiation for retinoblastoma. Because of their age, children with retinoblastoma who are treated with enucleation, irradiation, or both typically have smaller orbital volumes [20]. Radiation retards the growth of orbital structures and causes atrophy. Secondary surgery is often necessary to allow the socket to accommodate a prosthesis as well as for cosmesis. Volume loss is common and results in enophthalmos, superior sulcus defects, and ptosis. The orbital volume can be augmented with grafts, fillers, or implants. However, all of these treatment options are more likely to be associated with complications in this setting because wound healing is impaired after radiation therapy.

Successful reconstruction of irradiated sockets using temporalis flaps has been reported [21]. In severely contracted sockets, more aggressive reconstruction may be necessary. Li and associates [22] reported socket reconstruction with radial forearm flaps in 22 patients, 14 of whom had retinoblastoma treated with enucleation followed by irradiation. This technique can provide a large volume of vascularized tissue, which may be necessary in irradiated areas. However, forearm flaps cause donor site scarring and may cause numbness and decreased blood flow to the hand.

22.4.2 Patients with Uveal Melanoma with Microscopic Extrascleral Extension

Another group in which radiation therapy may be indicated after enucleation is patients with uveal melanoma with microscopic extrascleral extension [23, 24]. In such patients, the anophthalmic socket becomes contracted after radiation therapy and cannot retain a prosthesis [25, 26]. In patients with such a contracted socket, a larger socket can be successfully reconstructed with the use of oral mucous membrane grafts [27, 28].

22.4.3 Patients with Head and Neck Cancer

Occasionally, in patients with head and neck cancer in the periocular region or paranasal sinuses, an eye must be removed because of severe radiation-induced damage [29] (Figs. 22.3, 22.4, and 22.5). In such patients, it may be wise to avoid placement of any implants or to use simple silicone implants to minimize the risks of implant exposure, infection, and extrusion, all of which are more common with porous orbital implants [10, 11].

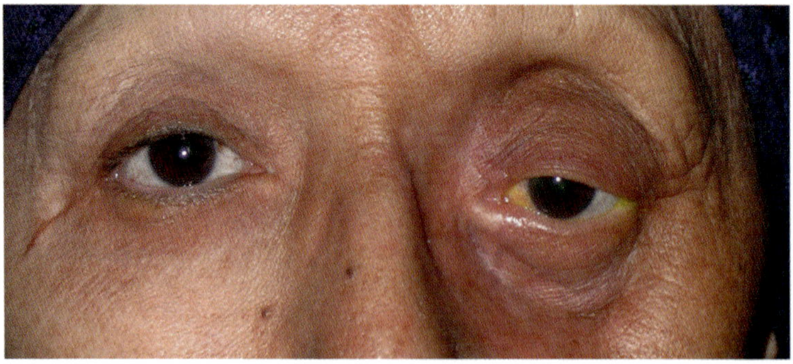

Fig. 22.3 Photograph of a patient with a maxillary sinus squamous cell carcinoma after a maxillectomy with loss of the floor of the orbit and radiation therapy. Note the loss of volume in the left orbit. The patient developed neovascular glaucoma and a blind painful eye, which necessitated an enucleation. Photo courtesy of Dr. Bita Esmaeli

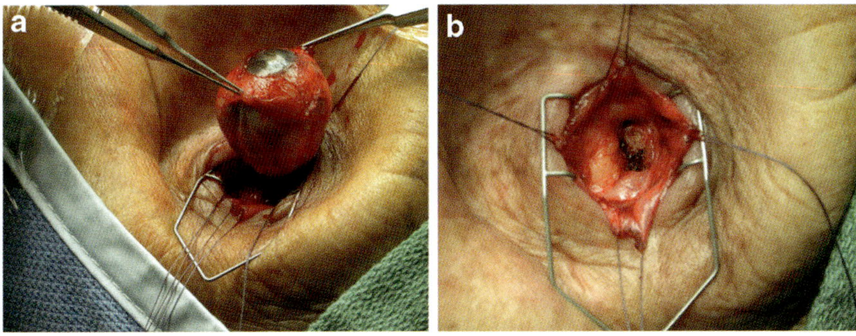

Fig. 22.4 Enucleation in the same patient as in Fig. 22.3. (**a**) The prephthisical globe was removed carefully without disruption of the posterior sclera. (**b**) View of the socket. A simple silicone implant was placed in the irradiated socket. Photos courtesy of Dr. Bita Esmaeli

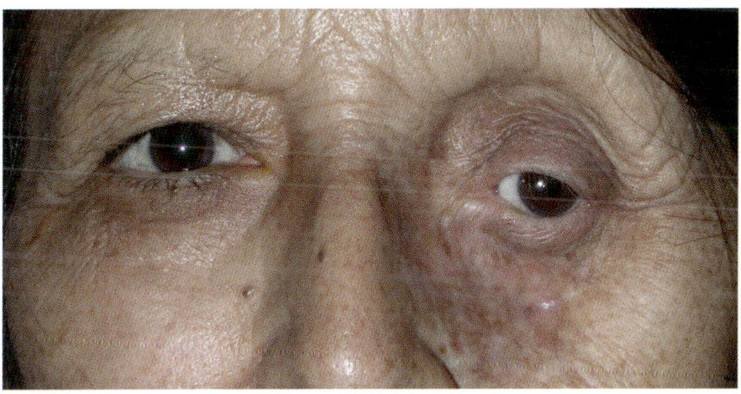

Fig. 22.5 Photograph showing the postoperative appearance in the same patient as in Fig. 22.3, after prosthesis fitting. Photo courtesy of Dr. Bita Esmaeli

22.5 Evisceration

There is considerable debate in the ophthalmic community and in the literature over the benefits of enucleation versus evisceration (removal of the contents of the eye but not the sclera) [30, 31]. The issues generally debated include the impact of surgery on implant motility and the risk of sympathetic ophthalmia. There is no question that enucleation is the appropriate choice when an eye is being removed because of an intraocular malignancy. Evisceration is not appropriate for the treatment of intraocular malignancies as this procedure may leave tumor behind. There have been instances of evisceration of eyes with previously undiagnosed intraocular malignancies [32, 33]. Before an evisceration is performed for another indication, it is extremely important to evaluate the eye to rule out the possibility of intraocular malignancy. The evaluation should include a dilated fundus examination. If the media is not clear enough to allow for a thorough assessment via ophthalmoscopy, B-scan ultrasonography should be performed.

There are situations in which evisceration is appropriate in cancer patients without intraocular malignancy. The most frequent such situation is a blind painful eye, often due to endogenous endophthalmitis, severe viral retinitis, or severe radiation damage.

References

1. Custer PL, Kennedy RH, Woog JJ, et al. Orbital implants in enucleation surgery: a report by the American Academy of Ophthalmology. Ophthalmology 2003;110(10):2054–61.
2. Magramm I, Abramson DH, Ellsworth RM. Optic nerve involvement in retinoblastoma. Ophthalmology 1989;96(2):217–22.
3. Abramson DH, Ellsworth RM. The surgical management of retinoblastoma. Ophthalmic Surg 1980;11(9):596–8.
4. Shields JA, Shields CL, De Potter P. Enucleation technique for children with retinoblastoma. J Pediatr Ophthalmol Strabismus 1992;29(4):213–5.
5. Havre DC. Obtaining long sections of optic nerve at enucleation. A new surgical technique based on the anatomy of the posterior fascia bulbi. Am J Ophthalmol 1965;60:272–7.
6. Myers RH. Revaluation of the snare technique for enucleation. Am J Ophthalmol 1950;33(7):1143–4.
7. Schiedler V, Dubovy SR, Murray TG. Snare technique for enucleation of eyes with advanced retinoblastoma. Arch Ophthalmol 2007;125(5):680–3.
8. Rubin PA, Popham JK, Bilyk JR, et al. Comparison of fibrovascular ingrowth into hydroxyapatite and porous polyethylene orbital implants. Ophthal Plast Reconstr Surg 1994;10(2): 96–103.
9. Remulla HD, Rubin PA, Shore JW, et al. Complications of porous spherical orbital implants. Ophthalmology 1995;102(4):586–93.
10. Nunery WR, Heinz GW, Bonnin JM, et al. Exposure rate of hydroxyapatite spheres in the anophthalmic socket: histopathologic correlation and comparison with silicone sphere implants. Ophthal Plast Reconstr Surg 1993;9(2):96–104.
11. Li T, Shen J, Duffy MT. Exposure rates of wrapped and unwrapped orbital implants following enucleation. Ophthal Plast Reconstr Surg 2001;17(6):431–5.
12. Colen TP, Paridaens DA, Lemij HG, et al. Comparison of artificial eye amplitudes with acrylic and hydroxyapatite spherical enucleation implants. Ophthalmology 2000;107(10):1889–94.
13. Lyle CE, Wilson MW, Li CS, et al. Comparison of orbital volumes in enucleated patients with unilateral retinoblastoma: hydroxyapatite implants versus silicone implants. Ophthal Plast Reconstr Surg 2007;23(5):393–6.
14. Sadiq SA, Mengher LS, Lowry J, et al. Integrated orbital implants—a comparison of hydroxyapatite and porous polyethylene implants. Orbit 2008;27(1):37–40.
15. Long JA, Tann TM 3rd, Bearden WH 3rd, et al. Enucleation: is wrapping the implant necessary for optimal motility? Ophthal Plast Reconstr Surg 2003;19(3):194–7.
16. Shields CL, Uysal Y, Marr BP, et al. Experience with the polymer-coated hydroxyapatite implant after enucleation in 126 patients. Ophthalmology 2007;114(2):367–73.
17. Smith B, Bosniak SL, Lisman RD. An autogenous kinetic dermis-fat orbital implant: an updated technique. Ophthalmology 1982;89(9):1067–71.
18. Heher KL, Katowitz JA, Low JE. Unilateral dermis-fat graft implantation in the pediatric orbit. Ophthal Plast Reconstr Surg 1998;14(2):81–8.
19. Mitchell KT, Hollsten DA, White WL, et al. The autogenous dermis-fat orbital implant in children. J AAPOS 2001;5(6):367–9.

20. Peylan-Ramu N, Bin-Nun A, Skleir-Levy M, et al. Orbital growth retardation in retinoblastoma survivors: work in progress. Med Pediatr Oncol 2001;37(5):465–70.
21. Foster JA, Castro E, Papay FA. Reconstruction of the irradiated contracted socket with an expanded superficial temporalis fascial flap. Am J Ophthalmol 1999;127(5):621–2.
22. Li D, Jie Y, Liu H, et al. Reconstruction of anophthalmic orbits and contracted eye sockets with microvascular radial forearm free flaps. Ophthal Plast Reconstr Surg 2008;24(2):94–7.
23. Hykin PG, McCartney AC, Plowman PN, et al. Postenucleation orbital radiotherapy for the treatment of malignant melanoma of the choroid with extrascleral extension. Br J Ophthalmol 1990;74(1):36–9.
24. Blanco G. Diagnosis and treatment of orbital invasion in uveal melanoma. Can J Ophthalmol 2004;39(4):388–96.
25. Macfaul PA, Bedford MA. Ocular complications after therapeutic irradiation. Br J Ophthalmol 1970;54(4):237–47.
26. Baylis HI, Call NB. Severe enophthalmos following irradiation of the anophthalmic socket: surgical approaches. Ophthalmology 1979;86(9):1647–54.
27. Karesh JW, Putterman AM. Reconstruction of the partially contracted ocular socket or fornix. Arch Ophthalmol 1988;106(4):552–6.
28. Bowen Jones EJ, Nunes E. The outcome of oral mucosal grafts to the orbit: a three-and-a-half-year study. Br J Plast Surg 2002;55(2):100–4.
29. Moshfeghi DM, Moshfeghi AA, Finger PT. Enucleation. Surv Ophthalmol 2000;44(4):277–301.
30. Walter WL. Update on enucleation and evisceration surgery. Ophthal Plast Reconstr Surg 1985;1(4):243–52.
31. Nakra T, Simon GJ, Douglas RS, et al. Comparing outcomes of enucleation and evisceration. Ophthalmology 2006;113(12):2270–5.
32. Eagle RC Jr, Grossniklaus HE, Syed N, et al. Inadvertent evisceration of eyes containing uveal melanoma. Arch Ophthalmol 2009;127(2):141–5.
33. Schefler AC, Abramson DH. Should evisceration ever be done in a blind, painful eye? Arch Ophthalmol 2009;127(2):211–2.

Chapter 23
Orbital Exenteration and Rehabilitation of the Exenterated Socket

Adam Hsu and Matthew M. Hanasono

Abstract Orbital exenteration is the surgical removal of orbital contents and periorbital structures. The majority of orbital exenterations are performed to remove malignant tumors, including primary epithelial tumors, rhabdomyosarcoma, retinoblastoma, and uveal melanoma. Other potential indications for orbital exenteration include severe and uncontrollable pain or deformity caused by extreme cases of sclerosing orbital pseudotumor, Graves' ophthalmopathy, neurofibromatosis, and socket contracture. Generally, orbital exenteration is subclassified into three types: standard, eyelid-sparing, and extended orbital exenteration. The type of exenteration performed, as well as the planned reconstruction, depends upon the extent of the oncologic defect. The primary goal of reconstruction is to line the orbital cavity with durable tissue and to exclude the nasal and/or sinus cavities when the medial or inferior orbital wall has been removed and to protect the brain when the orbital roof has been removed. The reconstructed orbit will need to be able to tolerate radiation therapy (if planned) and to accommodate an orbital prosthesis if one is desired by the patient.

23.1 Definition

Orbital exenteration is the surgical removal of orbital contents and periorbital structures. The exact amount of surgical ablation is highly individualized based on disease involvement. Orbital exenteration may include removal of periorbital skin, adnexal soft tissue, periorbita, extraocular muscles, orbital fat, the globe, the optic nerve, one or more of the bony orbital walls, and the paranasal sinuses.

A. Hsu (✉)
Section of Ophthalmology, Department of Head and Neck Surgery, The University of Texas M.D. Anderson Cancer Center, Houston, TX, USA
e-mail: ayhsu@yahoo.com

B. Esmaeli (ed.), *Ophthalmic Oncology*, M.D. Anderson Solid Tumor Oncology Series 6, DOI 10.1007/978-1-4419-0374-7_23,

23.2 Indications

The majority of orbital exenterations are performed to remove malignant tumors, including primary epithelial tumors, such as squamous cell carcinoma, basal cell carcinoma, melanoma, and sebaceous carcinoma, which can arise from eyelid skin, conjunctiva, or the sinonasal cavities. Malignancies arising from the lacrimal gland, such as adenoid cystic carcinoma, are also treated with orbital exenteration. Finally, rhabdomyosarcoma and other rare orbital cancers, as well as intraocular tumors such as retinoblastoma and uveal melanoma with extrascleral orbital invasion, may necessitate orbital exenteration. Once these tumors have gained access to the compartmentalized orbit and have invaded orbital fat, it becomes difficult if not impossible to perform local excision with negative margins without removing the whole orbital unit or a large part of it. Aggressive orbital infection by mucormycoses may also require radical debridement and orbital exenteration. These fungi predispose patients to arterial thrombosis and impede the effective delivery of intravenous antifungal medication to the infected orbit. Other potential indications for orbital exenteration include severe and uncontrollable pain or deformity caused by extreme cases of sclerosing orbital pseudotumor, Grave's orbital disease, neurofibromatosis, and socket contracture.

23.3 Preoperative Evaluation

Preoperative evaluation for orbital exenteration includes a comprehensive review of the patient's medical and surgical history. In cases involving cancer, pertinent questions regarding potential manifestations of metastatic disease are addressed. Likewise, physical examination should include inspection for locoregional and metastatic processes rather than focusing only on the orbital disease. Radiographic studies are performed to understand the anatomic extent of the disease process. Histologic examination of the biopsy specimen, when available, can further provide important information about the biologic behavior of the tumor prior to surgery. Both radiographic and histologic studies can influence surgical decision making with regard to the extent of surgical excision and options for reconstruction. However, for some primary ocular adnexal tumors, the exact extent of disease involvement may remain uncertain, despite thorough preoperative evaluation, until intraoperative assessment of the surgical specimen by frozen section histologic analysis.

Patients need to be fully informed about their disease, proposed treatment plan, including the possibility of more radical ablation, and alternatives to orbital exenteration, if any. The preoperative discussion should address psychological aspects of disfigurement resulting from orbital exenteration as well as quality-of-life issues due to loss of vision and facial disfigurement after surgery. The possibility of rehabilitation with an orbital prosthesis should be carefully considered by the clinician and discussed with the patient. Family members and others close to the patients often are included in the discussion since the surgery can be a psychologically traumatic experience for them as well as for the patients themselves. Showing patients post-operative pictures of patients who have previously undergone orbital exenteration, with and without prosthetic rehabilitation, helps to ease the anxiety experienced by some patients. Depending on the reconstruction planned, a discussion about the appropriate reconstructive flap or graft procedure should also be included.

Orbital exenteration requires the patient to undergo general endotracheal anesthesia. A preanesthetic medical evaluation is conducted to ensure the suitability of the patient to undergo the exenteration procedure as well as the reconstructive procedure. Information about coagulation and cardiopulmonary status, as well as history of allergic reactions, is obtained from the patient's primary or specialty care physicians if necessary.

23.4 Surgical Techniques of Orbital Exenteration

Generally, orbital exenteration is subclassified into three types: standard, eyelid sparing, and extended orbital exenteration. In standard exenteration, both eyelids and at least the anterior part of the orbit are removed. This technique is used for many adnexal cancers involving the eyelid with orbital extension. In eyelid-sparing exenteration, the anterior lamella of the eyelid (skin or musculocutaneous layer) is spared and used for coverage of the orbital defect. This technique is used when the eyelid skin and orbicularis muscles are not involved in the cancerous process, such as in some palpebral conjunctival and orbital cancers. Extended orbital exenteration is a more radical surgical ablation in which one or more bony orbital walls and neighboring structures, such as the sinuses and facial skin, are resected. This form of exenteration is used for cancers of the paranasal sinuses, nasal cavity, and periorbital and facial soft tissue extending to the orbit. Malignant lacrimal gland cancers, such as adenoid cystic carcinoma, are frequently found to have grossly or, based on intraoperative frozen section analysis, microscopically invaded the bony orbit. In these cases, extended orbital exenteration may be indicated to clear the disease or to remove high-risk tissues near the tumor to decrease the local tumor recurrence rate.

Orbital exenteration itself starts with marking of the planned incisions on the skin. For a standard exenteration, the orbital rim is outlined. For eyelid-sparing exenteration, the incision mark is made a few millimeters beyond the lash lines on the superior and inferior eyelid skin. Modifications to the incision line are made as needed to ensure a disease-free margin. Next, 4-0 silk traction sutures are placed at the upper and lower eyelid margins. These sutures allow better manipulation and facilitate separation of the orbit from adjacent structures while maintaining the integrity of the surgical specimen. For better hemostasis, lidocaine with epinephrine is injected into the marked lines before skin incision using either a fine-tip cautery or a scalpel.

The initial incision is extended down to the orbital rim with monopolar electrocautery to minimize bleeding. For the eyelid-sparing procedure, the dissection spares only eyelid skin or skin with orbicularis muscles, and these tissues are separated from the remaining deep and posterior structures with scissors. The dissection is carried out from the skin incision to the orbital rim, with care taken to avoid "buttonholing" the skin flap, and then continues with cutting electrocautery deep down to bony orbital rim.

The periosteum at the orbital rim is incised to gain access to the periorbita with a sharp scalpel or a fine-tip electrocautery. The periosteum is then carefully separated from the orbital bony walls with a periosteal elevator. To avoid excessive and potentially difficult-to-control bleeding, orbital vessels exiting anterior ethmoidal, posterior ethmoidal, and zygomaticotemporal foramina should be carefully identified. These vessels are first cauterized—preferably with bipolar cautery—or ligated before they are severed. The periosteum can be separated with relative ease except for areas of firm attachment between the periosteum and the bony wall at the orbital fissures, medial canthal tendon, and lateral tubercle, where separation often requires using a scalpel or a cutting electrocautery. The nasolacrimal duct is excised distal to the lacrimal sac. Extra caution is exercised while working on the thin medial and inferior orbital walls. Unnecessary violation of the bony orbital walls may lead to sino-orbital fistula, causing chronic infection and/or a nonhealing wound. In cases of extended orbital exenteration, removal of the orbital walls may be intentional and may necessitate reconstruction.

Once the dissection reaches the desired posterior limit at the orbital apex and the orbital content is free of any residual anterior attachment, the orbital specimen can be removed with an appropriate pair of heavy scissors while gentle pulling pressure is applied on the eyelid traction sutures. Although preclamping the orbital apex with a curved clamp before severing the orbital content is an option aimed at achieving good hemostasis, it is not utilized by our team because of the risk of creating crushing artifact at the posterior surgical margin, thereby adversely affecting microscopic study. As soon as the specimen is released posteriorly, the orbital cavity is packed with surgical gauze soaked with cold normal saline or thrombin solution. Light pressure is applied to the packing to facilitate hemostasis. The orbital specimen is then carefully oriented and sent for intraoperative frozen section histologic examination of the surgical margins. Depending on results of the frozen section exam, more resection may be required until a tumor-free margin is obtained.

After a tumor-free margin is established, the orbital cavity is inspected for any gross residual diseased tissue and bleeding. Any bleeding must be adequately controlled with further cauterization of the blood vessels, absorbable hemostatic packing material such as Surgicel (Ethicon Endosurgery, Cincinnati, OH), or bone wax for bone-perforating blood vessels. Additional resection beyond the orbit, as in extended exenteration, is executed according to the tumor location and size and often involves bone removal. Extended resection is frequently performed in collaboration with a head and neck surgeon when the exenteration includes resection of the paranasal sinuses or facial soft tissues or with a neurosurgeon when tumors invade the orbital roof or the orbital apex.

The optimal balance between achieving the best chance for complete tumor resection and preserving tissue to optimize cosmesis is judged in a highly individualized way. It may be impossible to surgically eradicate all tumor cells, such as in the case of perineural invasion by tumor cells. In such cases, adjuvant postoperative radiation therapy can be utilized to minimize the chances of locoregional cancer recurrence. In patients with short life expectancy, the goal of orbital exenteration may not be to completely resect the tumor but to achieve palliation.

23.5 Reconstructive Options

When considering available options for reconstructing the exenterated orbit, the reconstructive surgeon must be knowledgeable about advantages and limitations of each technique. The primary goal of reconstruction is to line the orbital cavity with durable tissue and to exclude the nasal or sinus cavities when the medial or the inferior orbital wall has been removed and protect the brain when the orbital roof has been removed. The reconstructed orbit will need to be able to tolerate radiation therapy if radiation therapy is planned and to accommodate an orbital prosthesis if one is desired by the patient. Ultimately, the extent of the oncologic defect as well as whether radiation therapy is planned (preoperatively or postoperatively) determines selection of the reconstructive technique. In addition, the patient's desire for prosthetic rehabilitation should be considered when planning the reconstruction as a deep cavity facilitates prosthetic fit, while a shallow cavity may not securely hold a prosthesis without osseointegrated implants or may cause the prosthesis to protrude unnaturally.

Healing by secondary intention and granulation may be the simplest treatment after tumor resection. The entire process will take 2–3 months and requires daily wound care with hydrogen peroxide solution and wet-to-dry dressing for infection prevention. The orbital cavity, when completely healed by secondary intention, is only slightly shallow because of granulation tissue, rendering inspection for local tumor recurrence relatively easy. It is our preference to accelerate wound closure by utilizing a meshed or an unmeshed split-thickness skin graft to line the orbital cavity. A bolster dressing is usually applied for 5–7 days after the skin graft is laid into the orbital cavity. Similar to healing by secondary intention, the split-thickness skin grafting of the orbital defect also allows excellent visualization of the orbital cavity for detecting local tumor recurrence. Because skin grafts are thin, skin graft reconstruction usually results in a deep orbital cavity that provides an excellent fit for an orbital prosthesis if one is desired by the patient (Figs. 23.1 and 23.2). When the patient has no history of prior irradiation and no postoperative radiation therapy is planned, a skin graft is usually successful, even on bare orbital bone.

If the orbital cavity is to be irradiated after surgery, thicker lining of the orbital cavity with soft tissue—rather than just spontaneous epithelialization or skin graft coverage—is necessary to prevent failure of the skin engraftment or osteoradionecrosis. Among local vascularized pedicled flaps used, the most common ones are the temporalis muscle flap and the temporoparietal fascia flap because of their proximity to the orbit. The temporalis muscle flap, based on the anterior

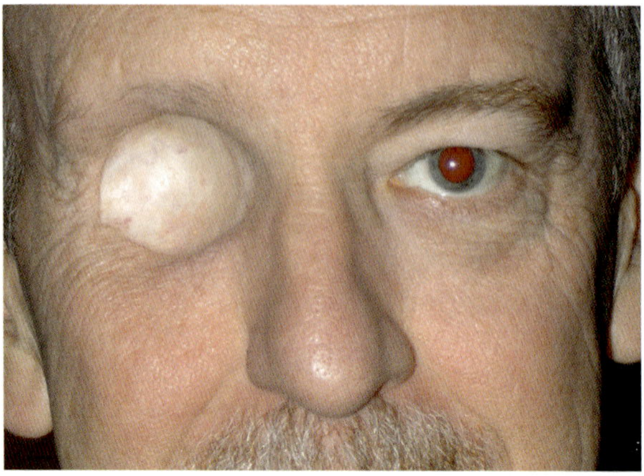

Fig. 23.1 Postoperative photograph following exenteration of the orbital cavity and reconstruction with a temporoparietal fascia flap and a full-thickness skin graft. Photo courtesy of Dr. Bita Esmaeli

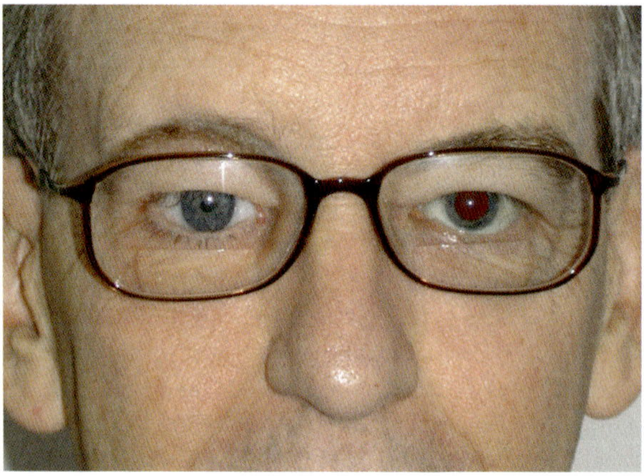

Fig. 23.2 The same patient as in Fig. 23.1 with his orbital prosthesis in place. Photo courtesy of Dr. Bita Esmaeli

and posterior deep temporal arteries arising from the internal maxillary artery, is thin enough to permit a reasonably secure fit for orbital prostheses, even without osseointegrated implants; however, this results in a depression at the donor site that may be cosmetically unsatisfactory to some patients. The temporoparietal fascia flap covered by a split-thickness skin graft may be preferable because there is no donor site deformity. In both cases, the reach of the flap may be limited, and it may be necessary to remove the lateral orbital wall in order to cover the medial orbital cavity. We tend to avoid large scalp or forehead flaps when other reconstructive options are available because of the donor site disfigurement associated with such flaps.

In extended orbital exenteration in which paranasal sinuses are resected, the size of the cavity usually necessitates soft tissue coverage larger than local or regional flaps can provide. Resection of the lateral orbital wall alone is usually inconsequential from a reconstructive standpoint. The orbital cavity may still be reconstructed with a skin graft or a regional flap. In addition, limited defects of the medial orbital wall can often still be reconstructed with a temporalis flap. For all other defects, we recommend reconstruction with a microvascular free flap.

Our preference is to reconstruct the cavity with a radial forearm fasciocutaneous free flap when the bony resection is limited (Fig. 23.3). This flap provides an adequate amount of tissue with relatively little bulk in nonobese patients that accommodates an orbital prosthesis without revision surgery. When the bony resection is more extensive—such as in the case of an orbitomaxillectomy—a larger, bulkier flap is preferred. The rectus abdominis muscle myocutaneous free flap and the anterolateral thigh free flap are good choices in this situation (Fig. 23.4). Both flaps may be designed such that muscle tissue obliterates the sinuses or creates a tight seal over any exposed dura, preventing infection with sinonasal bacterial flora. Bulkier flaps such as these are required to restore midfacial volume and preserve cheek contour.

Microvascular reconstructions are usually time consuming, and the patient must be a suitable candidate from a medical standpoint for this more extensive surgery. Postoperative hospitalization for 5 or more days is generally required to monitor flap viability. The risk for flap failure is usually highest during this time period. Early

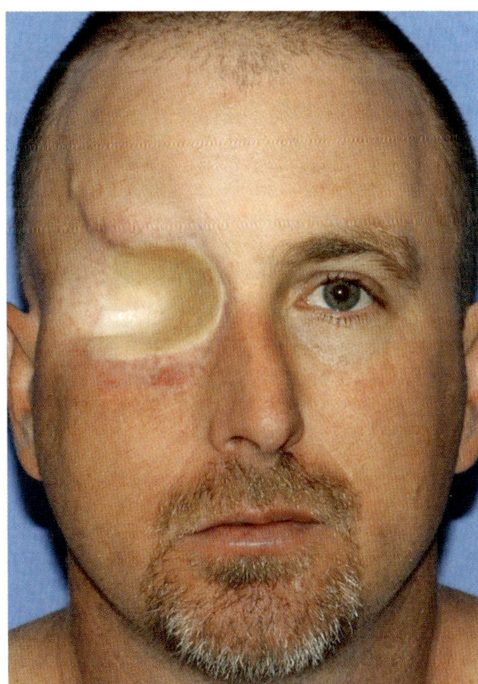

Fig. 23.3 Postoperative photograph following orbital exenteration and reconstruction with a radial forearm fasciocutaneous free flap in a patient who received postoperative radiation therapy. Photo courtesy of Dr. Bita Esmaeli

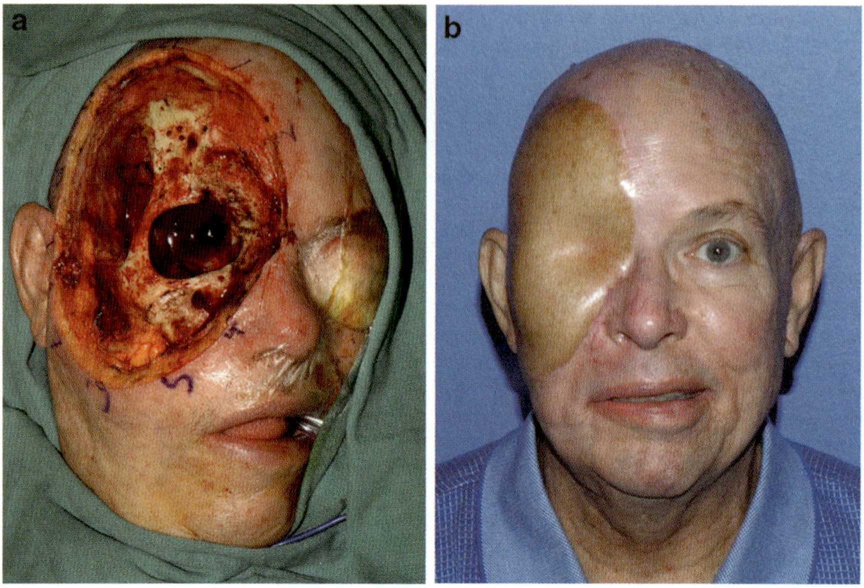

Fig. 23.4 (**a**) Photograph of the large surgical defect following an orbital exenteration. (**b**) Postoperative appearance after reconstruction with an anterolateral thigh free flap

detection of arterial or venous insufficiency and a rapid return to the operating room may allow salvage of the free flap. Whether free flap reconstruction masks local recurrence and leads to a delayed diagnosis is a subject of controversy. Patients with free flap reconstruction are usually followed with periodic imaging studies, such as computed tomography or magnetic resonance imaging, at intervals appropriate for their specific disease.

23.6 Surgical Complications

Postoperative complications of orbital exenteration include bleeding, infection, skin graft or flap failure, sino-orbital fistula, morbidity associated with the skin graft or tissue flap donor site, and unsatisfactory rehabilitation with an orbitofacial prosthesis. Prevention of hematoma and infection increases the skin engraftment rate. Sino-orbital fistula can be avoided by employing a careful surgical approach that does not violate the orbital walls. In extended orbital exenterations after which the orbit is reconstructed with flaps, sino-orbital fistula may be prevented by placing a nasal trumpet into the ipsilateral nostril during the healing period, preventing air escape through the suture line. Small fistulae are usually asymptomatic and may heal spontaneously. Larger ones may necessitate further surgery. In the case of bulky flaps, revision by suction-assisted lipectomy or direct excision of tissue may improve the cosmetic appearance of the patient.

23.7 Rehabilitation After Orbital Exenteration

Custom-made orbitofacial prostheses are widely used for rehabilitation after orbital exenteration. For complex defects, high-resolution computed tomography modeling systems can further improve fitting of the prosthesis. Polymethylmethacrylate prostheses are biocompatible and well tolerated, and the aesthetic result is pleasing, especially when the prosthesis is camouflaged by use of eyeglasses. Options for retention include the use of adhesive or osseointegrated titanium implants, which are placed into the bony orbital margins. Bone must be at least 4 mm thick to accommodate the implants, which are then covered with skin and soft tissue. After allowing several months for osseointegration to occur, the implants are exposed, and abutments, which protrude above the level of the skin, are attached to the implants. Finally, the prosthesis is coupled to the abutments via magnetic attachments.

Multistaged prosthetic rehabilitation demands significant motivation from the patient. Using an eye patch or dark glasses may be satisfactory for some patients. As mentioned, a bulky flap may limit accommodation of an orbital prosthesis or may cause the prosthesis to protrude excessively compared to the contralateral side. In some cases, the fit and appearance of an orbital prosthesis can be improved by debulking or recontouring of the reconstructive flap. Limitations of prostheses include the inability of the eye to move and the lids to close. Also, several fittings may be needed, and prostheses, which can be costly, need to be replaced periodically because of normal wear and tear. Regardless of the degree of aesthetic rehabilitation, monocular precautions, including constant eye protection and regular ophthalmologic exams, are emphasized to all patients to better protect the remaining functional eye.

Suggested Readings

1. Ben Simon GJ, Schwarcz RM, Douglas R, et al. Orbital exenteration: one size does not fit all. Am J Ophthalmol 2005;139:11–17.
2. Goldberg RA, Kim JW, Shorr N. Orbital exenteration: results of an individualized approach. Ophthal Plast Reconstr Surg 2003;19:229–36.
3. Groth MJ, Bhatnagar A, Clearihue WJ, et al. Long-term efficacy of biomodeled polymethyl methacrylate implants for orbitofacial defects. Arch Facial Plast Surg 2006;8:381–9.
4. Levin PS, Dutton JJ. A 20-year series of orbital exenteration. Am J Ophthalmol 1991;112:496–501.
5. Limawararut V, Leibovitch I, Davis G, et al. Sino-orbital fistula: a complication of exenteration. Ophthalmology 2007;114:355–61.
6. Looi A, Kazim M, Cortes M, et al. Orbital reconstruction after eyelid- and conjunctiva-sparing orbital exenteration. Ophthal Plast Recontr Surg 2006;22:1–6.
7. Menon NG, Girotto JA, Goldberg NH, et al. Orbital reconstruction after exenteration: use of a transorbital temporal muscle flap. Ann Plast Surg 2003;50:38–42.
8. Mohr C, Esser J. Orbital exenteration: surgical and reconstructive strategies. Graefes Arch Clin Exp Ophthalmol 1997;235:288–95.
9. Nassab RS, Thomas SS, Murray D. Orbital exenteration for advanced periorbital skin cancers: 20 years experience. J Plast Reconstr Aesthet Surg 2007;60:1103–9.

10. Nerad JA, Carter KD, LaVelle WE, et al. The osseointegration techniques for the rehabilitation of the exenterated orbit. Arch Ophthalmol 1991;109:1032–8.
11. Rahman I, Cook AE, Leatherbarrow B. Orbital exenteration: a 13 year Manchester experience. Br J Ophthalmol 2005;89:1335–40.
12. Reese A. Exenteration of the orbit with transplantation of the temporalis muscle. Am J Ophthalmol 1958;45:386–90.
13. Shields JA, Shields CL, Demirci H, et al. Experience with eyelid-sparing orbital exenteration: the 2001 Tullos L. Coston lecture. Ophthal Plast Reconstr Surg 2001;17:355–61.
14. Taylan G, Yildirim S, Akoz T. Reconstruction of large orbital exenteration defects after resection of periorbital tumors of advanced stage. J Reconstr Microsurg 2006;22:583–9.
15. Hanasono MM, Lee JC, Yang JS, Skoracki RJ, Reece GP, Esmaeli B. An algorithmic approach to reconstructive surgery and prosthetic rehabilitation after orbital exenteration. Plast Reconstr Surg 2009;123:98–105.

Chapter 24
Periorbital Surgical Rehabilitation After Facial Nerve Paralysis

Heather Chang, Mehryar Taban, and Tanuj Nakra

Abstract Facial nerve paralysis can result from a number of causes, including neoplasms, Bell's palsy, infections, trauma, congenital conditions, and idiopathic processes. Both the medical and social consequences of facial nerve paralysis can be distressing for patients. The most significant ophthalmic consequence of facial nerve paralysis is loss of function of the orbicularis oculi muscle. The complete assessment of a patient with facial nerve paralysis includes clinical evaluation of the resting tone and active function of the facial muscles, as well as determination of the extent of dry eye and the function of the lacrimal gland and lacrimal drainage system. The goal of medical therapy is symptomatic relief of dry eye and exposure keratopathy. Botulinum toxin can also be employed to treat other symptoms, such as synkinesis, hypertonicity, and spasms. The goal of surgical therapy is improved protection of the cornea, as well as a more symmetric static and dynamic appearance. Lagophthalmos and exposure keratopathy can be addressed with procedures such as surgical closure of the eyelids, known as tarsorrhaphy, or other alternatives, such as placement of an alloplastic gold weight in the upper eyelid, injection of hyaluronic acid gel into the upper eyelid, or palpebral springs. Ectropion also commonly results from facial nerve paralysis and can be improved with lateral or medial canthal procedures. Reanimation of the midface can be accomplished by any of several surgical techniques; some provide static support for the midface, while others attempt to restore dynamic movement to the paralyzed face.

24.1 Introduction

Facial nerve paralysis can result from a number of causes, including neoplastic processes, Bell's palsy, infections, trauma, congenital conditions, and idiopathic processes. Tumors can lead to facial nerve paralysis directly by mass effect or

---

H. Chang (✉)
Jules Stein Eye Institute, UCLA Medical Center, Los Angeles, CA, USA
e-mail: hkwon88@yahoo.com

B. Esmaeli (ed.), *Ophthalmic Oncology*, M.D. Anderson Solid Tumor Oncology Series 6, DOI 10.1007/978-1-4419-0374-7_24,

nerve infiltration; facial nerve paralysis can also occur following tumor resection [1]. Tumors can impact the facial nerve centrally, at the cerebellopontine angle (e.g., acoustic neuromas and meningiomas), and peripherally (e.g., parotid gland tumors).

Facial nerve paralysis can be distressing for patients and has both medical and social consequences. Periocular sequelae of paralysis, such as exposure keratopathy and paralytic ectropion, can cause significant discomfort and morbidity. Activities of daily living, such as eating and speaking, are often affected, and this can cause the patient emotional distress. Facial nerve paralysis can be accompanied by synkinesis, in which attempted voluntary movements lead to involuntary and undesired movements of other facial muscles, which is another potential source of emotional distress. Patients with facial nerve paralysis often reduce their participation in social activities, which negatively affects their mental health [2].

The treatment of facial nerve paralysis includes both medical and surgical management. The goal of medical therapy is symptomatic relief of dry eye and exposure keratopathy. Botulinum toxin can also be employed to treat synkinesis, hypertonicity, and spasms [3]. The goal of surgical therapy is a more symmetric static and dynamic appearance, as well as protection of the cornea. Surgical therapy can address lagophthalmos, ectropion, brow ptosis, and facial droop.

24.2 Relevant Anatomy

The facial nerve, the seventh cranial nerve, has multiple functions. It provides motor innervation to the muscles of facial expression, the throat muscles, the posterior belly of the digastric muscle, and the auricular, stylohyoid, and stapedius muscles. It also provides parasympathetic innervation to the lacrimal and salivary glands, along with sensory innervation to the external ear and the anterior two-thirds of the tongue. The course of the facial nerve is complex (Fig. 24.1). Four nuclei within the brainstem supply the facial nerve, which exits the brainstem laterally at the cerebellopontine angle and travels with the eighth cranial nerve to enter the internal auditory canal. The nerve then travels within the temporal bone and gives off the greater and lesser superficial petrosal nerves, as well as the nerve to the stapedius muscle and the chorda tympani. The facial nerve courses through the stylomastoid foramen, exits the temporal bone, passes through the parotid gland, and then finally divides into the temporal, zygomatic, buccal, mandibular, and cervical branches, which, in turn, innervate the corresponding facial muscles (Fig. 24.1).

The most significant ophthalmic consequence of facial nerve paralysis is loss of function of the orbicularis oculi muscle. This muscle's major function is to close the palpebral aperture, opposing the action of the levator palpebrae superioris muscle. In addition, the orbicularis oculi powers the "lacrimal pump": the simultaneous

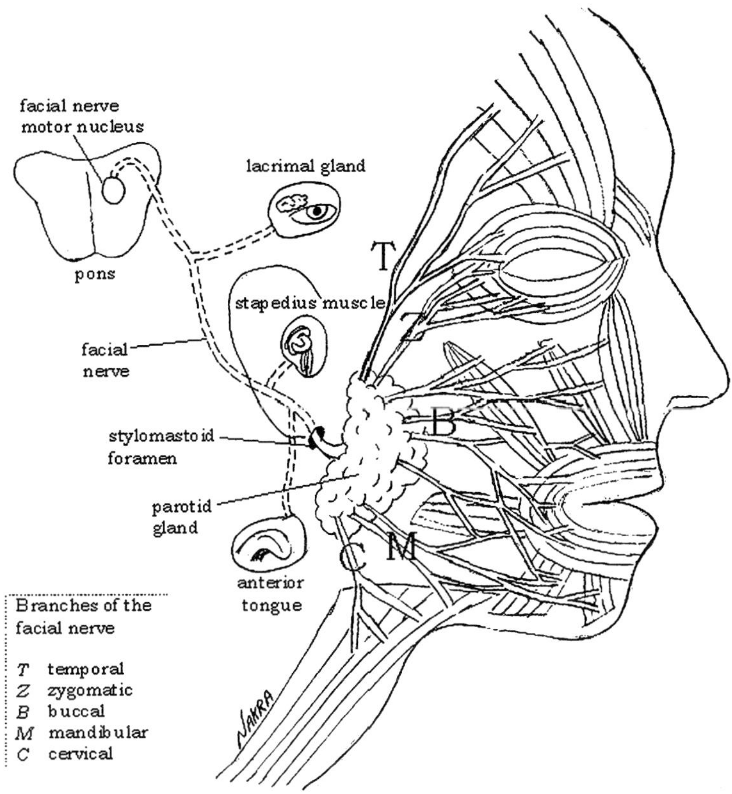

Fig. 24.1 Anatomy of the facial nerve. The facial nerve begins in the pons and provides parasympathetic innervation to the lacrimal and salivary glands. The nerve branches to innervate the stapedius muscle and anterior tongue and then exits the temporal bone through the stylomastoid foramen to innervate the parotid gland. Within the gland, the facial nerve divides into the temporal, zygomatic, buccal, mandibular, and cervical branches that provide motor innervation to the muscles of facial expression

contraction of the deep pre-tarsal head of the orbicularis oculi (Horner's muscle), which pulls the eyelid nasally and posteriorly, and the preseptal orbicularis oculi, which pulls the lacrimal sac laterally. This coordinated contraction compresses the canaliculi, pumping tears into the lacrimal sac. Subsequent relaxation of the orbicularis oculi then creates negative pressure in the canaliculi, thereby drawing tears in for the next pump cycle. Paralysis of the orbicularis oculi can result in lagophthalmos and paralytic ectropion, which places the ocular surface at risk of exposure and breakdown and can also result in epiphora.

Paralysis of other facial muscles can affect both voluntary and involuntary movements along with facial symmetry (Fig. 24.2). Decreased function of the frontalis muscle can lead to brow ptosis. The function of the dilator nasi muscle can be

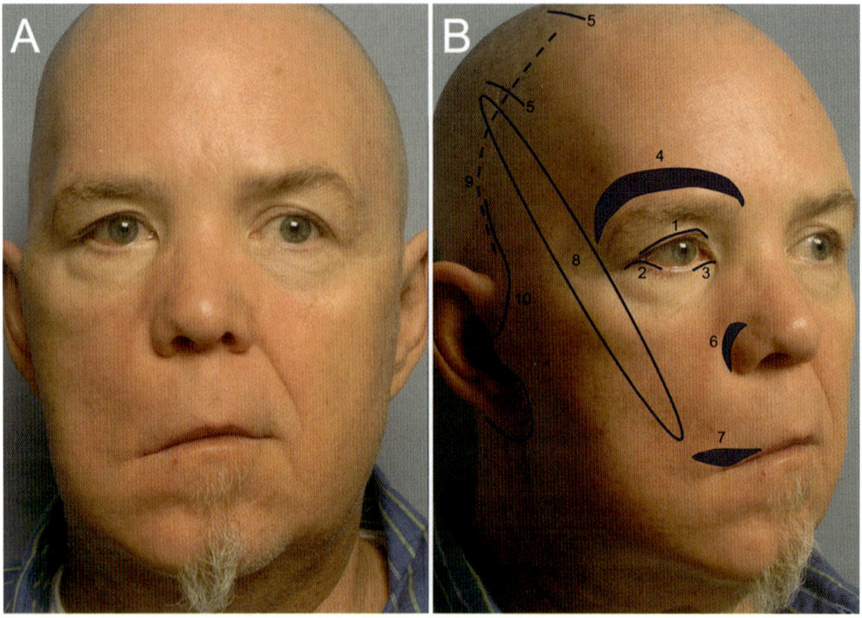

Fig. 24.2 Typical findings of facial nerve palsy and surgical approaches. (**a**) A 50-year-old man with right facial nerve paralysis after excision of a right acoustic neuroma. Note the paralytic right brow ptosis, mechanical dermatochalasis, lower eyelid ectropion, medial canthal laxity, nasolabial fold attenuation, alar collapse, lateral oral commissure droop, lower facial droop, and midfacial droop. (**b**) Composite photograph of the same patient illustrating the locations of various surgical approaches for comprehensive rehabilitation, including (1) insertion of an upper eyelid weight, (2) lateral canthoplasty and/or creation of a static lower eyelid sling, (3) medial canthopexy, (4) direct brow lift, (5) endoscopic forehead lift, (6) direct alar lift, (7) oral commissure lift, (8) midface lift, (9) temporalis muscle transfer or temporalis fascia sling, and (10) deep plane rhytidectomy and neck lift

affected, leading to nasal obstruction. Dysfunction of the orbicularis oris, risorius, or depressor anguli oris muscles contributes to asymmetry and can lead to problems with speech along with drooling and biting of the oral mucosa. Loss of function of the zygomaticus major and minor muscles leads to flattening of the nasolabial fold, increasing facial asymmetry, and potentially an increase in the patient's emotional distress.

24.3 Clinical Evaluation

The complete assessment of a patient with facial nerve paralysis includes clinical evaluation of the resting tone and the active function of muscles as well as determination of the extent of dry eye and the function of the lacrimal gland and lacrimal drainage system.

24.3.1 Evaluation of Muscle Function

The evaluation begins with the patient at rest with careful observation of involuntary movements and resting facial symmetry. Asking the patient to voluntarily contract the various muscle groups can further elucidate the pattern of loss of innervation. Electrophysiology testing—electromyography, electroneurography, maximal stimulation test, and nerve excitability test—can be used to further clarify the amount of degeneration of the facial nerve. Grading scales to grade the severity of the impairment of facial nerve function have been developed and emphasize the muscles of facial expression [2, 4].

As previously mentioned, loss of orbicularis oculi function is the most significant ophthalmic consequence of facial nerve paralysis and can result in lagophthalmos and paralytic ectropion, placing the ocular surface at risk for exposure and breakdown. The strength of the orbicularis oculi can be evaluated by observing the degree of lagophthalmos and the presence of Bell's phenomenon at rest and with gentle and then forceful blinking. Orbicularis oculi tone can be further evaluated by asking the patient to close his/her eyes while the clinician tries to manually force open the patient's eyelids. The cornea should be evaluated for both sensation and signs of exposure. The eyelid position should be assessed for the presence of laxity and for the presence of paralytic ectropion.

Evaluating frontalis muscle function can be especially helpful in determining whether facial nerve palsy is central or peripheral. Central facial nerve palsy spares frontalis muscle function as the forehead has bilateral upper motor neuron innervation. In contrast, peripheral facial nerve palsy affects ipsilateral frontalis muscle innervation, and the patient is unable to wrinkle the ipsilateral forehead, resulting in brow ptosis.

Evaluation of midfacial muscle function is also an important part of the clinical examination. The nasolabial fold is created by the zygomaticus major and minor, levator labii superioris, and levator labii superioris alaeque nasi muscles, and this fold may be effaced or absent with facial nerve palsy. The nasal ala may appear collapsed because of loss of levator labii superioris alaeque nasi function and support of the internal nasal valve. The zygomaticus major, which draws the angle of the mouth laterally, and the zygomaticus minor, which elevates and everts the upper lip, can be assessed by asking the patient to attempt to smile. The orbicularis oris muscle narrows the orifice of the mouth, purses the lips, and plays an important role in speech and oral competence. Difficulty in speech, along with the presence of drooling, lip laxity, and biting of the oral mucosa, can indicate involvement of the facial nerve branches innervating the zygomaticus and orbicularis oris muscles.

24.3.2 Evaluation of Lacrimal Gland and Lacrimal Drainage System Function

Both lacrimal gland function and the lacrimal drainage system can be compromised in patients with facial nerve palsy. The parasympathetic innervation for the secretomotor function of the lacrimal gland travels with the proximal part of the facial nerve. Thus, facial nerve paralysis can lead to decreased lacrimal gland function and decreased tear production, which can exacerbate exposure keratopathy. Decreased function of the lacrimal gland is particularly common with facial nerve paralysis resulting from acoustic neuromas or other central nervous system tumors. Lacrimal gland function is evaluated using the Schirmer test without anesthesia: less than 10 mm of wetting on a filter paper strip in 5 minutes can indicate that the proximal facial nerve is damaged. Patients with facial nerve paralysis can also be affected by lower eyelid ectropion and decreased function of the lacrimal pump, leading to epiphora and worsening of corneal exposure.

24.4 Medical Management

The first step in managing facial nerve palsy is supportive treatment to stabilize and protect the cornea. Maintaining the health of the cornea is crucial, as exposure keratopathy and corneal abrasions can result in serious corneal infections, corneal perforation, and even blindness. Artificial tears and lubricating ointments are mainstays of treatment. Preservative-free artificial tear preparations can be employed when frequent administration is required. In more severe cases, moisture chambers that are designed to slow the evaporation of tears from the surface of the eye can be used during sleep. These range from chambers created with a cellophane cover taped over the eyes to customized moisture goggles. Even the simple application of tape can be used to force the palpebral fissure closed during sleep; however, this needs to be done cautiously as the tape itself can be a source of corneal abrasion if it loosens during sleep. In patients with some remaining lacrimal pump function, punctal plugs can be useful in the treatment of dry eye. When corneal abrasions do occur, bandage contact lenses and pressure patching with ointment can help promote corneal healing.

Botulinum toxin can be useful in treating both exposure keratopathy and facial spasms. If the patient has a good Bell's phenomenon, injection of botulinum toxin into the levator palpebrae superioris at the upper border of the tarsus can produce ptosis and protect the cornea, although the patient's vision is obviously affected and some patients experience diplopia [4]. However, this procedure is a minimally invasive and temporary measure that still allows the cornea to be easily examined.

Another application of botulinum toxin in facial nerve paralysis is the treatment of facial muscle spasms and synkinesis. Hypertonicity of facial muscles often occurs during recovery after facial nerve trauma, and aberrant regeneration of the facial nerve branches can lead to involuntary spasms and involuntary muscle movements. Botulinum toxin can be selectively injected to target the hypertonic muscles and prevent involuntary muscle movements [3, 4].

In cancer patients, facial nerve paralysis can be caused by involvement of the facial nerve by leptomeningeal disease from hematologic malignancies or invasion of the facial nerve from metastases from solid tumors. In these cases, systemic or intrathecal chemotherapy may lead to resolution of facial nerve paralysis.

24.5 Surgical Management

When medical therapy insufficiently addresses the medical and social/emotional consequences of facial nerve paralysis, surgical therapy may be indicated. Occasionally, urgent surgical intervention is indicated for cases of impending ocular surface damage. The soft tissue changes that occur in facial nerve paralysis, such as lower eyelid ectropion, brow ptosis, and facial droop, can be ameliorated with surgical interventions (Fig. 24.2).

24.5.1 Treatment of Lagophthalmos and Exposure Keratopathy

Lagophthalmos and exposure keratopathy can be addressed with surgical closure of the eyelids, known as tarsorrhaphy. As a first step, application of cyanoacrylate glue to the eyelashes or placement of a nonabsorbable suture can create a temporary partial tarsorrhaphy. A temporary tarsorrhaphy may be preferable in cases of recent paralysis that may improve spontaneously over time. A partial tarsorrhaphy preserves some visual function and allows access to the cornea for examination. However, for patients without adequate Bell's phenomenon, a permanent tarsorrhaphy (either partial or complete) is a more effective treatment. A permanent tarsorrhaphy can be performed for established cases of severe palsy. A permanent tarsorrhaphy is accomplished by de-epithelializing the upper and lower eyelid margins and then approximating the upper tarsus and lower tarsus with mattress sutures.

Another option to address lagophthalmos is the placement of an alloplastic weight in the upper eyelid (Fig. 24.3). Gold and platinum are commonly used and aid passively in eyelid closure by exerting a gravitational effect while the levator palpebrae superioris muscle relaxes. The weight is especially useful in patients with exposure keratopathy accompanied by decreased tear production and poor Bell's phenomenon. Preoperative application of tester weights can facilitate selection of the weight that allows the greatest eyelid closure while also allowing adequate eyelid opening in primary gaze. Once the proper weight is selected, it is then secured to the upper border of the tarsus deep to the orbicularis oculi through an eyelid crease incision. Some surgeons choose to wrap the weight in a Dacron (terephthalate fiber) mesh to allow fibrosis around the weight to stabilize its position. Potential complications of alloplastic weight placement are persistent inflammation, extrusion, and eyelid distortion. For temporary facial nerve paralysis, personalized external weights that are secured to the skin of the upper eyelid with adhesive tape are commercially available and can lead to patient satisfaction.

Another alternative for the treatment of lagophthalmos resulting from temporary facial nerve weakness is the injection of hyaluronic acid gel into the upper eyelid [5]. A 30-G needle is used to perform multiple injections of small amounts of hyaluronic acid gel in sites across the length of the upper eyelid into the pre-tarsal and prelevator aponeurosis regions (Fig. 24.4). The hyaluronic acid gel is layered using

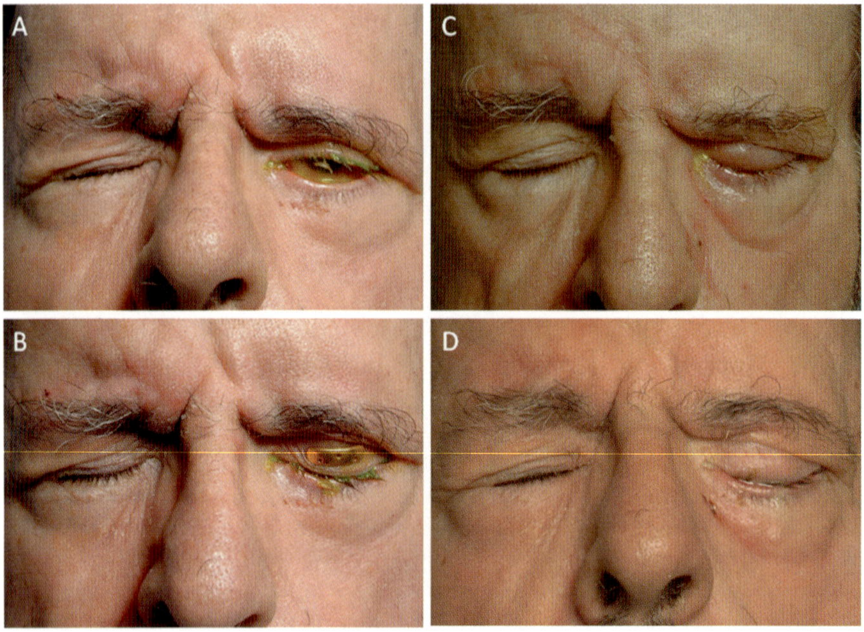

Fig. 24.3 Upper eyelid gold weight in a 60-year-old man with left paralytic lagophthalmos. (**a**) Degree of lagophthalmos before weight placement. (**b**) Fitting the patient with a trial weight preoperatively and having the patient test it by attempting to close the eyelid, which facilitates appropriate weight selection to avoid undercorrection or overcorrection. (**c**) Photograph taken 1 week after insertion of a 1.4-g gold weight into the left upper eyelid and medial canthopexy. (**d**) Photograph taken 1 year after placement of the gold weight, showing stable resolution of lagophthalmos

multiple thread-like injections that are placed deep to the orbicularis oculi muscle. Among the advantages of this technique is that it is temporary and that its effect can be reduced if necessary with hyaluronidase. Hyaluronic acid gel injections can also be used as an adjunct to previous gold weight placement when lagophthalmos persists, and these injections offer an alternative for patients who are poor surgical candidates.

Palpebral springs made of stainless steel can also be used in the treatment of lagophthalmos. These springs can restore a natural-appearing blink with full closure of the eyelid and do not rely on gravity. However, the process of adjusting the spring shape and tension for the individual patient is complex and requires frequent adjustments after the initial surgery. The size and shape of the spring are modified before implantation to follow the eyelid curvature. After exposure of the tarsus via an eyelid crease incision, the tarsal limb of the spring is wrapped in Dacron mesh and then secured to the tarsus, and the fulcrum of the spring is secured to the lateral orbital periosteum. The remaining limb of the spring is then sutured to the periosteum of the superior orbit. Potential complications include extrusion, spring malfunction, and the need for frequent readjustment. Because of these problems,

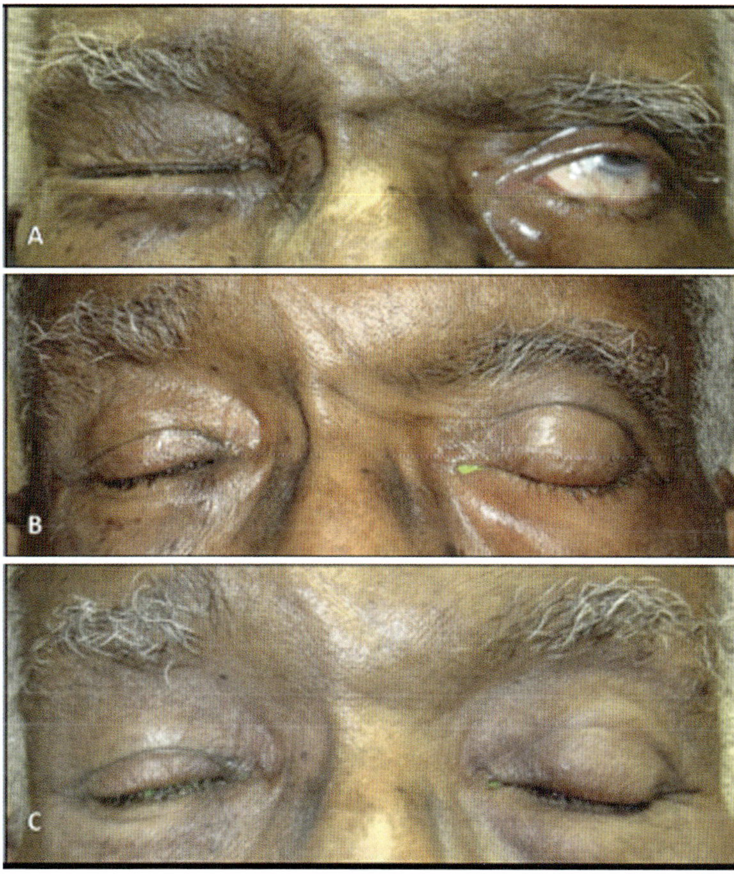

Fig. 24.4 Upper eyelid hyaluronic acid gel weight in a 90-year-old man with left paralytic lagophthalmos due to Bell's palsy. (**a**) Degree of lagophthalmos before injection. (**b**) Attempted closure immediately after injection of hyaluronic acid gel (Juvederm Ultra; Allergan, Inc., Irvine, CA) into the left upper eyelid. (**c**) Attempted closure at 5-month follow-up. Note the resolution of lagophthalmos. From Mancini R, Taban M, Lowinger A, et al. Use of hyaluronic gel in the management of paralytic lagophthalmos: the hyaluronic acid gel "gold weight." Ophthal Plast Reconstr Surg 2009;25:23–26. Reprinted with permission

very few centers currently use palpebral springs as first-line treatment for surgical rehabilitation of eyelids in facial nerve paralysis.

24.5.2 Treatment of Lower Eyelid Laxity and Ectropion

The midface extends from the lower eyelid margin to the oral commissure. The management of facial nerve palsy in this region is complex owing to the complex interplay of soft tissue gravitational effects and the loss of multiple vectors of muscular pull on the soft tissue. As with surgical options for treatment of lagophthalmos and exposure keratopathy, surgical therapy for lower eyelid laxity and ectropion begins with procedures designed to protect the ocular surface. Ectropion can be addressed with lateral or medial canthal procedures depending on whether the eyelid laxity is most apparent laterally or medially.

The lateral tarsal strip procedure can be useful in cases of severe laxity or ectropion and involves horizontal eyelid shortening to improve lower eyelid tone and position. The lower eyelid is horizontally shortened and is then reattached more tightly to the periosteum of the lateral orbital rim. However, this procedure is associated with drawbacks, including medial canthal distortion and limited efficacy in patients with prominent globes.

To address medial ectropion or punctal eversion, a medial canthopexy can be performed. The procedure may include excision of skin and/or conjunctiva to advance the lower eyelid superiorly and medially while paying close attention to the integrity of the canalicular system.

When there is laxity of the medial canthal tendon, a static eyelid sling can be created using autologous material, such as temporalis fascia, to further support the lower eyelid. In this procedure, the temporalis fascia is harvested via a posttrichial incision, and the lower eyelid tarsus is exposed along with the lateral and medial canthal tendons via an infralash incision. The fascia is secured to the medial canthal tendon and the tarsus and is then attached to the superficial periosteum of the lateral orbit [4, 6]. This procedure can be combined with the lateral canthal shortening procedures to correct ectropion.

24.5.3 Reanimation of the Midface

Reanimation of the midface in facial nerve paralysis can be addressed by any of several surgical techniques, some of which provide static support for the midface and others of which attempt to restore dynamic movement to the paralyzed face.

24.5.3.1 Static Reanimation

Static midface lifting can correct drooping caused by palsy of the midface muscles. Several different techniques can be utilized, but the goal is to restore the ptotic cheek to a more normal position and also to recruit tissue volume that can support the lower eyelid and ameliorate ectropion.

The classic midface lift is a subperiosteal lift via a lateral canthotomy and transconjunctival lower eyelid incision [7–9]. Another midface repositioning technique is creation of a temporalis fascia sling. In this technique, via a hemicoronal incision, the fascia overlying the temporalis muscle is released and hinged on its inferior–medial border and then brought into the midface as a static sling suspension [6, 10, 11]. A less invasive option is the subperiosteal midface dissection via a temporal and oral incision, along with fixation using a suture, harvested fascia lata, or commercially available midface suspension kit. Another, even less invasive,

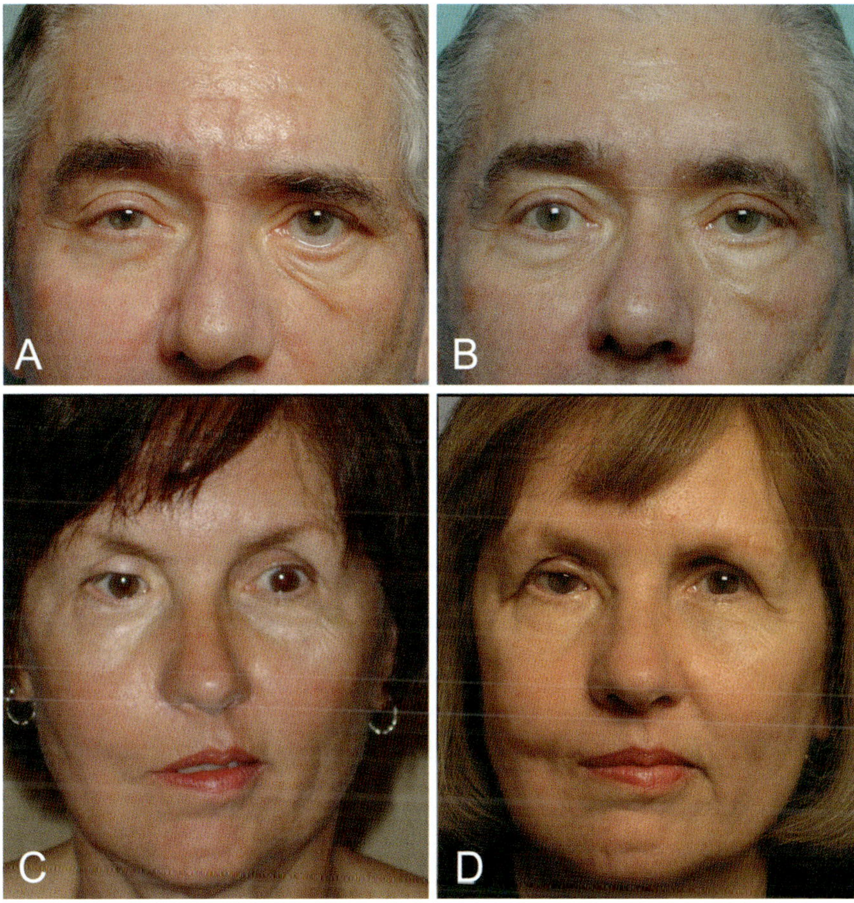

Fig. 24.5 Midface lift. Cable midface resuspension. (**a**) Profound complete left facial nerve palsy with ectropion in a 54-year-old man. (**b**) Photograph taken 1 year after lateral tarsal strip ectropion repair and minimally invasive midface resuspension with multiple 2-0 silk sutures anchored to the deep temporalis fascia. Note resolution of the ectropion. (**c**) Marked right facial nerve palsy in a 46-year-old woman. (**d**) Photograph taken 3 years after minimally invasive midface resuspension with multiple 2-0 silk sutures anchored to the deep temporalis fascia

option is the cable suspension technique, in which long sutures anchored in the midface are suspended to the temporalis fascia [12] (Fig. 24.5).

24.5.3.2 Dynamic Reanimation

Dynamic reanimation of the midface can be performed by muscle transfer and/or nerve grafting. Temporalis muscle transfer can help improve dynamic voluntary facial movement in the paralyzed face and is indicated for patients with chronic facial nerve palsy. Via a hemicoronal incision, the anterior and central portions of the temporalis muscle and fascia are developed into a muscular flap and dissected inferiorly toward the temporalis insertion [13–18]. The muscle segment is left attached inferiorly, but the flap is divided and sutured to the orbicularis oculi muscle and upper and lower lips, thereby creating a dynamic multiple sling suspension. The patient can then learn to close the eyelid voluntarily by attempting a chewing motion. However, while this procedure is effective in reanimating the lower face, it is also associated with complications including persistent facial droop, facial scarring, and unnatural facial movement.

Several dynamic reanimation techniques involving nerve grafting are available. Following traumatic injury to the facial nerve, such as during tumor resection, direct nerve repair can be attempted. However, during tumor resection, nerve grafting is often required to replace the sacrificed section of the facial nerve. Commonly used donor nerves include the sural nerve and the various cervical nerve branches [19–21]. Cross-face nerve grafting utilizes nerves from the nonparalyzed side of the face to provide innervation to the paralyzed side by incorporating sural nerve grafts [21, 22]. The nerve crossover technique takes advantage of nearby nerves, such as the ipsilateral glossopharyngeal and hypoglossal nerves, to serve as an autograft to the facial nerve [11, 20, 23]. While these procedures can offer some dynamic reanimation to the paralyzed face, their widespread use is prevented by limitations including graft-harvest-induced paralysis, and the complex nerve grafting surgery has the potential to be unsuccessful or result in uncoordinated movements. It also takes at least 6–12 months for the beneficial effect of nerve grafting to become apparent and, in general, nerve grafting is more effective for the lower facial branches of the facial nerve than for the upper facial (periocular) branches.

24.5.4 Options for Correction of Brow Ptosis

Brow ptosis in the paralyzed face can lead to mechanical ptosis, extreme dermatochalasis, and obstruction of the superior visual field. The direct-incision brow lift is the most effective and simplest surgical rehabilitation option. The amount of lift needed is measured with the patient sitting upright with the brows relaxed, and then the eyebrow is elevated to the desired position. The skin and subcutaneous tissue are then dissected to the level of the frontalis muscle and excised using an incision superior to the lateral two-thirds of the eyebrow. While this procedure is very effective, its disadvantages include the occasional unappealing scar and rare sensory nerve damage.

A more cosmetically sensitive approach to the brow lift utilizes endoscopic techniques via an incision hidden in the hairline and is associated with a lower rate of postoperative numbness and paresthesia [24, 25]. The dissection proceeds caudally in either a subperiosteal or preperiosteal plane. The corrugator and procerus muscles may be resected to reduce the action of brow depression. The elevated brow is then fixed posterior to the hairline with any one of various absorbable or nonabsorbable fixation devices. Potential complications of the endoscopic brow lift for elevating a paralytic brow include malposition of the brow and alopecia at the location of fixation; in addition, the endoscopic brow lift can result in a less robust lift than that achieved with the direct technique. In non-facial nerve palsy cases, the most serious complication of this procedure is damage to the temporal branch of the facial nerve.

24.5.5 Additional Procedures for Management of Facial Droop

Additional procedures for management of facial droop include rhytidectomy, lateral oral commissure lift, and lateral alar lift (Fig. 24.2). Rhytidectomy may be performed in conjunction with a midface lift and periocular reconstruction. Options for rhytidectomy via a preauricular incision are the superficial musculo-aponeurotic system lift and the deep plane lift. In patients with facial nerve paralysis, the usual concerns about damage to the facial nerve during the deep plane facelift do not apply, allowing for a more aggressive approach and making the deep plane rhytidectomy the preferred approach for resuspending the midface and lower face in such patients. Drooping of the corner of the mouth can be addressed with a lateral oral commissure lift, in which slings are used to suspend the orbicularis oris to either the orbital rim or the zygomatic arch. A simple variation is to perform a direct excision of skin and subcutaneous tissue along the lateral superior vermillion border; the open approach allows direct plication of the orbicularis oris. A lateral alar lift can correct collapse of the internal nasal valve; a direct curvilinear incision and skin resection can elevate the ala and open the nasal vestibule.

24.6 Special Circumstances in Cancer Patients with Facial Nerve Paralysis

Many patients with head and neck cancer who undergo a parotidectomy develop facial nerve paralysis either due to direct mechanical compression of the nerve by tumor or due to the necessary sacrifice of the facial nerve during cancer-ablative surgery. In the majority of these patients, postoperative adjuvant radiation therapy is planned within 4–6 weeks after head and neck surgery. In these patients, we prefer not to perform periocular surgical rehabilitation during the primary ablative procedure as this type of "one-size-fits-all" approach would lead to less than ideal outcomes [1]. Instead, we prefer to evaluate the patient after the ablative head and neck surgery to assess the facial tone, the size of gold weight needed, and the degree of paralytic ectropion and lagophthalmos before we plan surgical rehabilitation of the periocular soft tissues. Periocular surgery can be done either during the week or two after the parotidectomy or a few weeks after radiation therapy is completed. An important consideration in planning the timing of periocular surgery is that although the radiation field in most cases does not include the periocular soft tissues, the mask used during daily head and neck irradiation can be uncomfortable in the immediate postoperative period after periocular surgery.

Another potential special circumstance in cancer patients is chemotherapy-induced pancytopenia due to recent chemotherapy. In patients with such pancytopenia, surgery should be delayed until hematologic parameters have normalized. Prophylactic use of antibiotics in the perioperative period is also appropriate in the majority of cancer patients undergoing surgical rehabilitation for periocular manifestations of facial nerve paralysis.

24.7 Conclusion

Management of facial nerve paralysis in cancer patients poses complex challenges. Spontaneous improvement of facial nerve paralysis in cancer patients is uncommon as the nerve is often sacrificed during tumor resection. However, function may be regained if the nerve is affected only indirectly by compression or is only traumatized during ablative surgery or due to mass effect. The prevention of ocular surface morbidity is of paramount importance in facial nerve paralysis. Medical therapy is the first step, but often surgical intervention is indicated. Surgical procedures can help minimize morbidity to ocular tissues, provide static support for ptotic facial tissues, and sometimes restore dynamic voluntary movements. Furthermore, improvements in both facial function and symmetry from surgery may mitigate the psychological burden to patients living with facial nerve paralysis. Future developments in static and dynamic reanimation will help to further address the challenges of facial nerve paralysis. The extent and timing of rehabilitative surgery in cancer patients with facial nerve paralysis should be individualized and depend on many factors, including age, facial muscle tone, timing of adjuvant radiation therapy and chemotherapy, and long-term prognosis.

References

1. Golio D, De Martelaere S, Anderson J, et al. Outcomes of periocular reconstruction for facial nerve paralysis in cancer patients. Plast Reconstr Surg 2007;119:1233–7.
2. Kahn JB, Gliklich RE, Boyev KP, et al. Validation of a patient-graded instrument for facial nerve paralysis: the FaCE scale. Laryngoscope 2001;111:387–98.
3. Mehta RP, Hadlock TA. Botulinum toxin and quality of life in patients with facial paralysis. Arch Facial Plast Surg 2008;10:84–7.
4. Lee V, Currie Z, Collin JR. Ophthalmic management of facial nerve palsy. Eye 2004;18: 1225–34.
5. Mancini R, Taban M, Lowinger A, et al. The use of hyaluronic acid gel in the management of paralytic lagophthalmos: the hyaluronic acid gel "gold weight." Ophthal Plast Reconstr Surg 2009;25(1):23–6.
6. Rose EH. Autogenous fascia lata grafts: clinical applications in reanimation of the totally or partially paralyzed face. Plast Reconstr Surg 2005;116:20–32.
7. Edelstein C, Balch K, Shorr N, et al. The transeyelid subperiosteal midface-lift in the unhappy postblepharoplasty patient. Semin Ophthalmol 1998;13:107–14.
8. Paul MD, Calvert JW, Evans GR. The evolution of the midface lift in aesthetic plastic surgery. Plast Reconstr Surg 2006;117:1809–27.

9. Baylis HI, Goldberg RA, Shorr N. The deep plane facelift: a 20-year evolution of technique. Ophthalmology 2000;107:490–5.
10. Neuhaus RW, Shorr N. Use of temporal fascia and muscle as an autograft. Arch Ophthalmol 1983;101:262–4.
11. Rosson GD, Redett RJ. Facial palsy: anatomy, etiology, grading, and surgical treatment. J Reconstr Microsurg 2008;24:379–89.
12. Ugurbas SH, Goldberg RA, McCann JD, et al. Suture midface suspension. Head Face Med 2006;2:35–9.
13. Cheney ML, McKenna MJ, Megerian CA, et al. Early temporalis muscle transposition for the management of facial paralysis. Laryngoscope 1995;105(9 pt 1):993–1000.
14. Frey M, Giovanoli P, Tzou CJ, et al. Dynamic reconstruction of eye closure by muscle transposition or functional muscle transplantation in facial palsy. Plast Reconstr Surg 2004;114:865–75.
15. May M, Drucker C. Temporalis muscle for facial reanimation. A 13-year experience with 224 procedures. Arch Otolaryngol Head Neck Surg 1993;119:378–82.
16. Tate JR, Tollefson TT. Advances in facial reanimation. Curr Opin Otolaryngol Head Neck Surg 2006;14:242–8.
17. Yoleri L, Songur E. Modified temporalis muscle transfer for paralytic eyelids. Ann Plast Surg 1999;43:598–605.
18. Boahene KD. Dynamic muscle transfer in facial reanimation. Facial Plast Surg 2008;24:204–10.
19. Lee EI, Hurvitz KA, Evans GR, et al. Cross-facial nerve graft: past and present. J Plast Reconstr Aesthet Surg 2008;61:250–6.
20. Shah SB, Jackler RK. Facial nerve surgery in the 19th and early 20th centuries: the evolution from crossover anastomosis to direct nerve repair. Am J Otol 1998;19:236–45.
21. Terzis JK, Konofaos P. Nerve transfers in facial palsy. Facial Plast Surg 2008;24:177–93.
22. Frey M, Giovanoli P, Michaelidou M. Functional upgrading of partially recovered facial palsy by cross-face nerve grafting with distal end-to-side neurorrhaphy. Plast Reconstr Surg 2006;117:597–608.
23. Atlas MD, Lowinger DS. A new technique for hypoglossal-facial nerve repair. Laryngoscope 1997;107:984–91.
24. De Cordier BC, de la Torre JI, Al-Hakeem MS, et al. Endoscopic forehead lift: review of technique, cases, and complications. Plast Reconstr Surg 2002;110:1558–68.
25. Steinsapir KD, Shorr N, Hoenig J, et al. The endoscopic forehead lift. Ophthal Plast Reconstr Surg 1998;14:107–18.

Chapter 25
Psychosocial Aspects of Orbitofacial Disfigurement in Cancer Patients

Alessandro Bonanno and Jin Young Choi

Abstract The idea of an attractive face is socially constructed through interaction. The face is a fundamental element in the definition of identity and behavior, and individuals endowed with an attractive face are treated better than others. Accordingly, orbitofacial cancer survivors who are disfigured because of their cancer or cancer treatment suffer from stigmatization and social exclusion. Patients with acquired facial disfigurement suffer more serious psychosocial consequences than do individuals with congenital facial disfigurement. However, among patients with acquired facial disfigurement, cancer patients experience less severe social and psychological problems than do trauma patients. With time, as patients' fear of dying of cancer diminishes, the process of dealing with facial disfigurement begins and affects both patients and their family members. Active forms of coping generate better results than do passive coping strategies. Women with facial disfigurement tend to report more stress than men, and partners may experience more stress than patients. Interaction with acquaintances and strangers originates different levels of stigmatization in different social settings. Because facial disfigurement will continue to occur as a result of successful treatment of cancer, surgeons should be educated regarding the psychosocial consequences of facial disfigurement, and the roles that partners and other social actors play in social interaction and stigmatization should be considered in the formulation of protocols.

25.1 Introduction

Advances in medicine are allowing individuals with orbital and periorbital cancer to survive for many years after the cancer is treated [1, 2]. Surgical removal of the malignancy is often required and leaves patients with alterations of their facial

---

A. Bonanno (✉)
Department of Sociology, Sam Houston State University, Huntsville, TX, USA
e-mail: soc_aab@shsu.edu

B. Esmaeli (ed.), *Ophthalmic Oncology*, M.D. Anderson Solid Tumor Oncology Series 6, DOI 10.1007/978-1-4419-0374-7_25,

appearance. Procedures to correct these alterations are common, and increasingly sophisticated facial prostheses are available [3]. Even so, however, the faces of survivors of orbital and periorbital cancer are often notably different from the "normal" face. Survivors' visible facial deformities are associated with stigma—a mark of social disgrace [3–12]. In short, as medicine has developed and allowed more patients to survive, these patients are having to confront the stigma associated with facial disfigurement [9]. This situation requires the attention of surgeons as survivors' quality of life depends not only on physical status but also on emotional and social well-being.

25.2 The Importance of the Face and Its Social "Construction"

People who possess an attractive face enjoy a number of social benefits that other, "less attractive" individuals do not have. People with an attractive face are not only considered physically pleasing but often viewed on the basis of their attractiveness as endowed with positive intellectual, ethical, and emotional characteristics [10, 13, 14]. Individuals with an attractive appearance are often judged to be intelligent, kind, likable, and highly moral, and these individuals are treated better than other, less attractive members of society [4]. This situation persists even in societies that formally stress the importance of moral and intellectual qualities in social living. The power of physical beauty is significant [10]. As we are fully clothed for virtually all of our social activities, the face represents one of the most notable physical attributes: "Beauty is perceived as residing principally in the face" [15–18].

While there is a tendency to consider beauty as universal, it is actually culturally based and socially constructed [4, 8, 19, 20]. Different cultures[1] tend to employ different standards to define beauty and emphasize different facial parts as primary features of a beautiful face. Even in the American-dominated Western world, the parts of the face that define beauty are constructed by the society in which the individual lives.

The face is also one of the standards used to distinguish between individuals who fit social expectations—how we expect someone to behave in a given circumstance—and those who deviate from them [7, 19]. The face is employed in the creation of our understanding of "normality" and ownership of socially desirable characteristics. In this context, the face is used as a significant source of social information both prior to and during social interaction [7, 8, 11, 16–18, 21]. Given this social importance of the face—"one's presentation to the world" [5, 8, 10–12, 18, 21]—facial disfigurement causes "a major upheaval in people's lives" [8] that is reflected not only in people's reactions to the abnormal face but also in the interaction between disfigured individuals and various groups in society [16, 22–24].

[1] Culture refers to the ways in which members of a society, such as the United States, normally carry out daily tasks such as eating, dressing, and addressing each other. Each society has its own culture as each long-existing group of people developed specific manners for conducting themselves.

Those who suffer from facial disfigurement are often stigmatized [4, 19]. In his now-classic work on social stigma, the renowned sociologist Erving Goffman indicated how blemishes of the face are conditions that almost inevitably lead to the creation of stigma [21]. For Goffman, stigma is not reserved to specific groups of people; rather, it is a "relational" phenomenon—that is, it exists because we interact with other people and in so doing judge them according to established cultural standards. Frances Macgregor describes the negative responses that facially disfigured individuals encounter in their everyday lives as follows:

> [They] are subjected to visual and verbal assaults and a level of familiarity from strangers not otherwise dared: naked stares, startled reaction, "double takes," whispering, remarks, fugitive looks, curiosity, personal questions, advice, manifestation of pity or aversion, laughter, ridicule and outright avoidance. Whatever form the behaviors may take, they generate feelings of shame, impotence, anger and humiliation in their victims [10].

25.3 State of the Psychosocial Research on Facial Disfigurement

Research on the psychosocial aspects of facial disfigurement remains sparse and attracts even less attention than the already limited research associated with other forms of deformity [25–27]. The research on facial disfigurement to date stresses that facial disfigurement can be approached from at least three different directions. First, facial disfigurement has functional implications: patients encounter limitations as they attempt to carry out normal activities, and these limitations signal to others that patients are different. Functional implications also have consequences in terms of how patients feel about themselves and how others feel about and/or respond to them [8, 10, 14]. Second, facial disfigurement can be viewed in terms of the individual's reactions to his or her disfigurement, including reactions such as stress, anxiety, and coping strategies. Most psychological studies of facial disfigurement focus on patients' reactions [28]. Third, facial disfigurement has social implications—implications regarding how disfigured individuals interact with others and how others interact with disfigured individuals in various social contexts [8, 11, 27]. This third approach to studying facial disfigurement stresses the importance of social settings—e.g., the workplace, the street, shopping malls, restaurants—and the manner through which these settings aid in the construction of collective perceptions and actions toward the facially disfigured.

25.3.1 Psychosocial Consequences of Facial Disfigurement Caused by Cancer and Cancer Treatment

Studies of the relationship between cancer and disfigurement in general point out that while the social perception of cancer has changed in recent decades, this disease engenders a wide variety of attitudes and responses that differentiate it from other pathological situations [29]. Often, these attitudes and responses are stigmatizing [30]. However, differences have been recorded between reactions to forms of cancer that are perceived as uncontrollable—such as breast cancer—and those that are perceived as controllable—such as lung cancer due to smoking. Because the latter are seen as deriving from the patient's voluntary actions, more stigmatizing reactions are expected [31]. In the case of cancer-generated facial disfigurement, patients tend to experience responses based on "sympathy" when it is clear that the disfigurement is cancer generated, but when disfigurement is not clearly cancer generated, stigmatization tends to occur [32].

A limited number of studies have examined facial disfigurement caused by cancer. In general, individuals with acquired facial disfigurement suffer psychosocial consequences that are different from and, at least to some degree, more pronounced than those experienced by individuals with congenital disfigurement [19, 27]. However, among individuals with acquired facial disfigurement, cancer patients experience less severe social and psychological problems than do individuals who have been disfigured because of trauma [33]. For cancer patients, "fear of dying is immense" [29, 34], and this situation affects their perception of disfigurement and the behavior of those who interact with them [35]—patients are initially preoccupied more with the evolution of their cancer than with the social consequences of the scars that it left on their faces [27]. However, as this fear of dying diminishes, the process of dealing with disfigurement begins and affects both patients and their family members [5, 32, 34].

25.3.2 Patient Factors Affecting the Psychosocial Impact of Facial Disfigurement

While works on stigma in general are numerous, works on stigma caused by facial disfigurement in particular are relatively rare [8, 14, 25–27]. The literature on facial disfigurement to date tends to approach disfigurement and stigma from the point of view of the patient and emphasizes the individual's subjective state of mind and the strategies that he or she employs to successfully adapt to disfigurement [9, 11, 34]. It is reported that patients who employ active forms of coping, such as seeking out social support, have a better quality of life than those who adopt passive coping strategies, such as denial or avoidance [35]. (Denial is the process by which patients refuse to accept their condition of being disfigured. Avoidance refers to attempts to cope with disfigurement by avoiding contacts with others.) Furthermore, patients with enhanced social skills and greater social support have better chances of coping with stigmatization [33]. Women with facial disfigurement tend to report more stress than do men, and partners may experience more stress than do patients [27].

Demographically, cancer-generated facial disfigurement is more common among middle-aged men, married individuals, and members of the working class than among other groups [8]. Given the stage of life of such patients (e.g., already in a relationship rather than looking for a partner), the social support available to them (e.g., from a spouse), and the greater focus on basic needs associated with membership in the working class, the negative effects of disfigurement on quality of life tend to be diminished in these patients [27].

25.3.3 Safe Settings for Patients with Facial Disfigurement: the Family and the Hospital

Society is generally viewed as the place that originates stigmatization. Among the few safe settings in society for the facially disfigured are the family and the hospital [8, 11]. In the case of the family, family members generally support and care for patients and offer a social environment free of stigmatization. However, the same literature reports that spouses often feel the negative consequences of stigmatization as they try to shield cancer patients from unwanted interaction [32]. Further, research indicates that spouses are not immune from the influence of society and therefore may display stigmatizing behaviors toward disfigured individuals [21].

The hospital also tends to be a safe setting for patients because of caregivers' knowledge, tolerance, and understanding [8, 10, 27]. Even so, however, the relationship between patients and caregivers may result in episodes of stigmatization. It has been reported that lack of cultural and sociological training on the part of surgeons and staff may lead surgeons to mistake culturally based behavior for psychological and adaptive disorders [11] and may generate stress in patients [27].

25.3.4 Impact of Group Social Interactions on Patients with Facial Disfigurement

Some patients with facial disfigurement are largely unaffected by stigmatizing situations arising from social interaction. However, a larger group of patients experiences problems when interacting in small and large groups, with the level of stigmatization differing according to the type of interaction. Such patients tend to feel comfortable when interacting with close friends and family members. However, they display differing outcomes when interacting with strangers and/or acquaintances. The three general types of stranger or acquaintance behavior that have been studied are (1) unsolicited attention, (2) unsolicited support, and (3) lack of special attention.

When strangers or acquaintances pay unsolicited attention to patients, ask unwanted questions, make unwelcome remarks, stare, or otherwise make their unspoken curiosity felt, patients feel uncomfortable regardless of whether they are interacting in a small or large group.

When strangers and acquaintances provide unsolicited "support" for patients, a number of outcomes are common. In small groups, display of support engenders comfortable interaction between disfigured patients and acquaintances. It also shapes positive interaction in large groups as it is employed to construct advantageous conditions for patients [36]. Instrumentally, support is used even in situations in which support is not needed. Patients feel uncomfortable when support suggests that disfigurement is a greater problem than it actually is and when support creates a situation in which the patient is accorded undeserved respect.

Finally, when interacting individuals do not pay particular attention to patients, both positive and stigmatizing outcomes are possible in small groups [36]. In large groups, patients are comfortable when others do not pay particular attention to them. A large group allows patients to pass unnoticed among strangers.

25.4 Conclusions and Recommendations

It is increasingly common for patients with orbitofacial cancer to be cured of their cancer, and patients who are cured have to spend the rest of their lives with the stigmatizing limitations associated with facial disfigurement. Maintaining a successful social existence is of paramount importance for the overall well-being of these survivors.

At present, surgeons treating patients with orbitofacial cancers have limited exposure during training and later in the development of their medical practices to the results of psychosocial studies on facial disfigurement. It is important, therefore, to increase the exposure of surgeons and other medical personnel to knowledge regarding the psychosocial aspects of cancer-generated facial disfigurement; to increase collaboration between surgeons and social scientists; and to develop protocols that could be incorporated into standard orbitofacial cancer treatment. These protocols should be designed to minimize the negative social consequences of acquired facial disfigurement by preparing patients and their family members to face reactions that they will receive from society.

It is also important to stress that the psychosocial consequences of cancer-generated facial disfigurement cannot be successfully addressed by targeting patients alone. Stigmatization is a complex process that is defined by the collective process of interaction and involves both patients and other social actors, such as family members, caregivers, and strangers. Further, the unfolding of social interaction and its outcomes are affected by a variety of factors, including the size of the group within which interaction takes place, the setting, and the attitudes and actions of interacting individuals. The role played by family members and, above all, spouses should be carefully considered in the development of pertinent protocols [36].

References

1. Mood DW. Cancers of the head and neck. In: Varricchio C, editor. A Cancer Source Book for Nurses. Atlanta, GA: American Cancer Society, 1997:271–83.
2. Davis K, Wingo P, Parker S. Cancer statistics by race and ethnicity. CA Cancer J Clin 1998;1:31–47.
3. Davis K, Roumanas ED, Nishimura RD. Prosthetic–surgical collaboration in the rehabilitation of patients with head and neck defects. Otolaryngol Clin North Am 1997;30:631–45.
4. Bull R, Rumsey N. The Social Psychology of Facial Appearance. New York, NY: Springer, 1988.
5. Callahan C. Facial disfigurement and sense of self in head and neck cancer. Soc Work Health Care 2004;40:73–87.
6. Dropkin MJ. Body image and quality of life after head and neck cancer surgery. Cancer Pract 1999;7:309–13.
7. Hawkesworth M. Disabling spatialities and the regulation of a visible secret. Urban Stud 2001;38:299–318.

8. Hughes M. The Social Consequences of Facial Disfigurement. Aldershot, England: Ashgate Publishing, 2001.
9. Kent G. Understanding the experiences of people with disfigurements: an integration of four models of social and psychological functioning. Psychol Health Med 2000;5: 117–29.
10. Macgregor F. Facial disfigurement: problems and management of social interaction and implication for mental health. Aesthetic Plast Surg 1990;14:249–57.
11. Macgregor F. Transformation and Identity: The Face and Plastic Surgery. New York, NY: Quadrangle, 1974.
12. Macgregor F. Some psycho-social problems associated with facial deformities. Am Sociol Rev 1951;16:629–38.
13. Feingold A. Good looking people are not what we think. Psychol Bull 1992;111:304–41.
14. Kish V, Lansdown R. Meeting the psychosocial impact of facial disfigurement: developing a clinical service for children and families. Clin Child Psychol Psychiatry 2000;5: 497–512.
15. Synnott A. Truth and goodness, mirrors, and masks—part I: a sociology of beauty and the face. Br J Sociol 1989;40:607–36.
16. Anderson RC, Franke KA. Psychological and psychosocial implications of head and neck cancer. Internet J Mental Health 2002;1:55–64.
17. Cole J. About Face. Cambridge, England: MIT Press, 1998.
18. Jackson L. Physical attractiveness: a sociocultural perspective. In: Cash TF, Pruzinsky T, editors. Body Image: A Handbook of Theory, Research, and Clinical Practice. New York, NY: Guilford Press, 2002:13–21.
19. Cash TF, Pruzinsky T, editors. Body Image: A Handbook of Theory, Research, and Clinical Practice. New York, NY: Guilford Press, 2002.
20. Furness P, Garrud P, Faulder A, et al. Coming to terms: a grounded theory of adaptation to facial surgery in adulthood. J Health Psychol 2006;11:453–66.
21. Goffman E. Stigma: Notes on the Management of Spoiled Identity. New York, NY: Simon & Schuster, 1963.
22. Gotay CC. The experience of cancer during early and advanced stages: the views of patients and their mates. Soc Sci Med 1984;18:605–13.
23. Mah MA, Johnston C. Concerns of families in which one member has head and neck cancer. Cancer Nurs 1993;16:382–7.
24. Newell RJ. Altered body image: a fear-avoidance model of psycho-social difficulties following disfigurement. J Adv Nurs 1999;30:1230–8.
25. Clarke A. Psychosocial aspects of facial disfigurement: problems, management, and the role of a lay-led organization. Psychol Health Med 1999;4:127–42.
26. Clarke A, Rumsey N, Collin JRO, et al. Psychological distress associated with disfiguring eye conditions. Eye 2003;17:35–40.
27. Pruzinsky T, Levine E, Persing JA, et al. Facial trauma and facial cancer. In: Sarwer DB, Pruzinsky T, Cash T, Goldwyn RM, Persing JA, editors. Psychological Aspects of Reconstructive and Cosmetic Plastic Surgery: Clinical, Empirical, and Ethical Perspectives. Philadelphia, PA: Lippincott Williams & Wilkins, 2006:125–43.
28. Hagedoorm M, Molleman E. Facial disfigurement in patients with head and neck cancer: the role of social self-efficiency. Health Psychol 2006;25:643–7.
29. Mosher C, Danoff-Burg S. Death anxiety and cancer related stigma: a terror management analysis. Death Stud 2007;31:855–907.
30. Berremberg JL. Attitudes towards cancer as a function of experience with the disease: a test of three models. Psychol Health 1989;3:233–43.
31. Weiner B, Perry RP, Magnusson J. An attributional analysis of reaction to stigma. J Soc Issues 1988;35:120–55.
32. Millsopp L, Brandom L, Humphris G, et al. Facial appearance after operations for oral and oropharyngeal cancer: a comparison of case notes and patient-completed questionnaire. Br J Oral Maxillofac Surg 2006;44:358–63.

33. Rybarczyk BD, Behel JM. Rehabilitation medicine and body image. In: Cash TF, Pruzinsky T, editors. Body Image: A Handbook of Theory, Research, and Clinical Practice. New York, NY: Guilford Press, 2002:387–93.
34. van Doorne JM, van Waas MA, Bergsma J. Facial disfigurement after cancer resection: a problem with an extra dimension. J Invest Surg 1994;7:321–6.
35. Dropkin MJ. Anxiety, coping strategies, and coping behaviors in patients undergoing head and neck cancer surgery. Cancer Nurs 2001;24:143–8.
36. Bonanno A, Esmaeli B, Fingeret MC, Nelson D, Weber R. Social challenges of cancer patients with orbitofacial disfigurement. Ophthal Plast Reconstr Surg 2010;26(1):18–22.

Part IV
Ocular Side Effects of Cancer Therapy

Section Editor: Bita Esmaeli

Chapter 26
Lacrimal and Canalicular Toxicity

M. Amir Ahmadi and Bita Esmaeli

Abstract The lacrimal drainage system, which is covered by a highly proliferative epithelium, is susceptible to the side effects of chemotherapy drugs, which are secreted in tears. Docetaxel, an antineoplastic agent widely used to treat patients with advanced breast cancer as well as other malignancies, is secreted in tears almost immediately after intravenous administration and thus may cause canalicular inflammation and tear drainage obstructions. 5-Fluorouracil (5-FU), another frequently used chemotherapeutic agent, commonly causes increased lacrimation. Stenosis of the punctum and canaliculi is a less common side effect of systemic 5-FU therapy. To prevent the need for dacryocystorhinostomy or placement of permanent Pyrex glass lacrimal drainage tubes, patients undergoing treatment with docetaxel or 5-FU should be closely monitored for punctal and canalicular stenosis.

26.1 Introduction

Chemotherapeutic agents work primarily by interfering with DNA synthesis and mitosis, thereby leading to cell death and a reduction in the number of tumor cells. For this reason, chemotherapy's major side effects are on normal, highly proliferative tissues like the epithelium of skin and internal organs. The lacrimal drainage system is covered by a highly proliferative epithelium; therefore, it is susceptible to chemotherapeutic agents' side effects. Furthermore, several studies have shown that systemic chemotherapeutic agents are secreted in tears by the lacrimal glands. This explains the direct effects of systemic chemotherapy on the lacrimal secretory and drainage system.

M.A. Ahmadi (✉)
Department of Ophthalmology, University of Illinois at Chicago, Chicago, IL, USA
e-mail: mamirahmadi@yahoo.com

B. Esmaeli (ed.), *Ophthalmic Oncology*, M.D. Anderson Solid Tumor Oncology Series 6, DOI 10.1007/978-1-4419-0374-7_26,

26.2 5-Fluorouracil

5-Fluorouracil (5-FU) was first used as a chemotherapeutic agent for gastrointestinal carcinomas in 1958 [1]. It is now widely used in the treatment of gastrointestinal, breast, and head and neck malignancies. 5-FU inhibits thymidylate synthetase and causes DNA strand breakage [2]. Like many other chemotherapeutic agents, it has its greatest effect on rapidly dividing cells, such as epithelial cells.

Increased lacrimation, which resolves after chemotherapy is completed, is common with 5-FU and has been widely documented in the literature [3, 4]. Stenosis of the punctum and canaliculi is a less common side effect of systemic 5-FU therapy. Stenosis of the lacrimal system in patients treated with intravenous administration of 5-FU was first described by Caravella et al. [5] in a report of four patients in 1981. Several subsequent studies have suggested that 5-FU administered intravenously can cause inflammation of the canalicular mucosa, which can lead to fibrosis of the canaliculi and resultant lacrimal outflow obstruction [6–8]. In a study of 58 patients who received systemic 5-FU, Eiseman et al. [9] reported a prevalence of tearing of 24.1% (14 patients). The average time to onset of tearing after treatment with 5-FU in those patients who experienced excessive tearing was 3 weeks (standard deviation, 0.9 weeks). Three of 14 patients with excessive tearing (5.2%) had punctal and/or canalicular abnormalities [9]. Other studies reported a similar prevalence of tearing associated with systemic 5-FU [4, 10].

Despite multiple reports of the ocular side effects of 5-FU, it has been difficult to prove that those effects have been solely related to the use of 5-FU since most patients studied in the published reports were receiving multiple chemotherapeutic medications at the same time.

Several factors have been suggested as being responsible for excessive tearing in patients receiving 5-FU treatment. One theory is that tearing is a reflex phenomenon secondary to the irritation caused by the ocular surface disturbance. Two studies have shown that 5-FU is secreted in tears after intravenous administration and can thus bathe the ocular surface in the toxic substance [10, 11]. This would explain punctal and canalicular stenosis in patients receiving intravenous 5-FU. Evidence that topically applied 5-FU causes ocular surface toxicity, which can lead to excessive tearing, can be found in the results of several other studies [12, 13]. One of these studies found that the application of topical 5-FU in a rabbit model decreased the mitotic rate of both corneal and conjunctival epithelial cells to 1% of the normal rate [12]. In another study, over half the patients who had glaucoma-filtering surgery and were treated with postoperative subconjunctival 5-FU injections developed corneal epithelial defects and often took several weeks to resolve [13]. Finally, eyelid malposition from dermatitis and cicatricial changes, with subsequent punctal eversion and compromise of the lacrimal pump, could also be a cause of excessive tearing [9].

26.3 S-1

S-1 is a prodrug that consists of the 5-FU prodrug tegafur combined with two modulators: 5-chloro-2,4-dihydroxypyridine and potassium oxonate [14]. S-1 is an oral medication and is reportedly less toxic, with fewer gastrointestinal side effects, than 5-FU administered intravenously [15, 16]. Although it is expected that S-1 will have the same lacrimal side effects as 5-FU, there are only a few reported cases of punctal or canalicular stenosis linked to S-1 in the literature [17]. This could be a result of the medication's novelty, and more cases will be reported as more patients are treated with this new chemotherapeutic agent. S-1 is approved for use in gastrointestinal cancer in Japan, but it is not yet approved by the United States Food and Drug Administration.

26.4 Docetaxel

Docetaxel (Taxotere) is an antineoplastic agent widely used for treatment of patients with advanced breast cancer as well as for treatment of patients with other malignancies [18–20]. Docetaxel belongs to a class of antineoplastic agents known as taxanes, which act by causing apoptotic cell death. Esmaeli et al. [21] initially reported three patients with metastatic breast carcinoma in whom epiphora and canalicular stenosis developed while the patients were undergoing weekly docetaxel treatment.

Subsequent studies showed evidence of secretion of docetaxel in tears almost immediately after intravenous administration of the medication [22]. The secretion of docetaxel in tears may be a mechanism for canalicular inflammation and tear drainage obstructions.

Docetaxel tends to cause more ocular side effects when administered every week versus every 3 weeks. In a prospective study, epiphora occurred in 64% of patients who received weekly docetaxel versus 39% of patients who received docetaxel every 3 weeks, even when the cumulative dose was the same as in the weekly group [23]. The mean interval between initiation of docetaxel and onset of epiphora was 2 months in patients who received docetaxel weekly and 3 months in patients who received docetaxel every 3 weeks. The median cumulative docetaxel dose at the onset of epiphora was 496.5 mg for patients in the weekly group and 420 mg for patients in the every-3-weeks group [23].

In patients who developed epiphora because of weekly docetaxel, half had mild symptoms that improved with the administration of topical steroids, but the other half developed moderate or severe canalicular stenosis. Two-thirds of the patients with moderate or severe canalicular stenosis needed surgical intervention. At the time of surgery, the median cumulative docetaxel dose was 889.5 mg, and the median duration of treatment was 16 weeks. All the patients in the every-3-weeks group who developed epiphora had mild disease, and the epiphora improved with probing and irrigation and administration of topical steroids [23].

Patients who needed surgical repair in the early stages of canalicular stenosis benefited from temporary silicone intubation. The silicone tube was removed after the end of the chemotherapy course, leaving behind no residual stenosis of the canaliculi. Patients with more severe forms of stenosis needed permanent Pyrex glass tube placement. The study showed that early temporary silicone intubation in symptomatic patients receiving weekly docetaxel can prevent further closure of the lacrimal drainage apparatus and obviate the more involved surgical intervention of permanent Pyrex glass tube placement [23, 24].

26.5 Epiphora Associated with Other Chemotherapeutic Drugs

We have observed temporary and mild epiphora in association with paclitaxel (Taxol) and capecitabine (Xeloda) but have not observed the anatomic correlate of punctal or canalicular stenosis associated with these drugs. To our knowledge, there has been one reported case of nasolacrimal duct blockage and canalicular stenosis in a patient who received paclitaxel, but this patient also received head and neck radiation therapy, which is by itself a risk factor for canalicular stenosis and nasolacrimal duct blockage; thus, it is unlikely that paclitaxel causes anatomic closure of canaliculi and nasolacrimal ducts [25, 26].

Similarly, imatinib mesylate can be associated with the onset of epiphora in patients with gastrointestinal stromal tumors or chronic myelogenous leukemia who take this drug on a long-term basis. However, in our experience, the epiphora from imatinib is not associated with the anatomic correlate of punctal and/or canalicular stenosis or nasolacrimal duct blockage [27]. We believe that epiphora in these patients is caused by fluid retention in the periorbital soft tissues and conjunctival chemosis, causing an inefficient blink and lacrimal pump. It can be treated with nonsurgical measures such as the use of systemic diuretics or topical steroids.

26.6 Conclusions

It is important to look for and recognize significant punctal and canalicular stenosis as side effects of treatment with 5-FU, S-1, and docetaxel in early stages so that the judicious use of topical steroids and silicone intubation can prevent the need for a more involved surgery, such as dacryocystorhinostomy or placement of permanent Pyrex glass lacrimal drainage tubes.

References

1. Curreri AR, Ansfield FJ, McIver FA, et al. Clinical studies with 5-fluorouracil. Cancer Res 1958;18:478–84.
2. Heidelberger C, Ansfield FJ. Experimental and clinical use of fluorinated pyrimidines in cancer chemotherapy. Cancer Res 1963;23:1226–43.

3. Fraunfelder FT, Meyer SM. Ocular toxicity of antineoplastic agents. Ophthalmology 1983;90:1–3.
4. Hamersley J, Luce JK, Florentz TR, et al. Excessive lacrimation from fluorouracil treatment. JAMA 1973;225:747–8.
5. Caravella LP Jr, Burns JA, Zangmeister M. Punctal–canalicular stenosis related to systemic fluorouracil therapy. Arch Ophthalmol 1981;99:284–6.
6. Haidak DJ, Hurwitz BS, Yeung KY. Tear-duct fibrosis (dacryostenosis) due to 5-fluorouracil. Ann Intern Med 1978;88:657.
7. Lee V, Bentley CR, Olver JM. Sclerosing canaliculitis after 5-fluorouracil breast cancer chemotherapy. Eye 1998;12:343–9.
8. Fezza JP, Wesley RE, Klippenstein KA. The treatment of punctal and canalicular stenosis in patients on systemic 5-FU. Ophthalmic Surg Lasers 1999;30:105–8.
9. Eiseman AS, Flanagan JC, Brooks AB. Ocular surface, ocular adnexal, and lacrimal complications associated with the use of systemic 5-fluorouracil. Ophthal Plast Reconstr Surg 2003;19:216–24.
10. Loprinzi CL, Love R, Garrity JA, et al. Cyclophosphamide, methotrexate, and 5-fluorouracil (CMF): induced ocular toxicity. Cancer Invest 1990;8:459–65.
11. Christophidis N, Lucas I, Vajda FJ, et al. Lacrimation and 5-fluorouracil. Ann Intern Med 1978;89:574.
12. Shapiro MS, Thoft RA, Friend J, et al. 5-Fluorouracil toxicity to the ocular surface epithelium. Invest Ophthalmol Vis Sci 1985;26:580–3.
13. Fluorouracil Filtering Surgery Study Group. Fluorouracil filtering surgery study one-year follow-up. Am J Ophthalmol 1989;108:625–35.
14. Van Groeningen CJ, Godefridus JP, Schornagel JH, et al. Phase I clinical and pharmacokinetic study of oral S-1 in patients with advanced solid tumors. J Clin Oncol 2000;18:2772–9.
15. Hoff PM, Saad ED, Ajani JA, et al. Phase I study with pharmacokinetics of S-1 on an oral daily schedule for 28 days in patients with solid tumors. Clin Cancer Res 2003;9:134–42.
16. Fukushima M, Shimamoto Y, Kato T, et al. Anticancer activity and toxicity of S-1, an oral combination of tegafur and two biochemical modulators, compared with continuous i.v. infusion of 5-FU. Anticancer Drugs 1998;9:817–23.
17. Esmaeli B, Golio D, Lubecki L, et al. Canalicular and nasolacrimal duct blockage: an ocular side effect associated with the antineoplastic drug S-1. Am J Ophthalmol 2005;140:325–7.
18. Valero V. Docetaxel as single agent therapy in metastatic breast cancer: clinical efficacy. Semin Oncol 1997;24(Suppl 13):11–18.
19. Picus J, Schultz M. Docetaxel (Taxotere) as monotherapy in the treatment of hormone-refractory prostate cancer: preliminary results. Semin Oncol 1999;26(Suppl 17):14–18.
20. Burris HA III. Single-agent docetaxel (Taxotere) in randomized phase III trials. Semin Oncol 1999;26(Suppl 9):1–6.
21. Esmaeli B, Valero V, Ahmadi MA, et al. Canalicular stenosis secondary to docetaxel (Taxotere): a newly recognized side effect. Ophthalmology 2001;108:994–5.
22. Esmaeli B, Ahmadi MA, Rivera E, et al. Docetaxel secretion in tears: association with lacrimal drainage obstruction. Arch Ophthalmol 2002;120:1180–2.
23. Esmaeli B, Amin S, Valero V, et al. Prospective study of incidence and severity of epiphora and canalicular stenosis in patients with metastatic breast cancer receiving docetaxel. J Clin Oncol 2006;24:3619–22.
24. Ahmadi MA, Esmaeli B. Surgical treatment of canalicular stenosis in patients receiving weekly docetaxel. Arch Ophthalmol 2001;119:1802–4.
25. McCartney E, Valluri S, Rushing D, et al. Upper and lower system nasolacrimal duct stenosis secondary to paclitaxel. Ophthal Plast Reconstr Surg 2007;23:170–1.
26. Savar A, Esmaeli B. Upper and lower system nasolacrimal duct stenosis secondary to paclitaxel. Ophthal Plast Reconstr Surg 2009;25:418–19.
27. Esmaeli B, Diba R, Ahmadi MA, et al. Periorbital edema and epiphora as ocular side effects of imatinib mesylate (Gleevec). Eye 2004;18:760–2.

Chapter 27
Orbital and Periorbital Side Effects of Chemotherapy

John D. Ng

Abstract In this chapter, the side effects of chemotherapeutic agents on the orbit and periorbital structures, such as the eyelids, cyelashes, eyebrows, and conjunctiva, are discussed. Chemotherapy can affect these structures when it is administered topically for local disease, via selective ophthalmic artery infusion for regional disease in the orbit, or systemically for more diffuse metastatic disease or as adjuvant treatment. Systemic administration of chemotherapy often affects the eye, as drugs commonly are secreted into the tears, thereby causing local affects directly. With the exception of a few better documented side effects, the majority of side effects listed in this chapter are from small case series and anecdotal case reports. This may be a result of the rarity of side effects or of underreporting, as there are often other side effects or issues that take precedence in cancer patients. Additionally, many chemotherapeutic regimens involve more than one agent, and in such cases it is difficult to determine which agent is responsible for side effects. One must also consider a possible synergistic effect of multiple drugs. The text of this chapter is organized by drug, whereas the tables are organized by side effect, to allow practitioners to look up clinically observed side effects and attempt to determine the offending agents.

27.1 Introduction

Cancer patients are treated with multiple modalities, including surgery, radiation therapy, and chemotherapeutic and immunomodulating drugs. In this chapter, we describe the reported orbital, periorbital, and orbital teratogenic side effects of drugs used for cancer treatment. Some side effects occur commonly, and others are quite rare.

J.D. Ng (✉)
Departments of Ophthalmology and Otolaryngology and Head and Neck Surgery, Casey Eye Institute and Devers Eye Institute, Oregon Health Sciences University, Portland, OR, USA
e-mail: ngj@ohsu.edu

B. Esmaeli (ed.), *Ophthalmic Oncology*, M.D. Anderson Solid Tumor Oncology Series 6, DOI 10.1007/978-1-4419-0374-7_27,

Cancer patients are often treated with multiple medications administered simultaneously, and in such cases, the offending agent may be difficult to isolate. Synergistic effects of multiple drugs must also be considered.

In general, any drug can cause an allergic reaction, and some of the reported side effects—including erythema, urticaria, and edema—may be manifestations of allergic reactions. Stevens–Johnson syndrome and toxic epidermal necrolysis, both of which are included among the side effects listed in this chapter, represent a severe form of allergic reaction.

Tables are used to present the information for easy reference in clinical practice. In Tables 27.1 and 27.2, we have divided the side effects into orbital and periorbital categories. However, some of the listed effects appear in both categories. For instance, ptosis appears in both the orbital and periorbital categories because with some drugs, ptosis is caused by fibrosis of the extraocular muscles in the orbit.

Table 27.1 Periorbital side effects

Side effect	Drug(s) implicated[a]
Allergic reaction	Carmustine, Mitomycin
Angioneurotic edema	Busulfan, cyclophosphamide, doxorubicin, interleukin, thiotepa[b]
Ankyloblepharon	Fluorouracil
Blepharoconjunctivitis	Carmustine, cyclophosphamide, fluorouracil, imatinib mesylate (maybe), methotrexate, mitomycin
Blepharospasm	Fluorouracil (maybe)
Blepharitis	Methotrexate
Blue-green pigmentation	Mitoxantrone hydrochloride
Chemosis	Capecitabine, carmustine, cisplatin, imatinib mesylate
Cicatricial ectropion	Fluorouracil administered systemically or by local injection
Conjunctival erythema	Capecitabine, cisplatin, cytarabine, doxorubicin
Conjunctival hemorrhage	Carmustine, cytarabine, interferon
Conjunctival hyperemia	Carmustine, cetuximab, cyclophosphamide, methotrexate
Conjunctivitis	Capecitabine, cetuximab, cisplatin, mitoxantrone hydrochloride
Depigmentation	Methotrexate, thiotepa[b]
Dermatitis	Fluorouracil
Desquamative rash	Interleukin
Ectropion	Docetaxel
Epiphora	Docetaxel, erlotinib
Erythema multiforme	Busulfan (maybe)
Exfoliative dermatitis	Busulfan (maybe), cetuximab (maybe)
Eyelash/eyebrow loss	Busulfan, cisplatin, doxorubicin, fluorouracil administered systemically, fluorouracil administered by local injection (maybe), methotrexate, vincristine
Eyelid edema	Cytarabine, docetaxel, fluorouracil, imatinib mesylate, mitoxantrone hydrochloride
Eyelid erythema	Docetaxel, doxorubicin, fluorouracil, methotrexate
Eyelid hyperpigmentation	Busulfan, carmustine, cytarabine, doxorubicin, mercaptopurine, methotrexate
Eyelid hypopigmentation	Imatinib mesylate (maybe)

Table 27.1 (continued)

Side effect	Drug(s) implicated[a]
Graves ophthalmopathy	Interferon
Icterus	Mercaptopurine
Keratinized eyelid margin	Fluorouracil
Macular erythema	Interleukin
Meibomian gland dysfunction	Methotrexate
Periorbital edema	Cisplatin administered by intracarotid injection, methotrexate
Periorbital erythema	Cisplatin administered by intracarotid injection, fluorouracil administered subcutaneously
Periorbital pallor	Plicamycin
Poliosis	Thiotepa[b]
Ptosis	Cisplatin, vincristine
Purpura	Cytarabine
Squamous blepharitis	Cetuximab
Stevens–Johnson syndrome	Cyclophosphamide (maybe), imatinib mesylate (maybe)
Subcutaneous lymphoma	Interleukin
Symblepharon	Mitomycin
Toxic epidermal necrolysis	Cyclophosphamide (maybe), cytarabine, imatinib mesylate (maybe)
Trichomegaly	Cetuximab (maybe), erlotinib, interferon
Urticaria	Cisplatin, cytarabine, doxorubicin, interleukin, methotrexate, thiotepa[b]

[a]Drugs are known to cause the indicated side effect when administered systemically, unless "(maybe)" appears after the drug name, in which case the drug is considered a possible cause of the side effect

[b]Administered topically

Since reports of side effects come from multiple specialties, different terms are found in the literature that may represent the same entity—for example, "blepharo-conjunctivitis" and "conjunctivitis." We have generally listed all the terms we found in the literature in case subtle differences in wording represent subtle differences in the reported effects.

Chapter 26 in this book is dedicated to canalicular and nasolacrimal duct blockage associated with chemotherapy, but when epiphora is a reported side effect of a drug, that fact is mentioned herein.

27.2 Orbital, Periorbital, and Orbital Teratogenic Side Effects by Individual Drug

The various chemotherapy drugs associated with orbital, periorbital, or orbital teratogenic side effects are discussed in alphabetical order in the following paragraphs. In addition, orbital and orbital teratogenic side effects and implicated drugs are listed

Table 27.2 Orbital and orbital teratogenic side effects

Side effect	Drug(s) implicated[a]
Orbital side effects	
Cavernous sinus syndrome	Cisplatin by IC injection
Diplopia	Busulfan (maybe), cisplatin, vincristine
Edema	Carmustine by IC injection, imatinib mesylate, methotrexate
Extraocular muscle paresis	Busulfan (maybe), vincristine
Graves-like ophthalmopathy	Interferon
Inflammation	Etoposide by IC injection
Internal ophthalmoplegia	Carmustine by IC injection
Ocular myasthenia	Busulfan, cisplatin, interferon (maybe)
Pain	Carmustine by IC injection, cisplatin by IC injection, interferon
Proptosis	Carmustine by IC injection, etoposide by IC injection
Ptosis	Busulfan, vincristine
Rectus muscle fibrosis	Carmustine by IC injection
Vasodilation	Carmustine by IC injection
Orbital teratogenic side effect	
Microphthalmia	Busulfan, mercaptopurine

IC, intracarotid
[a]Drugs are known to cause the indicated side effect unless "(maybe)" appears after the drug name, in which case the drug is considered a possible cause of the side effect

in Tables 27.1 and 27.2. Much of the information on chemotherapy-related side effects was gleaned from the Web site of the National Registry of Drug-Induced Ocular Side Effects [1].

27.2.1 Busulfan

Busulfan (Busulfex, Myleran) is an alkylating agent most often used for treatment of granulocytic leukemia and other blood dyscrasias. Its use has been associated with keratitis sicca, eyelid hyperpigmentation, angioneurotic edema, and loss of eyelashes and eyebrows. Other possible side effects include myasthenia-like paresis of extraocular muscles causing diplopia and ptosis; exfoliative dermatitis; and erythema multiforme [2]. Possible teratogenic effects include microphthalmia [3, 4].

27.2.2 Capecitabine

Capecitabine (Xeloda) is a fluoropyrimidine antimetabolite most often used for treatment of metastatic breast cancer and colorectal cancer. Its use has been associated with chemosis, conjunctival erythema, and nonspecific conjunctivitis [2]. While epiphora can be seen in association with capecitabine, the experience at

The University of Texas M.D. Anderson Cancer Center suggests that there is no anatomic correlate of canalicular or nasolacrimal duct blockage with this symptom (B. Esmaeli, personal communication).

27.2.3 Carmustine

Carmustine (BiCNU, Gliadel) is a nitrosourea most often used to treat central nervous system tumors. Its use has been associated with blepharoconjunctivitis, chemosis, conjunctival hyperemia, and conjunctival hemorrhage. Allergic reactions and skin hyperpigmentation have also been noted [2].

Intracarotid injections of carmustine have been associated with vasodilation, proptosis, pain, and edema of the orbit. Additionally, rectus muscle fibrosis and internal ophthalmoplegia have occurred [2, 5–7].

27.2.4 Cetuximab

Cetuximab (Erbitux) is a monoclonal antibody that binds to epidermal growth factor receptors and has been used to treat metastatic colorectal cancers and cancers of the head and neck. Its use has been associated with squamous blepharitis and conjunctival hyperemia and conjunctivitis [7]. There is also a possible association between cetuximab and exfoliative dermatitis and eyelash trichomegaly. Trichomegaly has been reported to develop after 10 weeks of treatment. It is speculated that trichomegaly is a result of epidermal growth factor receptor inhibition causing increased terminal differentiation of eyelash follicles [8–10]. Eyelashes return to normal 1 month after cessation of cetuximab therapy [10].

27.2.5 Cisplatin

Cisplatin (Platinol, Platinol-AQ) is most commonly used to treat metastatic testicular, ovarian, and bladder carcinomas. Its use has been associated with conjunctivitis, eyelid and conjunctival erythema and edema, urticaria, and loss of eyelashes and eyebrows. Orbital pain has also been reported. There is possible myasthenia-like neuromuscular blockade causing diplopia and ptosis from paresis of extraocular muscles [2].

Intracarotid injections of cisplatin have been associated with ipsilateral orbital pain, periorbital erythema and edema, and cavernous sinus syndrome. Injection into the distal ophthalmic artery was reported to cause massive orbital edema within days of administration. There was accompanying uveal effusion, retinal detachment, ophthalmoplegia, and blindness [11]. Another report described extreme facial/periorbital edema, proptosis, and chemosis, also followed by irreversible vision loss. Since there were multiple agents involved, it is unclear which agent was the main factor responsible for these findings [2, 4, 11].

27.2.6 Cyclophosphamide

Cyclophosphamide (Cytoxan, Neosar) is an alkylating agent most often used to treat lymphoma, myeloma, and other tumors. Its use has been associated with conjunctival hyperemia, angioneurotic edema, blepharoconjunctivitis, and keratitis sicca [2, 3]. There have also been reported cases of possible Stevens–Johnson syndrome and toxic epidermal necrolysis [2–5].

27.2.7 Cytarabine

Cytarabine (Cytosar-U, DepoCyt) is most commonly used to treat acute granulocytic leukemia and polycythemia vera. Its use has been associated with conjunctival hemorrhage, conjunctival erythema, eyelid hyperpigmentation, urticaria, eyelid edema, purpura, and toxic epidermal necrolysis [2–5].

27.2.8 Docetaxel

Docetaxel (Taxotere) is an antimitotic chemotherapeutic agent that is most commonly used to treat advanced breast and prostate cancer but is also effective against ovarian, lung, and renal cancer. A very common side effect is epiphora due to canalicular stenosis, which is discussed in detail in Chapter 26. Acute erythema, eyelid edema (Fig. 27.1), and secondary mechanical ectropion have occurred as soon as 2 hours after delivery of docetaxel [12].

27.2.9 Doxorubicin

Doxorubicin (Doxil, Rubex) is an antibiotic used in the treatment of sarcomas, lymphomas, and leukemia. Its use has been associated with conjunctival and eyelid erythema, angioneurotic edema, urticaria, eyelid hyperpigmentation, and loss of eyelashes and eyebrows [2, 4, 5].

27.2.10 Erlotinib

Erlotinib (Tarceva) is an irreversible epidermal growth factor receptor inhibitor used for the treatment of glioblastoma multiforme, non-small cell lung cancer, head and neck cancer, and esophageal, ovarian, and hepatocellular carcinomas. Its use has

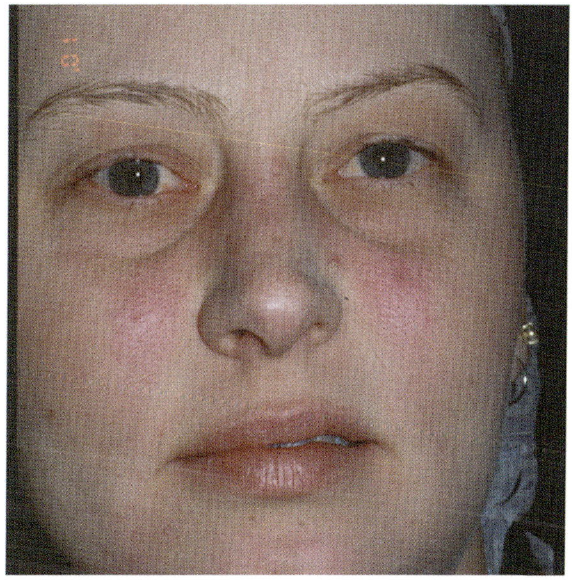

Fig. 27.1 Periorbital erythematous rash on lower eyelid skin and cheek in a patient with breast cancer treated with docetaxel. Photo courtesy of Dr. Bita Esmaeli

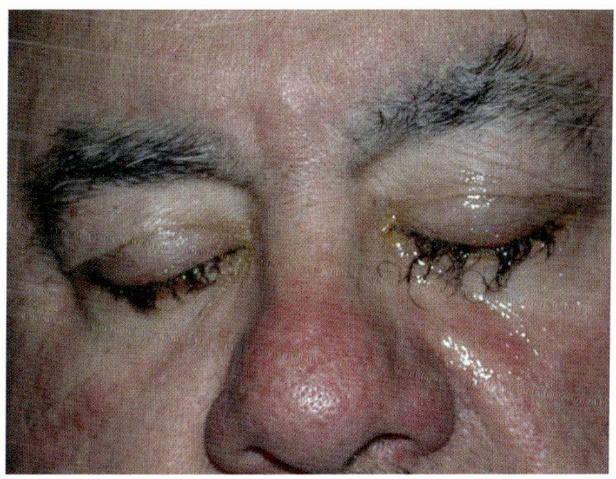

Fig. 27.2 Trichomegaly associated with erlotinib in a patient with glioblastoma multiforme. The eyelashes had to be trimmed every 3 months to keep the patient comfortable and prevent visual obstruction. Photo courtesy of Dr. Bita Esmaeli

been associated with epiphora and trichomegaly of the eyelashes and eyebrows with coarse, brittle, irregular eyelash growth (Fig. 27.2). Secondary corneal ulcerations due to eyelash–corneal contact have also been reported [13, 14].

27.2.11 Etoposide

Etoposide (Vepesid) is used to treat multiple systemic malignancies and also irreversibly inhibits *Cytomegalovirus* replication. Its intracarotid administration has caused orbital inflammation and proptosis [2, 15].

27.2.12 Fluorouracil

Fluorouracil (Carac, Efudex, Fluoroplex) is a fluorinated pyrimidine used for treatment of colon, rectal, breast, stomach, and pancreatic cancer. It is also used topically for treatment of actinic keratoses and for glaucoma surgery. Its systemic use has been associated with cicatricial ectropion, blepharoconjunctivitis, conjunctival erythema and edema, ankyloblepharon, dermatitis, keratinized eyelid margins, and loss of eyelashes and eyebrows. It may also induce blepharospasm [2–4, 16].

Subconjunctival injection of fluorouracil has caused periorbital edema. Local injection into the eyelid also causes cicatricial ectropion and may cause loss of eyelashes [2, 5, 17].

27.2.13 Imatinib Mesylate

Imatinib mesylate (Gleevec) selectively inhibits bcr-abl and platelet-derived growth factor receptor tyrosine kinase and is used as targeted therapy for myelogenous leukemia and gastrointestinal stromal tumors [2]. Its use has been associated with edema of the orbit, eyelids, and conjunctiva. Periorbital edema associated with imatinib rarely requires surgical intervention [18]. Most cases can be managed conservatively with occasional judicious use of diuretics. Imatinib may also cause chemosis, eyelid hypopigmentation, blepharoconjunctivitis, Stevens–Johnson syndrome, and toxic epidermal necrolysis [2, 18–21]. Epiphora has also been reported in association with imatinib, but with no associated anatomic narrowing of the canaliculi or nasolacrimal ducts [22, 23].

27.2.14 Interferons

Interferons (Actimmune, Alferon N, Avonex, Betaseron, Infergen, Intron A, PEGASYS, PEG-Intron, Rebif, Roferon-A) are used to treat chronic viral infections, chronic blood dyscrasias, and multiple sclerosis. Their use has been associated with orbital pain, subconjunctival hemorrhage, trichomegaly [24], and possibly Graves ophthalmopathy [25]. Ocular myasthenia-like findings have also been mentioned in a patient treated with 12 weeks of low-dose interferon alpha 2b therapy. There was no resolution of the myasthenia years after cessation of treatment [2, 26].

27.2.15 Interleukin-2, Interleukin-3, and Interleukin-6

Interleukin-2 (Proleukin), interleukin-3, and interleukin-6 are used for treatment of metastatic renal cell carcinoma and melanoma. Administration of these interleukins has been associated with eyelid pruritus, macular erythema, desquamative rash, angioneurotic edema, urticaria, and transient subcutaneous lymphoma [2, 27].

27.2.16 6-Mercaptopurine

6-Mercaptopurine (Purinethol) is a purine analog used to treat acute and chronic leukemia. Its use has been associated with eyelid hyperpigmentation and icterus. It may also be associated with microphthalmia as a teratogenic effect [2, 28].

27.2.17 Methotrexate

Methotrexate is a folic acid antagonist used in treating neoplasms, rheumatoid arthritis, psoriasis, and uveitis. Its use has been associated with eyelid erythema, blepharoconjunctivitis, seborrheic blepharitis depigmentation of the eyelids, eyelid hyperpigmentation, urticaria, and loss of eyelashes and eyebrows [2, 5]. Orbital edema has also been reported. Periorbital edema, blepharitis, and conjunctival hyperemia occur in up to 25% of patients receiving methotrexate [1, 2]. Findings may be related to change in metabolism of the meibomian glands [2–5, 23].

27.2.18 Mitomycin C

Mitomycin C (Mutamycin, Mitozytrex) is mostly used topically for treatment of conjunctival intraepithelial neoplasia or primary acquired melanosis with atypia. It can cause allergic reactions and blepharitis. Symblepharon formation is also a common finding with prolonged use [2]. Punctal and canalicular stenosis have also been reported in association with topical mitomycin C [2].

27.2.19 Mitoxantrone Dihydrochloride

Mitoxantrone (Novantrone) is used to treat acute leukemias and breast and ovarian cancer. Its use has been associated with eyelid edema, conjunctivitis, and, interestingly, blue-green pigmentation of the eyelid [2, 29, 30].

27.2.20 Plicamycin

Plicamycin (Mithracin) is used to treat testicular cancer. Its use may be associated with periorbital pallor [2, 4, 5].

27.2.21 Thiotepa

Thiotepa is used to treat breast and ovarian carcinomas, lymphomas, Hodgkin disease, and some sarcomas. Topical use of thiotepa has been associated with angioneurotic edema, urticaria, and depigmentation of the eyelids [1, 2, 31]. Thiotepa may also be associated with poliosis if the eyelashes are directly exposed to the drug [2, 31].

27.2.22 Vincristine

Vincristine is a vinca alkaloid used to treat Hodgkin disease, lymphosarcoma, reticulum cell sarcoma, rhabdomyosarcoma, neuroblastoma, and Wilms tumor. Its use has been associated with ptosis, extraocular muscle paresis with diplopia, and loss of eyelashes and eyebrows [2, 4, 5].

27.3 Summary

Chemotherapeutic agents causing orbital and periorbital side effects have been presented in a format for easy reference in a clinical setting. In order to better determine which agents truly cause orbital and periorbital side effects, reporting of such side effects, whether proven or potential, will need to continue. An excellent central repository of such information for reference and reporting is the National Registry of Drug-Induced Ocular Side Effects at http://www.eyedrugregistry.com/ [1].

Unfortunately, many of the orbital and periorbital side effects of chemotherapy are unavoidable and are expected consequences of current necessary treatment for life-threatening diseases. Management in general consists of being aware of potential side effects and stopping medications that cause serious side effects if stopping will not jeopardize the overall treatment. Supportive treatment such as topical lubrication, eyelid hygiene, and delayed secondary repair of residual effects such as ectropion, symblepharon, strabismus, and ptosis may also be required.

References

1. National Registry of Drug-Induced Ocular Side Effects. http://www.eyedrugregistry.com/. Accessed November 2008.
2. Fraunfelder FW, Fraunfelder FT. Drug-induced ocular side effects: oncolytic agents. In: Fraunfelder FT, Fraunfelder FW, Chambers WA, editors. Clinical Ocular Toxicology. Philadelphia, PA: Elsevier, 2008:199–221.
3. Fraunfelder FT, Meyer SM. Ocular toxicity of antineoplastic agents. Ophthalmology 1983;90:1–3.
4. Imperia PS, Lazarus HM, Lass JH. Ocular complications of systemic chemotherapy. Surv Ophthalmol 1989;34(3):209–30.
5. Schmid KE, Kornek GV, Scheithauer W, et al. Update on ocular complications of systemic cancer chemotherapy. Surv Ophthalmol 2006;51:19–40.
6. Chrousos GA, Oldfield EH, Doppman JL, et al. Prevention of ocular toxicity of carmustine (BCNU) with supraophthalmic intracarotid infusion. Ophthalmology 1986;93:1471–5.

7. Miller DF, Bay JW, Lederman RJ, et al. Ocular and orbital toxicity following intracarotid injection of BCNU (carmustine) and cisplatinum for malignant gliomas. Ophthalmology 1985;92:402–6.
8. Dueland S, Sauer T, Lund-Johansen F, et al. Epidermal growth factor receptor inhibition induces trichomegaly. Acta Oncol 2003;42:345–6.
9. Bouche' O, Brixi-Benmansour H, Bertin A, et al. Trichomegaly of the eyelashes following treatment with cetuximab. Ann Oncol 2005;16:1711–2.
10. Giuseppe T, Vicenzi B, Santini D, et al. Ocular toxicity related to cetuximab monotherapy in an advanced colorectal cancer patient. J Natl Cancer Inst 2005;97:606–7.
11. Margo CE, Murtagh FR. Ocular and orbital toxicity after intracarotid cisplatin therapy. Am J Ophthalmol 1993;116(4):508–9.
12. Kaya AO, Buyukberber S, Coskun U, et al. Acute erythema and edematous skin reaction and ectropion following docetaxel in a patient with non-small cell lung cancer. Cutan Ocul Toxicol 2008;27:327–31.
13. Marquez G, Herrera-Acosta E, Vidal I, et al. A case of trichomegaly of the eyelashes and facial hypertrichosis induced by erlotinib (Tarceva). Int J Dermatol 2009;48(1):97–8.
14. Lane K. Goldstein SM. Erlotinib-associated trichomegaly. Ophthal Plast Reconstr Surg 2007;23(1):65–66.
15. Lauer AK, Wobig JL, Shults WT, et al. Severe ocular and orbital toxicity after intracarotid etoposide phosphate and carboplatin therapy. Am J Ophthalmol 1999;127(2):230–3.
16. Forbes JE, Brazier DJ, Spittle M. 5-Fluorouracil and ocular toxicity. Br J Ophthalmol 1993;77(7):465–6.
17. Hurwitz BS. Cicatricial ectropion: a complication of systemic fluorouracil. Arch Ophthalmol 1993;111:1608–9.
18. Esmaeli B, Prieto VG, Butler CE, et al. Severe periorbital edema secondary to STI571 (Gleevec). Cancer 2002;95:881–7.
19. Grossman WJ, Wilson DB. Hypopigmentation from imatinib mesylate (Gleevec). J Pediatr Hematol Oncol 2004;26:214.
20. Fraunfelder FW, Solomon J, Druker BJ, et al. Ocular side effects associated with imatinib mesylate (Gleevec). J Ocul Pharmacol Ther 2003;19:371–5.
21. Schaich M, Schakel K, Illmer T, et al. Severe epidermal necrolysis after treatment with imatinib and consecutive allogeneic hematopoietic stem cell transplantation. Ann Hematol 2003;82:303–4.
22. Esmaeli R, Diba R, Ahmadi MA, et al. Periorbital oedema and epiphora as ocular side effects of imatinib mesylate (Gleevec). Eye 2004;18(7):760–2.
23. Fraunfelder FW, Solomon J, Druker BJ, et al. Ocular side-effects associated with imatinib mesylate (Gleevec). J Ocul Pharmacol Ther 2003;19:371–5.
24. Foon KA, Dougher G. Increased growth of eyelashes in a patient given leukocyte A interferon. N Engl J Med 1984;111:1259.
25. Deng-Huang S, Ying-Chun C, Shu-Lang L, Tien Chun C. Lanreotide treatment in a patient with interferon-associated Graves' ophthalmopathy. Graefes Arch Clin Exp Ophthal 2005;243(3):269–72.
26. Borgia G, Reynaud L, Gentile I, et al. Myasthenia gravis during low dose IFN alpha therapy for chronic hepatitis C. J Interferon Cytokine Res 2001;21:469–70.
27. Gaspari AA, Lotze MT, Rosenberg SA, et al. Dermatologic changes associated with interleukin 2 administration. J Am Med Assoc 1987;258(12):1624–9.
28. Polifka JE, Friedman JM. Teratogen update: azathioprine and 6-mercaptopurine. Teratology 2008;65(5):240–61.
29. Kumar K, Kochipillai V. Mitoxantrone induced hyperpigmentation. N Z Med J 1990;103:55.
30. Leyden MJ, Sullivan JR, Cheng ZM, et al. Unusual side effect of mitoxantrone. Med J Aust 1983;2(10):514.
31. Berkow JW, Gills JP, Wise JB. Depigmentation of eyelids after topically administered thiotepa. Arch Ophthalmol 1969;82:415–20.

Chapter 28
Ocular and Orbital Infections in the Immunocompromised Cancer Patient

Viet H. Ho and Hao H. Ho

Abstract Significant progress has been made in the treatment of cancer patients, and the proportion of cancer patients achieving complete remission and longer survival has increased in recent years. However, a significant proportion of patients still do not achieve complete remission, and infection remains a frequent cause of treatment failure, particularly in patients with hematologic malignancies. Ocular and orbital infections are particularly important, not only because of their frequency but also because of the associated local and systemic morbidity. Opportunistic infections can be found in all areas in and around the eye: in extraocular locations (neuro-ophthalmic, orbital, ocular adnexa), in the anterior segment (cornea and conjunctiva), and in the posterior segment (retina and choroid). All opportunistic infections of the eye have their origin in suppression of the host's immune system. Immune suppression can be acquired as a result of immunosuppressive therapy in solid organ transplant recipients or chemotherapy in patients with myeloproliferative disorders or solid tumors. Neutropenia remains the most important factor predisposing patients to infections.

28.1 Introduction

Cancer is one of the leading causes of death in developed countries. Cancer can be subdivided into two main categories: solid tumors and hematologic malignancies, which include leukemias, lymphomas, and multiple myeloma. Solid tumors account for more than 90% of all new cancer cases and hematologic malignancies for the remaining 5–10% [1]. Over the past decades, advances have resulted in substantial improvements in the prevention, early detection, and treatment of cancer, and the proportion of cancer patients achieving complete remission and longer survival has

---

V.H. Ho (✉)
Danville San Ramon Eye Medical Corp., Danville, CA, USA
e-mail: viethuyho@yahoo.com

B. Esmaeli (ed.), *Ophthalmic Oncology*, M.D. Anderson Solid Tumor Oncology Series 6, DOI 10.1007/978-1-4419-0374-7_28,

increased. Solid tumors are frequently treated with combinations of surgery, radiotherapy, and chemotherapy. In contrast, in patients with hematologic malignancies, chemotherapy is the cornerstone of treatment [1]. New therapeutic options, such as immunotherapy and gene therapy, are being developed. However, a significant proportion of patients still do not achieve complete remission, and infection remains a frequent cause of treatment failure, particularly in patients with hematologic malignancies. Ocular and orbital infections are particularly important, not only because of their frequency but also because of the associated local and systemic morbidity.

Many factors increase the risk of infection in cancer patients: poor clinical and nutritional status, mechanical obstruction of natural passages, damage to anatomic barriers (as a result of surgery or use of prosthetic and intravascular devices), and defects of humoral and cell-mediated immunity that are either associated with disease or secondary to radiotherapy or chemotherapy [1–4]. Cytotoxic agents exert their effects on both malignant cells and normally replicating progenitor cells and thus also cause major damage to normal tissues with high cell turnover (i.e., bone marrow and mucous membranes), resulting in myelosuppression and alteration of physiological barriers [1, 5]. Historically, hemorrhage and infections have been major complications of chemotherapy and leading causes of chemotherapy-related mortality [1]. In the 1960s, both the severity and duration of granulocytopenia were identified as major determinants of infectious complications [1, 2, 5]. In the early 1970s, prompt empirical antibiotic treatment became the cornerstone of management of febrile neutropenia, resulting in drastic reduction of the mortality of bacterial infections [1, 2, 5]. Since then, major progress has been made in the understanding of the pathogenesis and treatment of infectious complications in cancer patients.

28.2 Epidemiology

The majority of infections in immunocompromised cancer patients are caused by microorganisms of the host's endogenous flora [1, 6]. However, exogenous airborne and foodborne pathogens can also cause infection.

28.2.1 Bacterial

Gram-positive and gram-negative bacteria are the predominant pathogens in immunocompromised cancer patients. Over the past four decades, most cancer centers have experienced major changes in the etiology of bacterial infections in neutropenic patients [2, 4]. From the late 1960s to the early 1980s, aerobic gram-negative bacilli (*Escherichia coli*, *Klebsiella* species, and *Pseudomonas aeruginosa*) were the predominant causative agents, and *P. aeruginosa* was the most common isolate in all centers [3, 4]. Empirical antibiotic regimens were developed that took account of this pattern [7–10]. In the mid-1980s, there was a steady increase in gram-positive infections, and eventually 60–70% of cases of single-organism bacteremia were caused by gram-positive cocci (predominantly coagulase-negative staphylococci, viridans streptococci, and *Staphylococcus aureus*) [4, 5]. Although several factors have been proposed as contributors to this change in the pattern of causative agents—including more severe mucositis due to very aggressive chemotherapeutic regimens, longer duration of neutropenia, widespread use of long-dwelling right-atrial catheters, use of H2-receptor antagonists, and fluoroquinolone prophylaxis against gram-negative organisms—the underlying reasons are not absolutely clear. In recent years, however, the number of cases of gram-negative bacteremia has risen again, perhaps because of more parsimonious use of fluoroquinolones [1, 2, 5].

Gram-positive bacteria isolated from immunocompromised cancer patients today include *S. aureus*, coagulase-negative staphylococci, *Enterococcus* species, and viridans streptococci [1–5]. Viridans streptococci are part of the normal microbial flora and prevail in the oral cavity but also reside in the upper respiratory tract, the female genital tract, all regions of the gastrointestinal tract, and occasionally the skin [1, 3–5].

28.2.2 Viral

The herpesviruses are the most important viral pathogens in patients with cancer. This group includes herpes simplex virus 1 (HSV 1) and HSV 2, cytomegalovirus (CMV), varicella zoster virus, Epstein–Barr virus, and human herpesvirus 6 [1, 2, 11]. These DNA viruses establish a latent phase after primary infection, during which the viral genome resides in target cells for life with the potential to reactivate. Host defense against these viruses is dependent on viral-specific helpers and cytotoxic T lymphocytes, and thus both the likelihood of reactivation and the severity of disease are augmented during immunosuppression [2, 11].

HSV predominantly affects patients during profound neutropenia. Over 90% of the general adult population demonstrates seropositivity for HSV antibodies, indicating previous exposure [11]. The incidence of HSV reactivation in patients with previous exposure is approximately 70% after chemotherapy for leukemia or conditioning for hematopoietic stem cell transplantation [2].

CMV is very prevalent worldwide. It is the most serious of the viral pathogens in hematopoietic stem cell transplant recipients, and seropositive recipients are at greatest risk for developing CMV disease. Before the widespread adoption of prophylaxis against CMV, approximately 30% of seropositive transplant recipients developed CMV disease [2].

Reactivation of latent varicella zoster virus infection is common in patients with hematologic malignancies, especially after chemotherapy or treatment with corticosteroids, and typically occurs 3 months to 1 year after transplantation [2, 11].

Highly immunosuppressive regimens used for treatment of cancer patients have also created a population at higher risk for a variety of other viral infections, such as those due to adenoviruses, polyomavirus, and community respiratory viruses [11]. The three most recently discovered human herpesviruses (human herpesviruses 6, 7, and 8), like other members of the family, may cause a primary infection, establish latent infection in a specific set of cells in the host, and then reactivate if conditions of altered immunity develop [2, 11].

28.2.3 Fungal

Fungal infections in cancer patients can be divided into three major categories: infections caused by the common opportunistic fungi (*Candida* species and *Aspergillus* species); infections caused by pathogenic fungi (*Cryptococcus neoformans*, *Histoplasma capsulatum*, and *Coccidioides immitis*, which commonly cause self-limiting infections in the normal host); and infections caused by relatively uncommon more recently discovered fungal pathogens (e.g., phaeohyphomycetes, hyalohyphomycetes, and zygomycetes) [11–14].

Fungal infections are a major threat to immunocompromised patients. The incidence of invasive fungal infections has increased substantially during the past 30 years, to the extent that fungal infections are now a common cause of morbidity and mortality in patients with leukemia [11, 12]. Disseminated mycoses have been demonstrated at autopsy in 10–40% of patients with hematologic malignancies and are especially common in patients who have been treated with broad-spectrum antibiotics and corticosteroids [11, 15, 16]. Neutropenia has long been known to be a risk factor for fungal infections in patients with hematologic malignancies. Other risk factors include previous fungal infections; environmental exposure; long-term use of broad-spectrum antibiotics, steroids, or chemotherapeutic agents; and use of indwelling venous catheters.

Eighty to ninety percent of fungal infections are caused by *Candida* species. The remaining 10–20% are caused by *Aspergillus* species and other emerging fungi, including *Fusarium*, *Pseudallescheria*, *Scedosporium*, *Rhizopus*, and *Mucor* species [2, 5, 11]. Azole-resistant non-*albicans Candida* species have emerged in some cancer centers, usually in conjunction with several predisposing factors, including fluconazole prophylaxis [11].

Invasive candidiasis is generally preceded by colonization of mucosal surfaces [11, 12]. It can be classified as acute disseminated or chronic disseminated (hepatosplenic). Patients with proven bacterial or viral infections have a particularly high risk of infection by *Candida* species, perhaps because bacteremia with low-virulence bacteria is an indicator of mucosal lesions that allow *Candida* species to reach deep tissues and blood [11]. A high degree of colonization by *Candida* species in the gastrointestinal tract and oral cavity also increases the risk of systemic candidal infection [2].

Aspergillosis in neutropenic patients is usually caused by *Aspergillus fumigatus* or *A. flavus*. In contrast to candidiasis, aspergillosis is invariably acquired through the respiratory tract [11, 17]. The most frequent clinical manifestation of aspergillosis is pneumonia, but aspergillosis may also occur as invasive rhinosinusitis, cerebral infection, or disseminated infection [11, 12, 17].

28.3 Pathogenesis and Host Defense

The risk of infection in patients with cancer is a function of balance between the integrity of host defense mechanisms and the intensity of exposure to potentially pathogenic microorganisms in the host's environment (especially hospital pathogens).

Microbial invasion and development of infection are facilitated by the presence of comorbidities, immunosuppression, cancer treatment, and damage to anatomic barriers caused by the cancer itself or induced by chemotherapy [5, 9, 18, 19]. Cytotoxic chemotherapy used to treat cancer has potent effects on both humoral and cellular immunities [1, 2]. Cytotoxic regimens used for treating Hodgkin's and non-Hodgkin's lymphomas, solid tumors of the breast, lung, or germ cells and cancer of the genitourinary tract are in most cases given in cycles lasting weeks to months [1, 2]. These actions damage the host's defense mechanisms, which are already compromised in many cases by factors related to the underlying cancer (particularly in patients with myeloma, lymphoma, and chronic lymphocytic leukemia). Weakened immune components include the complement cascade and immunoglobulin production, T lymphocytes, monocytes/macrophages, neutrophils, and skin and mucous membranes [1, 2]. Patients with cancer are therefore highly susceptible to almost any type of infection.

Neutropenia is the main immune defect of cancer patients, and the inverse relationship between absolute neutrophil count and infection risk has been known since the 1960s [2]. However, neutropenia is not the only factor influencing the risk of infection. As new chemotherapy regimens and new antibiotics are developed and introduced for therapy or prophylaxis, the pattern of infection risk changes. For example, use of new purine analogues such as fludarabine in patients with chronic lymphocytic leukemia has been associated with an increase in infections with *Listeria monocytogenes* and *Pneumocystis carinii*, both associated with T lymphocyte dysfunction, and prophylaxis with trimethoprim–sulfamethoxazole and ciprofloxacin during severe mucositis has led to bacteremia with viridans streptococci [2, 5].

Additionally, underlying conditions such as obstruction of the lumen of a natural body passage (e.g., urinary, biliary, respiratory, digestive tract, or nasolacrimal duct) by cancer impairs the flow of body fluids and secretions, creating conditions that promote microbial growth [1–5, 18]. Cytotoxic chemotherapy damages the epithelial tissue lining, resulting in loss of the integrity of the mucous membrane barrier. Development of mucositis therefore predisposes to infection by the patient's endogenous commensal flora and colonizing pathogens [2, 5].

28.4 Ocular and Orbital Manifestations of Infection

28.4.1 Bacterial

Most systemic bacterial infections that affect the eye do so through bacteremia via hematogenous seeding. Ocular manifestations of bacteremia may be suppurative or nonsuppurative. Suppurative findings include endophthalmitis, subretinal abscess, and preseptal and orbital cellulitis, while nonsuppurative findings include nonspecific retinal lesions (e.g., cotton-wool spots) and uveitis [20, 21]. Conventional methods of culture of blood or vitreous are usually successful in diagnosing suppurative ocular complications of acute systemic infections, while molecular diagnostic techniques are proving useful in diagnosing nonsuppurative ocular complications of indolent systemic infections [20].

The ocular manifestation of an acute systemic bacterial infection, such as endocarditis or liver abscess, is usually acute endophthalmitis, while the ocular manifestation of a chronic systemic infection, such as tuberculosis or syphilis, is often a subacute uveitis [22–24]. Intraocular findings in patients with acute bacteremia include cotton-wool spots, superficial retinal hemorrhages, white-centered retinal hemorrhages (Roth spots), and endogenous endophthalmitis [20–23].

Orbital infections in the immunocompromised host are most commonly caused by bacteria, and a wide spectrum of bacteria are associated with orbital disease [23]. Infection reaches the orbit by one of three methods: implantation, local extension, or hematogenous spread. Specific anatomic features of the midface place the orbit at risk of infection. Implantation, which may occur in patients with an orbital foreign body, results from trauma to the periorbital area or sinuses. Local extension most often occurs as spread from a contiguous sinus, and hematogenous spread may occur from a multiplicity of distant sites in immunocompromised patients. Coagulase-negative staphylococci, *S. aureus*, viridans streptococci, and enterococci are now the major gram-positive pathogens. *E. coli*, *Klebsiella* species, and *P. aeruginosa* are the most common gram-negative pathogens causing initial fever [20–22].

Systemic immunosuppression may predispose patients to the development of infectious crystalline keratopathy, a distinct clinical entity characterized by intrastromal noninflammatory bacterial colonization seen morphologically as gray-white, needle-like branching opacities occurring commonly in the anterior or midcorneal stroma in an otherwise relatively quiet eye [25]. Alpha-hemolytic streptococci are the common causative organism, though other bacteria and even fungi have also been reported to cause infectious crystalline keratopathy. An immunocompromised state is a common predisposing factor. Infectious crystalline keratopathy is typically seen in a patient with an epithelial defect with or without a history of penetrating keratoplasty who is using topical steroids [25].

Concurrent orbital cellulitis and panophthalmitis have been reported by Jain and Garg [26], Tabbara et al. [27], Hornblass et al. [28], and Li et al. [29]. Additionally, a case of concurrent orbital cellulitis and suppurative panophthalmitis with associated ecthyma gangrenosum in an immunocompromised patient with *Pseudomonas* septicemia was described by Maccheron et al. [30].

Infections involving *Nocardia* organisms represent an increasingly recognized problem among patients with immunosuppression. It is estimated that at least 1000 new cases occur every year in the United States [2, 31]. *Nocardia* organisms are aerobic, soil-dwelling actinomycetes involved in the decay of organic matter. Nocardiosis is a multisystem disease that has high mortality and ocular morbidity rates. The choroid seems to be the site in the eye most commonly affected, followed by the cornea and sclera [31]. Lakosha et al. [31] have reported choroidal abscess development in a patient with chronic myeloid leukemia due to *Nocardia farcinica*.

Bartonella henselae is a gram-negative bacilli that causes the majority of cases of cat-scratch disease. The vast majority of cases of cat-scratch disease occur in children who present with local infection at the inoculation site followed by tender regional lymphadenopathy. In contrast, cat-scratch disease in immunosuppressed patients and those who have undergone organ transplantation can disseminate from the lymph nodes and cause neuroretinitis and chorioretinitis. *Bartonella* organisms responsible for cutaneous bacillary angiomatosis of the anterior orbit, eyelid, and conjunctiva have been described [32]. Patel et al. [33] reported an atypical presentation of *B. henselae* infection: bilateral chorioretinitis in an immunocompromised patient.

A rarely described bacterium, gram-negative *Providencia rettgeri*, has been responsible for dacryocystitis, conjunctivitis, keratitis, and endophthalmitis in patients with an immunocompromised state [34].

Disseminated toxoplasmosis is a well-known complication of immunodeficiency, including immunodeficiency induced by cancer, steroid therapy, cytotoxic drug therapy, and AIDS. When ocular toxoplasmosis occurs in an immunodeficient host or when immunosuppressive therapy is administered to a patient with active toxoplasmosis, widespread tissue destruction by proliferating organisms may result [20]. Ocular toxoplasmosis in an immunocompromised host presents difficult problems in diagnosis and management. There may be a variety of clinical lesions, including single foci of retinochoroiditis in one or both eyes, multifocal lesions, or diffuse areas of retinal necrosis [20, 35]. The majority of lesions do not arise from the borders of preexisting scars, which suggest that they result from acquired infection or dissemination of organisms from nonocular sites of disease [20]. In immunocompromised patients, *Toxoplasma gondii* may infect the iris, choroids, and vitreous tissues, which are not usually infected in immunocompetent hosts [35]. In patients with disseminated toxoplasmosis, ocular lesions appear to respond to standard antiparasitic drug therapies, but in the most immunocompromised patients, continued treatment is probably necessary to prevent reactivation of disease [20].

Mycobacterium haemophilum is an increasingly recognized pathogen in immunocompromised patients [36–39]. This nontuberculous mycobacterium has been isolated from specimens of skin, synovial fluid, bone, lung tissue, sputum, bronchoalveolar lavage fluid, lymph nodes, blood, and bone marrow [36]. Cutaneous and subcutaneous manifestations are the most frequently reported presentation of *M. haemophilum* infection. *M. haemophilum* infection presenting as filamentary keratopathy can occur in immunocompromised patients [37]. Chronic granulomatous iridocyclitis progressing to endophthalmitis has been reported [38].

Mycobacterium fortuitum infection masquerading as an orbital mass causing diplopia was reported by Ali et al. [39].

28.4.2 Viral

Despite significant advances in our ability to diagnose and treat viral infections, viruses continue to be a significant cause of both systemic and ocular illnesses.

Primary infection with HSV results from direct contact with infected secretions, typically from the mucosal surface of an infected person. The incubation period ranges from 2 to 12 days [11, 40]. Primary gingivostomatitis, which is most common in children but also occurs in adults, presents with a prodrome of fever, malaise, and pharyngitis, followed by the onset of small intraoral vesicles that coalesce to form painful ulcers [11, 41]. These lesions frequently involve the pharyngeal and buccal mucosa, soft palate, and gums and may extend to the posterior pharynx, tonsils, or lips [41]. Occasionally, spread to other cutaneous sites such as the face and eyelids is observed. Primary ocular involvement results in follicular conjunctivitis, which is typically unilateral with regional adenopathy, vesicular blepharitis, and epithelial keratitis [41]. Dacryoadenitis associated with HSV conjunctivitis can also result [42].

In severely immunocompromised patients, herpes zoster can present with unusual manifestations and can cause potentially life-threatening complications such as atypical generalized herpes zoster or abdominal herpes zoster. Ocular manifestations of varicella zoster virus infections are protean and include dermatitis, episcleritis, keratitis with neurotrophic ulceration and stromal scarring, uveitis, iris atrophy, retinitis, and optic nerve involvement [43]. Patients who are immunocompromised are particularly susceptible to these complications, which frequently occur without typical cutaneous dermatomal eruptions [41–43]. Simultaneous involvement of the retina and optic nerve by varicella zoster virus in acute retinal necrosis syndrome is well documented [43]. Greven et al. [44] reported a case of simultaneous involvement of the retina, optic nerve, and optic chiasm with varicella zoster virus. Optic disc edema with associated optic neuropathy and retrobulbar optic neuritis due to varicella zoster virus has been described in immunocompromised patients [45, 46].

Herpetic necrotizing retinitis is caused by the herpesvirus group of viruses: HSV, varicella zoster virus, CMV, and Epstein–Barr virus [20, 23, 47]. Progressive outer retinal necrosis is described as a distinct form of varicella zoster virus necrotizing chorioretinitis and is found almost exclusively in patients with AIDS. However, a few cases in non-AIDS patients have been reported. These patients were immunocompromised owing to therapy for idiopathic thrombocytopenic purpura, cutaneous non-Hodgkin's lymphoma, rheumatoid arthritis, renal transplantation, or allogeneic stem cell transplantation [47–49]. Typical features of progressive outer retinal necrosis include retinal lesions that are multifocal, coalescing, and beginning in the peripheral retina; rapid progression of these lesions; lack of response to treatment;

and lack of prominent inflammatory reaction in the vitreous and anterior chambers [47, 48, 50].

Acute retinal necrosis is a clinical syndrome consisting of peripheral necrotizing retinitis, occlusive retinal vasculitis, and notable anterior chamber and vitreous inflammation resulting from infection of the retina by certain members of the Herpesviridae family [50–53]. CMV retinitis is a well-recognized complication of immunodeficiency. It has been described as an early, small, opaque lesion with a white granular area of retinal necrosis that spreads in a centrifugal, brushfire-like manner, with vascular sheathing and intraretinal hemorrhages [51, 54, 55].

28.4.3 Fungal

The fungal infections most likely to have systemic manifestations involving the eye are presented here.

28.4.3.1 *Candida* Species

Candidiasis occurs worldwide. *Candida* species are normal commensals of humans and are commonly found in the oropharynx, the gastrointestinal tract, and the vagina and on the skin [12, 14]. Predisposition to candidiasis has become more common with the advent of antibiotics, which destroy the normal inhibitory bacterial flora and inhibit neutrophil phagocytosis, and with the use of cytotoxic chemotherapy; immunosuppressive agents, such as corticosteroids; and implantation of prosthetic devices, such as catheters, cardiac valves, and artificial hearts [12, 14, 16, 56].

Most cases of disseminated candidiasis are due to *Candida albicans* or *Candida tropicalis*. Patients typically present with fever and toxic effects but few localizing findings. When *Candida* disseminates, multiple organs are usually affected; renal, cerebral, cardiac, and ocular involvements are the most common, followed by hepatic and splenic involvement and, less frequent, pulmonary, gastrointestinal, cutaneous, bone, and endocrine involvements [12, 16].

Some patients with disseminated candidiasis have *Candida* endophthalmitis with single or multiple raised, white, fluffy, cotton-ball-like chorioretinal lesions in the presence or absence of overlying vitreous haze [12, 57, 58]. Lesions are usually in the macular area and may extend rapidly into the vitreous humor. Less common findings include hemorrhages, Roth spots, hypopyon, anterior chamber inflammation, and iritis [58]. Patients may complain of orbital pain, blurred vision, floating scotomas, or opacities in the visual fields. The presence of endophthalmitis serves as a major clue to the diagnosis of hematogenously disseminated candidiasis and is a potential cause of permanent blindness [58].

28.4.3.2 *Aspergillus* Species

Aspergillus species are often nonpathogenic residents of normal body flora as well as common contaminants in bacteriology laboratories and in unfiltered outside air.

Aspergillus species are ubiquitous in the environments of most countries of the world [12, 14]. The fungus grows well on a variety of substrates, including stored hay or grain, compost piles, dead leaves, soil, and dung [12, 14]. Aspergillosis is usually acquired by inhalation of airborne spores (conidia) that reach alveoli or paranasal sinuses. Among immunosuppressed patients, aspergillosis is second only to candidiasis as an opportunistic mycosis [12, 14, 16].

In severely immunosuppressed patients, skin or corneal trauma may be a nidus for *Aspergillus* infection [14]. The most common cause of aspergillosis is *A. fumigatus*. *A. flavus* is the second most common cause and assumes importance in immunosuppressed patients and in patients with nasal or paranasal sinus disease [14, 16, 17]. Host defense against aspergillosis relies primarily on cell-mediated immunity (neutrophils, monocytes, and macrophages) and not on antibodies or lymphocytes [16, 17]. Macrophages are responsible for killing conidia, whereas neutrophils attack mycelia. The complement cascade facilitates neutrophil damage to hyphae and monocyte killing of conidia and also provides a source of chemotactic factor [14–17].

Aspergillus species can infect and invade multiple organ systems, including the ear, sinuses, eye, lung, central nervous system, heart, gastrointestinal tract, skin, and bone [12]. A hyphal ball may form in a chronically obstructed paranasal sinus without tissue invasion. Fibrosing granulomatous inflammation with scanty *Aspergillus* hyphae within tissue may begin in the sinus and slowly invade the orbit and brain [58]. Clinically, patients with *Aspergillus* sinusitis may develop head or sinus pain, proptosis, or monocular blindness. In severely neutropenic patients, mucosal invasion beginning in the nose or sinus can spread rapidly to contiguous structures, causing vascular invasion and necrosis. *A. flavus* is particularly common in isolates from invasive aspergillosis of the nose and the paranasal sinuses. Invasive pulmonary aspergillosis occurs most commonly in patients who have a hematologic or lymphoreticular malignancy and patients who have undergone organ transplantation and are receiving high doses of corticosteroids, cytotoxic agents, or both [12, 14]. de O Machado et al. [59] reported a case of bilateral *Aspergillus* endophthalmitis in a patient with chronic lymphocytic leukemia.

Aspergillus endophthalmitis is a relatively rare condition that has a devastating course, with blindness as its usual outcome [58, 59]. Manifestations include cloudy vision, redness of the conjunctivae, and pain. Hypopyon with severe exudation into the anterior and posterior chambers may develop. *Aspergillus* keratitis may be caused by minor trauma to the eye, allowing deep stromal invasion by the fungus [12, 58]. Finally, *Aspergillus* infection may be a source of orbital cellulitis.

28.4.3.3 Other Fungal Species

Mucormycosis is the common name given to infection by any of several different fungi of the order Mucorales. Mucormycosis is best known for its ability to rapidly invade arterial vessels and for its rapid, destructive, and often fatal course

[12]. Members of the order Mucorales are ubiquitous worldwide and are common inhabitants of the soil and decaying organic debris [14, 16]. Inhalation of conidia must be fairly common, yet colonization and infection are infrequent, attesting to their low virulence and the importance of normal host defenses [12]. Mucormycosis tends to be limited to patients with immunosuppression, trauma, or diabetes mellitus, in whom mucormycosis is particularly common in patients with ketoacidosis [2, 12].

The fungus typically gains entrance to the body through the respiratory tract. The spores deposit on the mucous membranes of the nasal turbinates, where they germinate and then may be inhaled into the pulmonary alveoli [12, 60, 61]. To cause disease, spores must overcome the host's natural immunity and specific humoral and cell-mediated immune mechanisms [2, 14]. Once the fungus begins to grow, the hyphae invade tissue, cause suppuration with little granulomatous response, and have a special affinity for blood vessels [60, 61]. Direct penetration and growth through the blood vessel walls explain the propensity for thrombosis, embolization, infarction, and tissue necrosis. Disease spreads by both direct and hematogenous extensions [2, 14, 60, 61].

In patients with neutropenia and leukemia, burns, or open wounds, mucormycosis leads to rhinocerebral, pulmonary, or disseminated disease [2, 12, 14, 60, 61]. These patients with rhinocerebral mucormycosis may have facial pain, headache, or both. Other manifestations include nasal stuffiness, blood-tinged nasal discharge, and facial swelling [60, 61]. An examination of the nasal mucosa reveals necrotic turbinates. Fever, facial cellulitis, palatal or nasal septal perforation, and signs of sinusitis may be present. Spread of infection to the orbit results in orbital cellulitis, loss of extraocular muscle function, and proptosis with failing vision [60, 61]. Ultimately, there is a full-blown orbital apex syndrome with destruction of cranial nerves III, IV, and VI; the ophthalmic branch of V; and blood vessels traversing the optic foramen and superior orbital fissure [60, 61]. Mucorales organisms may also invade the cavernous sinus and internal carotid artery, causing thrombosis; cerebral infarction as a result of vascular compromise is common [60, 61].

Alternaria species are ubiquitous fungi known to be soil saprobes and plant pathogens. Ocular manifestations include keratitis and cutaneous involvement [12]. *Pseudallescheria boydii*, a fungus frequently isolated from soil, can cause a wide range of fungal diseases, including corneal ulcers and endophthalmitis [12].

Cases of *Fusarium* keratitis and endophthalmitis have been reported [57, 58, 62]. *Scedosporium apiospermum* is an opportunistic fungus usually found in soil. Orbital involvement by this organism is very rare [63]. In immunocompromised hosts, aggressive spread is common [64]. In 1977, Gluckman et al. [65] reported orbital extension of pansinusitis due to *S. apiospermum* in a diabetic patient. In 1984, Anderson et al. [66] described successful treatment of an orbitocranial infection due to this organism. And in 1999, Jones et al. [67] described a case of subperiosteal abscess in a leukemic patient. *S. apiospermum* was also found in a case of osteomyelitis of the orbit in an immunocompromised patient [63].

28.5 Conclusion

Patients with cancer vary both in terms of underlying malignancy and in terms of the level of immunosuppression. Multiple predisposing factors may exist, increasing the spectrum of likely pathogens. The recognition and treatment of infection in immunocompromised patients are very important. Collaboration between different specialties is crucial in managing patients with orbital or ocular infection. Not only can the visual outcome of ocular and orbital infection be poor, but associated systemic involvement and septicemia may be life-threatening.

References

1. Marchetti O, Calandra T. Infections in the neutropenic cancer patient. In: Cohen J, Powderly WG, editors. Infectious Diseases, second edition. New York, NY: Mosby, 2004:1077–93.
2. Segal BH, Walsh TJ, Gea-Banacloche J, et al. Infections in the cancer patient. In: DeVita VT Jr, Hellman S, Rosenberg SA, editors. Cancer Principles and Practice of Oncology, seventh edition. Philadelphia, PA: Lippincott Williams & Wilkins, 2005:2461–2511.
3. Bannister B, Gillespie S, Jones J. Infections in immunocompromised patients. In: Infection Microbiology and Management. Oxford: Blackwell, 2006:431–42.
4. Rolston KV. Infection in the neutropenic patient. In: Kantarjuan HM, Wolff RA, Koller CA, editors. The M. D. Anderson Manual of Medical Oncology. New York, NY: McGraw-Hill, 2006:957–66.
5. Vento S, Cainelli F. Infections in patients with cancer undergoing chemotherapy: aetiology, prevention, and treatment. Lancet 2003;4:595–604.
6. Easty DL. Infection in the compromised eye. Trans Am Ophthalmol Soc 1986;105:61–8.
7. Bal AM, Gould IM. Empirical antimicrobial treatment for chemotherapy-induced febrile neutropenia. Int J Antimicrob Agents 2007;29:501–9.
8. Oken MM, Pomeroy C, Weisdorf D, et al. Prophylactic antibiotics for the prevention of early infection in multiple myeloma. Am J Med 1996;100:624–8.
9. Noskin GA. Prevention of infection in immunocompromised hosts. In: Management of Infectious Complications in Cancer Patients. Boston: Kluwer, 1998:223–46.
10. Kowalski RP, Karenchak LM, Romanowski EG. Infectious disease: changing antibiotic susceptibility. Ophthalmol Clin North Am 2004;16:1–9.
11. Bodey GP, Chamaly RF, Kontoyiannis DP. Fungal and viral infections in cancer patients. In: Kantarjuan HM, Wolff RA, Koller CA, editors. The M. D. Anderson Manual of Medical Oncology. New York, NY: McGraw-Hill, 2006:967–92.
12. Samonis G, Bafaloukos D. Fungal infections in cancer patients: an escalating problem. In Vivo 1992;6:183–94.
13. Powles RL. Systemic fungal infections: major problems in cancer patients. Indian J Cancer 1994;31:180–4.
14. Mays SR, Bogle MA, Bodey GP. Cutaneous fungal infections in the oncology patient. Am J Clin Dermatol 2006;7:31–43.
15. Cornely OA, Bohme A, Reichert D, et al. Risk factors for breakthrough invasive fungal infection during secondary prophylaxis. J Antimicrob Chemother 2008;61:939–46.
16. Anaissie E. Opportunistic mycoses in the immunocompromised host: experience at a cancer center and review. Clin Infect Dis 1992;14:S43–53.
17. Herbrecht R, Denning DW, Patterson TF. Voriconazole versus amphotericin B for primary therapy of invasive aspergillosis. N Engl J Med 2002;347:408–15.
18. Rolston KV, Bodey GP, Safdar A. Polymicrobial infection in patients with cancer: an underappreciated and underreported entity. Clin Infect Dis 2007;45:228–33.

19. Jack MK, Hicks JD. Ocular complications in high-dose chemoradiotherapy and marrow transplantation. Ann Ophthalmol 1981;13:709–11.
20. Lynn WA, Lightman S. The eye in systemic infection. Lancet 2004;364:1439–50.
21. Khan A, Okhravi N, Lightman S. The eye in systemic sepsis. Clin Med 2002;2:444–8.
22. Mahajan VM. Acute bacterial infections of the eye: their aetiology and treatment. Br J Ophthalmol 1983;67:191–4.
23. Guembel HOC, Ohrloff C. Opportunistic infections of the eye in immunocompromised patients. Ophthalmologica 1997;211:53–61.
24. Bialasiewicz AA, Knospe V, Richard G. Ocular infections in the immunocompromised host. Dev Ophthalmol 1999;30:203–19.
25. Sridhar MS, Laibson PR, Rapuano CJ, et al. Infectious crystalline keratopathy in an immunosuppressed patient. CLAO J 2001;27:108–10.
26. Jain ML, Garg AK. Metastatic endophthalmitis in a patient with major burns: a rare complication. Burns 1995;21:72–3.
27. Tabbara KF, Juffali F, Matossian RM. Bacillus laterosporus endophthalmitis. Arch Ophthalmol 1977;95:2187–9.
28. Hornblass A, To K, Coden DJ, et al. Endogenous orbital cellulites and endogenous endophthalmitis in subacute bacterial endocarditis. Am J Ophthalmol 1989;108:196–7.
29. Li S, Perlman JI, Edward DP, et al. Unilateral blastomyces dermatitidis endophthalmitis and orbital cellulites. Ophthalmology 1998;105:1466–70.
30. Maccheron LJ, Groeneveld ER, Ohlrich SJ, et al. Orbital cellulitis, panophthalmitis, and ecthyma gangrenosum in an immunocompromised host with *Pseudomonas septicemia*. Am J Ophthalmol 2004;137;176–8.
31. Lakosha H, Pavlin CJ, Lipton J. Subretinal abscess due to Nocardia farcinica infection. Retina 2000;20:269–74.
32. Tsai PS, DeAngelis DD, Spencer WH, et al. Bacillary angiomatosis of the anterior orbit, eyelid, and conjunctiva. Am J Ophthalmol 2002;134:433–4.
33. Patel SJ, Petrarca R, Shah SM, et al. Atypical bartonella henselae chorioretinitis in an immunocompromised patient. Ocul Immunol Inflamm 2008;16:45–9.
34. Koreishi AF, Schechter BA, Karp CL. Ocular infections caused by Providencia rettgeri. Ophthalmology 2006;113:1463–6.
35. Hoerni B, Vallat M, Durand M, et al. Ocular toxoplasmosis and Hodgkin's disease. Arch Ophthalmol 1978;96:62–3.
36. Shah MK, Sebti A, Kiehn TE, et al. Mycobacterium haemophilum in immunocompromised patients. Clin Infect Dis 2001;33:330–7.
37. Millar MJ, Bulliard C, Balachandran C, et al. Mycobacterium haemophilum infection presenting as filamentary keratopathy in an immunocompromised adult. Cornea 2007;26:764–6.
38. Modi D, Pyatetsky D, Edward DP, et al. Mycobacterium haemophilum, a rare cause of endophthalmitis. Retina 2007;27:1148–51.
39. Ali S, Sivak-Callcot JA, Khakoo R, et al. Mycobacterium fortuitum infection masquerading as an orbital mass. Ophthal Plast Reconstr Surg 2007;23:327–9.
40. Bansal R, Tutrone WD, Weinberg JM. Viral skin infections in the elderly. Drugs Aging 2002;19:503–14.
41. Khan BF, Pavan-Langston D. Clinical manifestations and treatment modalities in herpes simplex virus of the ocular anterior segment. Int Ophthalmol Clin 2004;44:103–33.
42. Foster WJ, Krause MD, Custer PL. Herpes simplex virus dacryoadenitis in an immunocompromised patient. Arch Ophthalmol 2003;121:911–12.
43. Lightman S, Marsh RJ, Powell D. Herpes zoster ophthalmicus: a medical review. Br J Ophthalmol 1981;65:539–41.
44. Greven CM, Singh T, Stanton CA, et al. Optic chiasm, optic nerve, and retinal involvement secondary to varicella-zoster virus. Arch Ophthalmol 2001;119:608–10.
45. Friedlander SM, Rahhal FM, Ericson L, et al. Optic neuropathy preceding acute retinal necrosis in acquired immunodeficiency syndrome. Arch Ophthalmol 1995;114:1481–5.

46. Lee MS, Cooney EL, Stoessol KM, et al. Varicella zoster virus retrobulbar optic neuritis proceeding retinitis in patients with acquired immune deficiency syndrome. Ophthalmology 1998;105:467–71.
47. Long HM, Dick A. Presumed CMV associated necrotizing retinopathy in a non-HIV immunocompromised host. Clin Exp Ophthalmol 2005;33:330–5.
48. Foster RE, Peterson MR, Neuss MN, et al. Progressive outer retinal necrosis syndrome in a lymphoma patient with good visual outcome. Am J Ophthalmol 2001;132:117–20.
49. Kalpoe JS, van Dehn CE, Bollemeijer JG, et al. Varicella zoster virus (VZV)-related progressive outer retinal necrosis (PORN) after allogeneic stem cell transplantation. Bone Marrow Transplant 2005;36:467–9.
50. Westeneng AC, Rothova A, De Boer JH, et al. Infectious uveitis in immunocompromised patients and the diagnostic value of polymerase chain reaction and Goldmann-Witmer coefficient in aqueous analysis. Am J Ophthalmol 2007;144:781–5.
51. Akpek EK, Kent C, Jakobiec F, et al. Bilateral acute retinal necrosis caused by cytomegalovirus in an immunocompromised patient. Am J Ophthalmol 1999;127:93–5.
52. Derzko-Dzulynsky LA, Berger AR, Berinstein NL. Cytomegalovirus retinitis and low-grade non-Hodgkin's lymphoma: case report and review of the literature. Am J Hematol 1998;57:228–32.
53. Duker JS, Blumenkranz MS. Diagnosis and management of the acute retinal necrosis syndrome (ARN). Surv Ophthalmol 1995;35:327–43.
54. Pollard RB, Egbert PR, Gallagher JG, et al. Cytomegalovirus retinitis in immunosuppressed hosts. I. Natural history and effects of treatment with adenine arabinoside. Ann Intern Med 1980;93:655–64.
55. Egbert PR, Pollard RB, Gallagher JG, et al. Cytomegalovirus retinitis in immunosuppressed hosts. II. Ocular manifestation. Ann Intern Med 1980;93:664–70.
56. Segal BH, Almyroudis NG, Battiwalla M, et al. Prevention and early treatment of invasive fungal infection in patients with cancer and neutropenia and stem cell transplant recipients in the era of newer broad-spectrum antifungal agents and diagnostic adjuncts. Clin Infect Dis 2007;44:402–9.
57. Thursky KA, Playford EG, Seymour JF, et al. Recommendations for the treatment of established fungal infections. Intern Med J 2008;38:496–520.
58. Hariprasad SM, Mieler WF, Lin TK, et al. Voriconazole in the treatment of fungal eye infections: a review of current literature. Br J Ophthalmol 2008;92:871–8.
59. de O Machado O, Goncalves R, Fernandes EM, et al. Bilateral aspergillus endophthalmitis in a patient with chronic lymphocytic leukaemia. Br J Ophthalmol 2003;87:1429–30.
60. Hilal AA, Taj-Aldeen SJ, Mirghani AH. Rhinoorbital mucormycosis secondary to Rhizopus oryzae: a case report and literature review. Ear Nose Throat J 2004;83:556–62.
61. Jeevanan J, Gendeh BS, Faridah HA, et al. Rhino-orbito-cerebral mucormycosis: a treatment dilemma. Med J Malaysia 2006;61:106–8.
62. Louie T, el Baba F, Shulman M, et al. Endogenous endophthalmitis due to fusarium: case report and review. Clin Infect Dis 1994;18:585–8.
63. O'Doherty M, Hannan M, Fulcher T. Voriconazole in the treatment of fungal osteomyelitis of the orbit in the immunocompromised host. Orbit 2005;24:285–9.
64. Wood GM, McCormack JG, Muir DB, et al. Clinical features of human infection with Scedosporium inflatum. Clin Infect Dis 1992;14:1027–33.
65. Gluckman SJ, Ries K, Abrutyn E. Allescheria (Petriellidium) boydii sinusitis in a compromised host. J Clin Microbiol 1977;5:481–4.
66. Anderson RL, Carroll TF, Harvey JT. Petriellidium (Allescheria) boydii orbital and brain abscess treated with intravenous miconazole. Am J Ophthalmol 1984;97:771–5.
67. Jones J, Katz SE, Lubow M. Scedosporium apiospermum of the orbit. Arch Ophthalmol 1999;117:27203.

Part V
Neuro-ophthalmic Manifestations of Cancer

Section Editor: Jade S. Schiffman

Chapter 29
Cranial Nerve III, IV, and VI Palsies in the Cancer Patient

Meghan S. Flemmons and Jade S. Schiffman

Abstract Cranial nerve III, IV, and VI palsies in cancer patients can be caused by primary cranial nerve neoplasms, direct extension from brain, brain stem and skull base tumors, direct extension or perineural spread from head and neck tumors, metastases from tumors at distant sites, leptomeningeal disease, and other conditions, including raised intracranial pressure, radiation effect, infection, paraneoplastic syndromes, and certain medications. Ophthalmologic findings in patients with cranial neuropathies depend on the cranial nerve III, IV and VI involved and the location of involvement. Primary cranial nerve neoplasms are most commonly schwannomas. Skull base tumors often result in cranial nerve involvement as well as primary tumors of the breast, lung, and prostate that metastasize to the skull base. Head and neck cancers travel through the skull base and result in cranial nerve involvement. Leptomeningeal disease is a common cause of deficits of cranial nerves II–VII. Other conditions–from treatment of the primary tumor to complications of chemotherapy and immunosuppression–can result in cranial neuropathies.

29.1 Introduction

The presence of cranial nerve (CN) III, IV, and VI paresis in a cancer patient is concerning and requires careful evaluation to determine which nerve is involved, the location of the lesion, and determination if the cranial neuropathy is in fact related to the cancer. Cranial neuropathies in cancer patients can be caused by primary cranial nerve neoplasms, direct extension from brain or brain stem tumors, direct extension or perineural spread from head and neck tumors, metastases from tumors at distant sites, leptomeningeal disease, and other conditions. Neuropathies of cranial nerves III, IV, and VI often present to the neuro-ophthalmology practice.

M.S. Flemmons (✉)
Department of Ophthalmology and Visual Sciences, The University of Texas Medical Branch, Galveston, TX, USA
e-mail: meghan.flemmons@duke.edu

B. Esmaeli (ed.), *Ophthalmic Oncology*, M.D. Anderson Solid Tumor Oncology Series 6, DOI 10.1007/978-1-4419-0374-7_29,

The various mechanisms of these cranial neuropathies in patients with cancer are discussed herein.

29.2 Ophthalmologic Findings with CN III, IV, and VI Palsies

Ophthalmologic findings in patients with cranial neuropathies depend on the cranial nerve involved and the location of involvement. New-onset binocular diplopia is an important symptom indicating the potential of a new cranial neuropathy. An isolated cranial nerve III palsy presents with ptosis, pupil dilation, and an eye that is "down and out"—i.e., an eye with limited motility in elevation, adduction, and depression. A cranial nerve IV palsy presents with subjective torsion, vertical diplopia, and a head tilt. A cranial nerve VI palsy causes horizontal diplopia, a head turn toward the side of the involved nerve, and limited abduction. If multiple cranial nerves are involved, a cavernous sinus lesion is likely, especially if there is involvement of the trigeminal nerve first and second divisions. Proptosis or chemosis may indicate a process involving the orbit or cavernous sinus. Table 29.1 summarizes the various causes of CN III, IV, VI palsies in cancer patients from direct effects of primary and secondary tumors, to those related to the side effects of treatment, immunologic and hypercoagulable states.

Table 29.1 Differential Diagnoses of CN III, IV, VI in cancer patients

I. Neoplasm related (direct)	
Primary Cranial Nerve tumor of III, IV, VI	Schwannoma, Neurofibroma, Hemangioma
Secondary Involvement of III, IV, VI	
Brain Tumor	
-Primary	Astrocytomas, Oligodendroglioma, PNET, Lymphoma
-Secondary	Breast, Lung, Melanoma
Brain Stem/Cerebellar Tumor	
-Primary	Ependymoma, medulloblastoma, germinoma, glioma
-Secondary	Breast, Lung, Melanoma
Skull Base Tumor	
-Primary	Meningioma, chordoma, Schwannoma, hemangiopericytomas sella/parasellar tumors (pituitary adenoma, craniopharyngioma)
-Secondary	Breast, Prostate, Lung, Thyroid, Ewings, Osteosarcoma, Neuroblastoma, Plasmacytoma, Leukemias
Head and Neck Tumor	
-Direct Invasion	Squamous Cell Carcinoma, Adenoid Cystic Carcinoma Adenocarcinoma, SNUC, Esthesioneuroblastoma, Melanoma, Lymphoma etc.

Table 29.1 (continued)

-Perineural Invasion	Squamous Cell Skin Cancer, SCC of sinonasal cavities, oral cavity, oropharynx and nasopharynx, masticator space Adenoid Cystic Carcinoma, rarely Melanoma/Lymphoma
Leptomeningeal Disease	From primary brain tumors; liquid tumors (leukemias and lymphomas) and solid tumors (breast, lung, melanoma, ovarian etc)

II. Treatment-related

-Spinal Fluid Pressure changes from intervention

i. raised intracranial pressure from intrathecal injections, CNS surgery with hematomas, subarachnoid blood, infection etc.
ii. reduced intracranial pressure from CSF leaks from spinal tap site or skull base/spinal surgery.

-Medications

i. Drug induced idiopathic intracranial hypertension syndromes (CN VI), See Chapter 35.2
ii. Chemotherapeutic drugs dependent on route given: intravenous chlorambucil and 5-fluorouracil can cause diplopia; intraarterial carboplatin and cisplatin can cause an orbital syndrome; and plant alkaloids have been reported to cause cranial neuropathies [19]. Including a III nerve paresis with vincristine.
iii. Posterior Reversible encephalopathy (PRES) is caused by certain Chemotherapeutic Agents as well as cyclosporine or tacrolimus and may rarely result in PRES involving the brainstem.
iv. Drug induced neuromuscular blocking effects and breaking down of phorias due to narcotics may be confused with a CN III, IV and VI process.

-Radiation/Chemotherapy effect CN III, IV, VI and neuromyotonia

-Secondary to Infection (from immunosuppression, surgery etc)

Orbital Cellulitis, Cavernous sinus thrombosis, Meningitis, Abscess, Epidural, Subdural empyema. Many organisms including bacteria (including listeria) and Fungus (Cryptococcosis, Aspergillosis, Fusarium, Candida, Mucor), Protozoa (Toxoplasmosis) and Viral (herpes zoster and HIV), TB and other infections.

III. Neoplasm related (indirect)

-Immune related

Paraneoplastic syndromes (involving brainstem)

-Hypercoagulable states

Venous sinus thrombosis syndromes (resulting in raised ICP from venous thrombosis of cerebral venous sinuses, and jugular veins), superior ophthalmic vein and cavernous sinus thrombosis resulting in more prominent CN III, IV VI and proptosis

29.3 CN III, IV, and VI Palsies due to Primary Cranial Nerve Neoplasms and Direct Extension from Primary Brain, Brain Stem, or Skull base Tumors

Primary cranial nerve neoplasms include schwannomas, which account for 85% of primary cranial nerve neoplasms, with neurofibromas, hemangiomas, and other, rare tumors accounting for the rest [1]. Schwannomas originate from the neural sheath and are most often benign, slow-growing tumors. Although the nerves most often affected are the vestibulocochlear, trigeminal, vagal, hypoglossal, and facial nerves, schwannomas may also affect CN III, IV, or VI. Neurofibromas are composed of axons, Schwann cells, and fibroblasts. Hemangiomas are rare lesions that do not often involve CN III, IV, and VI but most commonly affect the vestibulocochlear nerve–facial nerve and optic nerve–optic chiasm complexes.

Supratentorial brain lesions, if confined in this space, will normally not be associated with CN III, IV, or VI paresis unless there is raised ICP causing a false localizing VI nerve paresis. Similarly obstructive hydrocephalus from a supratentorial lesion as in the III ventricle can lead to increased intracranial pressure and CN VI paresis. If the tumor is associated with mass effect it could result in uncal herniation, which may be associated with an ipsilateral CN III paresis, which is usually but not always associated with alteration in consciousness.

Some supratentorial tumors straddle between the supratentorial space and the skull base/brainstem region (eg thalamic tumor and hypothalamic tumors). Thalamic tumors may grow into the infratentorial space by growing directly into the mesodiencephalon and be associated with CN III and IV paresis in addition to components of Parinauds syndrome. Hypothalamic tumors may grow in the suprasellar/retrosellar region and may reach CN III and IV via involvement of the cisterns around the midbrain as well as occasional involvement of the cavernous sinus region.

Infratentorial lesions, intraaxial lesions (e.g., gliomas) can lead to paresis of CN III, IV, and VI nerves and other associated signs.

Skull base tumors often result in cranial nerve involvement (see Chapter 30). Lesions in the petrous portion of the temporal bone and clivus most often manifest with cranial nerve VI palsy [2]. Chordomas are often found in this location and may cause bilateral cranial nerve VI palsies [3]. Sellar and parasellar lesions, such as pituitary tumors, meningiomas or craniopharyngiomas may be associated with neuropathies involving cranial nerves III, IV, V, and VI. Cavernous sinus lesions (e.g., meningiomas) may affect cranial nerves III and IV, the ophthalmic division of cranial nerve V, and cranial nerve VI.

29.4 CN III, IV, and VI Palsies due to Metastasis to the Brain, Brain, Stem and Skull Base from Distant Sites

Metastases to brain, brainstem and skull base result in CN palsies may also result in cranial neuropathies. The primary solid tumors that most commonly metastasize to the brain and brainstem include breast, lung, melanoma among others mentioned below. These later tumors may also metastasize to the skull base along with the following tumor types which may have a predilection to the skull base, including prostate,colon, renal, thyroid, lymphoma, leukemias, plasmacytoma, Ewings, osteosarcoma, neuroblastoma and others skull base are breast, lung, and prostate tumors [5, 6].

29.5 Cranial Nerve III, IV, and VI Palsies due to Head and Neck Cancers

Head and neck cancers may cause cranial nerve deficits either by direct extension into the orbit, cavernous sinus, or skull base or by perineural spread (see Chapter 30).

Direct extension of head and neck tumors into the orbit, cavernous sinus, or skull base may result in cranial nerve deficits. The head and neck tumor that most commonly causes cranial neuropathies is squamous cell carcinoma, which accounts for greater than 90% of head and neck cancers. Squamous cell carcinoma commonly affects the maxillary sinus, nasal cavity and ethmoid sinus as well as nasopharynx. Nasopharyngeal carcinoma, may invade the sphenoid sinus, cavernous sinus, clivus and orbit to cause and middle cranial fossa to cause palsies of cranial nerves II–VI [7]. The frequency of cranial nerve involvement in nasopharyngeal carcinoma is 8–29% and is an important prognostic factor [8–10]. Adenocarcinoma, sarcoma, melanoma, lymphoma, and adenoid cystic carcinoma are other head and neck tumors that can extend into the orbit or skull base and cause cranial neuropathies. Not infrequently the entire central skull base may be involved, including the cavernous sinus, sphenoid, and clivus, leading to these multiple nerve palsies.

Perineural spread from head and neck tumors is well documented and most commonly occurs with squamous cell carcinoma and adenoid cystic carcinoma [7, 11, 12]. Perineural spread most commonly involves cranial nerve V (all three divisions may be involved) and may be retrograde (toward the brain) or anterograde (toward the orbit) [1, 7, 12]. Most often the tumors that infiltrate small branches of V1 and V2 go retrograde and involve the cavernous sinus and therefore will present with cavernous sinus signs of III, IV, and VI and any combination of these. Tumors on V3 go retrograde to Meckels cave and continue on to the brain stem where CN VI paresis may occur most commonly. On the other hand, tumors on V3 once they reach Meckels cave may travel anterograde to involve the cavernous sinus. Cranial nerve VII is the second most common cranial nerve affected by perineural invasion [1]. Perineural spread of cutaneous neoplasms such as squamous cell carcinoma and desmoplastic melanoma may affect any branch of cranial nerve V, depending on the location of the malignancy. Perineural spread from mucosal tumors such as squamous cell carcinoma and adenoid cystic carcinoma of the salivary glands often affects the second (maxillary) and third (mandibular) branches of cranial nerve V [1, 7, 11, 12]. Nasopharyngeal tumors may spread via the pterygopalatine fossa to the maxillary branch of cranial nerve V [9] and from there go into the cavernous sinus and cause CN III, IV, or VI. Malignant primary and secondary parotid gland tumors may be associated with perineural spread along cranial nerve VII and the mandibular branch of cranial nerve V, the latter getting into Meckel's cave and leading to either brain stem or cavernous sinus involvement [1]. Perineural tumor extension is also seen in lymphoma, melanoma rhabdomyosarcoma, and malignant nerve sheath tumors [1].

29.6 Cranial Nerve III, IV, and VI Palsies due to Leptomeningeal Disease

Leptomeningeal disease is a common cause of deficits of cranial nerves III, IV and VI. These palsies may be extremely subtle such that one does not see a restriction in ductions, therefore they can only be measured in extremes of gaze. Other cranial neuropathies are common including II, V, VII, VIII as well as the lower CN. Leptomeningeal disease may occur with solid tumors, hematogenous tumors, or primary central nervous system tumors. Please see Chapter 32 for a more detailed discussion of the causes and management of leptomeningeal disease.

29.7 Other Causes of CN III, IV, and VI Palsies in Cancer Patients

Other causes of cranial III, IV and VI palsies in cancer patients include those related to intracranial pressure, medications due to various mechanisms, radiation/chemotherapy effects, infections of orbit and CNS as well as paraneoplastic and hypercoagulable states see Table 29.1 for more detail.

Intracranial hypertension may result from many mechanisms (see 29.3 above and Chapter 35.2). In the setting of raised ICP without an associated mass, this may cause a unilateral or bilateral cranial nerve VI palsy, leading to diplopia. In this scenario, cranial nerve VI palsy may be a false localization sign. Intracranial hypotension can also result in unilateral or bilateral CN VI paresis most commonly. This can be a result of spinal taps, skull base tumor repairs or spinal tumor repairs with CSF leaks.

Medications can cause CN III, IV, VI paresis by its effect on ICP, direct effects, evoking PRES. Medication effects may result in diplopia but not do to CN issues but rather neuromuscular blockade effects and other mechanisms described in Table 29.1.

Radiation therapy can cause cranial nerve palsies. Although optic nerve enhancement on T1-weighted MR imaging from radiation necrosis may occur, enhancement of cranial nerves III, IV, and VI is not described as a common finding from radiation necrosis [1, 13, 14]. A few cases of isolated cranial nerve deficits following radiation therapy have been reported. These include deficits of cranial nerves VI and XII. One study evaluating tolerance of cranial nerves III, IV, V, and VI following stereotactic radiosurgery for lesions within or near the cavernous sinus demonstrated new cranial neuropathies in 12 of 62 patients [15]. We have seen enhancement of CN III in a patient with radiation necrosis of adjacent temporal lobe after treatment of an aggressive pituitary adenoma. We have also seen a patient with a temporal lobe glioma treated with radiation and gliadel wafers plus develop CN III paresis and enhancement of this nerve. Both of these patients also developed concomitant neuromyotonia of CN III.

Cranial nerve III enhancement due to radiation necrosis along with evidence of cranial nerve palsy with or without ocular neuromyotonia [16]. Ocular neuromyotonia is characterized by brief episodes of diplopia secondary to persistent spasm of one or more extraocular muscles induced by sustained gaze in the field of action of the affected muscle. This condition has clearly been demonstrated following radiation therapy. It most commonly involves cranial nerve III but has also been reported to involve cranial nerve VI [17]. Most cases involve radiation therapy for parasellar and sellar tumors affecting cranial nerve III; cases may occur years after irradiation. In the cases reported to involve cranial nerve VI, radiation therapy was applied to tumors in areas other than the parasellar or sellar area [17]. A related syndrome of acquired oculomotor nerve paresis with cyclic spasms also occurs post-radiation [16]. Herein patients present with spasms of hyperactivity and hypoactivity of CN III.

Infections can also cause cranial neuropathies. Infections are common in patients with cancer because the cancer and its treatment can lead to immunodeficiency. Infections of the orbit, with or without cavernous sinus thrombosis, meningitis, abscesses, epidural or subdural empyema are all potential types of infections that may cause CN III, IV and VI paresis depending on the site of the lesion and mass effect. A number of these can occur endogenously, relate to sinus infections or relate to prior, surgical procedures on the brain, brainstem or skull base.

Paraneoplastic syndrome refers to dysfunction of the nervous system secondary to a neoplasm via mechanisms other than metastasis, infection, treatment side effects, or vascular consequence. Paraneoplastic syndromes may present with nystagmus, horizontal or vertical gaze palsies, skew deviation, cranial neuropathy, or other neurologic signs. Paraneoplastic cerebellar degeneration is most frequently associated with Hodgkin disease and cancers of the lung, ovary, and breast and has been associated with nystagmus, ocular dysmetria, saccadic pursuit, saccadic intrusions and oscillation, skew deviation, and cranial nerve VI palsies [18]. In paraneoplastic brain stem encephalitis, the patient may complain of diplopia and may have findings of vertical nystagmus, horizontal gaze paresis, internuclear ophthalmoplegia, skew deviation, and cranial nerve III, V, and VI palsies [18]. Paraneoplastic syndrome associated with testicular carcinoma may cause oculomotility defects that mimic CN III, IV, and VI paresis.

29.8 Conclusion

New onset of a cranial nerve III, IV, and VI paresis in a cancer patient demands particular attention to the mechanism of the palsy in order to guide management. Direct tumor involvement, from both primary CNS vs metastatic tumors of the brain, brain stem, skull base direct or perineural spread from head and neck cancer, leptomeningeal disease, and other conditions may result in cranial neuropathies.

References

1. Borges A Casselman J. Imaging the cranial nerves: part II: primary and secondary neoplastic conditions and neurovascular conflicts. Eur Radiol 2007;17(9):2332–44.

2. Ayberk G, Ozveren MF, Yildirim T, et al. Review of a series with abducens nerve palsy. Turk Neurosurg 2008;18(4):366–73.
3. St Martin M Levine SC. Chordomas of the skull base: manifestations and management. Curr Opin Otolaryngol Head Neck Surg 2003;11(5):324–7.
4. Sethi DS. Isolated sphenoid lesions: diagnosis and management. Otolaryngol Head Neck Surg 1999;120(5):730–6.
5. Hall SM Buzdar AU, Blumenschein GR. Cranial nerve palsies in metastatic breast cancer due to osseous metastasis without intracranial involvement. Cancer 1983;53(1):180–4.
6. Ransom DT, Dinapoli RP, Richardson RL. Cranial nerve lesions due to base of the skull metastases in prostate carcinoma. Cancer 1990;65(3):586–9.
7. Ginsberg LE. MR imaging of perineural tumor spread. Magn Reson Imaging Clin North Am 2002;10(3):511–25, vi.
8. Chang JT Lin CY, Chen TM, et al. Nasopharyngeal carcinoma with cranial nerve palsy: the importance of MRI for radiotherapy. Int J Radiat Oncol Biol Phys 2005;63(5):1354–60.
9. Li JC Mayr NA, Yuh WT, Wang JZ, Jiang GL. Cranial nerve involvement in nasopharyngeal carcinoma: response to radiotherapy and its clinical impact. Ann Otol Rhinol Laryngol 2006;115(5):340–5.
10. Liu L Liang S, Li L, et al. Prognostic impact of magnetic resonance imaging-detected cranial nerve involvement in nasopharyngeal carcinoma. Cancer 2009;115(9):1995–2003.
11. Nemec SF Herneth AM, Czerny C. Perineural tumor spread in malignant head and neck tumors. Top Magn Reson Imaging 2007;18(6):467–71.
12. Ojiri H. Perineural spread in head and neck malignancies. Radiat Med 2006;24(1):1–8.
13. Danesh-Meyer HV, Savino PJ, Sergott RC. Visual loss despite anticoagulation in radiation-induced optic neuropathy. Clin Exp Ophthalmol 2004;32(3):333–5.
14. Hudgins PA Newman NJ, Dillon WP, Hoffman JC, Jr. Radiation-induced optic neuropathy: characteristic appearances on gadolinium-enhanced MR. AJNR Am J Neuroradiol 1992;13(1):235–8.
15. Tishler RB, Loeffler JS, Lunsford LD, Duma C, Alexander E, 3rd, Kooy HM, Flickinger JC. Tolerance of cranial nerves of the cavernous sinus to radiosurgery. Int J Radiat Oncol Biol Phys 1993;27(2):215–21.
16. Miller NR, Lee AG. Adult-onset acquired oculomotor nerve paresis with cyclic spasms: relationship to ocular neuromyotonia. Am J Ophthalmol 2004;137(1):70–6.
17. Ela-Dalman N, Arnold AC, Chang LK, Velez FG, Lasky JL, 3rd. Abducens nerve ocular neuromyotonia following non-sellar or parasellar tumors. Strabismus 2007;15(3):149–51.
18. Ko MW, Dalmau J, Galetta SL. Neuro-ophthalmologic manifestations of paraneoplastic syndromes. J Neuroophthalmol 2008;28(1):58–68.
19. Schmid KE, Kornek GV, Scheithauer W, Binder S. Update on ocular complications of systemic cancer chemotherapy. Surv Ophthalmol 2006;51(1):19–40.

Chapter 30
Skull Base Tumors

Anitha Raghunath and Jade S. Schiffman

Abstract Ocular manifestations are not infrequent in the presence of skull base tumors because of the crucial visual and oculomotor pathways traversing the skull base. Because familiarity with the intricate skull base anatomy is imperative for accurately diagnosing and effectively managing skull base tumors, this chapter provides a description of the anatomy of the skull base and a discussion of imaging techniques. Numerous types of tumors and their neuro-ophthalmologic correlations are also discussed, including esthesioneuroblastomas, chordomas, craniopharyngiomas, meningiomas, sinonasal tumors, schwannomas, pituitary tumors, myelomas, paragangliomas, and metastases.

30.1 Introduction

Skull base tumors account for 25.2% of cranial neoplasms [1]. Ocular manifestations are common in the presence of skull base tumors because of the crucial visual and oculomotor pathways traversing the skull base. A primary tumor of the skull base can directly spread to the orbit or cause cranial neuropathies by compressing or infiltrating cranial nerves along their course. Visual sensory symptoms can be due to involvement of the visual apparatus in the orbit, optic canal, chiasm, or retrochiasmal pathway. Visual motor symptoms can be due to involvement of the orbit, superior orbital fissure, or cavernous sinus and/or subarachnoid involvement of cranial nerves III, IV, or VI. The skull base is also a frequent site of direct spread of periorbital tumors (e.g., tumors of sinonasal structures) through bony walls and foramina. Additionally, sinonasal tumors and masticator space tumors can be associated with indirect perineural spread along the trigeminal and facial nerve branches, which introduce these tumors from the sinuses, often through skull base foramen into the intracranial aspect of the skull base. Familiarity with the intricate skull base

A. Raghunath (✉)
Section of Ophthalmology, Department of Head and Neck Surgery, The University of Texas M.D. Anderson Cancer Center, Houston, TX, USA
e-mail: anitha.raghunath@gmail.com

B. Esmaeli (ed.), *Ophthalmic Oncology*, M.D. Anderson Solid Tumor Oncology Series 6, DOI 10.1007/978-1-4419-0374-7_30,

anatomy and interconnections with knowledge of the nuances of radiologic imaging are helpful for accurate diagnosis and multidisciplinary management of skull base tumors.

30.2 Anatomy of the Skull Base

The skull base is the floor of the cranial cavity on which the brain rests and is important in terms of the various foramina through which the nerves, vessels, and medulla–spinal cord junction pass. The skull base can be divided into anterior, middle, and posterior cranial fossae.

The anterior fossa is formed by the frontal bone, ethmoid bone, and body and lesser wing of the sphenoid bone. The cribriform plate (part of the ethmoid bone) allows passage of olfactory fila and ethmoidal vessels. The planum sphenoidale forms the posterior boundary of the anterior fossa.

The middle cranial fossa is formed mainly by the sphenoid bone and the temporal bone. The body of the sphenoid bone in the anteromedial aspect houses the optic canal and, laterally, the superior orbital fissures, which are formed between the lesser and greater wings of the sphenoid bone. The optic canal transmits the optic nerve, while the superior orbital fissure transmits cranial nerves III and IV; the ophthalmic division of cranial nerve V (V_1); cranial nerve VI; and the superior ophthalmic vein. The central portion of the middle fossa contains the sella turcica, which houses the pituitary gland and stalk; the parasellar region includes the cavernous sinuses, which contain the internal carotid artery and cranial nerves III and IV, the V_1 and V_2 (maxillary division) branches of cranial nerve V, and cranial nerve VI. Postganglionic sympathetic fibers traveling on the internal carotid artery transfer to V_1 within the cavernous sinus before entering the orbit. Inferomedial to the superior orbital fissure is the foramen rotundum, which transmits V_2 extracranially. Posterolateral to the foramen rotundum is the foramen ovale, which transmits the mandibular division (V_3) of the fifth cranial nerve.

The clivus forms the anterior portion of the posterior cranial fossa. The clivus is composed of the sphenoid bone and the occipital bone. The sphenoid sinus anteriorly and clivus posteriorly forms the sloped roof of the nasopharynx which lies below these structures.

The posterior cranial fossa contains the midbrain, pons, medulla, and cerebellum, which are important structures that contain the cranial nerve nuclei and their interconnections.

Some extracranial structures are extremely important in that disease within these locations can result in intracranial spread. The infratemporal fossa is an extracranial space that extends from the inferior orbital fissure anteriorly to the jugular foramen posteriorly. The pterygopalatine (also known as sphenopalatine) fossa is a deep recess bound anteriorly by the maxilla, medially by the palatine bone, and posteriorly by the pterygoid process. The lateral aspect of the pterygopalatine fossa connects with the pterygomaxillary fissure. Superior to the pterygopalatine fossa is the opening into the orbital apex through the inferior orbital fissure. This fossa contains the pterygopalatine ganglion, which is a major junction for the V_2 division passing from the foramen rotundum. The vidian canal also connects to the fossa inferomedial to the foramen rotundum and transmits the vidian nerve. Lateral to the pterygopalatine ganglion is the masticator space that contains V3.

30.3 Imaging and Diagnosis of Skull Base Tumors

The skull base is best evaluated by neuroimaging techniques. Computed tomography (CT) and magnetic resonance imaging (MRI) have complementary roles in evaluation of skull base tumors.

As the skull base is an undulating surface of limited thickness oriented in the axial plane, CT scans of the skull base must always include sections in at least two different planes and slices approximately 3 mm thick [2]. Use of iodinated contrast agent is necessary in most cases to delineate tumor margins and adjacent vascular structures. CT seems well suited for studying the bony skull base and the effect of the tumor on adjacent bone, which helps characterize a tumor's aggressive or benign nature [2].

MRI is useful in the study of intracranial tumors and intracranial spread and the detection of dural, leptomeningeal, and cranial nerve involvement. MRI can also discriminate between secretions and tumor in sinonasal cavities as well as depict bone marrow invasion [2–8]. T1-weighted images are best used for the depiction of bone marrow invasion. As bone marrow normally has high-intensity signal due to its fat content, invasion of the marrow is seen as low to intermediate signal intensity. To discriminate between tumor and retained secretions, it is best to use a combination of T1-weighted, T2-weighted, and contrast-enhanced T1-weighted sequences, as secretions do not enhance. For depicting meningeal invasion and perineural spread of the disease, gadolinium enhancement is essential [7–9]. Gadolinium-enhanced, fat-suppressed images are routinely used to detect enhancing tumors close to fat-containing spaces, such as the orbit, neurovascular channels and openings. This technique is also useful for the skull-based structures of the clivus and petrous bone where marrow with fat exists. Gadolinium-enhanced skull base imaging must be used with caution [10] because failure of fat suppression near bone–air or bone–fat interfaces may mimic tumor enhancement [11].

Positron emission tomography using fluorodeoxyglucose has proven useful in follow-up to differentiate between posttreatment changes and recurrence but not as useful in the primary evaluation of tumors.

Orbital invasion occurs most commonly through the lamina papyracea medially. If the tumor has not penetrated the periorbita, a smooth convex protrusion of the wall can be seen with fat separating this line from the medial rectus muscle, which allows sparing of the orbital contents during tumor resection. Orbital invasion may also occur when lesions in the maxillary sinus or pterygopalatine ganglion invade into the floor of the orbit or when frontal sinus or frontal lobe tumors invade through the roof of the orbit.

Less commonly, tumors invade the lateral aspect of the orbit. Tumors can also spread to the pterygopalatine fossa and retromaxillary fat through the posterior wall of the maxillary sinus or sphenopalatine foramen [2–5]. The pterygopalatine fossa also houses the pterygopalatine ganglion, which is a major junction for tumors spreading along the V_2 division of the fifth cranial nerve. Upward spread through the inferior orbital foramen allows tumors direct access to the inferior extraconal space and apex of the orbit. Certain malignant tumors transgressing and particularly those extending into the orbital apex may require orbital exenteration [10] because tumors in the orbital apex can easily spread into the middle cranial fossa. Additionally, sinonasal tumors that result in perineural spread may require orbital exenteration to prevent the tumor from reaching the intracranial structures, e.g., the cavernous sinus (V_1 and V_2) or gasserian ganglion (V_3). The floor of the anterior and middle cranial fossa, orbits, pterygopalatine fossa, and palate are critical areas of tumor extension that alter surgical and radiation treatments and thus should be given special attention [2–4].

30.4 Skull Base Tumors and Neuro-ophthalmic Correlations

30.4.1 Esthesioneuroblastoma

Esthesioneuroblastoma, also known as olfactory neuroblastoma, is an uncommon malignant tumor arising from the olfactory epithelium in the nasal cavity. It can grow superiorly to involve the anterior cranial fossa through the cribriform plate and the adjacent orbits laterally. Esthesioneuroblastoma has a peak incidence of presentation in the second to fifth decades, with a slightly higher preponderance in males [12]. However, this tumor has been reported in 1- and 2-year-old children who experienced sudden blindness in one eye [13]. Patients may present with general symptoms of nasal obstruction or congestion, epistaxis, anosmia, or headache; when orbital involvement occurs, patients may manifest diplopia, proptosis, epiphora, or blindness. Motility may be compromised, depending on the extent of orbital involvement. If the tumor has involved the anterior skull base, including the planum sphenoidale, the optic nerve can be compressed on one or both sides, giving rise to blindness and optic atrophy. Rarely, the tumor can also cause leptomeningeal disease, with raised intracranial pressure manifesting as papilledema.

CT and MRI are good techniques for delineating areas of intraorbital and intracranial spread. Esthesioneuroblastoma, like other neuroectodermal tumors, expresses somatostatin receptors; hence, octreotide radionuclide scanning can also be used for imaging [14]. Definitive diagnosis requires biopsy and immunohistochemical analysis of markers specific for tissues of neural origin, such as neuron-specific enolase, synaptophysin, and chromogranin [15].

Management of esthesioneuroblastoma includes anterior craniofacial surgery with partial orbital resection as indicated, followed by radiation therapy. Orbital exenteration may be required. Chemotherapy is generally used either as an induction therapy or combined with radiation therapy following surgery; chemotherapy is rarely used alone. Follow-up after definitive treatment is essential in managing postsurgical ocular motility defects as well as effects of chemotherapy and radiation therapy. Optic nerve injury can occur during surgery or as a result of radiation therapy. Radiation-induced optic neuropathy can be diagnosed by gadolinium enhancement of the affected nerve on gadolinium-enhanced MRI [16].

30.4.2 Chordoma

Chordoma is a slow-growing tumor of notochordal origin commonly found at either end of the axial skeleton—50% of chordomas are found at the sacrum and 35% at the clivus. Chordomas, which are known to recur and cause local invasion, are primarily extradural in origin, but dural invasion can occur. Chordomas can occur at any age, though one study reported a mean age at presentation of 46 years [17].

An intracranial chordoma is most often located in the clivus, where tumors can cause significant symptoms. As the tumor erodes through the bone, it can cause simultaneous or consecutive bilateral sixth cranial nerve palsies, compression of the brain stem, and affect structures in the cavernous sinus laterally. The tumor may grow antero-superiorly to cause chiasmal compression or pituitary disturbances [18]. It may even erode inferiorly through the sphenoid sinus and present as a nasopharyngeal mass or through the foramen magnum and present with late signs of long-tract palsy and palsies of cranial nerves VIII–XII. Metastasis of sacral chordoma to lungs, skin [19], and even to the orbit has been reported [20].

The most common symptom of chordoma is diplopia due to sixth nerve palsy; other symptoms include increasing in frequency or intensity the following: headaches, visual disturbances (including bitemporal hemianopsia), ataxia, and persistent pain [21]. Signs of ischemia may be seen in the brain stem due to basilar artery compression at the clivus [18]. When the tumor compresses the brain stem, several critical structures of the oculomotor pathway are affected including nuclei of cranial nerve VI and VII, the pontine paramedian reticular formation, and medial longitudinal fasciculus in the pons. When the cavernous sinus is involved, the third, fourth, fifth, and sixth cranial nerves can become involved by tumor, and when in this location, this usually is a contraindication to extensive surgery. The presence of diplopia in patients with chordoma was associated with longer survival [17], probably because of the earlier time of diagnosis as well as the anterior location of the tumor [21]. As this tumor often involves the bone, appropriate thin-cut CT scans through the skull base and contrast-enhanced dynamic MRI are useful [22].

The primary treatment for chordoma is surgical resection, which is often difficult and incomplete due to the location and involvement of adjacent critical structures. In patients with significant cavernous sinus involvement, an aggressive surgical approach is contraindicated because of the procedure's related morbidity [21]. New endoscopic approaches are achieving high rates of success and this approach may be less invasive compared with intracranial surgery [23, 24]. Different approaches for management of residual chordoma include stereotactic radiosurgery and proton beam (charged-particle) radiation therapy.

30.4.3 Craniopharyngioma

Craniopharyngiomas account for 2–4% of all intracranial tumors [25]. There is a bimodal incidence peak—tumors are most often diagnosed in patients 5- to 14-years-old and patients 50- to 60-years-old. The most common location for these tumors is the suprasellar region, where they grow from the squamous epithelium derived from the Rathke pouch on the undersurface of the brain. Craniopharyngiomas are mostly slow-growing tumors that are usually both calcified and cystic in nature. In children, craniopharyngiomas are the most common tumors in the suprasellar area (54% of suprasellar tumors in children are craniopharyngiomas); in adults, craniopharyngiomas are the second most common suprasellar tumor after pituitary adenoma [26].

Because of their close proximity to the optic nerves, optic chiasm, and optic tract, craniopharyngiomas cause compression of the visual apparatus leading to visual field defects in 40–70% of patients. The classical visual field defect caused by craniopharyngioma is bitemporal hemianopia or inferior bitemporal quadrantanopia. This may be accompanied by central scotoma if optic nerve compression is also present. Other presentations of craniopharyngioma include homonymous hemianopia, unilateral temporal field defects, generalized constriction, or normal fields. Pleomorphism (defined as change from one type of visual field defect to another) may occur with time. This has been attributed to intermittent emptying of cyst fluid into the ventricular system but may be a sign of recurrence, too [25, 27]. Improvement in visual fields following treatment is seen in one-third of patients [25].

The clinical presentation is usually insidious, and visual symptoms are often preceded by neuropsychological symptoms, headache, and/or endocrine dysfunction. In children, the extent of visual loss is often not appreciated until systemic symptoms become apparent. Blurred vision is the most common visual symptom, and headache is the most common systemic complaint. Headaches and visual disturbances are more common in children than in adults. Children under the age of 6 years presenting with visual symptoms have an unfavorable visual prognosis due to a late diagnosis [25]. Visual deterioration resulting in frequent falls may be attributed to clumsiness and ignored by parents. Headache may be due to raised intracranial pressure secondary to hydrocephalus or compression of sellar dura mater. About 66–90% of patients have some degree of endocrine dysfunction; hypothyroidism is the most common. Funduscopy demonstrates optic nerve involvement in the form of optic atrophy accompanied by relative afferent pupillary defect and deterioration in color vision. Papilledema is more common in children due to hydrocephalus [26]. Chiasmal compression may lead to bow–tie atrophy due to loss of nasal maculopapular bundle fibers and nasal retinal fibers. If raised intracranial pressure occurs following the presence of bow–tie atrophy, edema of the remaining fibers in the superior and inferior poles of the optic dis results in "twin-peak papilledema," [28]. Occasionally the tumor may start in the suprasellar region but grow posterior to the sella and down the brainstem leading to diplopia as well as other posterior fossa signs.

Neuroimaging by CT demonstrates a calcified cyst, a hallmark of craniopharyngioma. Contrast enhancement of the cyst helps delineate the lesion further. MRI is useful for defining the local anatomy, especially in adults (since calcification is less common in adults than in children), for surgical planning and long-term follow-up. Treatment consists of surgical resection with adjunctive radiation therapy. Children with hydrocephalus may require shunting also. The adamantinomatous type of craniopharyngioma occurs more frequently in children, while the squamous type occurs more frequently in adults; the squamous type of craniopharyngioma seems to be less aggressive and has a lesser incidence of visual field defects. Improvement in visual fields is seen following treatment in one-third of patients [25]. However, compared to pituitary adenoma, craniopharyngioma has a poorer visual outcome as a result of delayed diagnosis and long-standing compression of visual structures. Postoperative complications include hypopituitarism, seizures, and paresis of the third and fourth cranial nerves. Radiation therapy may result in visual field changes that may not be reflected on MRI. Recurrences of tumor occur more commonly in children, who may have more than one episode of recurrence, the mean period of 8 years [25]. Sometimes cystic recurrences are very difficult to treat. There has been few reports of injections within the cyst with agents as interferon with variable results. The duration of symptoms prior to recurrence may be as short as 2 weeks, and symptoms may be similar to those at the initial presentation; blurred vision is the most common symptom. Since the risk of local recurrence is high, MRI is useful for long-term monitoring, but detailed neuro-ophthalmic testing with visual fields is most important for early detection of recurrence [25].

30.4.4 Meningioma

Meningiomas are the most common nonglial primary intracranial tumors and are often discovered in adults in their fourth to sixth decades of life. The incidence is higher in older individuals, in African Americans, and in females (female to male ratio of 2:1) [29]. Ninety percent of all meningiomas occur in the supratentorial compartment, where the parasagittal region and over the convexity are the most common locations [29, 30]. The incidence of skull base meningiomas is 9.3%, according to the National Cancer Data Base (1985–1994) statistics. Meningiomas may be multiple and may be part of a familial autosomal-dominant inherited syndrome, neurofibromatosis type 2 and meningiomatosis [31–33]. Meningiomas originate from arachnoid cap cells commonly found in association with arachnoid villi at the dural venous sinuses and veins [30, 34]. About 1–2% of meningiomas arise from extradural sites, including primary intraosseous meningioma, which arises from the bone [35]. Treatment is determined primarily by the World Health Organization classification system, a three-tiered system comprised of three grades—meningioma, atypical meningioma, and anaplastic (malignant) meningioma [29].

About 90% of meningiomas are considered histologically benign; the remaining are considered atypical or malignant [36]. The major risk factor for developing meningioma, apart from increased age, is exposure to ionizing radiation, including therapeutic radiation therapy for head and neck neoplasia. The majority of asymptomatic meningiomas can be followed safely with serial brain imaging until the tumor either enlarges significantly or becomes symptomatic [37].

Clinical presentation of a meningioma depends on the tumor's location. Gradually evolving new-onset headache and an insidious personality change may lead to a long latency before the diagnosis is made and depicts the slow-growing nature of the tumor. Meningiomas may be associated with clinical syndromes of neuro-ophthalmic interest; depending on the size and location of the tumor, meningiomas in the posterior parasagittal region can cause homonymous hemianopia, and if there is impingement of the superior sagittal sinus, there may be raised intracranial pressure with papilledema; sphenoid wing tumors can cause visual loss, trigeminal dysfunction, and/or ophthalmoplegia; suprasellar tumors can cause bitemporal hemianopia and optic atrophy; and olfactory groove meningioma can cause Foster-Kennedy syndrome usually with loss of smell. Cavernous sinus meningiomas may result in proptosis, diplopia, or primary aberrant oculomotor regeneration [29, 30]. Skull base intraosseous meningiomas are usually slow growing and painless, with symptoms present for months to years prior to diagnosis. These symptoms can include cranial nerve deficits, ophthalmoplegia, visual field problems, proptosis (sometimes proptosis is present only as a result of hyperostosis of the orbital bones) and deformity [35].

Primary optic nerve sheath meningiomas (ONSMs) arise from the optic nerve sheath, intraorbital or intracanalicular optic nerve, or intracranial optic nerve. (Optic nerve tumors are covered in detail in Chapter 31.)

Secondary ONSM is an extension of intracranial meningioma into the orbit. Secondary ONSMs are much more common than primary ONSMs, but the unqualified term "optic nerve sheath meningioma" ordinarily refers to primary ONSM. ONSM is an important cause of visual loss [38]. Occasionally, bilateral or multifocal meningioma and meningiomatosis is seen, with neurofibromatosis type 2 and almost all of these patients also harbor bilateral acoustic neuromas.

Secondary ONSMs arise intracranially from the dura at locations other than the orbit, e.g., sphenoid bone (including the anterior clinoid), on or near the planum sphenoidale, olfactory groove, cavernous sinus, and other locations that spread toward the orbit and within the confines of the optic nerve sheath through the optic canal, compromising function by impairing blood supply to the nerve and interfering with axon transport [38]. The majority of secondary ONSMs are unilateral; however, bilateral cases may occur as a result of spread of a planum sphenoidale meningioma to both optic canals or of a unilateral secondary ONSM across the planum to the contralateral side. Similar to other meningiomas, all types of ONSMs are associated with neurofibromatosis type 2. The presenting feature is a slowly progressive optic neuropathy and variable visual loss, disturbances of color vision, visual field defects, pain, double vision, and transient visual obscuration, which is almost always associated with optic disc swelling [38]. The triad of visual loss, optic atrophy, and optociliary shunts is almost pathognomonic for ONSM, though this may occur late in the course [39].

Both CT and MRI with contrast are useful for imaging of meningioma. Precontrast CT is superior in detecting calcification within the tumor, which is said to indicate slow growth and adjacent hyperostotic bone changes [40, 41]. MRI is better for detecting intracanalicular ONSM because of the absence of bone signal [41]. MRI is superior in determining if cavernous sinus meningiomas are entering the orbit through the superior orbital fissue/orbital apex. MRI is superior than CAT scan in determining if a optic nerve meningioma is primary or secondary because of the finer detail that can be seen with MRI in the region of the planum, anterior clinioid, optic canal, orbital apex region.

30.4.5 Sinonasal and Nasopharyngeal Tumors

Tumors that involve the paranasal sinuses, nasal cavity, and nasopharynx are often clinically silent at early stages and, thus, at diagnosis may involve a wide area of the adjacent skull base vital structures. Paranasal sinus tumors are most frequently located in the maxillary sinuses, whereas nasal cavity tumors most often arise from the nasal septum [42]. Maxillary sinus spreads through the roof into the inferior orbit, through the posterior wall into the pterygopalatine fossa, and upward through the inferior orbital fissure to the orbital apex or posterolaterally into the infratemporal fossa. Tumors in the ethmoid sinuses can spread laterally into the medial orbit through the thin lamina papyracea. Frontal sinuses antero-superiorly and the sphenoid sinus postero-superiorly have only a bony wall separating them from the orbit, and this bony wall can be breached by tumor spread. Sphenoid body tumors can compress the optic nerve in the canal during expansion in a medial direction.

Nasopharyngeal carcinoma (NPC) is usually a squamous cell carcinoma that arises from the epithelium and, in some populations, is related to Epstein–Barr virus. NPC frequently arises behind the medial crura of the eustachian tube opening (Rosenmueller fossa) in the nasopharynx and may extend laterally into the parapharyngeal space through the sinus of Morgagni, a natural defect in the lateral wall. The nasopharynx is surrounded posteriorly and laterally by a tough pharyngobasilar fascia that can occasionally be invaded by NPC to involve the clivus. The skull base can be destroyed by superior extension of NPC into the sphenoid sinus or cavernous sinus or lateral extension into the foramen ovale and/or foramen lacerum [42].

Sinonasal tumors and NPC often present with vague symptoms, and affected patients are frequently treated for sinusitis or other maladies before a suspicion of cancer arises. Patients may have unilateral nasal obstruction with a blood-tinged discharge, auditory tube dysfunction with conductive deafness and tinnitus, or, more commonly, painless neck masses due to lymph node involvement. Patients with NPC quite frequently have advanced disease at the time of diagnosis [42].

Patients with sinonasal tumors and NPC may present with ophthalmic symptoms at onset or during the course of the disease because of the proximity of these tumors to the orbit and their ability to spread perineurally. Diplopia is a common complaint due to either direct orbital spread or indirect perineural spread along trigeminal nerve branches, involving the skull base and intracranial cavity, including the cavernous sinus. Perineural spread may be both retrograde (toward the brain) and antegrade (toward the face) (Figs. 30.1 and 30.2). Patients often have complaints of unilateral paresthesia or hypesthesia along the distribution of the fifth cranial nerve because of perineural spread. Blurring of vision, visual field defects, and, rarely, blindness may occur because of compromise of the optic nerve in the orbital apex or optic canal as a result of tumor spread. Orbital apex involvement can occur because of tumor spread via the inferior orbital fissure upward or in an anterograde manner from the cavernous sinus through the superior orbital fissure. The patient may have involvement of some or all branches of cranial nerves III, IV, and VI with varying ocular motility manifestations. Intractable headache may be seen when the skull base or dura is involved as well as when the trigeminal nerve is infiltrated. Extensive involvement of the orbit may necessitate orbital exenteration or may be considered inoperable if the lesion has progressed to the cavernous sinus.

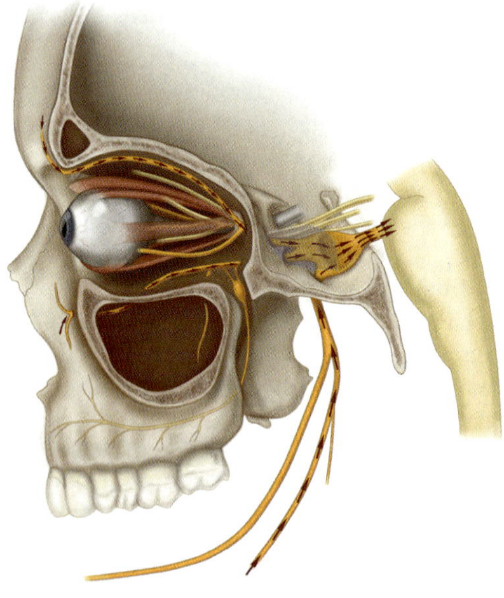

Fig. 30.1 Retrograde routes of perineural spread along V_1, V_2, or V_3 branches of cranial nerve V from the periphery to the brain stem

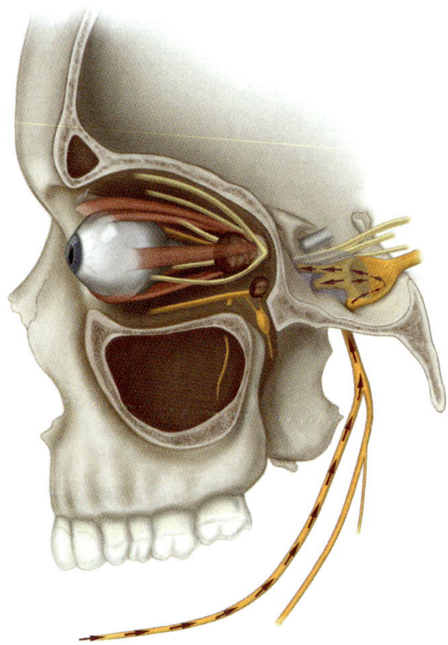

Fig. 30.2 Antegrade perineural spread tracking anteriorly from the Meckel cave through the cavernous sinus en route to the orbit

CT and MRI are complimentary for the diagnosis of sinonasal and NPC. Skull base erosion is more easily appreciated on CT scan, while perineural spread is better delineated on MRI, which is also more effective in monitoring recurrence. Positron emission tomography is used to detect distant metastasis [42].

30.4.6 Schwannoma

Schwannomas are benign tumors of the cranial nerves and account for 8% of primary brain tumors. Schwannomas can arise from any of the cranial nerves except the optic nerves, which lack Schwann cells, and rarely in the olfactory nerve (see below). Schwannomas arise most commonly from the vestibular division of the eighth nerve, followed by the trigeminal nerve sheath, facial nerves, and lower cranial nerves [43]. Schwannomas are more common in females in most anatomic locations. Vestibular tumors are usually isolated, but approximately 5% are associated with neurofibromatosis, mainly type 2. Patients with neurofibromatosis type 2 have bilateral tumors in more than 90% of cases [43]. Trigeminal schwannomas are rare, accounting for only 2–3% of intracranial schwannomas [44]. Trigeminal schwannomas can arise from the trigeminal nerve root, gasserian ganglion, or one of the three peripheral branches and may have a complicated pattern in the middle cranial fossae. They have also been found in the infratemporal fossa and orbit [45]. Though rare, a few cases of olfactory groove schwannomas have been reported in young males. The origin of these tumors is not known, but theories have pointed to embryonic terminal nerves, peripheral nerves in close proximity, such as the anterior ethmoidal nerve, or ectopic foci of Schwann cells [44]. Vidian nerve schwannoma is very rare and located in the retromaxillary space. It can grow silently and become extremely large by the time symptoms present and the diagnosis is made [46].

Jugular foramen schwannomas can arise from any of the lower cranial nerves and pass through the jugular foramen and identification of the involved nerve is often difficult. The tumor may be predominantly intracranial, predominantly extracranial, both intracranial and extracranial, or located mainly in the canal [43]. In a study of 53 patients with jugular foramen schwannomas, the most common deficits observed were deficits of the vagus nerve, followed by deficits of the vestibular/cochlear nerve and glossopharyngeal nerve. In vestibular schwannomas as well as other prepontine schwannomas, the lesions grow toward the cerebello-pontine angle, and the facial–acoustic complex is affected early, manifesting as hearing loss that may be followed by hoarseness and absence of the gag reflex [47]. On examination, absent corneal reflex, nystagmus, sensorineural deafness, and cerebellar signs, such as ataxia and pyramidal tract involvement in the form of hemiparesis, may be seen due to distortion of the brain stem. Patients rarely display facial weakness even when a schwannoma is closely associated with the seventh nerve [43].

Motor nerve schwannomas of the third, fourth, sixth, and twelfth cranial nerves are rare and have a long duration of symptoms [48]. Patients may present with headache, nausea, and vomiting due to raised intracranial pressure and diplopia. Neuro-ophthalmic examination may reveal anisocoria, ptosis, and papilledema. Other complaints may include facial numbness or burning pain, dysphagia and dysarthria, tinnitus, numbness of the tongue, and taste disturbance due to involvement of lower cranial nerves. These symptoms may be accompanied by findings of hemiparesis, hemianesthesia, dysmetria, and ataxia, indicating long tract as well as cerebellar compression [49]. Occasionally, pathological laughter and aggressive behavior have been described with fourth cranial nerve palsy [48, 50, 51]. In the case of lesions traversing the base of skull foramina, CT may reveal enlargement of foramina, and T1-weighted MRI may show isointense lesions with dense enhancement after contrast administration [52].

30.4.7 Pituitary Tumors

Pituitary tumors are usually benign neoplasms located in the sella turcica and are the third most common primary intracranial neoplasm, accounting for 9.5% of primary intracranial neoplasms (Central Brain Tumor Registry of the United States, 2007). Nonfunctional pituitary adenomas occur more frequently than hormone-secreting adenomas, namely, prolactin-secreting and growth hormone-secreting adenomas. Compared with their hormone-secreting counterparts, the nonfunctional pituitary adenomas go undetected for a longer time since there are no alerting symptoms and grow to larger sizes before becoming symptomatic due to compression of normal pituicytes or visual disturbances. Patients with pituitary tumors may present with hormonal disturbances (either under- or over-secretion), headache, or gradual visual disturbances. However, the extent of visual loss may not correlate with the duration of symptoms as patients may not notice a gradual loss of peripheral vision. Visual field defects were found in half of the patients with a histologically proven pituitary tumor. Bitemporal hemianopia was the most common visual defect (seen in 17.2% of patients) [53]. Visual loss in patients with pituitary tumors occurs as a result of long-standing compression of the adjacent visual apparatus due to suprasellar extension of the tumor [53]. Compression of the optic chiasm gives rise to bitemporal hemianopia. If the chiasm is prefixed, the patient may manifest with signs of optic tract compression; if the chiasm is postfixed, the patient may present with signs of optic nerve compression. Optic tract compression causes homonymous field defects, and optic nerve compression causes optic nerve visual field defects. Patients may have a compressive optic neuropathy, causing visual acuity to be affected. Additionally, if the patient has significant chiasmal compression, affecting not only the nasal crossing fibers but also the temporal fibers that do not cross, vision can be compromised in both eyes [53]. Diplopia occurs by involvement of one or both cavernous sinuses when the tumor expands laterally through the dura. Third to sixth cranial nerve dysfunction may be a sign of tumor growth, tumor recurrence, or pituitary apoplexy.

Pituitary apoplexy refers to a sudden expansion in intrasellar contents that results in a sudden expansion of the mass. This is usually due to hemorrhage or infarction of a preexisting adenoma but has also been reported, rarely, in the normal pituitary gland in pregnancy [54]. In 60–80% of cases, pituitary apoplexy is the first presentation of a pituitary tumor, which can be misdiagnosed as meningitis or a subarachnoid hemorrhage because of its abrupt onset and similar signs. Precipitating factors for apoplexy have been reported in 25–30% of cases, such as closed-head trauma, hypotension, hypertension, anticoagulant therapy, and use of dopamine agonists [54–57]. Though more common in nonfunctional pituitary adenomas all types of pituitary adenomas are at risk of apoplexy.

Headache is the most consistent symptom of pituitary apoplexy; headache in such cases is sudden and severe; can be retro-orbital, frontal, or occipital; and is often accompanied by nausea or vomiting [54]. Patients can also manifest with sudden onset or worsening of visual field defects and partial or total loss of vision due to upward compression of the optic structures. Ophthalmoplegia, Horner syndrome, or stroke may be seen due to compression of cranial nerves, the sympathetic branch, or the internal carotid artery within the cavernous sinus. These features help differentiate pituitary apoplexy from meningitis or aneurysmal rupture, wherein fever and meningismus develop fairly early. Hypopituitarism, usually that of the anterior pituitary hormones, often results in significant morbidity and mortality, especially adrenocorticotropic hormone deficiency that leads to acute adrenal insufficiency [54]. It is important to perform visual acuity and visual field examinations as early as possible if the patient is alert, and changes should be monitored regularly. Cerebrospinal fluid studies are not conclusive. MRI is the technique of choice, particularly in determining optic apparatus or cavernous sinus extension. It is also much more useful in subacute or chronic stages of gland hemorrhage for which a CT scan is less specific. It is important to keep a high level of suspicion for pituitary apoplexy when a patient has new onset of diplopia or visual field defects even with negative CT findings, as CT is usually the first modality used in emergency rooms. It would also be helpful to obtain pituitary hormone levels to confirm the diagnosis as low levels are corroborative. If an aneurysm cannot be excluded, computed tomography angiography, magnetic resonance angiography, or conventional angiography are helpful [54, 58]. Prompt diagnosis of an acute case vastly improves the prognosis when the condition is managed with corticosteroid administration, supportive hemodynamic measures, or urgent surgical management. Immediate surgical decompression is mandatory when vision loss is severe, as the rapid loss of vision, if not promptly reversed, can result in irreversible changes. Conservative measures, such as steroid administration, have also been reported to be helpful in visual and neurologic recovery in less symptomatic, stable patients [54].

30.4.8 Myeloma

Plasma cell myeloma encompasses a wide spectrum of tumors, ranging from benign solitary plasmacytoma to extremely malignant multiple myeloma [59]. Multiple myeloma is a rare cause of mass lesions at the skull base and cavernous sinus; a study of 273 cases of multiple myeloma revealed that only 3% of patients had cranial or intracranial tumors [60]. Sixth nerve palsy, in isolation or in combination with other cranial neuropathies, may be the initial presenting feature of multiple myeloma; however, this presentation is rare [61, 62]. Clival lesions may cause unilateral or bilateral compression of the sixth cranial nerve [61], while a combination of cranial neuropathies occurs with involvement of the cavernous sinus, sphenoid sinus, or orbital apex [63]. Rarely, plasma cell tumors in the intrasellar area can present with symptoms and signs indistinguishable from those of nonfunctioning adenoma. Fourteen patients with pituitary area plasmacytomas have been described, with the most common presenting symptoms being headache, diplopia, and visual loss (in that order). Cranial nerve involvement (seen in 12 of the 14 patients) can present with atypical symptoms that should arouse suspicion, including sensorineural deafness, visual loss, or unexpected preservation of anterior pituitary function. CT or MRI is helpful in the diagnosis of skull base myeloma, which is seen as an extracranial or intracranial mass with homogeneous enhancement, smooth margins, and bone remodeling [64].

30.4.9 Paraganglioma

Paragangliomas are a group of tumors that arise from extra-adrenal neural crest derivatives and are similar to pheochromocytomas. Paragangliomas can arise in various locations of sympathetic chain ganglia. Among the skull base paragangliomas, carotid body tumors are the most common, accounting for 60% of all lesions [42]. Paragangliomas may also present as part of the multiple endocrine neoplasia syndrome. The presence of such tumors at the carotid bifurcation may give rise to Horner syndrome [65]. Glomus jugulare tumors involve the jugular bulb and tympanic cavity. These tumors often involve the lower cranial nerves in the vicinity; massive tumors may cause raised intracranial tension due to pressure on the outflow tract and can manifest with transient obscuration of vision with papilledema [66, 67]. Arterial hypertension may be seen because of the capacity of these tumors to secrete catecholamines. In cases of late diagnosis, chronic hypertension may give rise to hypertensive retinopathy findings and, occasionally, loss of vision in the case of malignant hypertension [68]. Paragangliomas can also be found in the sellar and parasellar regions; when these regions are affected, visual symptoms may include oculomotor paresis with or without endocrine dysfunction [69, 70]. Orbital paragangliomas are extremely rare and present with proptosis, papilledema, and loss of vision [71]. They may extend to the middle skull base and may be mistaken for the more common meningioma [72]. Imaging of paragangliomas can be done with either MRI or CT, and the diagnosis is confirmed by histology and immunohistochemistry [42].

30.4.10 Metastases

The skull base is a common site of bone metastasis. Bone metastasis has been reported to occur in about 4% of cancer patients, and the primary tumors that most frequently metastasize to bone are breast (40%), lung (14%), and prostate (12–38%) [73, 74]. Metastasis to the skull base may also occur in colon, renal, or thyroid cancers, lymphoma, melanoma, and neuroblastoma. Skull base metastasis usually occurs late in the course of cancer, and the complicated anatomy of the skull base makes accurate interpretation of imaging difficult. The diagnosis is even more difficult when the skull base metastasis is the first sign of cancer, which occurred in 28% of patients in one review [73]. Most skull base metastases are due to hematogenous spread. Clinical manifestations of skull base metastases have been classified into five clinical syndromes—orbital (7%), parasellar and sellar (29%), middle fossa (35%), jugular foramen (16%), and occipital condyle [74]. However, another presentation includes the "hemibasis syndrome" or Garcin syndrome, which is characterized by progressive ipsilateral paralysis of the cranial nerves in the absence of raised intracranial pressure or other neurological signs [75]. In the orbital syndrome, frontal headache, diplopia, blurred vision, first-division trigeminal sensory loss, and proptosis may be seen. Parasellar syndrome is due to metastases in the cavernous sinus, a common site for lymphoma metastases that affects oculomotor function as well as divisions of the fifth cranial nerves [76]. Sellar metastases in the pituitary gland have been noted to cause diabetes insipidus, occurring more commonly than anterior hypopituitarism or visual loss [77]. Middle fossa involvement includes the gasserian ganglion, which involves the second and third divisions of the trigeminal nerve, and gives rise to sensory as well as motor weakness [73]. The sixth nerve may be involved with petrous ridge spread. Jugular foramen and occipital condyle metastases manifest with neuralgia and paralysis of lower cranial nerves IX–XII. Rarely, the jugular vein or transverse sinus may get compressed, giving rise to syncope or papilledema due to raised intracranial pressure.

MRI with and without gadolinium administration is the best method to detect skull base metastases [78, 79]. On MRI without gadolinium administration, bone metastases typically appear as substitution of the usual hyperintense fat signal by a hypointense lesion; with gadolinium administration, variable enhancement is typically seen. Imaging of suspected lytic lesions is better on CT with bone windows and orbital views [80]. The prognosis when skull base metastasis occurs is generally poor because of the late stage of disease; the longest survival has been seen in breast carcinoma (60 months) and shortest in colon carcinoma (1.5 months) [73]. Symptomatic relief and improvement in cranial neuropathies may be seen with early radiation therapy, which is the standard treatment for skull base metastases; radiation treatment may be complemented with surgery, chemotherapy, or radiosurgery.

References

1. Davis FG, McCarthy BJ, Berger MS. Centralized databases available for describing primary brain tumor incidence, survival, and treatment: Central Brain Tumor Registry of the United States; Surveillance, Epidemiology, and End Results; and National Cancer Database. Neuro Oncol 1999;1(3):205–11.
2. Durden DD, Williams DWI. Radiology of skull base neoplasms. Otolaryngol Clin North Am 2001;34(6):1043–64.
3. Atlas SW. Magnetic Resonance Imaging of the Brain and Spine, Vol 2, third edition. Baltimore, MD: Lippincott Williams & Wilkins, 2002.
4. Som PM, Curtin HD. Head and Neck Imaging, fourth edition. St Louis, MO: Mosby, 2003.
5. Lufkin R, Borges A, Villablanca P. Teaching Atlas of Head and Neck Imaging, first edition. New York, NY: Thieme, 2000.
6. Chong VF, Fan YF, Tng CH. Pictorial review: radiology of the sphenoid bone. Clin Radiol 1998;53(12):882–93.
7. Fischbein NJ, Kaplan MJ. Magnetic resonance imaging of the central skull base. Top Magn Reson Imaging 1999;10(5):325–46.
8. Tomura, Hirano H, Sashi R, et al. Comparison of MR imaging and CT in discriminating tumor infiltration of bone and bone marrow in the skull base. Comput Med Imaging Graph 1998;22(1):41–51.
9. Williams L. Advanced concepts in the imaging of perineural spread of tumor to the trigeminal nerve. Topics Magn Reson Imaging 1999;10(6):376–83.
10. Borges A, Casselman J. Skull base tumours part I: imaging technique, anatomy, and anterior skull base tumours. Eur J Radiol 2008;66(3):338–47.
11. Borges AR, Lufkin RB, Huang AY, Farahani K, Arnold AC. Frequency-selective fat suppression MR imaging. Localized asymmetric failure of fat suppression mimicking orbital disease. J Neuroophthalmol 1997;17(1):12–7.
12. DeAngelis L. Current diagnosis and treatment of leptomeningeal metastasis. J Neurooncol 1998;38:245–52.
13. de Champs C, Demeocq F, Merie P, et al. Olfactory neuroblastoma disclosed by blindness in a 9-month-old girl [in French]. Arch Fr Pediatr 1985;42(2):119–21.

14. Ramsay HA, Kairemo KJ, Jekunen AP. Somatostatin receptor imaging of olfactory neuroblastoma. J Laryngol Otol 1996;110(12):1161–3.
15. DeAngelis LM, Gutin PH, Leibel SA, Posner JB. Intracranial Tumors: Diagnosis and Treatment, first edition. London, UK: Martin Dunitz, 2002.
16. Guy J, Mancuso A, Beck R, Moster ML, Sedwick LA, Quisling RG, Rhoton AL, Jr., Protzko EE, Schiffman J. Radiation-induced optic neuropathy: a magnetic resonance imaging study. J Neurosurg 1991;74(3):426–32.
17. Forsyth PA, Cascino TL, Shaw EG, Scheithauer BW, O'Fallon JR, Dozier JC, Piepgras DG. Intracranial chordomas: a clinicopathological and prognostic study of 51 cases. J Neurosurg 1993;78(5):741–7.
18. Miller SJ. Ocular signs of chordomas. Proc R Soc Med 1972;65(6):522–3.
19. Agrawal PP, Bahadur AK, Mohanta PK, et al. Chordoma: 6 years' experience at a tertiary centre. Australas Radiol 2006;50(3):201–5.
20. Konuk O, Pehlivanli Z, Yirmibesoglu E, Erkal HS, Erekul S, Unal M. Compressive optic neuropathy due to orbital metastasis of a sacral chordoma: case report. Ophthal Plast Reconstr Surg 2005;21(3):245–7.
21. Lanzino G, Dumont AS, Lopes MB, Laws ER, Jr. Skull base chordomas: overview of disease, management options, and outcome. Neurosurg Focus 2001;10(3):E12.
22. Ikushima I, Korogi Y, Hirai T, Hamatake S, Takahashi M, Ushio Y. Chordomas of the skull base: dynamic MRI. J Comput Assist Tomogr 1996;20(4):547–50.
23. Dehdashti AR, Karabatsou K, Ganna A, Witterick I, Gentili F. Expanded endoscopic endonasal approach for treatment of clival chordomas: early results in 12 patients. Neurosurgery 2008;63(2):299–307; discussion 307–309.
24. Hong Jiang W, Ping Zhao S, Hai Xie Z, Zhang H, Zhang J, Yun Xiao J. Endoscopic resection of chordomas in different clival regions. Acta Otolaryngol 2009;129(1):71–83.
25. Chen C, Okera S, Davies PE, Selva D, Crompton JL. Craniopharyngioma: a review of long-term visual outcome. Clin Exp Ophthalmol 2003;31(3):220–8.
26. Repka MX, Miller NR, Miller M. Visual outcome after surgical removal of craniopharyngiomas. Ophthalmology 1989;96(2):195–9.
27. Kennedy HB, Smith RJ. Eye signs in craniopharyngioma. Br J Ophthalmol 1975;59(12):689–95.
28. Paul TO, Hoyt WF. Funduscopic appearance of papilledema with optic tract atrophy. Arch Ophthalmol 1976;94(3):467–8.
29. Rockhill J, Mrugala M, Chamberlain MC. Intracranial meningiomas: an overview of diagnosis and treatment. Neurosurg Focus 2007;23(4):E1.
30. De Monte F. Current management of meningiomas. Oncology (Williston Park) 1995;9(1). 83–91, 96.
31. Antinheimo J, Sankila R, Carpen O, Pukkala E, Sainio M, Jaaskelainen J. Population-based analysis of sporadic and type 2 neurofibromatosis-associated meningiomas and schwannomas. Neurology 2000;54(1):71–6.
32. Gutmann DH, Aylsworth A, Carey JC, Korf B, Marks J, Pyeritz RE, Rubenstein A, Viskochil D. The diagnostic evaluation and multidisciplinary management of neurofibromatosis 1 and neurofibromatosis 2. JAMA 1997;278(1):51–7.
33. King A, Gutmann DH. The question of familial meningiomas and schwannomas: NF2B or not to be? Neurology 2000;54(1):4–5.
34. Wilson CB. Meningiomas: genetics, malignancy, and the role of radiation in induction and treatment. The Richard C. Schneider Lecture. J Neurosurg 1994;81(5):666–75.
35. Elder JB, Atkinson R, Zee CS, et al. Primary intraosseous meningioma. Neurosurg Focus 2007;23(4):E13.
36. Barnholtz-Sloan JS, Kruchko C. Meningiomas: causes and risk factors. Neurosurg Focus 2007;23(4):E2.
37. Olivero WC, Lister JR, Elwood PW. The natural history and growth rate of asymptomatic meningiomas: a review of 60 patients. J Neurosurg 1995;83(2):222–4.

38. Berman DM, Miller NR. New concepts in the management of optic nerve sheath meningiomas. Ann Acad Med Singapore 2006;35(3):168–74.
39. Hollenhorst RW Jr, Hollenhorst RW Sr, MacCarty CS. Visual prognosis of optic nerve sheath meningiomas producing shunt vessels on the optic disk: the Hoyt-Spencer syndrome. Trans Am Ophthalmol Soc 1977;75:141–63.
40. Saeed P, Rootman J, Nugent RA, et al. Optic nerve sheath meningiomas. Ophthalmology 2003;110(10):2019–30.
41. Moster ML. Detection and treatment of optic nerve sheath meningioma. Curr Neurol Neurosci Rep 2005;5(5):367–75.
42. Hao SP, Ngan MT, Kupferman ME. Nasopharyngeal carcinoma. In: Practical Head and Neck Oncology. Petruzzelli GJ, editor. San Diego, CA: Plural Publishing, 2009:640.
43. DeMonte F, Gilbert MR, Mahajan A, McCutcheon IE. Tumors of the Brain and Spine, first edition. New York, NY: Springer, 2007.
44. Sabel LH, Teepen JL. The enigmatic origin of olfactory schwannoma. Clin Neurol Neurosurg 1995;97(2):187–91.
45. Zhang L, Yang Y, Xu S, Wang J, Liu Y, Zhu S. Trigeminal schwannomas: a report of 42 cases and review of the relevant surgical approaches. Clin Neurol Neurosurg 2009;111(3):261–9.
46. Honda K, Asato R, Tanaka S, Endo T, Nishimura K, Ito J. Vidian nerve schwannoma with middle cranial fossa extension resected via a maxillary swing approach. Head Neck 2008;30(10):1389–93.
47. Zhao H, Li X, Lv Q, Yuan Y, Yu H. A large dumbbell glossopharyngeal schwannoma involving the vagus nerve: a case report and review of the literature. J Med Case Reports 2008;2:334.
48. Ohba S, Miwa T, Kawase T. Trochlear nerve schwannoma with intratumoral hemorrhage: case report. Neurosurgery 2006;58(4):E791; discussion E791.
49. Boggan JE, Rosenblum ML, Wilson CB. Neurilemmoma of the fourth cranial nerve. Case report. J Neurosurg 1979;50(4):519–21.
50. Nadkarni TD, Goel A. Trochlear nerve neurinoma presenting as pathological laughter. Br J Neurosurg 1999;13(2):212–3.
51. Shenouda EF, Ghosh A, Coakham HB. Trochlear nerve schwannoma removed by combined petrosal approach. Br J Neurosurg 2002;16(6):600–4.
52. Bulsara KR, Sameshima T, Friedman AH, Fukushima T. Microsurgical management of 53 jugular foramen schwannomas: lessons learned incorporated into a modified grading system. J Neurosurg 2008;109(5):794–803.
53. Wang H, Sun W, Fu Z, Si Z, Zhu Y, Zhai G, Zhao G, Xu S, Pang Q. The pattern of visual impairment in patients with pituitary adenoma. J Int Med Res 2008;36(5):1064–9.
54. Nawar RN, AbdelMannan D, Selman WR, Arafah BM. Pituitary tumor apoplexy: a review. J Intensive Care Med 2008;23(2):75–90.
55. Randeva HS, Schoebel J, Byrne J, Esiri M, Adams CB, Wass JA. Classical pituitary apoplexy: clinical features, management and outcome. Clin Endocrinol 1999;51(2):181–8.
56. Knoepfelmacher M, Gomes MC, Melo ME, Mendonca BB. Pituitary apoplexy during therapy with cabergoline in an adolescent male with prolactin-secreting macroadenoma. Pituitary 2004;7(2):83–7.
57. Nagarajan DV, Bird D, Papouchado M. Pituitary apoplexy following anticoagulation for acute coronary syndrome. Heart 2003;89(1):10.
58. Semple PL, Webb MK, de Villiers JC, Laws ER, Jr. Pituitary apoplexy. Neurosurgery 2005;56(1):65–72; discussion 72–73.
59. Higurashi M, Yagishita S, Fujitsu K, Kitsuta Y, Takemoto Y, Osano S. Plasma cell myeloma of the skull base: report of two cases. Brain Tumor Pathol 2004;21(3):135–41.

60. Silverstein A, Doniger DE. Neurologic complications of myelomatosis. Arch Neurol 1963;9:534–44.
61. Kanemura N, Tsurumi H, Hara T, Yamada T, Sawada M, Moriwaki H. [Multiple myeloma complicated by bilateral abducens nerve palsy due to a tumor in the clivus]. Rinsho Ketsueki 2001;42(3):218–20.
62. Movsas TZ, Balcer LJ, Eggenberger ER, Hess JL, Galetta SL. Sixth nerve palsy as a presenting sign of intracranial plasmacytoma and multiple myeloma. J Neuroophthalmol 2000;20(4):242–5.
63. Miyazaki T, Taguchi J, Obana T, Yamaji S, Koharazawa H, Fujimaki K, Kanamori H, Ishigatsubo Y. [Multiple myeloma presenting as cavernous sinus syndrome]. Rinsho Ketsueki 2006;47(10):1393–5.
64. Willinsky RA, Cooper PW, Kassel EE. CT of myeloma involving the skull base. J Can Assoc Radiol 1985;36(4):328–31.
65. Moyer JS, Bradford CR. Sympathetic paraganglioma as an unusual cause of Horner's syndrome. Head Neck 2001;23(4):338–42.
66. Angeli SI, Sato Y, Gantz BJ. Glomus jugulare tumors masquerading as benign intracranial hypertension. Arch Otolaryngol Head Neck Surg 1994;120(11):1277–80.
67. Hierons R, Meadows SP. Glomus jugulare tumour presenting with papilloedema and obscurations of vision. Proc R Soc Med 1954;47(4):298–9.
68. Venkatesh P, Verma L, Tewari H. Decreased vision as presenting feature in childhood paraganglioma. Indian Pediatr 2002;39(7):681–4.
69. Voulgaris SG, Partheni M, Tzortzidis F, Ravazoula P, Pessach IS, Papadakis N, Polyzoidis KS. Suprasellar and intrasellar paragangliomas. Clin Neuropathol 2006;25(5):221–6.
70. Peltier J, Fichten A, Lefranc M, Grunewald P, Thelu F, Toussaint P, Desenclos C, Le Gars D. [Paraganglioma of the cavernous sinus. Case report]. Neurochirurgie 2007;53(5):391–4.
71. Sharma MC, Epari S, Gaikwad S, Verma A, Sarkar C. Orbital paraganglioma: report of a rare case. Can J Ophthalmol 2005;40(5):640–44.
72. Venkataramana NK, Kolluri VR, Kumar DV, Rao TV, Das BS. Paraganglioma of the orbit with extension to the middle cranial fossa: case report. Neurosurgery 1989;24(5):762–4.
73. Laigle-Donadey F, Taillibert S, Martin-Duverneuil N, Hildebrand J, Delattre JY. Skull-base metastases. J Neurooncol 2005;75(1):63–9.
74. Greenberg HS, Deck MD, Vikram B, Chu FC, Posner JB. Metastasis to the base of the skull: clinical findings in 43 patients. Neurology 1981;31(5):530–7.
75. Mubaidin SI, Sunna JB, Beiruti MA, Shennak MM, Ayoub MS. Renal cell carcinoma presenting as Garcin's syndrome. J Neurol Neurosurg Psychiatry 1990;53(7):613–4.
76. Julien J, Ferrer X, Drouillard J, Philippe JC, Desbordes P. Cavernous sinus syndrome due to lymphoma. J Neurol Neurosurg Psychiatry 1984;47(5):558–60.
77. Aung TH, Po YC, Wong WK. Hepatocellular carcinoma with metastasis to the skull base, pituitary gland, sphenoid sinus, and cavernous sinus. Hong Kong Med J 2002;8(1):48–51.
78. Johnston JL. Parasellar syndromes. Curr Neurol Neurosci Rep 2002;2(5):423–31.
79. Reiter R, Allert M, Knuchel R, Strutz J. [Sinugenic metastasis of bilateral renal cell carcinoma (hypernephroma)]. HNO 2002;50(2):165–8.
80. Post MJ, Mendez DR, Kline LB, Acker JD, Glaser JS. Metastatic disease to the cavernous sinus: clinical syndrome and CT diagnosis. J Comput Assist Tomogr 1985;9(1):115–20.

Chapter 31
Optic Nerve Pathway Gliomas and Optic Nerve Meningiomas

Sonali Singh and Jade S. Schiffman

Abstract Optic pathway gliomas are intrinsic slow-growing brain tumors that are the most common primary neoplasms of the optic pathways. Optic pathway gliomas are associated with neurofibromatosis type 1; the incidence of optic nerve glioma in patients with this syndrome varies from 8% to 31%. Sporadic optic pathway gliomas present with visual symptoms, the most common of which is decreased visual acuity, but only half of patients with syndromic tumors develop tumor-related signs or symptoms. The optimal treatment of optic pathway gliomas is controversial; options include observation; surgery with clear margins; radiotherapy; and chemotherapy. In general, optic pathway gliomas tend to be low grade and slow growing and associated with long patient survival. Optic nerve sheath meningiomas represent 1% to 2% of all meningiomas and are seen in approximately one quarter of patients with neurofibromatosis type 2. Only 10% of optic nerve sheath meningiomas are primary (arising from the arachnoid villi surrounding the intraorbital or intracanalicular portions of the optic nerves); the remaining 90% are secondary (arising intracranially). The hallmark of optic nerve sheath meningiomas is slowly progressive vision loss. Treatment is conservative, because these tumors usually grow very slowly. Meningiomas are compatible with good vision for many years and are not life threatening

31.1 Optic Pathway Gliomas

Optic pathway gliomas (OPGs) are intrinsic slow-growing brain tumors that are the most common primary neoplasms of the optic pathways. These tumors represent 1% of all brain tumors and up to 5% of all brain tumors in children [1]. OPGs can arise anywhere in the optic pathway and are typically described by locations, from

S. Singh (✉)
Department of Ophthalmology, Veterans Hospital, Temple, TX, USA
e-mail: sonalis25@gmail.com

B. Esmaeli (ed.), *Ophthalmic Oncology*, M.D. Anderson Solid Tumor Oncology Series 6, DOI 10.1007/978-1-4419-0374-7_31,

just behind the globe, through the chiasm, optic tracts, and hypothalamus, all the way to the geniculate body. Some of these tumors originate in the walls of the third ventricle and infiltrate optic pathways anteriorly and laterally; others arise in the chiasm and infiltrate the hypothalamus posteriorly. Tumors confined to the optic nerve and/or chiasm are categorized as anterior OPGs while tumors that extend beyond the chiasm to the hypothalamus and/or optic tracts are defined as posterior OPGs [2]. There have been case reports of OPGs involving the optic radiations in addition to the pregeniculate optic pathways [3].

The most common syndrome associated with OPG is neurofibromatosis type 1 (NF1) (see Chapter 34). The reported incidence of NF1 among patients with optic nerve or chiasmal gliomas ranges from 10 to 70% while the remaining are sporadic. The incidence of optic nerve glioma in patients with NF1 varies from 8 to 31% [4]. There are rare case reports associating OPG with other syndromes like Turcot syndrome (familial intestinal polyposis and primary neuroepithelial tumors). OPGs have been reported in patients with hybrid phacomatosis, for example, the combined disease of both NF1 and tuberous sclerosis.

In the following discussion of OPGs, we highlight differences between sporadic and syndromic tumors.

31.1.1 Demographics and Presentation

Patients with OPG may be asymptomatic or may present with symptoms that vary depending on the location. Patients with an optic glioma of the optic nerve within the orbit often present with slow, painless, unilateral visual loss, optic disc swelling and/or atrophy, proptosis, and strabismus. Rarely patients with optic nerve gliomas may develop a central retinal vein occlusion, iris rubeosis with neovascular glaucoma. Patients with more posterior intracranial gliomas involving the hypothalamic/third ventricle/optic chiasmal region can present with bilateral visual loss, endocrine/hypothalamic disturbance, spasmus nutans, and obstructive hydrocephalus [5].

NF1-associated OPG is more common in females and presents at an earlier age compared with sporadic OPG. Sporadic OPG presents with visual symptoms, while only half of the patients with syndromic OPG ever develop signs or symptoms related to the OPG. Therefore, a significant number of patients with NF1 may have an asymptomatic OPG. In symptomatic OPG, decreased visual acuity is the most common clinical feature with greater incidence among patients with sporadic OPG.

On ophthalmological examination, optic atrophy has been reported as the most common manifestation in sporadic as well as syndromic OPG; however, optic disc edema, optociliary shunts, relative afferent pupillary defects, and visual field defects may also present.

Exophthalmos is more common in NF1 patients while features of raised intracranial pressure are more likely to occur in patients with sporadic OPG [1]. Grill et al. [6] found that in their series of cases, proptosis was significantly more frequent in patients with NF1 (21.5%) than in those without (5.5%), whereas patients without NF1 were more likely to present with nystagmus and hydrocephalus [6].

31.1.2 Histopathology

OPGs are typically low-grade juvenile pilocytic astrocytomas, although fibrillary astrocytomas have been reported. Pilocytic astrocytomas have a biphasic pattern with characteristic Rosenthal fibers and eosinophilic granular bodies. Pilomyxoid astrocytomas are a relatively new group of OPGs which demonstrate piloid cells in a loose fibrillary myxoid background and lack Rosenthal fibers and rarely show eosinophilic granular bodies. Pilomyxoid astrocytomas present at an earlier age than pilocytic astrocytomas and have more aggressive behavior.

OPG can exhibit either a perineural or an intraneural growth pattern. Patients with NF1 are more likely to have perineural pattern, whereas patients without NF1 predominantly have an intraneural growth pattern [5].

31.1.3 Imaging and Lesion Location

Lesions in patients with the sporadic form predominantly have a chiasmatic location and are cystic in morphology and deform the normal shape of the optic nerve pathways, while patients with NF1 have gliomas most commonly located in the orbital optic nerve although they may continue intracranially. They rarely have a cystic component and have no effect on the shape of the optic nerve. Cystic morphology is clinically significant, accounting for more than 50% of the tumor size in patients with cystic OPGs. The larger tumor size in the sporadic group is probably responsible for the symptomatic status of these patients compared with syndromic patients.

Patients with the sporadic form commonly have gliomas that extend beyond the optic pathways and cause hydrocephalus [1].

Computerized tomography (CT) demonstrates enlargement of the optic nerve or chiasm which has imaging characteristics as isodense with the normal brain. Contrast enhancement is variable, from imperceptible to moderate, but generally less than with optic nerve sheath meningiomas. Typically optic nerve gliomas show a well-outlined, fusiform enlargement of the optic nerve (Fig. 31.1), but occasionally it may be more rounded or even multilobular. Chiasmal lesions appear as an enlargement of the chiasm or as a suprasellar mass (Fig. 31.2), occasionally with a cystic component, and are seen best on coronal images. Cystic spaces within the lesion usually correspond to areas of mucinous accumulation. Calcification is rare and can differentiate the intraaxial OPGs from optic nerve meningiomas, which frequently calcify. Chiasmal glioma can rarely calcify [7].

Although CT is excellent for orbital optic glioma, magnetic resonance imaging (MRI) has proven to be superior to CT for imaging optic nerve glioma

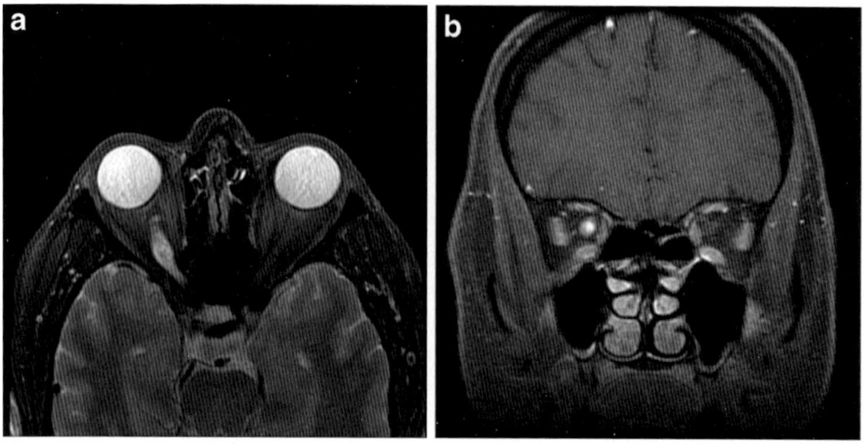

Fig. 31.1 MRI glioma optic nerve OD: (**a**) axial and (**b**) coronal

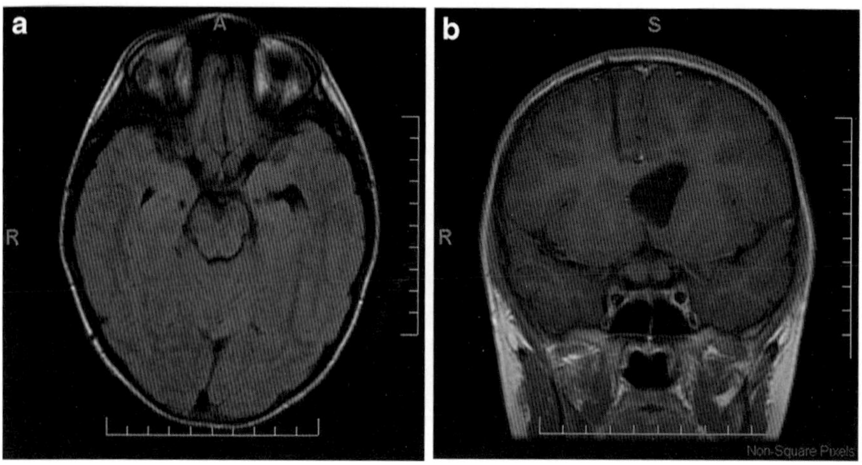

Fig. 31.2 MRI glioma optic chiasm: (**a**) axial and (**b**) coronal

posterior extension, including involvement of the intracanalicular portions of the nerve, because of elimination of bone artifacts. MRI is superior to CT for evaluation of chiasmal, hypothalamic, and optic tract lesions due to improved contrast enhancement resulting from subtle differences in fat contents and hydration of neural tissues [8].

On MRI, gliomas show normal to slightly prolonged T1 relaxation times which image isointense to slightly hypointense to cerebral white matter on T1-weighted sequence while areas of necrosis or mucinous degeneration are hypointense. The T1 image is best for characterization of tissue composition. The T2 relaxation time is prolonged, giving gliomas a hyperintense image on T2-weighted sequence. This best delineates the tumor margins. Contrast enhancement with gadolinium can be homogenous or heterogeneous, and contrast-enhanced T1- or T2-weighted images are the best for visualizing posterior extension into the tracts. In patients with NF1 there is almost always a fusiform enlargement of the optic nerve with a clear-cut margin produced by the intact dural sheath. In patients with sporadic optic nerve gliomas the nerve is more irregular and tends to show both kinking and buckling as well as low-density areas within the nerve [7].

31.1.4 Differential Diagnosis

In a patient with neurofibromatosis and optic nerve or chiasmal enlargement on MRI, the diagnosis is straightforward. However, in patients without NF1 the differential diagnosis of vision loss and optic nerve or chiasmal and hypothalamic enlargement includes malignant optic glioma of adulthood and optic nerve meningioma. In cases where there is chiasmal/hypothalamic presentation, the differential diagnosis includes chiasmal glioma, craniopharyngioma, dysgerminoma, sarcoidosis, and others.

31.1.5 Management

Because of the low incidence of OPG in the general population, its highly variable growth rate, and the variety of treatment plans proposed by different groups, optimal treatment plans are controversial. As these lesions are low grade and generally do not undergo malignant transformation and are often considered as hamartomas, some suggest that treatment of these tumors has no better outcome than the natural history of these lesions. Additionally, documented cases of tumor regression without treatment and with or without improvement in visual function occur. Therefore, treatment considerations are dependent on a number of variables including age at diagnosis, tumor location, severity of the neuroendocrine deficit, and the rate of disease progression as well as the presence or absence of NF1 [9]. When tumor is confined to the optic nerve, chiasm, or optic tracts, prognosis for life is excellent.

Anteriorly placed tumors within the orbit need to be treated if they produce unsightly proptosis, particularly if vision is significantly compromised [2]. While tumor remains confined to the optic nerve, treatment by complete surgical excision with clear margins of resection is curative. However, many of these children may retain useful vision for some time, and conservative management with close observation is reasonable. Such patients should be followed with serial MRI scans for evidence of posterior extension since visual stability or even improvement is not a reliable indicator of nonprogression.

In cases of tumor progression when surgery is not primarily indicated, the choice of therapy differs depending on if the case involves sporadic or syndromic

OPGs. Radiotherapy has been used as primary or postsurgical adjuvant therapy for both syndromic and sporadic OPGs in patients older than 5 years. However, complications were more prevalent in patients with NF1 and included cerebrovascular occlusion in a phenomenon known as moyamoya syndrome (characterized by stenosis or occlusion of the internal carotid artery and/or the proximal portion of the anterior cerebral or middle cerebral arteries, resulting in cerebral infarction and associated with radiotherapy to the brain early in life) and poorer intellectual function.

Once tumor extends to the optic chiasm the eventual threat to life from hypothalamic or third ventricle involvement rises to 28%. Surgical intervention at this point does not improve survival and is associated with significant visual morbidity and patient mortality. Similarly treatment with radiotherapy does not appear to alter the ultimate prognosis for life, but in some cases it may lead to temporary improvement in vision. However, the central nervous system complications of radiotherapy especially in very young children, should not be overlooked.

Once chiasmal tumors invade adjacent hypothalamus and/or third ventricle, the prognosis for life changes markedly with a 15-year mortality rate of more than 50%. Radiotherapy does not alter the final outcome but may possibly prolong life for several years and therefore be justified in such advanced cases. Surgical intervention is recommended only for control of hydrocephalus [7].

Chemotherapy has typically been reserved for children younger than 5 years of age requiring treatment. Chemotherapy is considered first-line therapy for OPGs that are symptomatic, such as with vision loss, pituitary dysfunction, and hypothalamic dysfunction. It can treat tumors that have gone beyond the observation age, even in young children, without the long-term cognitive and neuroendocrine sequelae seen with surgery and radiation therapy [1].

Given the data surrounding the unacceptable risks of radiotherapy in patients with NF1, chemotherapy is now regarded as the primary modality in those with progressive, nonsurgical NF1-associated OPGs. Nevertheless, such treatment carries its own risk of neuropsychological complications. The most common regimen is carboplatin/vincristine combination therapy. Other antineoplastic drugs such as temozolamide alone or lomustine are active against these tumors, but such alkylating agents have induced secondary malignancy in NF1 mouse models and thus have contraindications. The use of these agents in sporadic OPGs may be an effective alternative in individuals who cannot tolerate carboplatin and vincristine or whose tumors are resistant to them [1].

31.1.6 Prognosis

The natural history of OPGs is highly variable and is based on the anatomical location, histological findings, presence or absence of NF1, and also differences in each patient. Overall OPGs tend to be low grade and slow growing with long patient survival. The presence of NF1 and an anterior location is associated with a more favorable prognosis, whereas younger age at presentation is associated with a poorer prognosis [5].

31.2 Optic Nerve Sheath Meningiomas

Meningiomas constitute approximately 20% of intracranial neoplasms and have a total annual incidence of 7.8 per 100,000. Optic nerve sheath meningiomas (ONSMs) represent 1–2% of all meningiomas. The frequency of ONSM among orbital tumors is 8–14% in larger series. After gliomas, these are the second most common type of optic nerve tumor. There is a relationship between optic nerve meningiomas and neurofibromatosis type 2 [10]. A study by Bosch et al. showed that 27% of patients with neurofibromatosis 2 developed optic nerve meningioma [11].

ONSMs can be divided into two types:

(i) Primary optic nerve meningiomas are those that arise from the meningothelial cells of the arachnoid villi surrounding the intraorbital or intracanalicular portions of the optic nerves. Primary meningiomas may grow intracranially to involve the optic chiasm, contralateral optic nerve, internal carotid artery, cavernous sinus, and sella tursica.
(ii) Secondary optic nerve meningiomas arise intracranially usually from the sphenoid ridge, tuberculum sellae, or olfactory groove, and later on invade the optic canal and orbit by extending between the dura and arachnoid of the optic nerve [10].

31.2.1 Incidence

Primary ONSMs represent only 10% of all ONSMs; the other 90% are secondary ONSMs. Of the primary ONSMs, it is estimated that approximately 96% are true primary ONSMs and only 4% are considered ectopic, i.e., those arising from ectopic arachnoid cells within the orbital interstitial tissues or along the orbital nerves [10].

Of all primary ONSMs 92% arise intraorbitally and only 8% intracanalicularly. Therefore, when one sees what appears to be an ONSM in the region of the optic canal, one should look carefully for a secondary ONSM, in that there may be the primary lesion in the region of the anterior clinoid or tuberculum or other. Most of these tumors are unilateral with 5% presenting bilaterally. There is no strong evidence for predilection for left or right laterality. Canalicular meningiomas have a higher incidence of bilaterality than ONSM within the orbit [12].

As with other intracranial meningiomas, primary ONSMs typically develop in middle-aged women with remarkably consistent gender ratio with the proportion of females in several series ranging from 70 to 80%. Males tend to present at a younger age, while the mean age at presentation in women is typically in their fourth to fifth decades; men present 10–15 years earlier. Primary ONSM can occur in children as well. Primary ONSM in children behave more aggressively, are characterized by faster growth, tend to be bilateral and show intracranial involvement, and exhibit a more invasive growth [10].

31.2.2 Histology and Pathophysiology

ONSMs arise from accumulations of meningothelial cells. Within the orbit, such accumulations of meningothelial cells are called the arachnoid villi. ONSM are regarded to arise from cap cells of these arachnoid villi. They grow within the subarachnoid space, the intact arachnoid and dura acting as a tumor "capsule." Their spread usually results in a mass encircling the optic nerve while respecting its dural sheath, exerting increasing pressure on the nerve itself as well as a progressive impairment of its vascular supply. Though the pattern of growth is mainly one of growth along the preexistent anatomic pathways, invasion of the optic nerve along fibrovascular septae and vessels has been shown on a histological basis. Infiltration of the dura and extension into the orbital tissue is a rare event. The tumor may extend from the globe to the optic canal and eventually exhibit continued growth into the middle cranial fossa and involve the chiasm or even the contralateral nerve. Whether cases of bilateral ONSM represent two separate tumors or continuous growth of tumor cells along the tuberculum sellae remains a matter of debate [10].

31.2.3 Clinical Presentation

The symptoms and signs of ONSM depend on whether they have arisen within the orbit, within the optic canal, or intracranially. Slowly progressive visual loss is the hallmark of an ONSM. A relative afferent pupillary defect and dyschromatopsia invariably are present. The optic disc may be swollen or atrophic, have an element of both, or be normal in appearance. The optic disc is usually swollen when the tumor surrounds or compresses the intraorbital portions of the optic nerve and rarely shows peripapillary hemorrhages. When the tumor originates at the apex of the orbit or within the optic canal, there is slowly progressive visual loss without orbital signs, usually with a normal-appearing optic disc, although atrophy or slight swelling of the nerve may be seen. With time the disc becomes pale. Optociliary collateral vessels and retinal and choroid folds may be evident on fundus examination. The triad of visual loss, optic atrophy, and optociliary shunt vessel is most commonly caused by meningiomas. In some cases the tumor may invade the optic nerve by growing along the fibrovascular septa. Extraocular motility dysfunction is present in at least half of the patients, but most patients may not notice diplopia as their vision is impaired [4].

31.2.4 Imaging

The diagnosis of meningioma is established by neuroimaging using high-resolution CT scanning or MRI. CT scan is an excellent imaging study for evaluating ONSM, particularly when performed both before and after administration of iodinated contrast medium. Thin sections (1.5–3 mm) are essential to visualize the tumor, its actual extent, and the presence of micro/macrocalcification. ONSM appears as well-defined tubular enlargement of the optic nerve or bulbous enlargement of the optic nerve at the apex with distal tubular enlargement. The borders of the enlarged optic nerve may enhance after administration of intravenous contrast, to leave a central, linear lucency within the optic nerve sheath known as the "tram-track sign" on the axial image (Fig. 31.3a). The tram-track sign on axial imaging and the "doughnut sign" on coronal imaging (Fig. 31.3b) are characteristically seen with meningiomas; however, these signs are not specific as this imaging pattern may be present with orbital pseudotumor, lymphomas, sarcoidosis, leptomeningeal disease, and perioptic neuritis among other differentials. Meningiomas surround the optic nerve, and thus the caliber of the nerve itself is attenuated within the surrounding tumor (Fig. 31.4a). This feature is best appreciated in coronal sections (Fig. 31.4b). This is in contrast to optic nerve gliomas, where the nerve itself appears expanded. Presence of calcification surrounding the optic nerve (present in 20–50%) is characteristic of meningiomas.

MRI remains the modality of choice for the imaging diagnosis of ONSM. On MRI, meningiomas can be seen as a localized diffuse or fusiform enlargement of the optic nerve sheath complex. MRI fat suppression and gadolinium can detect and demarcate precisely the degree of intracanalicular and intracranial extensions of ONSMs. The majority of intraorbital and intracranial meningiomas are detected by

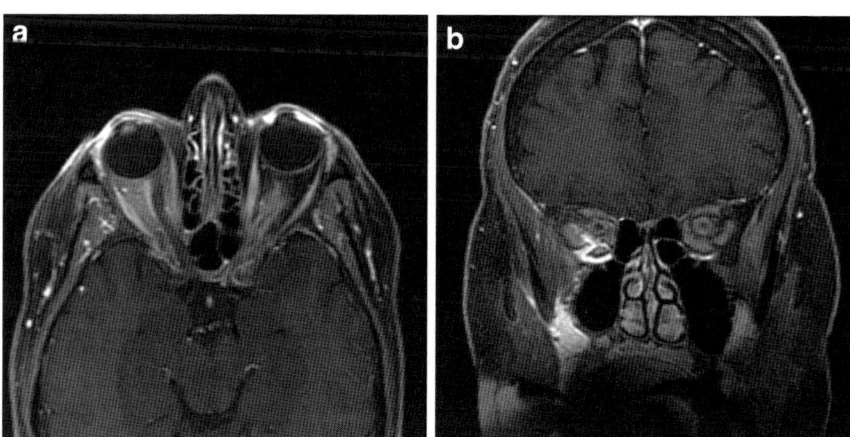

Fig. 31.3 MRI meningioma OS (post-gadolinium): (**a**) axial, tram-track sign and (**b**) coronal, doughnut sign

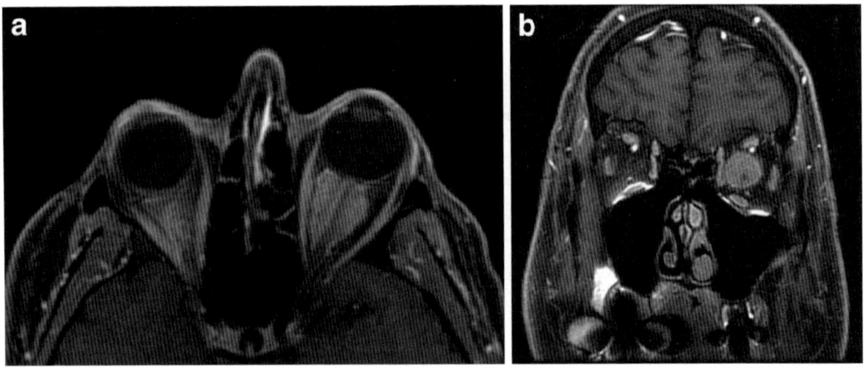

Fig. 31.4 MRI meningioma OS (post-gadolinium): (**a**) axial and (**b**) coronal

CT scans, but only gadolinium-enhanced MRI reliably demonstrates a meningioma that involves the intracanalicular optic nerve, and MRI shows the intracranial portion with more accuracy, especially around bony structures. T1-weighted MRI obtained following intravenous injection of gadolinium-based contrast material demonstrates moderate to marked contrast enhancement of meningiomas. Post-contrast-enhanced fat suppression T1 MRI is most valuable for defining the extent of the optic nerve pathology. Studies with high-quality MRI demonstrate that, even with small tumors, intracranial extension is the rule rather than the exception [13].

31.2.5 Treatment

Treatment of ONSM is conservative, because these tumors usually grow very slowly. Observation, serial automated visual fields, and regular MRI scans with gadolinium enhancement are appropriate for patients who have good vision and no evidence of intracranial or intracanalicular extension of tumor. An undisputed decline in visual function or any intracranial extension often results in treatment of the ONSM. The treatment of choice for a tumor confined to the orbit is stereotactic fractionated radiation. Stereotactic fractionated radiation uses multiple small doses of radiation using tight margins. A reasonable alternative, three-dimensional conformal fractionated radiation uses CT guided planning but usually requires wider margins [14]. Proton radiotherapy has also been used at our center for treatment of ONSM and is a particularly attractive option for younger patients, given the more focused delivery of radiation with proton therapy and theoretically fewer expected side effects in the surrounding intracranial structures such as the pituitary axis (see Chapter 32). Conventional radiation uses much wider margins and would not be recommended for the treatment of ONSM. The radiation can be administered during 5–6 weeks in 28 daily fractions of 1.8–2 Gy/fraction to a total of 50.4–56 Gy. Many patients have improvement or stabilization of their visual function. Gamma knife radiosurgery does not have a role in ONSM because the required dose is toxic to the optic nerve. A tumor that extends intracranially may be treated with fractionated radiation if any vision remains. Surgical excision can be considered for significant intracranial extension, but this often leads to complete vision loss in the ipsilateral eye. A blind, disfigured eye also may be treated with en bloc surgical resection of the meningioma.

When there is evidence of significant intracranial spread of tumor across the planum sphenoidale in a patient with primary ONSM and useful vision, removal of the intracranial portion of the tumor by craniotomy to prevent tumor spread to the contralateral optic nerve should be considered. Documented intracanalicular or intracranial progression of tumor growth warrants neurosurgical removal of the tumor. Patients who have blind eyes and severe exophthalmos may benefit from removal of intraorbital and intracranial tumor.

Meningiomas of the optic nerve sheath are compatible with good vision for many years and are not life-threatening. The prognosis for life is excellent, with an overall tumor-related mortality of near zero.

References

1. Shamji MF, Benoit BG. Syndromic and sporadic pediatric optic pathway gliomas: review of clinical and histopathological differences and treatment implications. Neurosurg Focus 2007;23(5):E3.
2. Hoffman HJ, Humphreys RP, Drake JM, Rutka JT, Becker LE, Jenkin D, Greenberg M. Optic pathway/hypothalamic gliomas: A dilemma in management. Pediatr Neurosurg 1993;19: 186–95.
3. Liu GT, Brodsky MC, Phillips PC, Belasco J, Janss A, Golden JC, Bilanuik LL, Burson T, Duhaime AC, Sutton LN. Optic radiation involvement in optic pathway gliomas in neurofibromatosis. Am J Ophthalmol 2004;137:407–14.
4. Miller NR. Primary tumours of the optic nerve and its sheath. Eye (Lond) 2004;18(11): 1026–37.
5. Binning MJ, Liu JK, Kestle JRW, Brockmeyre DL, Walker ML. Optic pathway gliomas: a review. Neurosurg Focus 2007;23(5):E2.
6. Grill J, Laithier V, Rodriguez D, Raquin MA, Pierre-Kahn A, Kalifa C. When do children with optic pathway tumours need treatment? An oncological perspective in 106 patients treated in a single centre. Eur J Pediatr 2000;159(9):692–6.
7. Dutton JJ. Gliomas of the anterior visual pathway. Surv Ophthalmol 1994;38(5):427–52.
8. Lee AG. Neuroophthalmological management of optic pathway gliomas. Neurosurg Focus 2007;25(5):E1.
9. Ahn Y, Cho B-K, Kim S-ki, et al. Optic pathway glioma: outcome and prognostic factors in a surgical series. Childs Nerv Syst 2006;22:1136–42.
10. Jeremić B, Pitz S. Primary Optic Nerve Sheath Meningiomas, first edition. New York, NY: Springer, 2004.
11. Bosch MM, Wichmann WW, Boltshauser E, Landau K. Optic nerve sheath meningiomas in patients with neurofibromatosis type 2. Arch Ophthalmol 2006;124(3):379–85.
12. Dutton JJ. Optic nerve sheath meningioma. Surv Ophthalmol 1992;37(3):167–183.
13. Yanoff M, Duker JS, editors. Prechiasmal pathways—compression by optic nerve and sheath tumors. In: Ophthalmology, second edition. St. Louis, MO: Mosby Elsevier, 2004.
14. Radhakrishnan S, Lee MS. Optic nerve sheath meningiomas. Curr Treat Options Neurol 2005;7:51–5.

Chapter 32
Leptomeningeal Disease

Gerardo D. Camoriano, Anitha Raghunath, and Jade S. Schiffman

Abstract Leptomeningeal disease (LMD) is an umbrella term used to refer to cancer involvement of the arachnoid and pia mater. Over the past four decades, the incidence of LMD has increased, largely as a result of new diagnostic modalities, improved therapies for systemic cancer, and increased clinical awareness. LMD can be divided into three categories: LMD resulting from solid tumors, LMD resulting from hematogenous tumors, and LMD resulting from primary brain tumors. Patients with LMD due to solid tumors usually present with a random and highly asymmetric distribution of symptoms. LMD due to hematogenous cancers is often identified during periods of remission or systemic disease inactivity and typically presents with a higher frequency of cranial nerve signs than is seen with LMD due to solid tumors. LMD arising from primary brain tumors usually occurs late in the course of the disease. The diagnostic gold standard for LMD is a positive cerebrospinal fluid cytology finding. Treatment of LMD is aimed at preventing neurologic deterioration and improving patient survival. Patients in the good-risk group may proceed to a cerebrospinal fluid flow study followed by initial intrathecal or intraventricular chemotherapy along with fractionated external-beam radiation therapy. Patients in the poor-risk group may benefit from more targeted fractionated external-beam radiation therapy delivered to symptomatic sites only, along with supportive care. Despite aggressive treatment protocols, the overall prognosis of patients with LMD remains poor; most studies report a median survival of 2–3 months.

32.1 Introduction

Leptomeningeal disease (LMD) is an umbrella term used to refer to primary or metastatic cancer involvement of the arachnoid and pia mater. LMD is also known by many other names, including carcinomatous meningitis, neoplastic meningitis,

G.D. Camoriano (✉)
Department of Ophthalmology and Visual Sciences, The University of Texas Medical Branch, Galveston, TX, USA
e-mail: gdcamori@utmb.edu

B. Esmaeli (ed.), *Ophthalmic Oncology*, M.D. Anderson Solid Tumor Oncology Series 6, DOI 10.1007/978-1-4419-0374-7_32,

lymphomatous meningitis, leukemic meningitis, leptomeningeal carcinomatosis, and leptomeningeal metastasis. To avoid confusion, we will refer to these entities collectively as LMD.

32.2 Epidemiology

The first reported case of LMD was reported by Eberth [1] in 1870. At that time, the condition was considered rare and was uncommonly diagnosed before death. Over the past four decades, the incidence of LMD has increased, largely as a result of new diagnostic modalities, improved therapies for systemic cancer, and increased clinical awareness [2]. LMD currently complicates the management of approximately 5% of patients with cancer [3, 4]. Several clinical series have estimated LMD to occur in 7–15% of patients with lymphoma, 5–15% of patients with leukemia, 4–15% of patients with solid tumors, 1–7% of patients with an unknown primary tumor, and 1–2% of patients with primary brain tumors [5–11]. The high incidence of LMD seen with solid tumors may reflect reporting bias rather than a true predisposition for leptomeningeal involvement, as solid tumors occur more frequently than hematologic malignancies [12].

32.3 Clinical Presentation

Three domains of leptomeningeal involvement have been described: the cerebral hemispheres, the cranial nerves, and the spinal cord and roots. Hemispheric symptoms may include headache and mental status change with attendant signs such as cognitive deficits, confusion, dementia, seizures, and hemiparesis. Patients may also develop stroke-like symptoms from tumor occlusion of the small pial blood vessels or symptoms of increased intracranial pressure with or without frank hydrocephalus [12]. Cranial nerve symptoms may include loss of vision, diplopia, facial weakness or numbness, and hearing loss. Signs of cranial nerve dysfunction include disc edema, extraocular muscle palsies, trigeminal and facial nerve palsies, and neurosensory hearing loss. Spinal symptoms and signs may include weakness (lower extremity more often than upper), dermatomal numbness, and radicular pain. In advanced cases, patients may also develop cauda equina syndrome or conus medullaris involvement [2, 3, 6, 10, 12–15].

Cancers can reach the leptomeninges by direct extension, migration along perivascular or perineural spaces, vascular extension (i.e., through the choroid plexus or Batson's venous plexus), or hematogenous spread [2]. Two growth patterns have been observed: sheet-like diffusion along the pial surface, sometimes associated with inflammation; and development of multiple nodules on the surface of the brain, ventricles, and cranial nerves [16]. Despite these limited routes of dissemination, LMD is a protean disease with multiple clinical manifestations arising from differences in tropism of the inciting cancer. In order to better understand these differences in clinical behavior, it is appropriate to divide LMD into three categories: LMD resulting from solid tumors, LMD resulting from hematogenous tumors, and LMD resulting from primary brain tumors.

32.3.1 LMD due to Solid Tumors

The solid tumors that most commonly spread to the leptomeninges are breast, lung, and head and neck cancers, melanoma, and gastric cancer. In the case of breast and lung cancers, the incidence of LMD appears to be increasing. However, this is likely due to better systemic therapies and increased survival in these patients. In addition, many of the first-line chemotherapeutic agents used to treat breast and lung cancers have poor penetration of the blood–brain barrier and are not effective against leptomeningeal disease [2, 17].

Patients with LMD due to solid tumors usually present with a random and highly asymmetric distribution of symptoms. This presentation is far more common than meningeal irritation; only 15% of patients have positive Kernig and Brudzinski signs [17]. In a series of 90 patients with solid tumor leptomeningeal metastases, the overall prevalence of cerebral and spinal symptoms and signs was higher than that of cranial neuropathies. The cranial neuropathies observed included ophthalmoplegia (30% of patients, with abducens more common than oculomotor and oculomotor more common than trochlear palsies), facial weakness (27%), hearing loss (13%), optic neuropathy (8%), trigeminal neuropathy (8%), and diminished gag reflex (5%) [5, 17, 18]. Hence, there should be a high index of suspicion of LMD in cancer patients who present with new onset of neurologic symptoms, including cerebral, spinal, and cranial neuropathies.

LMD generally presents late in the disease course in patients with solid tumor metastases; up to 90% of patients with LMD have advanced disease burden at diagnosis [10]. Approximately two-thirds of these patients have multifocal symptoms at presentation. Patients with LMD who present with unifocal and/or nonlocalizing symptoms or signs represent a diagnostic challenge and often experience delays in diagnosis [15, 18].

32.3.2 LMD due to Hematogenous Tumors

With the notable exception of primary central nervous system (CNS) lymphoma, the leukemias and lymphomas reach the leptomeninges almost exclusively by hematogenous spread. As opposed to LMD due to solid tumors, LMD due to hematogenous cancers is often identified during periods of remission or systemic disease inactivity and typically presents with a higher frequency of cranial nerve signs [10, 12, 15, 19–23].

In a series of 37 patients with chronic lymphocytic leukemia and leptomeningeal involvement compiled from cases reported over the past three decades, the most frequent presenting signs were cranial nerve abnormalities (54% of patients), including optic neuropathy (28%), mental status changes (28%), headache (23%), lower extremity weakness (23%), and cerebellar signs (18%) [22].

In a series of 24 patients with LMD due to non-Hodgkin's lymphoma, 15 patients (63%) presented with cranial nerve palsies, most commonly localized to the facial nerve (10 of 15 patients, or 75%) [19]. Similarly, in another series of 24 patients with non-Hodgkin's lymphoma, 17 patients (71%) had cranial nerve involvement. In this series as well, the facial nerve was also the most commonly affected cranial nerve, followed by the abducens and oculomotor nerves [20]. Review of seven reported cases of CNS lymphoma with cranial nerve III palsy as the initial presentation of LMD revealed pupil involvement in four patients (57%) [21].

Primary CNS lymphomas appear to behave like systemic non-Hodgkin's lymphoma with respect to leptomeningeal involvement. In a series of five consecutive patients with T-cell CNS lymphoma and LMD, all five patients presented with symptoms of cranial nerve involvement. Clinical presentations included papilledema and unilateral abducens palsy, bilateral oculomotor palsy, mononeuritis multiplex and hearing loss, bilateral facial nerve palsy, unilateral hearing loss, and the presence of bilateral uveitis, which is usually lacking in systemic lymphomas that present with LMD [23]. A large retrospective series of 45 patients with primary T-cell CNS lymphoma reported by the International Primary CNS Lymphoma Collaborative Group found one patient with exclusive leptomeningeal involvement presenting with cranial nerve palsies but no obvious intracranial lesions [24]. The same happens with the more common B-cell primary CNS lymphoma.

32.3.3 LMD due to Primary Brain Tumors

LMD arising from primary brain tumors is rare and usually occurs late in the course of the disease. In a review of 52 patients with malignant gliomas, 11 patients (21%) were found to have leptomeningeal involvement at autopsy. Of these, ten patients had hydrocephalus, nine patients had tumor invasion of the lateral ventricles, eight patients had spinal subarachnoid seeding with involvement of the cauda equina, and three patients had symptomatic compression at the thoracic or lumbar level [25]. In general, gliomas have a predilection for the ventricles and may drop along the CNS to involve the spinal nerve roots. Cranial nerve lesions occur less frequently than in solid or hematogenous tumors. For glioblastoma multiforme, LMD manifestations have included optic neuropathy and oculomotor, abducens, and facial nerve palsies; there have been no reports in the literature of trochlear nerve palsies [25–27].

32.4 Diagnosis

The fact that autopsy studies consistently show incidences of LMD exceeding those in clinical series indicates that many cases of LMD go undiagnosed. The Memorial Sloan-Kettering Cancer Center review of 2375 autopsies of patients with cancer found an 8% incidence of LMD, compared to 5% reported in most clinical studies [12, 13].

Similarly, the National Cancer Institute study of small cell lung cancer showed an 11% incidence of LMD antemortem compared to 25% postmortem [14].

Multiple factors contribute to the difficulty of early diagnosis of LMD, including nonlocalizing signs and symptoms, which are frequently ascribed to the primary tumor or to a side effect of the medical treatment. Also, cerebrospinal fluid (CSF) analysis may be challenging. In a study by Glass et al. [28], 41% of patients with negative CSF cytology antemortem were found to have LMD at autopsy. This finding was supported by Wasserstrom et al. [9] and Murray et al. [29], who independently demonstrated variable yields of malignant cells at different levels in the CNS, with the highest concentrations localizing to the cisternal and ventricular compartments. More specifically, Wasserstrom et al. [9] identified a subgroup of approximately 5% of patients with negative lumbar punctures who had positive cytology findings only from CSF derived from the ventricles or cisterna magna. Another subgroup of approximately 9% of patients had consistently negative CSF cytology findings despite radiographically unequivocal disease [9]. It follows that the optimal number of samples necessary to diagnose patients with LMD by cytology has not been established. While some authors have noted a significant increase in sensitivity with repeat testing in initially cytologically negative cases [2, 10, 30], others have reported no added diagnostic benefit from conducting more than two lumbar punctures [4, 9]. Of interest is that despite the high rate of false-negative cytology findings (up to 50% in some series), a completely normal lumbar puncture is associated with LMD in fewer than 5% of cases [9, 31]. Abnormalities in CSF on initial lumbar puncture in patients with LMD have been reported to include a high opening pressure (>160 mmH_2O; 50% of lumbar punctures), high protein level (>50 mg/dl; 81%), hypoglycorrachia (<40 mg/dl; 31%), and pleocytosis (>5 white blood cells/mm^3; 57%) [9].

Although a positive CSF cytology finding is the diagnostic gold standard for LMD [30], other ancillary biochemical CSF markers have been described in the literature, in particular for LMD due to solid and hematogenous tumors. These include carcinoembryonic antigen, α-fetoprotein, gastrin-releasing peptide, β-human chorionic gonadotropin, β_2-microglobulin, β-glucuronidase, soluble CD27, LDH isoenzyme-5, glucose-6-phosphate isomerase, and various types of monoclonality. The latter include immunoglobulin gene rearrangements identified by flow cytometry or polymerase chain reaction. In patients with negative CSF cytology findings, positive surface markers support the diagnosis of LMD. These ancillary markers may also be used to monitor treatment response [12, 32–38].

32.4.1 Radiographic Imaging

Radiographic modalities useful in the diagnosis and staging of LMD include cranial-enhanced computed tomography (CT), CT myelography, brain and spine magnetic resonance imaging (MRI), and radionuclide CSF flow studies. Cranial-enhanced CT is abnormal in approximately 25% of patients with LMD. The abnormalities observed include parenchymal volume loss, ependymal or subependymal enhancement, subarachnoid enhancing nodules (less common in hematologic malignancies), sulcal–cisternal enhancement or obliteration, intraventricular enhancing nodules, communicating hydrocephalus, and irregular tentorial enhancement [4]. Brain MRI has a greater sensitivity (up to 76%) than cranial-enhanced CT but lower reported sensitivity for hematologic tumors (55%) than for solid tumors (90%) [16, 39]. Brain MRI is the imaging modality of choice for the diagnosis of intracranial LMD. Findings on brain MRI in patients with LMD include leptomeningeal, subependymal, dural, or cranial nerve enhancement. Table 32.1 outlines the differential diagnosis of cranial nerve enhancement and Fig. 32.1 shows examples of MRI findings in LMD, superficial cerebral lesions, and communicating hydrocephalus [40]. While CT and MRI are more useful for identifying bulky CNS disease, CSF flow studies provide information regarding the functional anatomy of CSF spaces. This allows for targeted treatment of areas with flow abnormalities. In addition, functional CSF status as determined by CSF flow studies has been correlated with patient survival [4, 7, 31, 41–44].

32.4.2 Optic Neuropathies in LMD

An isolated optic neuropathy may be the presenting sign of LMD in cancer patients. Among patients with leptomeningeal optic nerve involvement, up to 44% experience

Table 32.1 Differential diagnosis of cranial nerve enhancement [42]

Infectious disorders	Granulomatoses
Bacterial	Neurosarcoidosis
Bacterial meningitis	Wegener's granulomatosis
Tuberculous meningitis	Tuberculosis
Lyme disease	Tolosa-Hunt syndrome
Neurosyphilis	Idiopathic hypertrophic cranial pachymeningitis
Viral	Neoplastic
Herpes simplex virus encephalitis	Perineural tumor spread
Varicella zoster virus encephalitis	Squamous cell carcinoma
Cytomegalovirus encephalitis	Adenoid cystic carcinoma
Fungal meningitis	Malignant schwannoma
Cryptococcal meningitis	Primary nerve tumors
Rhinocerebral mucormycosis	Schwannomas/meningiomas
Parasitic	Hemangiomas
Neuroschistosomiasis	Leptomeningeal disease
Postinfectious and demyelinating disorders	Solid tumors
Bell's palsy	Hematogenous tumors
Ramsay Hunt syndrome	Primary brain tumors
Multiple sclerosis	Other
Optic neuritis	Postradiation neuritis
Guillain–Barré syndrome	Ophthalmoplegic migraine
Miller-Fisher syndrome	Moyamoya disease
Charcot–Marie–Tooth disease	

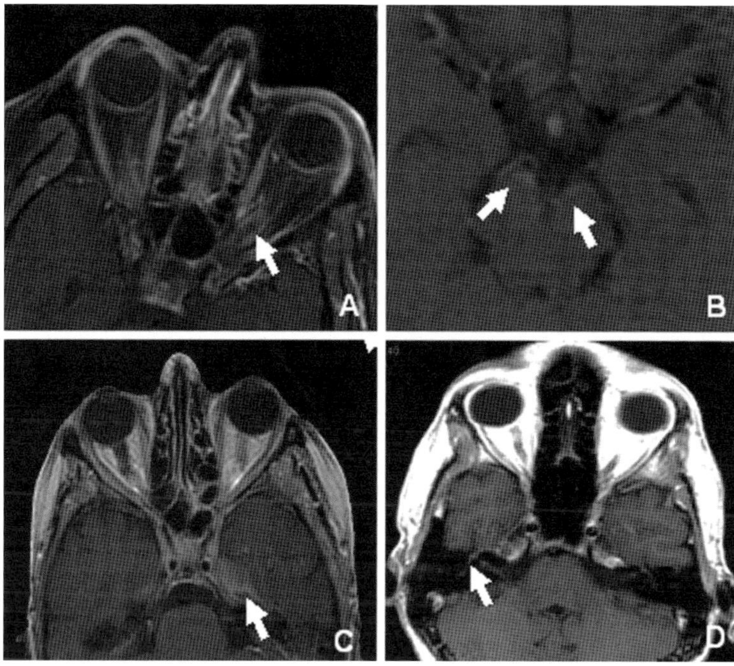

Fig. 32.1 Cranial nerve involvement in four cases of LMD. Contrast-enhanced axial T1-weighted images show enhancement and involvement of cranial nerves: (**a**) left optic nerve sheath (*arrows*); (**b**) oculomotor nerves (*arrows*); (**c**) left Meckel's cave (*arrows*); and (**d**) right facial nerve (*arrows*)

visual loss [43]. However, patients may have normal vision at the time of their initial assessment. An almost constant finding in these cases is a relative afferent pupillary defect. The magnitude of this defect as measured by neutral density filters may be used to clinically follow these patients. Color vision is likewise affected early, resulting in confusion of the red–green axis on Hardy–Rand–Ritter or Ishihara color plate testing. Visual field changes may include a central scotoma, diffuse depression, or nonspecific visual field changes. Dilated fundus examination may reveal no abnormality; it may also reveal optic disc edema due to raised intracranial pressure and/or optic nerve infiltration, optic disc hemorrhages, optic disc pallor or atrophy, retinal or vitreous hemorrhages, or engorged retinal vasculature. A diagnostic quartet of leptomeningeal optic nerve infiltration has been proposed by McFadzean et al. [44] involving the combination of headaches typical of raised intracranial pressure, blindness, sluggish or absent pupillary reflexes, and normal-appearing optic discs. Although long-standing papilledema may lead to post-stasis optic atrophy, optic nerve damage usually results from infiltration of the tumor in the optic nerve sheath. This may cause a compartment syndrome resulting in posterior segment ischemia. In this situation, patients may experience rapid and profound visual loss to blindness within a matter of 48 h. MRI in this setting may be unrevealing and, as such, leptomeningeal optic neuropathy remains a clinical diagnosis. Even in the acute setting, treatment with radiation therapy and intravenous steroids has been largely disappointing [44, 45].

32.5 Treatment

Treatment of LMD is aimed at preventing neurologic deterioration and improving patient survival. The National Comprehensive Cancer Network clinical practice guidelines stratify patients with LMD for treatment purposes into good-risk and poor-risk groups. The good-risk group comprises patients with minimal neurologic deficits and minimal systemic disease as evidenced by a high Karnofsky performance status score (60 or above). The poor-risk group is characterized by multiple, serious neurologic deficits, extensive systemic disease, bulky CNS disease, encephalopathy, and a low Karnofsky performance status score. Patients in the good-risk group may proceed to a CSF flow study followed by initial intrathecal or intraventricular chemotherapy along with fractionated external-beam radiation therapy. The CSF flow study identifies areas of poor CSF distribution or obstruction that may resolve with focused radiation therapy, thus allowing for a more homogeneous distribution of subsequent intrathecal chemotherapy. Patients in the poor-risk group may benefit from more targeted fractionated external-beam radiation therapy delivered to symptomatic sites only, along with supportive care [41].

Chemotherapy regimens for LMD have focused on four drugs: methotrexate, cytarabine, sustained-release cytarabine (depo-Cyt), and thiotepa. These agents have classically been administered intrathecally through a subcutaneous reservoir and ventricular catheter (i.e., Ommaya reservoir) or by lumbar puncture. They are highly effective for small leptomeningeal deposits or tumor cells suspended in CSF and have decreased penetration in bulky disease or sequestered deposits in perineural and Virchow–Robin spaces. Given the fragile neurologic status of patients with LMD, care must be taken to remove isovolumetric amounts of CSF prior to infusing chemotherapy to avoid increasing the total CSF volume. These samples can be sent for cytologic and other studies. Side effects of the four drugs commonly used to treat LMD include leukoencephalopathy and myelosuppression. In addition, increased intracranial pressure has been associated with the use of cytarabine and depo-Cyt [32].

Treatment strategies on the horizon include the use of other chemotherapeutic agents (dacarbazine, diaziquone, mafosfamide, nitrosoureas, busulfan, trimetrexate, melphalan, and topotecan), immunomodulatory drugs (intrathecal interleukin-2 and interferon-α), monoclonal antibody therapy (intravenous rituximab or radiolabeled monoclonal antibodies), and gene therapy (adenoviral vector delivery of herpes simplex virus-thymidine kinase to leptomeningeal metastases followed by systemic administration of ganciclovir) [2, 33].

32.6 Prognosis

Despite aggressive treatment protocols, the overall prognosis of patients with LMD remains poor; most studies report a median survival of 2 months (range, 2–3 months) [2, 46, 47]. Survival appears to be dependent on the primary tumor type. Reported median survival rates for breast cancer-related LMD range from 2.6 to 7.2 months, while those for lung cancer-related LMD range from 1 to 3 months. For the hematogenous tumors, survival after a diagnosis of LMD has likewise been dismal—median survival times of 6.0 and 2.3 months have been reported for the leukemias and lymphomas, respectively [4]. Interestingly, in one study patients with primary brain tumor-related LMD were diagnosed at a younger age and had a slightly longer median survival (not statistically significant, however) than patients with primary brain tumors without leptomeningeal involvement [25, 27].

In a study of 85 patients with solid tumors, the following predictors of good prognosis were identified on univariate analysis: female gender, LMD as the first relapse site, an interval of more than 1 year between diagnosis of the primary tumor and diagnosis of LMD, and good performance status. However, on multivariate regression analysis, only performance status and the extent of leptomeningeal involvement on CT or MRI achieved statistical significance [47].

Another commonly cited prognostic factor is CSF flow status, which, as mentioned previously, also guides treatment decisions. In a study of 31 patients with solid tumor-, hematologic tumor-, or primary brain tumor-related LMD, survival was significantly longer among patients with initially normal and abnormal but correctable CSF flow than among those with uncorrectable CSF flow (6.9, 13.0, and 0.7 months, respectively; $P < 0.001$) [48].

Finally, neurologic status at presentation and the extent of systemic cancer play an important role in determining clinical outcomes. In this regard, patients with encephalopathy secondary to hydrocephalus may respond well to symptomatic measures, while those with more focal neurologic deficits may be more resistant to treatment [17].

32.7 Conclusion

LMD currently complicates the management of approximately 5–8% of cancer patients, and the incidence of LMD is expected to continue to increase in the future as a result of new diagnostic modalities, improved therapies for systemic cancer, and increased clinical awareness. Recognizing LMD requires a high index of suspicion for new neurologic complaints, a comprehensive neurologic and neuro-ophthalmic examination with attention to the three domains of involvement (the cerebral hemispheres, the cranial nerves, and the spinal cord and roots), and a multidisciplinary approach. An excellent history and physical examination are instrumental in guiding imaging, particularly in cases with negative CSF cytology. Patient stratification based on Karnofsky performance status score, radiographic extent of disease, and CSF flow studies allows for the implementation of more compassionate and cost-effective treatment strategies. Treatment is aimed at preventing neurologic deterioration and improving patient survival. Unfortunately, despite aggressive treatment, prognosis remains poor in most cases. New therapies may allow for extended survival in patients with LMD.

References

1. Eberth C. Zur entwicklung des epitheliomas dur pia under der lung. Virchows Arch 1870;49:51–63.
2. Grossman SA, Krabak MJ. Leptomeningeal carcinomatosis. Cancer Treat Rev 1999;25: 103–19.
3. DeAngelis L. Current diagnosis and treatment of leptomeningeal metastasis. J Neurooncol 1998;38:245–52.
4. Chamberlain MC, Nolan C, Abrey LE. Leukemic and lymphomatous meningitis: incidence, prognosis and treatment. J Neurooncol 2005;75(1):71–83.
5. Olson M, Chernik N, Posner J. Infiltration of the leptomeninges by systemic cancer. A clinical and pathologic study. Arch Neurol 1974;30:122–37.
6. Little J, Dale A, Okazaki H. Meningeal carcinomatosis clinical manifestations. Arch Neurol 1974;30:138–43.
7. Shapiro WR, Posner JB, Ushio Y, Chemik NL, Young DF. Treatment of meningeal neoplasms. Cancer Treat Rep 1977;61(4):733–43.
8. Theodore W, Gendelman S. Meningeal carcinomatosis. Arch Neurol 1981;38:696–9.
9. Wasserstrom W, Glass J, Posner J. Diagnosis and treatment of leptomeningeal metastases from solid tumors: experience with 90 patients. Cancer 1982;49:759–72.
10. Kaplan JG, DeSouza TG, Farkash A, Shafran B, Pack D, Rehman F, Fuks J, Portenoy R. Leptomeningeal metastases: comparison of clinical features and laboratory data of solid tumors, lymphomas and leukemias. J Neurooncol 1990;9(3):225–9.
11. Chamberlain M. Leptomeningeal metastases: 111indium-DTPA CSF flow studies. Neurology 1991;41:1765–9.
12. Chamberlain M. Leptomeningeal metastases: a review of evaluation and treatment. J Neurooncol 1998;37:271–84.
13. Posner JB, Chernik NL. Intracranial metastases from systemic cancer. Adv Neurol 1978;19:579–92.
14. Rosen ST, Aisner J, Makuch RW, Matthews MJ, Ihde DC, Whitacre M, Glatstein EJ, Wiernik PH, Lichter AS, Bunn PA, Jr. Carcinomatous leptomeningitis in small cell lung cancer: a clinicopathologic review of the National Cancer Institute experience. Medicine (Baltimore) 1982;61(1):45–53.
15. van Oostenbrugge R, Twijnstra A. Presenting features and value of diagnostic procedures in leptomeningeal metastases. Neurology 1999;53:382–5.
16. Maroldi R, Ambrosi C, Farina D. Metastatic disease of the brain: extra-axial metastases (skull, dural, leptomeningeal) and tumor spread. Eur J Radiol 2004;15:617–26.
17. Taillibert S, Laigle-Donadey F, Chodkiewicz C, Sanson M, Hoang-Xuan K, Delattre JY. Leptomeningeal metastases from solid malignancy: a review. J Neurooncol 2005;75(1):85–99.
18. Balm M, Hammack J. Leptomeningeal carcinomatosis. Presenting features and prognostic factors. Arch Neurol 1996;53:626–32.
19. Law IP, Dick FR, Blom J, Bergevin PR. Involvement of the central nervous system in non-Hodgkin's lymphoma. Cancer 1975;36(1):225–31.
20. Levitt LJ, Dawson DM, Rosenthal DS, Moloney WC. CNS involvement in the non Hodgkin's lymphomas. Cancer 1980;45(3):545–52.

21. Bhatti M, Schmalfuss I, Eskin T. Isolated cranial nerve III palsy as the presenting manifestation of HIV-related large B-cell lymphoma: clinical, radiological, and postmortem observations: report of a case and review of the literature. Surv Ophthalmol 2005;50: 598–606.
22. Lange CP, Brouwer RE, Brooimans R, Vecht Ch J. Leptomeningeal disease in chronic lymphocytic leukemia. Clin Neurol Neurosurg 2007;109(10):896–901.
23. Levin N, Soffer D, Grissaru S, Aizikovich N, Gomori JM, Siegal T. Primary T-cell CNS lymphoma presenting with leptomeningeal spread and neurolymphomatosis. J Neurooncol 2008;90(1):77–83.
24. Shenkier TN, Blay JY, O'Neill BP, Poortmans P, Thiel E, Jahnke K, Abrey LE, Neuwelt E, Tsang R, Batchelor T, et al. Primary CNS lymphoma of T-cell origin: a descriptive analysis from the international primary CNS lymphoma collaborative group. J Clin Oncol 2005;23(10):2233–9.
25. Yung W, Horten C, Shapiro W. Meningeal gliomatosis: a review of 12 cases. Ann Neurol 1980;8:605–8.
26. Reifenberger G, Bostrom J, Bettag M, Bock WJ, Wechsler W, Kepes JJ. Primary glioblastoma multiforme of the oculomotor nerve. Case report. J Neurosurg 1996;84(6):1062–6.
27. Trivedi RA, Nichols P, Coley S, Cadoux-Hudson TA, Donaghy M. Leptomeningeal glioblastoma presenting with multiple cranial neuropathies and confusion. Clin Neurol Neurosurg 2000;102(4):223–6.
28. Glass JP, Melamed M, Chernik NL, Posner JB. Malignant cells in cerebrospinal fluid (CSF): the meaning of a positive CSF cytology. Neurology 1979;29(10):1369–75.
29. Murray JJ, Greco FA, Wolff SN, Hainsworth JD. Neoplastic meningitis. Marked variations of cerebrospinal fluid composition in the absence of extradural block. Am J Med 1983;75(2):289–94.
30. Glantz MJ, Cole BF, Glantz LK, Cobb J, Mills P, Lekos A, Walters BC, Recht LD. Cerebrospinal fluid cytology in patients with cancer: minimizing false-negative results. Cancer 1998;82(4):733–9.
31. Reuler J, Meier D. Leptomeningeal carcinomatosis with normal CSF features. Arch Intern Med 1979;139:237–8.
32. Chowdhary S, Chamberlain M. Leptomeningeal metastases: current concepts and management guidelines. J Natl Compr Canc Netw 2005;3:693–703.
33. Kara I, Sahin B, Gunesacar R. Levels of serum and cerebrospinal fluid soluble CD27 in the diagnosis of leptomeningeal involvement of hematolymphoid malignancies. Adv Ther 2007;24:741–7.
34. Schold SC, Wasserstrom WR, Fleisher M, Schwartz MK, Posner JB. Cerebrospinal fluid biochemical markers of central nervous system metastases. Ann Neurol 1980;8(6):597–604.
35. Ernerudh J, Olsson T, Berlin G, von Schenck H. Cerebrospinal fluid immunoglobulins and beta 2-microglobulin in lymphoproliferative and other neoplastic diseases of the central nervous system. Arch Neurol 1987;44(9):915–20.
36. Klee GG, Tallman RD, Goellner JR, Yanagihara T. Elevation of carcinoembryonic antigen in cerebrospinal fluid among patients with meningeal carcinomatosis. Mayo Clin Proc 1986;61(1):9–13.
37. Schipper HI, Bardosi A, Jacobi C, Felgenhauer K. Meningeal carcinomatosis: origin of local IgG production in the CSF. Neurology 1988;38(3):413–6.
38. Newton HB, Fleisher M, Schwartz MK, Malkin MG. Glucosephosphate isomerase as a CSF marker for leptomeningeal metastasis. Neurology 1991;41(3):395–8.
39. Freilich R, Krol G, Deangelis L. Neuroimaging and cerebral spinal fluid cytology in the diagnosis of leptomeningeal metastasis. Ann Neurol 1995;38:51–7.
40. Saremi F, Helmy M, Farzin S, Zee CS, Go JL. MRI of cranial nerve enhancement. AJR Am J Roentgenol 2005;185(6):1487–97.
41. Network NCC. NCCN Clinical Practice Guidelines in Oncology. National Comprehensive Cancer Network, Vol 1, Jenkintown, PA, 2008:23–6.

42. Shapiro W, Young D, Mehta B. Methotrexate: distribution in CSF fluid after intravenous, ventricular, and lumbar injections. N Engl J Med 1975;293:161–6.
43. Katz J, Valsamins M, Jampel R. Ocular signs in diffuse carcinomatous meningitis. Am J Ophthalmol 1961;76:672–9.
44. McFadzean R, Brosnahan D, Doyle D, Going J, Hadley D, Lee W. A diagnostic quartet in leptomeningeal infiltration of the optic nerve sheath. J Neuroophthalmol 1994;14(3):175–82.
45. Losa F, Montes A, Arruga J, Mesía R, Cardenal F. Meningeal carcinomatosis as a cause of partially reversible blindness. Clin Transl Oncol 2000;2(6):320–1.
46. Jayson G, Howell A. Carcinomatous meningitis in solid tumors. Ann Oncol 1996;7:773–86.
47. Waki F, Ando M, Takashima A, Yonemori K, Nokihara H, Miyake M, Tateishi U, Tsuta K, Shimada Y, Fujiwara Y, et al. Prognostic factors and clinical outcomes in patients with leptomeningeal metastasis from solid tumors. J Neurooncol 2009;93(2):205–12.
48. Glantz MJ, Hall WA, Cole BF, Chozick BS, Shannon CM, Wahlberg L, Akerley W, Marin L, Choy H. Diagnosis, management, and survival of patients with leptomeningeal cancer based on cerebrospinal fluid-flow status. Cancer 1995;75(12):2919–31.

Chapter 33
Paraneoplastic Visual Syndromes

Anitha Raghunath and Jade S. Schiffman

Abstract A paraneoplastic visual syndrome is a syndrome of cancer-related ocular dysfunction that is not due to either direct effects of primary or metastatic tumor or treatment or treatment-related complications. Paraneoplastic visual syndromes are thought to be principally autoimmune conditions in which the tumor expresses a neuronal antigen that triggers an immune response against cross-reacting ocular antigens. Carcinoma-associated retinopathy (CAR), the most common paraneoplastic visual disorder, results in visual loss that is usually bilateral, rapid, and painless, with both cone and rod dysfunction. The carcinoma-associated cone dysfunction syndrome, part of the CAR spectrum, is very rare; patients with this syndrome have antibodies primarily directed against cones. Melanoma-associated retinopathy is distinguished by symptoms such as sudden shimmering and night blindness; usually, there is near normal color vision, visual acuity, and central vision. Paraneoplastic optic neuropathy is a syndrome of visual loss that is usually characterized by bilateral optic disc swelling, nerve fiber layer hemorrhages, and vitritis; sometimes there are abnormal findings on electroretinography. Treatments that have been tried in patients with paraneoplastic visual syndromes include immunotherapies and mono clonal antibodies. Though temporary improvement in vision has been reported, a progressive decline to severe visual loss is the usual course, even with treatment.

33.1 Introduction

Paraneoplastic visual syndrome is the term used to refer to cancer-related ocular dysfunction that is not due to either direct effects of primary or metastatic tumor or treatment or treatment-related complications. Paraneoplastic visual syndromes include paraneoplastic retinopathies and paraneoplastic optic neuropathy.

A. Raghunath (✉)
Section of Ophthalmology, Department of Head and Neck Surgery, The University of Texas M. D. Anderson Cancer Center, Houston, TX, USA
e-mail: anitha.raghunath@gmail.com

B. Esmaeli (ed.), *Ophthalmic Oncology*, M.D. Anderson Solid Tumor Oncology Series 6, DOI 10.1007/978-1-4419-0374-7_33,

Paraneoplastic retinopathies are retinal disorders that present with a constellation of symptoms, few if any ocular signs, abnormal findings on electroretinography (ERG), and usually circulating antiretinal antibodies. The diagnosis is often missed initially, particularly in the absence of an established history of malignancy. *Carcinoma-associated retinopathy* is the term used for an autoimmune retinopathy associated with a cancer other than melanoma. *Melanoma-associated retinopathy* is the term used for an autoimmune retinopathy associated specifically with melanoma. Paraneoplastic optic neuropathy is a rare disorder characterized by painless visual loss, most commonly associated with optic disc edema. Occasionally there is also retinal dysfunction.

Evidence supports an autoimmune basis for the ocular dysfunction associated with paraneoplastic visual syndromes, which are characterized by the presence of circulating autoantibodies and a lack of obvious cancer metastasis causing the structural and functional damage to the retina or nerve [1, 2].

Paraneoplastic neurologic and ophthalmologic syndromes affect the eye as well as other parts of the nervous system, including the cerebellum, limbic system, and peripheral nerves. These syndromes may become apparent before the oncologic diagnosis. Many of these syndromes have antibodies associated with a specific malignancy, which allows targeting the workup to specific organs and/or tissue types. Paraneoplastic neurologic and ophthalmologic syndromes often cause severe and permanent neurologic and ocular morbidity. In general, it is not uncommon for more than one paraneoplastic neurologic syndrome and antibody to coexist in the same patient. However, paraneoplastic retinopathies usually occur without other neurologic autoimmune syndromes and, therefore, the presentation is usually that of vision loss alone. In contrast, paraneoplastic optic neuropathy is commonly associated with cerebellar, cognitive, and other neurological deficits.

33.2 Pathogenesis

Paraneoplastic visual syndromes are thought to be principally autoimmune conditions in which the tumor expresses a neuronal antigen that triggers an immune response against cross-reacting ocular antigens. Antibodies implicated in causing central nervous system paraneoplastic phenomena have been well described and include antineuronal nuclear antibody (ANNA-1 (anti-Hu) and ANNA-2 (anti-Ri)), to name just a couple.

However, in paraneoplastic retinopathy, although a large number of antiretinal antibodies have been reported, only two antibodies have been well characterized [3–5]: antibodies against recoverin (a 23-kDa protein found in rod and cone photoreceptors) and alpha-enolase (a 46-kDa protein). In addition to these, several other antibodies have been suggested as pathogenic in carcinoma-associated retinopathy (CAR)—including tubby-like protein, heat shock cognate protein (hsc70), and 22-, 35-, 40-, and 70-kDa proteins—but their exact location and function in the retina are still being investigated [6–9]. While a few protein antigens, such as mitofilin and titin, have been implicated in melanoma-associated retinopathy (MAR), the immune response characteristically involves antigens within the bipolar cell layer [10].

In paraneoplastic optic neuropathy, CRMP-5 (anti-CV2) has frequently been isolated from the optic nerve [11]. A 22-kDa antigen has also been implicated in paraneoplastic optic neuropathy [6].

33.3 Carcinoma-Associated Retinopathy

CAR is the most common paraneoplastic visual disorder and is most often associated with small cell lung carcinoma and less often associated with carcinoma of the endometrium, ovary, cervix, or breast; hepatocellular carcinoma; gastric cancer; thymoma; colon cancer; and prostate cancer [12–22].

CAR results in visual loss that is usually bilateral, rapid, and painless, with both cone and rod dysfunction. CAR must be suspected in patients who complain of positive visual phenomena like flashing lights, flickering, smoky or swirling vision, transient visual dimming, loss of color vision, and nyctalopia. CAR usually presents after the diagnosis of a malignancy, but in some cases, CAR precedes the cancer diagnosis. On examination, in the early stages of CAR, visual acuity may be preserved, or there may be central vision loss or scotoma, dyschromatopsia, and mild anterior or posterior uveitis; there are few if any fundus changes in the early stages of the disease. Later examinations may reveal retinal vascular attenuation, retinal pigment epithelium loss, and, rarely, optic disc pallor. These findings are usually bilateral, though they may be asymmetric. CAR is associated with abnormalities of a- and b-waves on ERG, signifying photoreceptor dysfunction.

In CAR, there is usually an autoantibody against a specific retinal antigen. Antibodies against recoverin and α-enolase are commonly detected. Anti-recoverin antibodies are almost always associated with a malignancy, whereas anti-enolase antibodies are associated with a malignancy in only about 40% of cases. This means that anti-enolase antibodies can be seen in a syndrome that looks like CAR but no cancer is detectable. In this situation we call the syndrome an autoimmune retinopathy (see Section 33.6) [23].

Recoverin is believed to be a product of a gene localized to the short arm of chromosome 17 at p13.1, close to the gene for the p53 tumor suppressor protein [24]. Recoverin is a 23-kDa calcium-binding protein with 202 amino acid residues. Recoverin can be found not only in rod and cone cells but also in pineal body, optic nerve, and optic tectum [5, 26]. It is known to play an important role in light and dark adaptation by regulating rhodopsin phosphorylation and dephosphorylation in a calcium-dependent manner. Recoverin has been found to be aberrantly expressed in cancer cells or cancer cell lines obtained from CAR patients, and this aberrant expression may trigger the autoimmune reaction, causing progressive retinal degeneration through apoptosis of retinal cells [21, 25]. Expression of recoverin was also found in 50% of cancer tissues from patients without visual symptoms of

CAR. To elucidate the functional roles of aberrant recoverin expression, investigators transfected recoverin into a lung adenocarcinoma cell line (A549) not originally expressing recoverin and found that this caused a slowdown in cell proliferation [21]. Further, the investigators found that recoverin-specific cytotoxic T lymphocytes exist in the peripheral circulation of CAR patients and that these cytotoxic T lymphocytes can recognize tumor that expresses recoverin.

These observations along with the identification of serum antiretinal antibodies point to the autoimmune nature of CAR, which may involve either cell-mediated or humoral immunity, and form the basis for utilizing autoimmune modulating therapies for this condition [26, 27].

33.4 Carcinoma-Associated Cone Dysfunction Syndrome

The carcinoma-associated cone dysfunction syndrome, part of the CAR spectrum, is a rare manifestation of a systemic malignancy, with only a few cases reported in the literature [28–30]. Patients with carcinoma-associated cone dysfunction syndrome have antibodies primarily directed against cones (the antibodies reported are against 23-, 40-, and 50-kDa retinal antigens [28–30]) and consequently have decreased central vision, achromatopsia, central scotomas, glare after light exposure, photosensitivity, positive photostress test, and ERG findings showing marked reduction in cone responses compared to rod responses. Multifocal ERG would be extremely helpful in diagnosing this entity. Histopathology shows loss of cones in the macula and infiltration by macrophages.

33.5 Melanoma-Associated Retinopathy

The other well-known paraneoplastic retinopathy is MAR. This syndrome usually occurs months to years after diagnosis of melanoma when there is advanced metastatic disease, including brain metastasis [31]. The earliest reports of MAR were associated with cutaneous melanoma and, in these cases, MAR was detected at the same time as metastases [32, 33]. While one study found an average time of 3.6 years from the diagnosis of melanoma to the onset of MAR [31], reports in the literature indicate that latency can range from 2 months to 23 years [31, 34].

MAR is distinguished by symptoms such as sudden shimmering and night blindness; usually, there is near normal color vision, visual acuity, and central vision. ERG typically shows markedly reduced or absent dark-adapted b-wave with sparing of a-wave. The fundus findings are initially unremarkable, but subtle abnormalities may be seen by the time a diagnosis is made. In a study of 51 patients with MAR by Keltner et al. [31], fundus findings were normal in 44% of patients; optic disc pallor was observed in 23%, retinal vessel attenuation in 30%, and vitreous cells in 30%. In addition, atypical findings such as serous macular detachment and nummular vitelliform lesions resembling Best vitelliform macular dystrophy have been described [34, 35].

The immune response involves antigens characteristically within the bipolar cell layer detected by immunohistochemistry. The bipolar cell antigens involved are very small quantities of proteins, proteoglycans, lipids, or carbohydrates [31]. Other antigens such as neuronal antigen (22 kDa), transducin β, Muller cell protein (35 kDa), mitofilin, and titin have also been implicated in MAR and can be detected by Western blotting [6, 10, 36, 37]. MAR has also been reported with uveal melanomas [34, 35, 38]. In two cases of MAR associated with uveal melanoma, a 120-kDa antiretinal antibody, anti-enolase (46 kDa), and bestrophin-1 (68 kDa) were isolated from the serum without any signs of bipolar reactivity.

Unfortunately, melanoma has usually metastasized to the central nervous system by the time of diagnosis of MAR, and therefore, patients with this condition usually have a poor prognosis for life.

33.6 Autoimmune Retinopathy

Autoimmune retinopathy is a diagnosis of exclusion established in patients who present with paraneoplastic retinal symptoms but have no malignancy detected after an extensive search. Autoimmune retinopathy has been reported in case reports in the literature [25, 39–42]. In a patient diagnosed with autoimmune retinopathy and a negative initial cancer workup, it is important to repeat the cancer evaluation again after a sufficient duration of follow-up since many patients present with visual symptoms months to years before a malignancy is diagnosed.

The symptoms are generally more subclinical and gradually progressive compared with CAR. However, some patients may have rapid deterioration of vision [27]. Autoimmune retinopathy appears to be self-limiting [42] and has rarely been reported to progress to total blindness as is often the case with CAR due to anti-recoverin [26]. Patients initially complain of central visual loss and photopsia; the periphery may gradually be involved as the condition progresses. Dyschromatopsia, relative afferent pupillary defect disproportionate to the loss of vision, visual field defects, and significant attenuation of amplitude on ERG together with isolation of one or more antiretinal antibodies support the diagnosis of autoimmune retinopathy.

Treatments with immunosuppressive agents are rarely effective in this condition. One reason may be that diagnosis is often delayed until there has been irreversible damage to the neurosensory layers of the retina.

33.7 Paraneoplastic Optic Neuropathy

Paraneoplastic optic neuropathy is a syndrome of visual loss that is usually characterized by bilateral optic disc swelling, nerve fiber layer hemorrhages, and vitritis; sometimes there are abnormal findings on ERG indicating there is also an associated retinopathy. CRMP-5 and anti-CV2 (62 kDa) immunoglobulin, anti-60-kDa, and antiretinal ganglion cell antibodies have been reported in association with this syndrome [11, 43, 44]. Neurological problems are often seen, such as mental status abnormalities, seizures, neuropathies, muscle weaknesses, chorea, hemiballismus, and cerebellar and autonomic abnormalities. Tumors associated with paraneoplastic optic neuropathy include small cell carcinoma of the lung and, less commonly, Hodgkin's disease, non-Hodgkin's lymphoma, neuroblastoma, and thymoma.

33.8 Diagnostic Testing

Given the usual paucity of findings on retinal examination, additional investigations are useful in establishing a diagnosis of paraneoplastic visual syndrome. Electrophysiologic investigations in the form of ERG, visual evoked potential, and sometimes electrooculography have been found to be useful [33]. Photopic and scotopic full-field ERG show extreme attenuation of the electrical response, or even nonrecordable response, but multifocal ERG is useful in demonstrating localized involvement, which is often central. In the conventional full-field ERG the response represents the summed response from different parts of the field; hence, localized defects can be missed. Particularly in cases in which the macula is involved almost exclusively, e.g., carcinoma-associated cone dysfunction, the full-field ERG may not show the extent of the abnormality whereas the multifocal ERG can isolate focal abnormalities in the latency and amplitude of the response. It also provides an alternative for patients who cannot reliably perform visual field tests. A decrease of visual evoked potential that is disproportionate to the decline in visual acuity

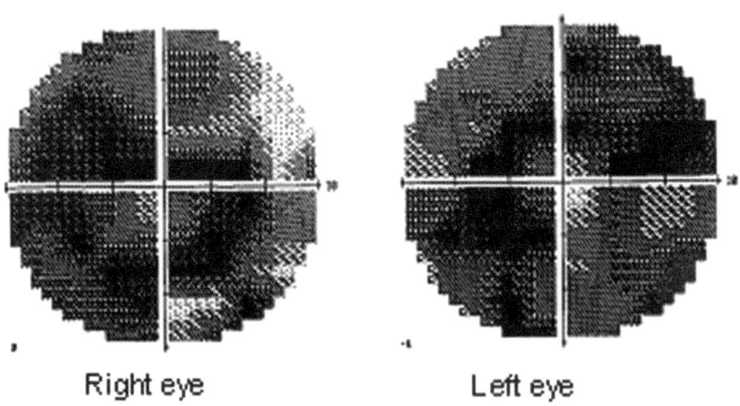

Fig. 33.1 Humphrey visual fields (30-2) showing severe scotoma in a 72-year-old woman. She was diagnosed with autoimmune retinopathy and was diagnosed 1 year later with neuroendocrine carcinoma of the right fallopian tube. From Raghunath A, Adamus G, Bodurka DC, et al. Cancer-associated retinopathy in neuroendocrine carcinoma of the fallopian tube. J Neuroophthalmol 2010;30:252–254. Reprinted with permission

suggests impairment of the macula or the optic nerve as seen in paraneoplastic syndromes [45]. Amsler's grid testing, computerized visual field testing, and ocular coherence tomography (showing thinning of the retina) are other noninvasive techniques that may aid diagnosis [46].

Computerized tomography, magnetic resonance imaging, and positron emission tomography are systemic investigations that are done to rule out the presence of a malignancy when the above investigations point to a diagnosis of paraneoplastic syndrome but no malignancy has previously been identified (Fig. 33.1) [47].

33.9 Differential Diagnosis

A paraneoplastic syndrome is rarely initially considered when a patient presents with symptoms of photopsia or visual loss. Bilateral retinal, bilateral optic nerve, as well as bilateral postchiasmal cortical visual loss should be considered in the differential diagnosis. The more common diagnoses to be considered are infectious diseases, collagen vascular disorders, sarcoid, vasculitis, uveitic syndromes, chemotherapy- or radiation-induced retinopathy, and retinal disorders such as acute zonal occult outer retinopathy (AZOOR) [48, 49]. AZOOR is seen most commonly in females with myopia [50]. It presents with photopsias and almost always involves the blind spot; therefore, AZOOR almost always manifests with enlargement of the blind spot as well as marked areas of visual loss adjacent to the blind spot. The etiology of AZOOR is unknown but may relate to an infectious agent that propagates from the optic disc to the peripapillary choroid.

33.10 Treatment and Prognosis

Visual deterioration in patients with paraneoplastic visual syndromes is believed to occur mainly because of photoreceptor and neuronal cell death by apoptosis, which is permanent once it occurs. This would explain why total recovery of vision has not been reported either spontaneously or with treatment. This also implies that early treatment is necessary for salvaging vision. Though temporary improvement in vision has been reported, a progressive decline to severe visual loss is the usual course, even with treatment.

Various immunotherapies have been tried in patients with paraneoplastic visual syndromes to help prevent deterioration of vision. Agents that have been administered in conjunction with antineoplastic therapy include oral and intravenous steroids, plasmapheresis, intravenous immunoglobulin, and cyclosporine; these have resulted in partial or no success in visual stabilization as reviewed by Chan et al. [51–54].

Other treatments that have been tried include monoclonal antibodies, such as alemtuzumab, which stabilized vision in a patient with chronic lymphocytic leukemia for 8 years [55]. We have used rituximab with mixed results in various syndromes. We had a patient with potential lymphoma-associated retinopathy who responded to rituximab and not steroids.

Anti-recoverin antibody, which is the antibody most commonly associated with CAR, is believed to localize to the photoreceptors and enhance rhodopsin phosphorylation in a calcium-dependent manner, which finally leads to apoptosis of the cell [56]. This prompted some investigators to experimentally use calcium channel blockers such as nilvadipine to reduce intracellular calcium levels and suppress retinal cellular apoptosis [57]. This approach has not yet been proven to be clinically effective [46].

33.11 Conclusion

In conclusion, not only are the paraneoplastic visual syndromes difficult to diagnose, they are also difficult to treat. There is no particular recommended treatment that would work for every patient. Patient tolerance, response to therapy, and titers of circulating antiretinal or anti-optic nerve antibodies could be used as guidelines to choose the best therapy for trying to limit the devastating visual loss seen with paraneoplastic visual syndromes.

References

1. Grunwald GB, Klein R, Simmonds MA, Kornguth SE. Autoimmune basis for visual paraneoplastic syndrome in patients with small-cell lung carcinoma. Lancet 1985;1(8430):658–661.
2. Thirkill CE. Cancer-induced, immune-mediated ocular degenerations. Ocul Immunol Inflamm 2005;13(2–3):119–31.
3. Adamus G, Amundson D, Seigel GM, Machnicki M. Anti-enolase-alpha autoantibodies in cancer-associated retinopathy: epitope mapping and cytotoxicity on retinal cells. J Autoimmun 1998;11(6):671–7.
4. Adamus G, Guy J, Schmied JL, Arendt A, Hargrave PA. Role of anti-recoverin autoantibodies in cancer-associated retinopathy. Invest Ophthalmol Vis Sci 1993;34(9):2626–33.
5. Adamus G, Machnicki M, Elerding H, Sugden B, Blocker YS, Fox DA. Antibodies to recoverin induce apoptosis of photoreceptor and bipolar cells in vivo. J Autoimmun 1998;11(5):523–33.
6. Keltner JL, Thirkill CE. The 22-kDa antigen in optic nerve and retinal diseases. J Neuroophthalmol 1999;19(2):71–83.
7. Ohguro H, Ogawa K, Nakagawa T. Recoverin and Hsc 70 are found as autoantigens in patients with cancer-associated retinopathy. Invest Ophthalmol Vis Sci 1999;40(1):82–9.
8. Takahashi K, Suzuki J, Ohguro H, Ohyachi H, Yoshida K, Takahashi H, Nakagawa T. [A case of paraneoplastic retinopathy with serum antibody against retinal soluble 70 kDa protein]. Nippon Ganka Gakkai Zasshi 1997;101(1):92–6.
9. Kikuchi T, Arai J, Shibuki H, Kawashima H, Yoshimura N. Tubby-like protein 1 as an autoantigen in cancer-associated retinopathy. J Neuroimmunol 2000;103(1):26–33.
10. Pfohler C, Preuss KD, Tilgen W, Stark A, Regitz E, Fadle N, Pfreundschuh M. Mitofilin and titin as target antigens in melanoma-associated retinopathy. Int J Cancer 2007;120(4):788–95.
11. Cross SA, Salomao DR, Parisi JE, Kryzer TJ, Bradley EA, Mines JA, Lam BL, Lennon VA. Paraneoplastic autoimmune optic neuritis with retinitis defined by CRMP-5-IgG. Ann Neurol 2003;54(1):38–50.

12. Adamus G, Amundson D, MacKay C, Gouras P. Long-term persistence of antirecoverin antibodies in endometrial cancer-associated retinopathy. Arch Ophthalmol 1998;116(2): 251–3.
13. Khan N, Huang JJ, Foster CS. Cancer associated retinopathy (CAR): an autoimmune-mediated paraneoplastic syndrome. Semin Ophthalmol 2006;21(3):135–41.
14. Chang PY, Yang CH, Yang CM. Cancer-associated retinopathy in a patient with hepatocellular carcinoma: case report and literature review. Retina 2005;25(8):1093–6.
15. Eltabbakh GH, Hoogerland DL, Kay MC. Paraneoplastic retinopathy associated with uterine sarcoma. Gynecol Oncol 1995;58(1):120–3.
16. Harmon JP, Purvin VA, Guy J, Aptsiauri N, Sutton GP. Cancer-associated retinopathy in a patient with advanced epithelial ovarian carcinoma. Gynecol Oncol 1999;73(3):430–2.
17. Harper DG, Arsura EL, Bobba RK, Reddy CM, Sawh AK. Acquired color blindness in an elderly male patient from recurrent metastatic prostate cancer. J Am Geriatr Soc 2005;53(7):1265–7.
18. Seles S, Lang GE. [CAR syndrome (carcinoma-associated retinopathy syndrome) associated with an adenocarcinoma of the cervix]. Klin Monbl Augenheilkd 2005;222(9):736–9.
19. Yamada G, Ohguro H, Aketa K, Itoh T, Shijubo N, Takahashi H, Fujiwara O, Satoh M, Ohtsuka K, Abe S. Invasive thymoma with paraneoplastic retinopathy. Hum Pathol 2003;34(7):717–9.
20. Yoon YH, Cho EH, Sohn J, Thirkill CE. An unusual type of cancer-associated retinopathy in a patient with ovarian cancer. Korean J Ophthalmol 1999;13(1):43–8.
21. Ohguro H, Odagiri H, Miyagawa Y, Ohguro I, Sasaki M, Nakazawa M. Clinicopathological features of gastric cancer cases and aberrantly expressed recoverin. Tohoku J Exp Med 2004;202(3):213–9.
22. Jacobson DM, Adamus G. Retinal anti-bipolar cell antibodies in a patient with paraneoplastic retinopathy and colon carcinoma. Am J Ophthalmol 2001;131(6):806–8.
23. Weleber RG, Watzke RC, Shults WT, Trzupek KM, Heckenlively JR, Egan RA, Adamus G. Clinical and electrophysiologic characterization of paraneoplastic and autoimmune retinopathies associated with antienolase antibodies. Am J Ophthalmol 2005;139(5):780–94.
24. McGinnis JF, Austin B, Klisak I, Heinzmann C, Kojis T, Sparkes RS, Bateman JB, Lerious V. Chromosomal assignment of the human gene for the cancer-associated retinopathy protein (recoverin) to chromosome 17p13.1. J Neurosci Res 1995;40(2):165–8.
25. Adamus G. Autoantibody-induced apoptosis as a possible mechanism of autoimmune retinopathy. Autoimmun Rev 2003;2(2):63–8.
26. Whitcup SM, Vistica BP, Milam AH, Nussenblatt RB, Gery I. Recoverin-associated retinopathy: a clinically and immunologically distinctive disease. Am J Ophthalmol 1998;126(2): 230–7.
27. Heckenlively JR, Fawzi AA, Oversier J, Jordan BL, Aptsiauri N. Autoimmune retinopathy: patients with antirecoverin immunoreactivity and panretinal degeneration. Arch Ophthalmol 2000;118(11):1525–33.
28. Jacobson DM, Thirkill CE. Paraneoplastic cone dysfunction: an unusual visual remote effect of cancer. Arch Ophthalmol 1995;113(12):1580–2.
29. Parc CE, Azan E, Bonnel S, Sahel JA, Kaplan J, Thirkill CE. Cone dysfunction as a paraneoplastic syndrome associated with retinal antigens approximating 40 kiloDalton. Ophthalmic Genet 2006;27(2):57–61.
30. Cogan DG, Kuwabara T, Currie J, Kattah J. [Paraneoplastic retinopathy simulating cone dystrophy with achromatopsia]. Klin Monbl Augenheilkd 1990;197(2):156–8.
31. Keltner JL, Thirkill CE, Yip PT. Clinical and immunologic characteristics of melanoma-associated retinopathy syndrome: eleven new cases and a review of 51 previously published cases. J Neuroophthalmol 2001;21(3):173–87.
32. Rougier MB, Hostyn P, Bret-Dibat C, Delaunay MM, Riss I, Le Rebeller MJ. [Paraneoplastic retinopathy associated with cutaneous melanoma. An update apropos of a case]. J Fr Ophthalmol 1995;18(5):396–403.

33. Weinstein JM, Kelman SE, Bresnick GH, Kornguth SE. Paraneoplastic retinopathy associated with antiretinal bipolar cell antibodies in cutaneous malignant melanoma. Ophthalmology 1994;101(7):1236–43.
34. Zacks DN, Pinnolis MK, Berson EL, Gragoudas ES. Melanoma-associated retinopathy and recurrent exudative retinal detachments in a patient with choroidal melanoma. Am J Ophthalmol 2001;132(4):578–81.
35. Eksandh L, Adamus G, Mosgrove L, Andreasson S. Autoantibodies against bestrophin in a patient with vitelliform paraneoplastic retinopathy and a metastatic choroidal malignant melanoma. Arch Ophthalmol 2008;126(3):432–5.
36. Flynn M, Fishman G, Adamus G. Antiretinal Muller cell antibodies in patients with melanoma associated and autoimmune retinopathy. Invest Ophthalmol Vis Sci 2000;41:S567.
37. Potter MJ, Adamus G, Szabo SM, Lee R, Mohaseb K, Behn D. Autoantibodies to transducin in a patient with melanoma-associated retinopathy. Am J Ophthalmol 2002;134(1): 128–30.
38. Sotodeh M, Paridaens D, Keunen J, van Schooneveld M, Adamus G, Baarsma S. Paraneoplastic vitelliform retinopathy associated with cutaneous or uveal melanoma and metastases. Klin Monbl Augenheilkd 2005;222(11):910–4.
39. Peek R, Verbraak F, Coevoct HM, Kijlstra A. Muller cell-specific autoantibodies in a patient with progressive loss of vision. Invest Ophthalmol Vis Sci 1998;39(10):1976–9.
40. Hargitai J, MacKay C, Behrens M, Odel JG, Hood DC, Gouras P. Auto-immune-like cone dystrophy. Doc Ophthalmol 2004;109(3):215–21.
41. Mizener JB, Kimura AE, Adamus G, Thirkill CE, Goeken JA, Kardon RH. Autoimmune retinopathy in the absence of cancer. Am J Ophthalmol 1997;123(5):607–18.
42. Mantel I, Ramchand KV, Holder GE, Ohbayashi M, Morohoshi K, Patel N, Toda M, Fitzke FW, Bird AC, Ono SJ. Macular and retinal dysfunction of unknown origin in adults with normal fundi: evidence for an autoimmune pathophysiology. Exp Mol Pathol 2008;84(2): 90–101.
43. Lieberman FS, Odel J, Hirsh J, Heinemann M, Michaeli J, Posner J. Bilateral optic neuropathy with IgGkappa multiple myeloma improved after myeloablative chemotherapy. Neurology 1999;52(2):414–6.
44. Luiz JE, Lee AG, Keltner JL, Thirkill CE, Lai EC. Paraneoplastic optic neuropathy and autoantibody production in small-cell carcinoma of the lung. J Neuroophthalmol 1998;18(3):178–81.
45. Matsui Y, Mehta MC, Katsumi O, Brodie SE, Hirose T. Electrophysiological findings in paraneoplastic retinopathy. Graefes Arch Clin Exp Ophthalmol 1992;230(4):324–8.
46. Mohamed Q, Harper CA. Acute optical coherence tomographic findings in cancer-associated retinopathy. Arch Ophthalmol 2007;125(8):1132–3.
47. Linke R, Schroeder M, Helmberger T, Voltz R. Antibody-positive paraneoplastic neurologic syndromes: value of CT and PET for tumor diagnosis. Neurology 2004;63(2):282–6.
48. Sadowski B, Kriegbaum C, Apfelstedt-Sylla E. Tamoxifen side effects, age-related macular degeneration (AMD) or cancer associated retinopathy (CAR)? Eur J Ophthalmol 2001;11(3):309–12.
49. Koestinger A, Guex-Crosier Y, Borruat FX. Autoimmune retinal dysfunction in sarcoid chorioretinopathy. Klin Monbl Augenheilkd 2006;223(5):428–30.
50. Gass JD. Acute zonal occult outer retinopathy. Donders Lecture: The Netherlands Ophthalmological Society, Maastricht, Holland, June 19, 1992. J Clin Neuroophthalmol 1993;13(2):79–97.
51. Guy J, Aptsiauri N. Treatment of paraneoplastic visual loss with intravenous immunoglobulin: report of 3 cases. Arch Ophthalmol 1999;117(4):471–7.
52. Klingele TG, Burde RM, Rappazzo JA, Isserman MJ, Burgess D, Kantor O. Paraneoplastic retinopathy. J Clin Neuroophthalmol 1984;4(4):239–45.
53. Chan JW. Paraneoplastic retinopathies and optic neuropathies. Surv Ophthalmol 2003;48(1):12–38.

54. Subhadra C, Dudek AZ, Rath PP, Lee MS. Improvement in visual fields in a patient with melanoma-associated retinopathy treated with intravenous immunoglobulin. J Neuroophthalmol 2008;28(1):23–6.
55. Espandar L, O'Brien S, Thirkill C, Lubecki LA, Esmaeli B. Successful treatment of cancer-associated retinopathy with alemtuzumab. J Neurooncol 2007;83(3):295–302.
56. Maeda T, Maeda A, Maruyama I, Ogawa KI, Kuroki Y, Sahara H, Sato N, Ohguro H. Mechanisms of photoreceptor cell death in cancer-associated retinopathy. Invest Ophthalmol Vis Sci 2001;42(3):705–12.
57. Ohguro H, Ogawa K, Maeda T, Maruyama I, Maeda A, Takano Y, Nakazawa M. Retinal dysfunction in cancer-associated retinopathy is improved by Ca(2+) antagonist administration and dark adaptation. Invest Ophthalmol Vis Sci 2001;42(11):2589–95.
58. Raghunath A, Adamus G, Bodurka DC, Liu J, Schiffman J. Cancer-associated retinopathy in neuroendocrine carcinoma of the fallopian tube. J Neuroopthalmol 2010;30(3):252–4.

Chapter 34
Neurofibromatosis: Tumors of the Optic Pathway

John M. Slopis and Jade S. Schiffman

Abstract Various tumors occur in patients with neurofibromatosis type 1. In this chapter, we discuss the clinical presentation and evaluation of four types of tumors affecting patients with neurofibromatosis type 1: periorbital and orbital neurofibroma, intraorbital optic nerve glioma, chiasmal and hypothalamic glioma, and intraparenchymal astrocytoma. Treatment options are also discussed.

34.1 Introduction

Neurofibromatosis (NF) is a common neurocutaneous disorder affecting approximately 1 in 4000 individuals [1]. NF is a group of genetic disorders that include NF type 1 (NF1), NF type 2 (NF2), and multiple schwannomatosis; each form of the disorder has different genetic mutations and pathologic bases. NF2 and multiple schwannomatosis are essentially disorders of the cranial nerves, peripheral nerves, and meningeal tissues and do not as commonly impact the optic pathway as NF1. This chapter will focus on NF1; therefore, NF2 and multiple schwannomatosis will be excluded from this discussion.

The *NF1* gene coding region is a large gene segment localized to chromosome 17 [2, 3]. The *NF1* gene is nearly ubiquitous in human tissues. The gene is expressed in fetal ectoderm, neuroectoderm, mesoderm, and neural crest tissues; thus, the *NF1* gene impacts virtually all organ systems, including all components of the optic pathway. The *NF1* gene codes the production of the protein neurofibromin, which is central to the growth and development of many tissues during fetal development and serves as a maintenance growth regulator for tissues after birth [4]. Mutations of this gene thus lead to congenital tumors and other structural malformations, as well as benign tumors of later onset that continue to grow throughout life.

The most common tumor caused by *NF1* mutation is the neurofibroma, a histologically benign tumor of the peripheral nerve sheath that often involves adipose

J.M. Slopis (✉)
Department of Neuro-Oncology, The University of Texas M.D. Anderson Cancer Center, Houston, TX, USA
e-mail: jmslopis@mdanderson.org

B. Esmaeli (ed.), *Ophthalmic Oncology*, M.D. Anderson Solid Tumor Oncology Series 6, DOI 10.1007/978-1-4419-0374-7_34,

or connective tissues and vascular structures. Periorbital and orbital neurofibromas are histologically and developmentally distinct from optic pathway gliomas. Craniofacial neurofibromas may develop within the neural, muscular, and osseous elements of the orbital wall.

The "benign" nature of neurofibroma endows it with resistance to conventional chemotherapy and radiation therapy. Although optic pathway gliomas in NF1 patients are presumed to result from the same gene mutation, optic pathway gliomas may be more amenable to current treatment methods, which will be discussed later. Subsets of optic nerve gliomas do remain resistant to treatment, and more effective medical regimens are needed. Localization of the *NF1* gene in 1970 and subsequent isolation of the neurofibromin protein in 1990 have led to the development of numerous strategies for treatment of *NF1* using modulators of intracellular cell signal transduction, but novel treatment trials are just beginning.

The diagnosis of NF1 is based on clinical findings. The diagnostic criteria for NF1 (see Table 34.1) are based on a consensus statement by the National Institutes of Health, developed in 1988 [5] and reaffirmed in 1997 [6], representing the most frequent clinical features of NF1. The diagnosis of NF1 is established when two or more features from this list are identified in the patient.

Table 34.1 Diagnostic criteria for NF1

1. Six or more cafe-au-lait spots greater than 5 mm in diameter in prepubertal children or greater than 15 mm in diameter in postpubertal individuals
2. Two or more neurofibromas of any form or one plexiform neurofibroma
3. Freckling in the axillary or inguinal regions
4. Optic glioma
5. Two or more Lisch nodules (iris hamartomas)
6. Distinctive osseous lesion, such as sphenoid dysplasia or thinning of the long bone cortex with or without pseudoarthrosis
7. A first-degree relative with NF1 by the above criteria

Note: The presence of two or more criteria constitutes a definitive diagnosis in an individual. If an individual has a first-degree relative with NF1, then only one additional criterion is required for the diagnosis

The most promising development in genetic testing for NF1 is DNA sequencing of the *NF1* coding region on chromosome 17. This technology has revealed great variability in DNA sequences in the *NF1* gene region, as might be expected in a disorder with great clinical variability. Several hundred distinct mutation patterns, including deletions and rearrangements, have been found in DNA samples from individuals who meet clinical diagnostic criteria.

34.2 NF1 and the Optic Pathway

We will be restricting our discussion hereafter to NF1 and the visual sensory pathway. Optic pathway tumors occur in approximately 15% of patients with NF1 [7]. The overwhelming majority of these tumors are asymptomatic, and symptomatic tumors usually present in childhood. A small number of tumors become symptomatic in early adulthood. These tumors develop anywhere along the optic pathway, with each location presenting unique challenges in clinical management. Although most discussions of NF1 and the visual pathway refer to tumors as "optic gliomas," several tumor types affect the visual pathways in NF1. We divide NF1-related tumors into four types related to their anatomic distribution: (1) periorbital and orbital neurofibroma, (2) intraorbital optic nerve glioma, (3) chiasmal and hypothalamic glioma, and (4) intraparenchymal astrocytoma.

Periorbital and orbital neurofibroma only rarely affects the orbital optic nerve; however, significant visual problems are created because of its amblyogenic potential (to be discussed below); therefore, we have included a discussion of this tumor in this chapter.

The *NF1* gene plays a dominant role in fetal tissue development, and the impact may be general or focal in nature. The sequence of events in embryogenesis that leads to development of the brain and eyes includes interactions between developing bone, muscle, skin, neural tissue, and neural crest tissue. For this reason, in many cases the resulting tumors are actually dysplastic growths of multiple tissue (neurofibromata), and in the case of periorbital neurofibroma, these lesions can cause distortion of the normal periorbital anatomy. In cases of optic nerve gliomas, this may be an isolated finding among otherwise normal-appearing anatomic structures.

When necessary for cosmetic and/or vision problems, periorbital and orbital neurofibromas of NF1 are most often managed by surgical means alone. Optic nerve gliomas are usually managed conservatively, and there is controversy on how to manage these tumors when and if progressive visual loss ensues. Some continue conservative management without intervention; others use chemotherapy and, rarely, surgery depending on the specific anatomy. Radiation therapy may be considered for optic nerve gliomas when all other modalities fail and the patient is developing progressive visual loss; however, this modality may have significant morbidity in patients with NF1.

34.3 Periorbital and Orbital Neurofibroma

34.3.1 Description and Clinical Issues

Periorbital and orbital neurofibromas are relatively uncommon and are challenging tumors to manage. Most often these tumors form as plexiform neurofibromas and usually affect patients with NF1 within the first year of life [8]. Periorbital and orbital neurofibromas affect the face and are among the most disfiguring and problematic of all lesions in NF1 patients. Tissues involved include periorbital skin, fascia, and muscle, which are dysplastic tissues and often involve the eyelid and anterior part of the orbit. Rarely do these tumors affect the optic nerve, but they often affect vision because of several amblyogenic factors associated with the tumor (see below). The slow growth of plexiform neurofibromas often remains a persistent problem after surgical resection, especially in the case of tumors involving the eyelid that are not fully resected and continue to grow. Frequently, continued growth of a neurofibroma leads to progressive obstruction of the visual axis by simple overgrowth or by induction of ptosis due to levator muscle dysfunction. Surgical resection of the neurofibroma is often complicated because the dysplastic nature of the tumor obscures normal anatomic tissue planes and clean margins of resection cannot be obtained. Connective tissues often become excessively elastic over time because of the presence of the *NF1* gene mutations, and slow regrowth of the tumor often leads to repeat surgical procedures throughout the patient's lifetime. Bony dysplasia, particularly seen in the sphenoid bone, can lead to massive proptosis and brain herniation (Fig. 34.1).

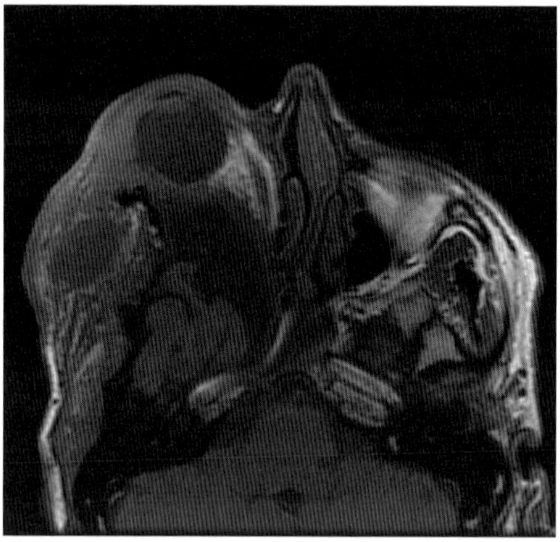

Fig. 34.1 MRI findings in a patient with NF1 with severe sphenoid wing dysplasia and herniation of the brain parenchyma (the right temporal lobe) into the orbit causing massive proptosis. There is also a periorbital and subcutaneous neurofibroma that extends into the infratemporal and pterygopalatine fossa. Figure courtesy of Dr. Bita Esmaeli

It is very rare for a plexiform neurofibroma of the eyelid or orbit to affect the ipsilateral optic nerve. Additionally, it is unusual for a child with a plexiform neurofibroma of the eyelid or orbit to have a concomitant optic nerve glioma in the same eye, but this scenario is sometimes encountered and makes identifying the cause of progressive visual loss more difficult.

34.3.2 Evaluation and Management

Preoperative assessment includes magnetic resonance imaging (MRI) of the face and orbit to determine the extent of the tumor in the periorbita and orbit. T1- and T2-weighted MRI sequences are helpful in delineating the margins of tumor amid distorted anatomic structures. Contrast enhancement offers little useful information, but special imaging sequences, including fat-suppressed MRI, may be helpful. Three-dimensional computed tomography (CT) with reconstruction is often useful in defining associated features resulting from NF1, such as bony dysplasia of the orbit and associated facial structures, when this information is required.

Routine ophthalmologic examination is mandatory. Periorbital and orbital neurofibromas can cause amblyopia due to one or more of the following three mechanisms: (1) Occlusion amblyopia caused by the lid covering the visual axis. (2) Anisometropic amblyopia caused by a ptotic, heavy lid creating a pressure-induced astigmatism in the affected eye. If this refractive error is left uncorrected, it leads to refractive amblyopia. This can happen without the visual axis being covered, leading to a false belief that amblyopia is not present because the visual axis is uncovered. (3) Strabismic amblyopia caused by an ocular muscle imbalance that often is not obvious and requires ophthalmic skill to detect. This problem can happen silently and may be missed if the patient is not properly examined. As stated before, plexiform neurofibromas do not usually involve the orbit to the extent that they cause optic neuropathy, but this is still a potential source of decreased vision.

Different from the periorbital and orbital plexiform neurofibroma described above, occasionally isolated orbital neurofibromas can develop that may cause proptosis or strabismus (with or without visual loss depending on its bulk) and may have amblyogenic potential and less likely compress the optic nerve. These tumors arise from nerves within the orbit and may involve the superior orbit, including the lacrimal gland, or the inferior orbit.

Periorbital and orbital neurofibromas include cutaneous and subcutaneous elements that can undergo malignant transformation; however, concern about malignant transformation is not the basis for considering intervention [9].

The risk of malignant transformation is about 7–10% for neurofibromas in patients with NF1, and transformation of an orbital neurofibroma to a soft tissue sarcoma may also be encountered [10].

It is therefore important to have an ophthalmologist experienced in amblyopia detection and management routinely evaluate those with periorbital and orbital neurofibromas to maintain the best possible vision by management of amblyopia. Additionally, plexiform neurofibromas in NF1 patients are sometimes associated with congenital glaucoma, and this needs to be examined for carefully by a trained ophthalmologist. There is up to a 50% chance of glaucoma on the side of the neurofibroma, and this glaucoma may present as buphthalmos with or without corneal edema. The risk of glaucoma is higher in patients with NF1 with ectropion uvea. Of course malignant degeneration needs to be looked for with a rapid growth phase.

Indications for surgical intervention vary from case to case. Apparent progression toward occlusive ptosis and facial disfigurement should be the primary indications for intervention. There is no specific age required for surgical intervention; however, surgery is usually delayed as long as possible because of the recurrent nature of these tumors. There is no predictable growth pattern of periorbital and orbital tumors, although some may progress more rapidly when children enter puberty and therefore this may not indicate malignant transformation.

34.4 Intraorbital Optic Nerve Glioma

34.4.1 Description and Clinical Issues

The term *intraorbital optic nerve glioma* refers to tumors of the optic nerve and includes juvenile pilocytic astrocytoma of the optic nerve proper. A number of optic nerve growths in NF1 patients are very stable and cause no visual loss; it is thought that many of these growths are actually dural ectasia (thickening of the optic nerve sheath) and are not really a dividing tumor. True optic nerve gliomas occur as early as the first year of life, and the incidence peaks between 4 and 6 years of age [7]. These tumors rarely progress if they are still asymptomatic when a patient reaches 6 years of age. As a group, these tumors all appear on MRI as abnormal thickening of the orbital component of the optic nerve.

Optic nerve gliomas may be detected because of the presence of proptosis, disorder of extraocular movement, visual loss, optic disc swelling and/or pallor, or asymptomatic incidental findings on MRI.

It is important to determine whether optic nerve gliomas are growing or stable. As mentioned above, many cases of optic nerve glioma are thought to represent simple dural ectasia, an asymptomatic lesion that does not affect the patient's vision and extraocular motility, representing an incidental finding on screening MRI or CT. Dural ectasias are nonprogressive and should not be treated. Some believe that the optic nerve glioma in NF1 is really a hamartoma. Some clinicians conclude that only symptomatic tumors actually require attention and that MRI of the orbit in patients with NF1 is indicated only in cases of disturbance of visual acuity or extraocular motility. This position has been formalized in some published principles of management for NF1 patients [6]. A second school of thought suggests that early detection leads to closer scrutiny of visual status in the affected child, making routine MRI for all children with NF1 more prudent. An additional argument in favor of MRI screening is that clinically silent features of NF1, such as glioma of the optic chiasm, hypothalamus, or other areas, may be detected as part of the screening process. Given the varying approaches to MRI screening, the exact ratio of asymptomatic to symptomatic tumors is unknown, but it is estimated to be about 10:1.

Many cases of symptomatic optic nerve glioma are histopathologically proven juvenile pilocytic astrocytoma. These cases are identified from tissue samples obtained during debulking of symptomatic mass lesions. The mechanism of visual loss is presumed to be invasion of the central core of the optic nerve with subsequent disruption of the axon bundles comprising the optic nerve. The slowly progressive nature of the visual loss caused by these tumors supports this idea. Proptosis—due to a dense mass effect of the thickened optic nerve or cystic accumulations of spinal fluid along the optic nerve—is present in some but not all cases of symptomatic intraorbital optic nerve glioma. Of note, a number of these gliomas actually involve the entire visual pathway, including the intracranial optic nerve, chiasm, and tract.

34.4.2 Evaluation and Management

Asymptomatic intraorbital optic nerve gliomas are generally diagnosed by a screening MRI; at the time of discovery, the tumors should be considered presymptomatic until proven otherwise. No specific protocol exists for clinical follow-up or routine imaging. A strong case can be made for yearly follow-up MRIs until the age of 6 years, accompanied by careful ophthalmologic examination every 6 months, then yearly thereafter. Formal visual field testing is perhaps the most sensitive and reproducible tool for measurement of visual impairment, but the early age of onset, e.g., 18–24 months, makes this approach untenable. Some children can do visual field testing reliably at age 3, but most cannot. Because many children with NF1 also have attention-deficit disorder, visual field testing may be unreliable even at older ages. Regular visual evoked response testing has been endorsed by some authors, but the utility of this procedure remains untested in large clinical trials [11]. We endorse careful ophthalmologic examination with attention to vision and visual function, confrontation visual field testing, and a careful pupil examination with quantification of afferent pupillary defects when possible.

Management options for optic glioma disorders depend on the loss of visual function and/or the development of proptosis. Some children with optic nerve gliomas develop a sensory esotropia or exotropia, and a component of the visual loss may be from amblyopia; however, in our experience, if there is a deviation of the eye from an optic nerve glioma, most of the visual loss is from the optic nerve problem and not due to the strabismus causing amblyopia. However, it is not unreasonable to try patching of the good eye to see if there is improvement in the eye with the optic glioma and strabismus. Management of progressive and severe proptosis may include surgical debulking, but this approach will not likely improve visual function.

Chemotherapy can be considered if possible, and radiation therapy should be considered as a last resort. Chemotherapy for optic nerve glioma has been studied in a trial at the Children's Cancer Group (CCG A9952). This trial included a comparison of response rates of optic nerve glioma in children with and without NF1. The response rate for the two clinical groups was similar and, to date, combination of cisplatin and vincristine remains the most commonly used regimen. The trial results are not formally available; however, the response rates were reportedly up to 50%. However, treatment of these benign-acting tumors still remains controversial, in that we do not know whether the natural history of vision loss with or without treatment is better. Also there are documented cases where vision improves without intervention.

Radiation therapy remains a highly controversial modality for patients with NF1. Although radiation produces excellent control in over 90% of patients, long-term secondary effects do occur, including secondary tumors and radiation injury to the optic nerve itself [12, 13]. Some reports indicate that the long-term outcome for vision may be improved following radiation treatment [14]. In the Children's Cancer Group trial, children with NF1 below the age of 2 years were not allowed to receive radiation therapy because of the general risk of radiation injury to the developing brain and the high risk of long-term secondary malignancy and vascular malformations. Secondary malignancies include meningioma formation within the orbit or base of the skull. Vascular malformations include progressive stenosis of the proximal middle cerebral artery at the junction of the internal carotid artery, also known as moyamoya disease [15]. Since the *NF1* gene is a growth regulator and tumor suppressor gene, radiation therapy is usually avoided when possible at any age, and it is used only when patients have a poor response to chemotherapy.

34.5 Chiasmal and Hypothalamic Glioma

34.5.1 Description and Clinical Issues

As previously mentioned, the incidence of optic pathway tumors in NF1 patients is 15%, but what proportion of those tumors are optic chiasm tumors is unknown. Tumors of the optic chiasm present with imaging features similar to those of intraorbital optic nerve glioma, and intraorbital tumors often extend through the optic canal to the chiasm and, sometimes, the optic tract. Symptoms associated with active chiasmal glioma are quite different from those of pure intraorbital tumors because of the bilaterality of visual loss. Symptomatic optic chiasmal gliomas are most often true juvenile pilocytic gliomas.

Visual symptoms of optic chiasm glioma include unilateral or, more often, bilateral optic nerve defects and bitemporal and homonymous visual field defects. Optic atrophy is often present, which is sometimes associated with a “bow–tie” pattern. Afferent pupillary defects are often present in the eye with the most visual field loss. Formal visual field testing is the preferred approach to clinical testing, but again, the early age of presentation makes this problematic.

34.5.2 Evaluation and Management

MRI demonstrates enlargement of the chiasm that is either symmetric or asymmetric [16]. The optic chiasm may enlarge sufficiently to merge with the hypothalamic structures just caudal to the chiasm, so high-resolution MRI with thin cuts through the chiasm, pituitary, and hypothalamus is usually the preferred modality. Progressive or active tumors frequently show enhancement on T1 postcontrast images. T2 flair images frequently show increased signal intensity of the chiasm and adjacent hypothalamic structures as well as the more distal regions of the optic pathway extending into the brain parenchyma to the region of the posterior thalamus. Positive response to treatment is judged by reduction of size of the chiasmal mass, stability of the chiasmal mass, or reduction of T1 postcontrast enhancement. T2 flair images may remain unchanged after treatment, and therefore flair changes are a less reliable sign of treatment response. Not infrequently, chiasmal gliomas grow into one or both of the optic tracts.

Therefore, careful ophthalmic follow-up with visual acuity testing, pupillary examination, and confrontation visual field testing with quantification (when possible) is important to determine whether there are signs of progression. No specific data are available regarding the use of visual evoked potentials to assess the status of vision with these tumors. Rarely, these tumors become large enough to occlude the third ventricle and cause obstructive hydrocephalus. Children with hydrocephalus may or may not have papilledema. The presence of papilledema is dependent on the degree of optic atrophy present. When optic atrophy is present, the optic nerves may not have enough axons to demonstrate optic disc swelling despite the presence of raised intracranial pressure in association with the hydrocephalus. (Please see discussion below about management of papilledema.) Other ophthalmic findings from hydrocephalus could include Parinaud syndrome and cranial nerve palsies, usually of cranial nerve VI.

Tumors of the optic chiasm are frequently associated with endocrine dysfunction, even when there is no clear involvement of the hypothalamic structures or pituitary [17]. Interestingly, optic chiasm glioma is associated with accelerated systemic growth and secondary sex characteristic development, also known as precocious puberty. Irradiation of the optic chiasm for treatment of progressive tumor induces hypopituitarism. Children treated with radiation therapy should thus be followed by pediatric endocrinologists [17]. This is yet another risk of radiation treatment, but it may be considered an acceptable risk in cases of a treatment-resistant tumor and progressive visual loss. Monitoring requires careful endocrinologic examinations. A major problem in patients with hypothalamic involvement is hypothalamic obesity, a problem that is extremely difficult to manage and is a major health risk.

Similar to the treatment of optic nerve gliomas, the treatment of optic chiasmal gliomas remains controversial, in that we do not know if the natural history of vision loss in children with these tumors is altered by treatment and there have been documented cases where vision improves without intervention.

34.6 Intraparenchymal Astrocytoma

34.6.1 Description and Clinical Issues

Tumors beyond the optic tract and within the brain parenchyma are usually low-grade tumors, specifically juvenile pilocytic astrocytoma. These tumors are sampled infrequently, primarily when tumors are resected following treatment failure or when tumor mass effect is producing secondary intracranial symptoms such as obstructive hydrocephalus. Symptoms of visual disturbance are variable, depending on the tumor location along the optic pathway from the lateral geniculate/posterior thalamus. Astrocytomas generally do not develop in the most posterior segments of the optic pathway beyond the thalamus to the calcarine cortex; instead, astrocytomas more often develop anteriorly. Posteriorly placed tumors cause visual disturbances which include field defects and disorders of visual higher cortical function, such as hemineglect syndromes [18]. Functional studies of vision in these locations are best assessed by formal visual field testing. Of note, when a tumor causes obstructive hydrocephalus, as might occur with a tumor of the posterior thalamus and/or midbrain, patients may develop hydrocephalus and papilledema and secondary visual loss from long-standing papilledema.

Cases of papilledema must be followed closely by an experienced ophthalmologist to determine if visual function is threatened, which would require intervention by shunt placement, third ventriculostomy, and/or optic nerve sheath fenestration. Visual function in children with papilledema may be difficult to follow, especially if the child is young, inattentive, and unable to perform automated visual field testing. Therefore, careful and detailed visual acuity examination, pupillary examination, and quantification of confrontation visual fields must be done with a frequency that is determined case by case, on the basis of the child's response and ability to quantitate the visual function. Other factors influencing management decisions include the amount of edema, presence or absence of impending postpapilledema optic atrophy, and change over time. When visual failure is threatening, a qualified multidisciplinary team of physicians should be involved in determining the correct procedure and medical management, which may be temporizing (e.g., acetazolamide). As visual failure from undertreated papilledema is usually not reversible, it is imperative to intervene early.

Disorders of higher cortical function secondary to tumor development must not be confused with specific higher cortical dysfunction syndromes commonly associated with NF1. These syndromes include visual spatial and visual motor dysfunction, which are present in approximately 40% of NF1 patients [19]. These syndromes are commonly expressed as various forms of dyslexia and/or dysgraphia and are usually first recognized as learning disabilities in children with NF1 [20]. These cognitive syndromes in NF1 have been well studied and appear to result from several forms of disordered brain development in utero [21–24]. These disorders are easily screened for with the judgement of line orientation test, and this technique should be utilized in assessment of all children with NF1 as part of the full neurocognitive assessment and screening for learning disability [25]. Likewise, a full neurocognitive assessment should be performed on all children prior to treatment of tumors within the brain parenchyma.

Although most tumors of the optic pathway are juvenile pilocytic astrocytomas, other tumor types may develop, including lower-grade and higher-grade tumors. Lower-grade tumors are referred to as hamartomas and are essentially regions of tissue dysplasia without neoplastic features. Unfortunately, mutation of the *NF1* gene may serve as a tumor growth promoter (failure of tumor suppressor gene function), causing some parenchymal mass lesions to evolve spontaneously or to recur at resection margins. Primary and recurrent tumors may develop as higher-grade astrocytomas, including anaplastic astrocytomas, glioblastomas multiforme, and glial sarcomas.

In patients with NF1, intraparenchymal astrocytomas of the brain stem and cerebellum may occur. Although these tumors are not technically in the sensory visual pathway, their growth leads to obstructive hydrocephalus, which can lead to visual involvement related to complications of hydrocephalus. These tumors can also lead to paralytic strabismus that, if not monitored, can lead to strabismic amblyopia.

34.6.2 Evaluation and Management

Assessment of tumors of the brain parenchyma includes an MRI of the brain, MR spectroscopy of specific lesions, neurological assessment, and neuro-ophthalmological assessment. MRI characteristics of juvenile pilocytic astrocytomas and higher-grade tumors include high signal intensity of the mass lesion on T1 postcontrast scans and high signal intensity in T2-flair sequences. MR spectroscopy may be helpful in delineating tumor grade through specific patterns of the creatine/choline and *N*-acetyl aspartate peaks derived from scanning the tumor and its margins. NF1 patients also show specific patterns of benign imaging "abnormalities" on MRI that are known as T2 hyperintensities. These findings include regions of T2 and T2-flair hyperintensities that occur in the optic pathway, mesial temporal lobe, basal ganglia, and deep white matter of the cerebellum among the years [26–28]. These findings occur in approximately 60% of children with NF1 and usually become less apparent with age. These findings are generally benign, stereotypically occur in the aforementioned locations, and must not be misinterpreted as indicating tumors of the central nervous system. Occasionally, children with NF1 can develop aqueductal stenosis without an obvious tumor, causing obstructive hydrocephalus.

Evaluation and management of parenchymal optic pathway tumors follow the same general principles outlined above for tumors of the optic chiasm. The primary differences arise in the treatment of tumors of higher grade; there is great variability in the response of such tumors to treatment, and an array of different chemotherapy protocols may be used after primary treatment modalities fail. These evaluation and management decisions are defined in "road map" plans per experimental protocol but usually follow very individual courses that are tailored as the clinical picture evolves with each patient. Further discussion of these protocols is beyond the scope of this chapter.

34.7 Conclusion

NF1 causes a genetic predisposition to tumor-related conditions that affect the visual pathways. Four major tumor types were presented in this review: periorbital and orbital plexiform neurofibroma, intraorbital optic nerve glioma, chiasmal and hypothalamic glioma, and intraparenchymal astrocytomas of the post-optic-tract region of the brain. The variety of these tumors reflects the potential impact of the *NF1* gene on many primitive tissues in fetal development. Ophthalmic examination and follow-up are important to determine the optimal timing and type of interventions.

References

1. Mulvihill JJ, Parry DM, Sherman JL, Pikus A, Kaiser-Kupfer MI, Eldridge R. NIH conference. Neurofibromatosis 1 (Recklinghausen disease) and neurofibromatosis 2 (bilateral acoustic neurofibromatosis). An update. Ann Intern Med 1990;113(1):39–52.
2. Wallace MR, Marchuk DA, Andersen LB, Letcher R, Odeh HM, Saulino AM, Fountain JW, Brereton A, Nicholson J, Mitchell AL, et al. Type 1 neurofibromatosis gene: identification of a large transcript disrupted in three NF1 patients. Science 1990;249(4965):181–6.
3. Viskochil D, Buchberg AM, Xu G, Cawthon RM, Stevens J, Wolff RK, Culver M, Carey JC, Copeland NG, Jenkins NA, et al. Deletions and a translocation interrupt a cloned gene at the neurofibromatosis type 1 locus. Cell 1990;62(1):187–92.
4. von Deimling A, Krone W, Menon AG. Neurofibromatosis type 1: pathology, clinical features and molecular genetics. Brain Pathol 1995;5(2):153–62.
5. Neurofibromatosis. Conference statement. In: National Institutes of Health Consensus Development Conference, Vol. 45, 1988/05/01 edn. Arch Neurol 1988:575–8.
6. Gutmann DH, Aylsworth A, Carey JC, Korf B, Marks J, Pyeritz RE, Rubenstein A, Viskochil D. The diagnostic evaluation and multidisciplinary management of neurofibromatosis 1 and neurofibromatosis 2. JAMA 1997;278(1):51–7.
7. Listernick R, Louis DN, Packer RJ, Gutmann DH. Optic pathway gliomas in children with neurofibromatosis 1: consensus statement from the NF1 Optic Pathway Glioma Task Force. Ann Neurol 1997;41(2):143–9.
8. Friedman JM. Neurofibromatosis 1: clinical manifestations and diagnostic criteria. J Child Neurol 2002 Aug;17(8):548–54; discussion 571–2, 646–51.
9. Evans DG, Baser ME, McGaughran J, Sharif S, Howard E, Moran A. Malignant peripheral nerve sheath tumours in neurofibromatosis 1. J Med Genet 2002;39(5):311–4.
10. Thomas C, Somani N, Owen LG, Malone JC, Billings SD. Cutaneous malignant peripheral nerve sheath tumors. J Cutan Pathol 2009;36(8):896–900.
11. Chang BC, Mirabella G, Yagev R, Banh M, Mezer E, Parkin PC, Westall CA, Buncic JR. Screening and diagnosis of optic pathway gliomas in children with neurofibromatosis type 1 by using sweep visual evoked potentials. Invest Ophthalmol Vis Sci 2007;48(6): 2895–902.
12. Montgomery AB, Griffin T, Parker RG, Gerdes AJ. Optic nerve glioma: the role of radiation therapy. Cancer 1977;40(5):2079–80.
13. Parker JC, Jr., Smith JL, Reyes P, Vuksanovic MM. Chiasmal optic glioma after radiation therapy. Neuro-ophthalmologic/pathologic correlation. J Clin Neuroophthalmol 1981;1(1):31–43.
14. Glaser JS, Hoyt WF, Corbett J. Visual morbidity with chiasmal glioma. Long-term studies of visual fields in untreated and irradiated cases. Arch Ophthalmol 1971;85(1):3–12.
15. Ullrich NJ, Robertson R, Kinnamon DD, Scott RM, Kieran MW, Turner CD, Chi SN, Goumnerova L, Proctor M, Tarbell NJ, et al. Moyamoya following cranial irradiation for primary brain tumors in children. Neurology 2007;68(12):932–8.
16. Aoki S, Barkovich AJ, Nishimura K, Kjos BO, Machida T, Cogen P, Edwards M, Norman D. Neurofibromatosis types 1 and 2: cranial MR findings. Radiology 1989;172(2):527–34.
17. Vassilopoulou-Sellin R, Klein MJ, Slopis JK. Growth hormone deficiency in children with neurofibromatosis type 1 without suprasellar lesions. Pediatr Neurol 2000;22(5):355–8.
18. Billingsley RL, Lang FF, Slopis JM, Schrimsher GW, Ater JL, Moore BD, 3rd. Visual-spatial neglect in a child following sub-cortical tumor resection. Dev Med Child Neurol 2002;44(3):191–9.
19. Mazzocco MMM, Turner JE, Bridge Denckla M, Hofman KJ, Scanlon DC, Vellutino FR. Language and reading deficits associated with neurofibromatosis type 1: evidence for a not-so-nonverbal learning disability. Dev Neuropsychol 1995;11(4):503–22.
20. Coude FX, Mignot C, Lyonnet S, Munnich A. Academic impairment is the most frequent complication of neurofibromatosis type-1 (NF1) in children. Behav Genet 2006;36(5): 660–4.

21. Balestri P, Vivarelli R, Grosso S, Santori L, Farnetani MA, Galluzzi P, Vatti GP, Calabrese F, Morgese G. Malformations of cortical development in neurofibromatosis type 1. Neurology 2003;61(12):1799–801.
22. Billingsley RL, Schrimsher GW, Jackson EF, Slopis JM, Moore BD, 3rd. Significance of planum temporale and planum parietale morphologic features in neurofibromatosis type 1. Arch Neurol 2002;59(4):616–22.
23. Itoh T, Magnaldi S, White RM, Denckla MB, Hofman K, Naidu S, Bryan RN. Neurofibromatosis type 1: the evolution of deep gray and white matter MR abnormalities. AJNR Am J Neuroradiol 1994;15(8):1513–9.
24. Kayl AE, Moore BD, 3rd, Slopis JM, Jackson EF, Leeds NE. Quantitative morphology of the corpus callosum in children with neurofibromatosis and attention-deficit hyperactivity disorder. J Child Neurol 2000;15(2):90–6.
25. Schrimsher GW, Billingsley RL, Slopis JM, Moore BD, 3rd. Visual-spatial performance deficits in children with neurofibromatosis type-1. Am J Med Genet A 2003;120A(3):326–30.
26. DiPaolo DP, Zimmerman RA, Rorke LB, Zackai EH, Bilaniuk LT, Yachnis AT. Neurofibromatosis type 1: pathologic substrate of high-signal-intensity foci in the brain. Radiology 1995;195(3):721–4.
27. Duffner PK, Cohen ME, Seidel FG, Shucard DW. The significance of MRI abnormalities in children with neurofibromatosis. Neurology 1989;39(3):373–8.
28. Sevick RJ, Barkovich AJ, Edwards MS, Koch T, Berg B, Lempert T. Evolution of white matter lesions in neurofibromatosis type 1: MR findings. AJR Am J Roentgenol 1992;159(1):171–5.

Chapter 35
Other Optic Nerve Maladies in Cancer Patients

Jade S. Schiffman, Anitha Raghunath, and Rosa Ana Tang

Abstract Many optic neuropathies in cancer patients are related to the direct effect of cancer on the optic nerve (e.g., orbital and parasellar skull base compressive lesions or infiltration of the optic nerve with leptomeningeal disease). However, a number of optic neuropathies occur unrelated to those mechanisms. Other mechanisms of optic neuropathy in cancer patients include those caused by raised intracranial pressure (ICP), nutritional deficiencies, drugs, and radiation injury. Optic neuropathy related to elevated ICP does not initially affect vision; therefore, early recognition of the underlying problem is important for visual preservation. In patients with nutritional or drug-related optic neuropathy, symptoms and signs usually present simultaneously and bilaterally with visual loss that is progressive and painless; color vision is affected early on, but pupil examination may remain normal. The nutritional deficiencies may present slowly and symmetrically, and potential deficiencies include vitamins B_{12}, folate, and thiamine B_1. Radiation-related optic neuropathy often manifests within about 18 months after radiotherapy and usually after cumulative radiation doses greater than 50 Gy or single doses greater than 10 Gy. Patients often do not have optic disc swelling, and they develop progressive visual loss over weeks to months, with bilateral sequential loss being more common; the end result is vision of 20/200 or worse. Rarely, paraneoplastic syndrome can result in an optic neuropathy.

35.1 Introduction

Optic neuropathy in cancer patients is often related to the anatomic site of the malignancy. Some tumors cause optic neuropathy directly, such as those in the eyeball, e.g., melanoma and retinoblastoma primary orbital lesions and metastatic orbital

J.S. Schiffman (✉)
Section of Ophthalmology, Department of Head and Neck Surgery, The University of Texas M.D. Anderson Cancer Center, Houston, TX, USA
e-mail: jschiffm@mdanderson.org

B. Esmaeli (ed.), *Ophthalmic Oncology*, M.D. Anderson Solid Tumor Oncology Series 6, DOI 10.1007/978-1-4419-0374-7_35,

implants. Additionally, lesions of the skull base in the sella and parasellar region can cause optic neuropathy; these include primary brain tumors (e.g., pituitary adenoma, meningioma, craniopharyngioma, germinoma), tumors arising from adjacent areas (e.g., head and neck tumors such as squamous cell carcinoma, esthesioneuroblastoma), and tumors metastatic to the skull base region (breast). Optic neuropathy due to leptomeningeal disease (LMD) can occur in patients with hematogenous tumors (e.g., leukemias), solid tumors (e.g., breast, lung, melanoma), and primary brain tumors (glioma, germinoma etc.). Paraneoplastic syndromes affecting vision usually involve the retina, but may also affect the optic nerve (e.g., CRMP 5). Optic neuropathy can also result from orbital cellulitis, a serious infection in immune-suppressed patients. Optic neuropathies in cancer patients may also be the result of infectious meningeal diseases (e.g., cryptococcal meningitis). In this chapter, we will concentrate on optic neuropathies that do not have an obvious direct compressive component and in which imaging, therefore, may not be helpful. We discuss optic neuropathies related to raised intracranial pressure (ICP), nutritional deficiencies, drugs, and radiation injury.

35.2 Optic Neuropathies Related to Elevated ICP

Optic neuropathies related to elevated ICP are not rare in cancer patients. Elevated ICP leads to papilledema, and chronic papilledema can lead to vision loss.

Optic neuropathy associated with elevated ICP does not initially affect vision; therefore, early recognition of its presence is important for visual preservation. Optic neuropathy associated with long-standing papilledema initially affects the peripheral visual field (inferonasal); central vision is affected late in the process, most commonly within 6 months but as soon as 2 weeks in cases of severe and acute ICP elevation. Also, papilledema may be present for months to years without affecting visual function. Patients may not note vision impairment until central vision becomes affected; therefore, patients may have significant visual field loss before they are found to have papilledema. The optic neuropathy of papilledema may be asymmetric, i.e., one eye may have significant visual field loss while the other eye is not symptomatic.

35.2.1 Causes of Elevated ICP

Large volume brain lesions: Intracranial masses (primary brain tumors or brain metastases from a primary tumor at another site) can cause elevated ICP as a result of displacement of space in the cranium, cerebral edema, and/or obstruction of cerebrospinal fluid (CSF) flow. Supratentorial tumors may compress the falx or vein of Galen. Infratentorial tumors often obstruct the aqueduct and/or fourth ventricle and lead to hydrocephalus.

Obstructive hydrocephalus: Elevated ICP can be caused by obstructive hydrocephalus, such as that occurring when a mass compresses the aqueduct of Sylvius (e.g., a pinealoma or intrinsic midbrain tumor).

Communicating hydrocephalus: Communicating hydrocephalus occurs when CSF outflow is affected beyond the fourth ventricle, as with obstruction of the foramina of Luschka and Magendie or involvement of the arachnoid granulations, often by disorders that are not detectable on imaging. Meningeal disease due to either cancer (e.g., LMD) or infection often results in infiltration of the arachnoid granulations, leading to impaired CSF resorption and communicating hydrocephalus. However, sometimes cancer cells and infectious and inflammatory products result in debris that leads to arachnoid granulation failure and poor CSF drainage without the presence of communicating hydrocephalus. The presence or absence of communicating hydrocephalus does not always predict if the ICP is elevated. Therefore, elevated ICP may not be predicted accurately based on neuroimaging clues alone.

Spinal cord tumors: Spinal cord tumors can produce high protein levels in the CSF, which in turn may result in elevated ICP due to impaired resorption of fluid from the arachnoid granulations. Also, spinal cord tumors can grow from the cervical region to compress the cerebellum and obstruct CSF egress from the foramina of Luschka and Magendie, leading to a communicating hydrocephalus.

Venous sinus thrombosis: Venous sinus thrombosis can result from compression by a dural-based tumor or other appropriately situated lesion affecting the cerebral venous outflow system. Venous sinus thrombosis can also be encountered in patients with a hypercoagulable state associated with some types of cancer or treatments for cancer. Not intuitive is that venous obstruction in areas remote from the central nervous system (CNS) may result in elevated ICP. For example, proximal thoracic lesions, such as lesions causing a superior vena cava syndrome or neck lesions affecting a jugular vein, can impair venous return and may result in elevated ICP. Iatrogenic causes of venous sinus thrombosis include ligation or occlusion of a jugular vein during surgery and thrombosis resulting from indwelling venous catheters placed for chemotherapy, which may in turn cause papilledema secondary to the elevated ICP obstructive mechanism. Similarly, catheter-induced subclavian vein thrombosis and radical neck dissection have been associated with elevated intracranial venous and CSF pressures. In these latter cases, papilledema usually gradually resolves as collateral veins form to shunt the CSF.

Drugs: Some drugs may induce a hypercoagulable state resulting in cerebral venous thrombosis, such as L-asparaginase [1] and retinoids [2]. Other drugs linked to elevated ICP resulting in secondary intracranial hypertension are corticosteroids, cyclosporine, cytarabine, doxycycline, tetracycline, and others.

35.2.2 Treatment of Elevated ICP

If vision and visual fields are not affected and there is frequent surveillance to ensure continued unaffected vision, treatment of elevated ICP is not mandatory, and treatment is aimed to symptoms, such as headaches. However, when elevated ICP is associated with visual field loss with or without visual acuity loss, elevated ICP must be treated to avoid continued damage to the optic nerve.

The treatment modality for elevated ICP depends on the cause. The goal must be reduction of ICP and/or reduction of pressure in the perioptic nerve sheath. The severity of the visual acuity loss and visual field loss determines the rapidity with which interventions need to be implemented. Specific treatment options include the following: tumor removal (for tumor-induced elevated ICP); treatment of underlying hydrocephalus or leptomeningeal disease; discontinuation of drugs (in the case of drug-induced elevated ICP); utilization of diuretics with or without steroids; shunting by means of a lumboperitoneal or ventriculoperitoneal shunt; optic nerve sheath fenestration; and chemotherapy or radiation therapy (if elevated ICP is related to a tumor or leptomeningeal disease).

Patients with severe visual field loss and involvement or fixation before initiation of treatment usually have irreversible damage. Routinely sending patients with any of the above potential causes of elevated ICP for ophthalmic examination is a way to identify the condition early and potentially stall vision loss.

35.3 Optic Neuropathies Caused by Nutritional Deficiencies

The nutritional deficiencies that most commonly affect the optic nerve are deficiencies of vitamin B_{12} (cobalamin), folate, and thiamine (B_1).

The symptoms and signs of an optic neuropathy related to nutritional deficiency are progressive symmetric painless visual loss affecting the central and the color vision early on with initially normal findings on pupil examination and central or cecocentral scotomas on visual field testing and late development of temporal disc pallor.

35.3.1 *Vitamin B_{12} Deficiency Optic Neuropathy*

Vitamin B_{12} deficiency optic neuropathy can occur in seemingly healthy individuals and is more common in males (80% of affected patients) than in females [3]. The risk of vitamin B_{12} deficiency and associated optic neuropathy is seen with partial or complete removal of the stomach, as in patients needing gastrectomy to remove malignant tumors, and patients who have undergone bariatric surgery, up to 40% of whom suffer from B_{12} deficiencies [4]. Vitamin B_{12} deficiency is also present in patients with pernicious anemia, an autoimmune condition that impairs the absorption of vitamin B_{12} in the ileum due to lack of intrinsic factor. Sometimes optic neuropathy is the first sign of pernicious anemia. The neurologic manifestations of this deficiency can be the earliest manifestations and include myelopathy affecting the posterior columns and cortical spinal tract, referred to as subacute combined degeneration, involving the cervical and upper thoracic posterior columns [4].

These patients can present with paresthesias and weakness [5]; rarely, sensory and autonomic disturbances [6] and neuropsychiatric manifestations such as memory problems, personality changes, and psychosis [4] can be seen as well as a megaloblastic anemia that develops slowly and can be severe.

Adenosine triphosphate (ATP) is thought to play a key role in optic neuropathy related to vitamin B_{12} deficiency [3]. The postulated mechanism is as follows: vitamin B_{12} deficiency increases the level of methyltetrahydrofolate, which in turn causes excessive depolarization and depletion of ATP. This ATP deficiency could be the explanation for the cecocentral scotoma characteristically seen in vitamin B_{12} deficiency optic neuropathy, because the parvoretinal ganglion cells of the papillomacular bundle require more energy than the magnoganglion cells [3].

In patients in whom vitamin B_{12} deficiency optic neuropathy is suspected, serum cobalamin, serum methylmalonate, and serum homocysteine levels should be checked [3]. Methylmalonate and homocysteine are metabolites of cobalamin, and if the serum cobalamin level is at low-normal or normal levels, these other metabolites can help establish a diagnosis of cobalamin deficiency. Once vitamin B_{12} deficiency has been established, a Schilling test should be done to determine the degree of cobalamin malabsorption.

Patients with vitamin B_{12} deficiency optic neuropathy are generally treated with cyanocobalamin 100 μg intramuscularly three times weekly for the first 2 weeks and then 500–1000 μg intramuscularly monthly [3]. Most patients must continue this therapy forever. Stopping maintenance therapy can result in the return of neurological symptoms. The earlier the therapy is instituted, the higher the likelihood that symptoms and signs will resolve.

35.3.2 Folate Deficiency Optic Neuropathy

Like B_{12}, folate is involved in methionine metabolism. Folate, in the form of methyltetrahydrofolate, donates a methyl group to homocysteine to form methionine and tetrahydrofolate. Tetrahydrofolate helps metabolize formate. Folate deficiency leads to the accumulation of formate, a toxic metabolite from methanol, causing optic neuropathy [4]. Folate deficiency also causes other neurological manifestations, such as polyneuropathy and even subacute combined degeneration of the spinal cord, that are many times indistinguishable from those caused by cobalamine deficiency.

In women of childbearing age who have epilepsy and are on anticonvulsant treatment, a daily dose of folate 0.4 mg is suggested to avoid future neural tube defects when these women have children [4].

Although folate deficiency often occurs with other nutrient deficiencies, isolated folate deficiency has been shown to cause optic neuropathy [7]. In the study by Hsu et al. [8], six patients with low folate levels but normal B_{12} levels developed bilateral visual loss, color defects, and central or cecocentral scotomas with optic discs that were normal or had temporal disc pallor. Measurement of erythrocyte folate was found to be more sensitive than measurement of serum folate in the early diagnosis of this disorder. With folate replacement therapy, patients' vision improved within 4–12 weeks of symptom onset [8].

35.3.3 Vitamin B_1 (Thiamine) Deficiency Optic Neuropathy

Thiamine acts as a coenzyme in the metabolism of carbohydrates, lipids, and some amino acids. Thiamine deficiency results in reduced synthesis of certain high-energy phosphates and the accumulation of lactate. Because of a short half-life, a thiamine-deficient diet may result in symptoms in a few days. Patients who are undergoing nasogastric feeding, total parenteral nutrition, bariatric surgery, and the so-called refeeding syndrome as well as those with recurrent vomiting, hyperthyroidism, gastric surgery, alcoholism, or extreme dieting are at risk of this deficiency [4].

Isolated vitamin B_1 deficiency can cause optic neuropathy as well as ataxia and polyneuropathy [4, 9].

The syndrome of Wernicke can develop in patients with a marginal thiamine diet and consists of a triad of (1) ocular abnormalities (diplopia and nystagmus due to brain stem manifestations), (2) gait ataxia, and (3) mental status changes [10].

About 80% of patients who survive Wernicke develop Korsakoff syndrome, which is an amnestic confabulatory syndrome [4].

Brain MRI findings in thiamine deficiency include increased T2 or proton density or FLAIR signal in the mamillary bodies, which is characteristic of Wernicke's. The signal abnormalities can partially resolve with treatment with resultant partially atrophic mamillary bodies. Also, this partial atrophy can affect the thalamus, hypothalamus, midbrain, pons, medulla, and cerebellum [4].

Low levels of serum transketolase (an indication of B_1 deficiency) and reduced serum and urinary thiamine levels as well as levels of RBC thiamine diphosphate can help in early diagnosis of deficiency [4].

Intravenous glucose infusion in patients with thiamine deficiency can precipitate acute Wernicke's and should be avoided by giving thiamine replacement first when needed. Suggested dose is 100 mg IV every 8 h for a few days followed by long-term oral maintenance of 50–100 mg of thiamine daily. The ocular signs improve quickly in hours, but the mental changes can take many days [4].

Other deficiencies that are less clinically significant in causing optic neuropathies are vitamin E and zinc. Copper deficiency is not linked to optic neuropathy but to myelopathy and is being recognized as a common problem in patients who have had bariatric surgery [4].

35.3.4 Vitamin E Deficiency Optic Neuropathy

Vitamin E deficiency can produce spinocerebellar syndrome with peripheral neuropathy, progressive ataxia, areflexia, ophthalmoplegia, and pigmentary retinopathy, with optic neuropathy being quite rare [4].

35.3.5 Zinc Deficiency Optic Neuropathy

Zinc is required for the metabolism of vitamin A in the eye. Zinc plays an important role in stabilizing microtubules for axonal transport. Zinc deficiency causes defective rapid axonal transport in vitro and therefore may contribute to the development of optic neuropathy but is quite rare [4].

35.4 Optic Neuropathies Caused by Drugs

A number of different drugs have been associated with optic neuropathy in cancer patients. Like the symptoms and signs of nutritional optic neuropathy, the symptoms and signs of drug-related ("toxic") optic neuropathy usually present simultaneously and bilaterally with visual loss that is progressive and painless; there is loss of high spatial frequency contrast sensitivity and color vision is affected early on (hence red Amsler grid testing is quite sensitive early on) with pupil examination being initially normal. Central visual field testing such as with the Amsler grid (preferably red color as well as white) and Humphrey VF-10-2 test is most helpful at the earliest stage.

As toxicity effect progresses, there is loss of axons, which can be documented using optical coherence tomography technology. Later optic disc pallor is seen mostly in the temporal aspect of the disc.

The mitochondria provide most of the ATP that the cells require for their metabolism. Defective mitochondrial function can affect the axonal transport and affect ATP production with predilection toward the retinal ganglion cell axons of the papillomacular bundle—this is a possible mechanism to explain toxic optic neuropathy [11].

Because cancer patients are often treated with combinations of chemotherapeutic agents, it is very often difficult to attribute optic neuropathy in a patient treated with chemotherapy to any one particular agent in isolation. In addition, in cancer patients treated with both chemotherapy and radiation therapy with the optic nerves included in the field, it can be difficult to distinguish between drug-related optic neuropathy and radiation-related optic neuropathy. Information about cancer drugs that can cause optic neuropathy mainly comes from retrospective case series and reports from Med Watch, the United States Food and Drug Administration, the World Health Organization, and the National Registry of Drug-Induced Ocular Side Effects databases [12].

The World Health Organization classification helps clinicians determine the likelihood that a particular drug is the culprit in vision loss and when to stop treatment with a given drug. The most important steps are rapid identification of the toxic agent and prompt withdrawal of the same [12].

Optic neuropathies caused by drugs can be classified according to whether they are associated with disc edema due to elevated ICP or disc edema due to direct toxic effect. Drugs can cause optic disc edema by raising the ICP ("intracranial hypertension"); less commonly, drugs can induce cerebral venous thrombosis resulting in elevated ICP with or without other focal findings. In addition, drugs can cause direct toxic optic neuropathy with associated optic disc edema, in which the disc edema is a prominent posterior pole finding and there is no significant visual dysfunction unless the condition is long-standing. In this type of direct toxic optic neuropathy, cessation of the suspected agent usually results in total or partial visual recovery. Finally, drugs can cause direct toxic neuropathy without associated optic disc edema, which is generally associated with significant visual loss, usually bilateral and progressive and early dyschromatopsia, which may or may not recover after the agent is stopped.

35.4.1 Optic Disc Edema Secondary to Drug-Induced Elevated ICP

A number of drugs have been associated with optic disc edema secondary to elevated ICP with an unknown underlying mechanism and are on the list of causes of idiopathic intracranial hypertension also known as pseudotumor cerebri. Oral, intravenous, or intrathecal administration of drugs may result in elevated ICP, depending on the particular drug.

35.4.1.1 Retinoids

Retinoids are used to arrest or reverse carcinogenesis. Retinoids and their synthetic and naturally occurring analogs, including all-*trans*-retinoic acid and isotretinoin (used in the treatment of recurrent glioblastoma multiforme), have been reported to cause increased ICP by causing elevation of the vitamin A levels in both adults and children after oral administration [2, 12, 13].

The problem resolves with discontinuation of the drug and normalization of the levels of vitamin A in the blood.

35.4.1.2 Imatinib Mesylate

Imatinib mesylate (Gleevec) is a tyrosine kinase inhibitor that has been reported to cause periorbital edema, optic disc edema, and retinal edema and elevated ICP with bilateral papilledema. Other less common side effects are headaches, confusion, and CNS hemorrhage [12].

35.4.1.3 Cyclosporine A

Cyclosporine A is used to prevent graft-versus-host disease in bone marrow transplant recipients, liver transplant recipients, recipients of other organ transplants, and patients with rheumatoid arthritis, autoimmune disorders, psoriasis, and atopic dermatitis.

Cyclosporine A is used in both intravenous and oral forms. Bilateral disc edema without elevated ICP was attributed to cyclosporine A in a patient who received prophylactic oral treatment with this drug for 6 months after bone marrow transplantation [14]. Following cessation of cyclosporine A, vision improved in 2 months and disc edema resolved over 6 months. The mechanism by which cyclosporine A causes optic neuropathy has been variously attributed to microangiopathy, direct toxic effects on optic nerve axons, and elevated ICP. Pseudotumor cerebri-type picture has been associated with the use of cyclosporine [15].

35.4.1.4 Cytarabine

Liposomal cytarabine (Depocyt), the long-acting form of cytarabine, is an alkylating agent that has been reported to cause neurological complications, including intracranial hypertension secondary to arachnoiditis (more common with intrathecal therapy), encephalopathy, seizures, cerebellar dysfunction, and cauda equina syndrome. Some of the reported ocular changes include macular edema, cotton wool spots, optic neuropathy, and retinal neovascularization [12].

35.4.2 Elevated ICP Secondary to Cerebral Venous Thrombosis

Both cisplatin and L-asparaginase with or without methotrexate can cause elevated ICP secondary to cerebral venous thrombosis [16].

35.4.2.1 Cisplatin

Cisplatin is a heavy metal compound used in the treatment of many pediatric and adult malignancies, such as germ cell tumors and brain tumors. Nephrotoxicity due to cisplatin administration is well documented, and impaired renal function can lead to significant increase in CNS levels of cisplatin. Not only can this lead to nerve demyelination and optic neuropathy, but also intravenous cisplatin has been reported to lead to dural sinus thrombosis because of its propensity to cause coagulation disorders and thrombosis [12, 17].

35.4.2.2 L-Asparaginase

L-asparaginase used in the treatment of acute lymphoblastic leukemia can cause superior sagittal sinus thrombosis and cerebral venous thrombosis. These conditions may occur when L-asparaginase is given in combination with methotrexate or when L-asparaginase is given as a single agent and generally occur a few weeks after therapy is initiated [12, 17].

Dural venous thrombosis can cause elevated ICP and manifest as neurological events such as seizures and papilledema, which are evident on fundus examination [1].

35.4.3 Optic Disc Edema Usually Without Elevated ICP

Some of the drugs that can cause optic disc edema usually without elevated ICP include cisplatin, carmustine, vincristine, fluorouracil, cyclosporine A, and tacrolimus.

35.4.3.1 Cisplatin

Toxic effects of cisplatin have been outlined above. Treatment with cisplatin can cause both an optic neuropathy and maculopathy leading to pale optic discs and granular pigmentation of the retina. The electroretinogram may be flat [12, 17].

Cisplatin in combination with other drugs has also been implicated in optic neuropathy. Degeneration of the optic nerve and tract has been reported after supraophthalmic internal carotid artery infusion of cisplatin and carmustine [12, 17].

35.4.3.2 Carboplatin

A related platinum compound, carboplatin, has been reported to cause "optic neuritis" and blindness after intravenous administration as well as peripheral neuropathy [17].

35.4.3.3 Carmustine

Carmustine, an alkylating agent, can be given intra-arterially or intravenously. It can penetrate the blood–brain barrier and cause retinal ischemia, central retinal artery occlusion, optic disc edema, optic neuropathy, and encephalopathy [17].

35.4.3.4 Vincristine

Vincristine, a microtubule inhibitor, is more commonly used in pediatric malignancies and is known to cause reversible peripheral neuropathy and sometimes also autonomic neuropathy as well as ataxia and headaches. The patient may also have seizures and cranial neuropathies.

35.4.3.5 5-Fluorouracil

This is a fluorine-substituted analog of the pyrimidine uracil. It is an antimetabolite that inhibits thymidylate synthetase, blocking DNA synthesis. It is also known to inhibit the S phase of the cell cycle. It is more commonly given intravenously by bolus injection and sometimes also intra-arterially or by direct injection. This agent crosses the blood-brain barrier and can cause toxicity to the CNS with preferential site being the cerebellum causing a subacute cerebellar syndrome with a triad of ataxia, dysarthria, and nystagmus. Rarely acute recurrent toxic optic neuropathy may occur following administration of 5-fluorouracil [17].

35.4.3.6 Cyclosporine A

Cyclosporine A can cause both elevated ICP with optic disc edema and secondary optic nerve fiber loss or a presumed direct effect [18].

35.4.3.7 Tacrolimus

Tacrolimus may directly affect the optic nerve and may also cause optic disc edema without associated increased intracranial pressure.

35.4.4 Optic Neuropathy Without Disc Edema

Drugs that can cause optic neuropathy without disc edema include fludarabine, tamoxifen, tacrolimus, paclitaxel, methotrexate, and cytarabine.

35.4.4.1 Fludarabine

Fludarabine is an antimetabolite that can cause delayed but significant ocular and neuro-ophthalmic morbidity including optic disc edema, optic neuropathy, and transient cortical visual loss with variable degrees of visual loss [17].

35.4.4.2 Tacrolimus

Tacrolimus is an immunosuppressive agent that is used following transplants such as bone marrow transplants, pancreas transplants, and liver transplants. Like other calcineurin inhibitors, tacrolimus has been linked to optic neuropathy and also to cortical visual loss.

35.4.4.3 Paclitaxel

Paclitaxel (Taxol) is a neurotubule stabilizer that can cause neurotoxicity with sensory and motor peripheral neuropathy and also myalgias. Rarely it has been linked to transient scotomas and optic neuropathy [17].

35.4.4.4 Methotrexate

Methotrexate is an antifolate metabolite used to decrease nucleic acid synthesis by limiting availability of reduced folate. It is given by various routes, including oral, parenteral, and intrathecal, for malignancies such as head and neck cancer, breast cancer, lymphoma, and others as well as for autoimmune diseases such as rheumatoid arthritis. High doses are linked to toxic neuro-ophthalmic problems such as optic neuropathy, optic nerve demyelination, retinal pigmentary mottling, and myelopathy as well as aseptic meningitis mostly with intrathecal administration [17].

35.4.4.5 Cytarabine

Intravenous cytarabine, an alkylating agent, is used in the treatment of leukemia and lymphoma, and intrathecal cytarabine is used for prevention or treatment of CNS lymphoma. Intrathecal cytarabine can cause neurotoxicity with arachnoiditis, cerebellar dysfunction, seizures, and encephalopathy. Optic neuropathy, macular edema, and cotton wool spots can also occur [17].

35.5 Optic Neuropathies Caused by Radiation

Optic neuropathy associated with radiation is an ischemic process presenting as a posterior ischemic optic neuropathy, on average about 18 months after radiotherapy and usually after cumulative radiation doses greater than 50 Gy or single doses greater than 10 Gy. However, the process can occur earlier or even years after radiotherapy. Optic disc swelling is usually absent. The patient experiences progressive visual loss over weeks to months, with bilateral sequential loss being more common, and the end result is vision of 20/200 or worse. The visual field may show altitudinal defect or central scotoma. The disc becomes pale in 4–6 weeks [19]. Magnetic resonance imaging is the study of choice to distinguish radiation-related optic neuropathy from recurrent tumor. In cases of radiation-related optic neuropathy, magnetic resonance imaging usually reveals the optic nerves to be slightly swollen but otherwise normal on unenhanced studies and demonstrates focal contrast enhancement of the optic nerves with TI-weighted Gd-DTPA images.

Radiation-related optic neuropathy is more often seen after radiotherapy for cancer of the paranasal sinuses and skull base, pituitary adenomas, and meningiomas [19]. Radiation dose per fraction, total dose, total duration of treatment, volume of tissue irradiated, and type of radiation (proton, electron, or neutron) can also affect the risk of developing radiation-induced optic neuropathy. Higher total dose, fraction size, and volume irradiated are associated with higher frequency of complications and shorter time to onset of complications. Preexisting medical disorders, such as diabetes and endocrinologic disturbances from Cushing syndrome or growth hormone-producing tumors, are additional risk factors. It is well known that patients who receive chemotherapy are at increased risk for radiation-induced optic neuropathies at radiation doses lower than those expected to cause optic neuropathy in patients not treated with chemotherapy.

There is no proven effective treatment for radiation-related optic neuropathy. Hyperbaric oxygen has been used with mixed results, but it has been found that early introduction of hyperbaric oxygen (e.g., within 72 h of symptoms) is more likely to be beneficial. Trental 400 mg tid and vitamin E 400 units daily are often given, although there is no definite proof of benefit. Although there are some anecdotal reports of its success in treating optic neuropathy due to radiotherapy, the role of anticoagulation in this disorder requires further investigation. Occasionally, systemic corticosteroids are successful. Their mechanism of action is not clear, but steroids may reduce overall tissue edema and retard demyelination.

Based on the experience to date with various treatments, some management strategies have evolved to help improve visual outcome. If one eye has been affected, serial eye examinations must be done over the 10- to 20-month period after treatment to monitor for any signs of recurrence in the other eye because bilateral sequential involvement is not uncommon. Serial magnetic imaging of the brain and orbits should be performed over the 20-month period after radiation therapy is completed.

The most common protocol for hyperbaric oxygen therapy: 30 sessions of therapy, with the patient breathing 100% oxygen at 2.4 atm absolute (ATA) for 90 min per session. At therapeutic pressure, ocular side effects of hyperbaric oxygen therapy include a transient myopic shift, cataract, and transient blindness (only in patients with a previous optic neuritis) and rarely seizures. Hyperbaric oxygen therapy is a safe and now proven technique used to treat various medical conditions, such as decompression sickness, anaerobic infections, postirradiation osteonecrosis, postirradiation cystitis, and complicated wounds.

References

1. Foroozan R. Ocular complications of sigmoid sinus thrombosis from L-asparaginase. J Pediatr Ophthalmol Strabismus 2005;42(2):117–9.
2. Schroeter T, Lanvers C, Herding H, Suttorp M. Pseudotumor cerebri induced by all-trans-retinoic acid in a child treated for acute promyelocytic leukemia. Med Pediatr Oncol 2000;34(4):284–6.
3. Chan JW. Optic Nerve Disorders: Diagnosis and Management, first edition. New York, NY: Springer, 2007.
4. Kumar N. Neurologic presentations of nutritional deficiencies. Neurol Clin 2010;28(1):107–70.
5. Healton EB, Savage DG, Brust JC, Garrett TJ, Lindenbaum J. Neurologic aspects of cobalamin deficiency. Medicine (Baltimore) 1991;70(4):229–45.
6. Puntambekar P, Basha MM, Zak IT, Madhavan R. Rare sensory and autonomic disturbances associated with vitamin B12 deficiency. J Neurol Sci 2009;287(1–2):285–7.
7. Golnik KC, Schaible ER. Folate-responsive optic neuropathy. J Neuroophthalmol 1994;14(3):163–9.
8. Hsu CT, Miller NR, Wray ML. Optic neuropathy from folic acid deficiency without alcohol abuse. Ophthalmologica 2002;216(1):65–7.
9. Adamolekun B. Thiamine deficiency and the etiology of tropical ataxic neuropathy. Int Health 2010;2(1):17–21.
10. Sechi G, Serra A. Wernicke's encephalopathy: new clinical settings and recent advances in diagnosis and management. Lancet Neurol 20076(5):442–55.
11. Sadun AA, Wang MY. Ethambutol optic neuropathy: how we can prevent 100,000 new cases of blindness each year. J Neuroophthalmol 2008;28(4):265–8.
12. Fraunfelder FW, Fraunfelder FT. Adverse ocular drug reactions recently identified by the National Registry of Drug-Induced Ocular Side Effects. Ophthalmology 2004;111(7):1275–9.
13. Friedman DI. Pseudotumor cerebri. Neurol Clin 2004;22(1):99–131, vi.
14. Walter SH, Bertz H, Gerling J. Bilateral optic neuropathy after bone marrow transplantation and cyclosporin A therapy. Graefes Arch Clin Exp Ophthalmol 2000;238(6):472–6.
15. Cruz OA, Fogg SG, Roper-Hall G. Pseudotumor cerebri associated with cyclosporine use. Am J Ophthalmol 1996;122(3):436–7.

16. Sung G. Acute treatment of cerebral venous thrombosis. Curr Treat Options Neurol 2002;4(4):319–22.
17. al-Tweigeri T, Nabholtz JM, Mackey JR. Ocular toxicity and cancer chemotherapy. A review. Cancer 1996;78(7):1359–73.
18. Apaydin C, Gur B, Yakupoglu G, Saka O. Ocular and visual side effects of systemic cyclosporine. Ann Ophthalmol 1992;24(12):465–9.
19. Markman M. Chemotherapy-induced peripheral neuropathy: underreported and underappreciated. Curr Pain Headache Rep 2006;10(4):275–8.

Part VI
Common Vitreoretinal Conditions in Cancer Patients

Section Editor: Bernard F. Godley

Chapter 36
Management of Endogenous Endophthalmitis

Kapil G. Kapoor, Gibran S. Khurshid, Garvin H. Davis, and Bernard F. Godley

Abstract Endogenous endophthalmitis is a potentially blinding ocular infection resulting from hematogenous spread from a remote primary source. Endogenous endophthalmitis accounts for only 2–8% of cases of endophthalmitis and usually occurs in the setting of at least a relatively immunocompromised state. Causes include both gram-positive and gram-negative bacteria and fungi. Streptococcal species are the most commonly implicated bacterial organisms; *Candida* species are the most commonly implicated fungal organisms. Endogenous mold endophthalmitis is rare and typically occurs in the setting of relative immunocompromise or intravenous drug use. Early diagnosis of endogenous endophthalmitis requires a high degree of suspicion and is critical if vision is to be preserved. Therapeutic management includes hospitalization and delivery of broad-spectrum systemic and intravitreal antibiotics. Vitrectomy may be appropriate in some cases. The prognosis of patients with endogenous endophthalmitis is disappointing; even with aggressive treatment, useful vision (i.e., ability to count fingers or better) is preserved in only about 40% of patients.

36.1 Introduction

Endogenous endophthalmitis is a potentially blinding ocular infection resulting from hematogenous spread from a remote primary source. Endogenous endophthalmitis is relatively uncommon compared to exogenous endophthalmitis (endophthalmitis associated with an extrinsic portal of entry), accounting for only 2–8% of cases of endophthalmitis [1]. It usually occurs in the setting of at least a relatively immunocompromised state, such as that seen in patients with diabetes

K.G. Kapoor (✉)
Department of Ophthalmology and Visual Sciences, The University of Texas Medical Branch, Galveston, TX, USA
e-mail: kgkapoor@utmb.edu

B. Esmaeli (ed.), *Ophthalmic Oncology*, M.D. Anderson Solid Tumor Oncology Series 6, DOI 10.1007/978-1-4419-0374-7_36,

mellitus (30.7% of cases of endogenous endophthalmitis), chronic obstructive airway disease (23.1%), end-stage renal disease (15.4%), or cancer (7.7%) [2]. Cancer patients are intrinsically immunocompromised because of the malignancy and are also iatrogenically immunocompromised because of cancer treatment, which can involve intensive chemotherapy, radiation therapy, and bone marrow transplantation with lifelong immunosuppressive therapy. Although each of these factors presumably leads to further immunocompromise and predisposition to endophthalmitis, the literature lacks a comprehensive study examining the cumulative insult delivered by these factors to cancer patients.

Endogenous endophthalmitis is relatively rare but may become more common in clinical practice because of the rapid advance of medical technology, a longer life span of patients with chronic diseases, and a rising prevalence of long-term intravenous access. It is important that oncologists be aware of endogenous endophthalmitis because early diagnosis and prompt aggressive treatment are imperative if significant vision loss is to be avoided. Many organisms (gram-positive bacteria, gram-negative bacteria, and fungi) have been reported to cause endogenous endophthalmitis. Risk factors include most causes of immune suppression [2, 3].

36.2 Epidemiology

Endogenous endophthalmitis can occur at any age and has no gender predilection. The right eye is involved twice as often as the left eye, because of the more proximal and direct blood flow to the right carotid artery. Bilateral involvement occurs in approximately 25% of cases. The population at greatest risk includes immunocompromised patients with leukemia, lymphoma, asplenia, or hypogammaglobulinemia and patients taking immunosuppressive therapy, including corticosteroids. Chronic diseases such as diabetes mellitus, renal insufficiency, and malignancies also increase the risk because of compromised immunity and increased likelihood of undergoing invasive procedures. Persons with AIDS may develop endogenous bacterial retinitis, but surprisingly few cases of endophthalmitis have been reported in AIDS patients. Alcoholics have an increased incidence of endogenous endophthalmitis. Intravenous drug use is specifically associated with *Bacillus cereus* infection and fungal endophthalmitis. Patients undergoing intravenous hyperalimentation are particularly predisposed to fungal endophthalmitis [4, 5]. One study demonstrated a mean interval between the start of intravenous hyperalimentation and the onset of disease of 11 days [5].

36.3 Microbiology

Etiologic agents of endogenous endophthalmitis are restricted to bacterial or fungal, as viruses and parasites infect the retina or uvea, leading to retinitis or uveitis, respectively. Bacterial endophthalmitis is the most common, followed by yeast and mold endophthalmitis [2].

36.4 Clinical Manifestations and Diagnosis

A high degree of suspicion is necessary to make an early diagnosis of endogenous endophthalmitis. Information about the risk factors mentioned above should be elicited, in addition to information about symptoms that suggest the presence of the primary infection.

Patients with endogenous endophthalmitis commonly complain of eye pain, blurring of vision, ocular discharge, and photophobia [6, 7]. Patients who present at a later stage in the disease may have obvious signs such as chemosis, proptosis, and hypopyon [7]. Earlier signs, such as retinal hemorrhages, Roth's spots (round, white retinal spots surrounded by hemorrhage), and retinal periphlebitis, can be seen using fundoscopy [8]. Slit-lamp examination and ocular ultrasonography should be performed to look for vitreous inflammatory cells and retinochoroidal thickening. A thorough systemic examination is required to identify the primary source of infection. Although these clinical markers are important, they occasionally have limited reliability in cancer patients, further emphasizing the need for a high degree of suspicion to make an early diagnosis of endogenous endophthalmitis. In cancer patients with endogenous endophthalmitis, the inflammatory markers and other clinical signs may be less evident given patients' immunosuppression and inability to mount an inflammatory response. Heightened awareness and careful examination are thus critical, particularly in cancer patients who are significantly immunocompromised or extremely ill and sedated, such as posttransplant patients and those in intensive care units.

In addition to initial diagnostic laboratory tests, testing for human immunodeficiency virus infection should be considered in otherwise healthy persons with endogenous endophthalmitis [9, 10]. Routine radiographs are warranted and may reveal a primary pulmonary infection. Echocardiography is also warranted to assess the possibility of endocarditis.

Other tests may be necessary, depending on the clinical presentation. Blood cultures and intraocular cultures obtained from both anterior and posterior chambers of the eye before institution of antimicrobial therapy have the highest yield for isolating the pathogen [11]. The direct inoculation of ocular specimens in blood culture bottles may increase the yield [12]. Cultures of specimens from other sites, including intravenous line catheter tips should be obtained when appropriate. Giemsa, Gomori methenamine silver, and periodic acid-Schiff staining should be done for direct examination of fungi. Polymerase chain reaction may be used for rapid diagnostic results and may aid in early differentiation between bacterial and fungal etiologies [13]. Gram stains of intraocular fluid may not be reliable. Immunologic tests for specific bacterial antigens can be performed in patients who have already received antibiotics; however, the utility of these tests has been challenged [14].

36.5 Treatment

Therapeutic management of endogenous endophthalmitis includes hospitalization and delivery of broad-spectrum systemic and intravitreal antibiotics in consultation with an infectious disease specialist and based on the proven or presumed infectious agent [15]. Small trials have suggested improved outcomes with intravitreal antibiotic administration and with vitrectomy, which provides the dual benefit of reducing infective load and supplying adequate diagnostic material, although both of these approaches are still controversial [16]. Topical cycloplegics and topical steroids, depending on the degree of anterior segment inflammation, may be used to supplement primary therapeutic options [17].

36.5.1 Bacterial Endophthalmitis

Endogenous bacterial endophthalmitis occurs in the setting of bacteremia secondary to endocarditis (40% of cases of endogenous bacterial endophthalmitis), urinary tract infections, abdominal abscesses, meningitis, indwelling catheters, organ transplantation, malignancy, and chemotherapy [1, 6].

The patient's risk factors may help the physician predict the etiologic agent or narrow the list of potential organisms. The most common bacterial pathogens are gram-positive organisms, especially the streptococcal species, including *Streptococcus pneumoniae*. *Staphylococcus aureus* is found more often in patients with diabetes mellitus, renal failure, cutaneous infections, or intravenous catheters [2]. Infected arteriovenous fistulae have also been reported as a source of staphylococcal infection [1, 18, 19]. In the past 10 years, *B. cereus* has become a common bacterial agent in intravenous drug users. It is an aggressive agent, leading to blindness if antibiotic therapy is not instituted very early [19].

Gram-negative organisms are also sometimes encountered. *Neisseria meningitidis* was the most common pathogen in the preantibiotic era [3]. The number of cases of endophthalmitis related to *Haemophilus influenzae* is expected to decrease with the advent of vaccination, paralleling the documented decrease in meningitis. Cases of endophthalmitis related to *Escherichia coli* and *Klebsiella* species have been associated with diabetes, liver disease, and urinary tract infections [2, 20].

One report on the bacteriology of endogenous bacterial endophthalmitis reported that streptococci caused 32% of cases, *S. aureus* caused 25%, and *E. coli* caused 18% [1]. *Klebsiella pneumoniae* invasive primary liver abscess syndrome can lead to systemic spread of infection in approximately 5–15% of cases [20].

Management of endogenous bacterial endophthalmitis includes broad-spectrum systemic antibiotics and intravitreal antibiotics covering gram-positive and gram-negative organisms. A standard regimen is vancomycin (systemic dose: 1.0 g intravenously every 12 h; intravitreal dose: 1.0 mg in 0.1 mL may repeat at 48–72 h) plus either ceftazidime (systemic dose: 2 g intravenously every 12 h; intravitreal dose: 2.2 mg in 0.1 mL may repeat at 48–72 h) or ciprofloxacin (500–750 mg by mouth twice daily). If the patient has severe or persistent inflammation, a second intravitreal injection (depending on culture results) may be considered at 48–72 hours.

Early intravenous antibiotic therapy remains the cornerstone of treatment. Although systemic antibiotics are not necessary in the treatment of exogenous endophthalmitis, endogenous endophthalmitis is particularly responsive to intravenous antibiotics. Systemic antibiotics also treat distant foci of infection and prevent continued bacteremia, thereby reducing the chances of invasion of the unaffected eye. Empiric broad-spectrum antibiotic therapy with vancomycin and an aminoglycoside (e.g., amikacin) or a third-generation cephalosporin (e.g., ceftazidime) is warranted.

The nature of the clinical presentation, as well as the presumed (or confirmed) source of infection, can be used to guide the decision about which antibiotic to use. Third-generation cephalosporins penetrate ocular tissues and are effective against gram-negative organisms. In cases of documented gastrointestinal or genitourinary infection, second- or third-generation cephalosporins and aminoglycosides are considered the drugs of choice. Vancomycin should be given to patients with a known history of drug abuse, covering the possibility of *Bacillus* infection. In the presence of wounds, oxacillin or a first-generation cephalosporin should be used.

Intravitreal antibiotic injections have revolutionized the treatment of exogenous endophthalmitis, but their utility in treating endogenous endophthalmitis is controversial. Similarly, surgical intervention (i.e., vitrectomy) is widely accepted in postsurgical and posttraumatic endophthalmitis, but its benefits in endogenous endophthalmitis have been debated [15, 21].

The roles of intravitreal antibiotics and vitrectomy are evolving, and these therapeutic modalities will likely become more widely accepted in the future.

Surgical intervention is generally recommended for patients infected with especially virulent organisms, visual acuity of 20/400 or less, or severe vitreous involvement. The outcome of posterior diffuse endophthalmitis or panophthalmitis is frequently blindness, regardless of treatment measures. Vitrectomy and intravitreal antibiotics may, however, prevent ocular atrophy or the need for enucleation. (For further details on the role of vitrectomy in cancer patients, see Chapter 38.)

Inflammatory mediators may also impart some damage. Steroids such as dexamethasone have been administered intravitreally, although their role is not clear. Topical steroids have been used empirically in patients with anterior focal or diffuse disease to prevent complications such as glaucoma and formation of posterior synechiae.

36.5.2 Fungal Endophthalmitis

Fungal endogenous endophthalmitis (Fig. 36.1) secondary to yeast is often treated successfully, whereas endogenous endophthalmitis secondary to mold often results in considerable visual loss. If the patient's history, stains, or culture results suggest a fungal infection, amphotericin B, fluconazole, or itraconazole should be included in the regimen.

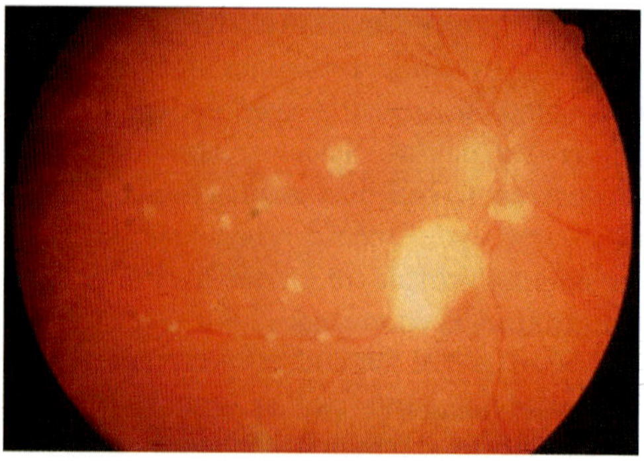

Fig. 36.1 Multifocal fungal chorioretinitis with snowball vitreous involvement

36.5.2.1 Yeast Endophthalmitis

In patients with endogenous endophthalmitis secondary to yeast, *Candida* species are the most common offending agent. Risk factors for candida endophthalmitis include central venous catheters, total parenteral nutrition, neutropenia, prior abdominal surgery, broad-spectrum antibiotic therapy, corticosteroid therapy, and intravenous drug use [22, 23]. Of the *Candida* species, *Candida albicans* is the most frequent offending agent, consistent with its higher virulence and higher incidence of candidemia.

One study examined fungal endophthalmitis in cancer patients specifically and confirmed *C. albicans* as the most frequent offending organism of the *Candida* species. A propensity of *Candida* to affect patients with solid tumors was also suggested, as 50% of those with *Candida* endophthalmitis had solid tumors [24].

Studies have shown that among patients with candidemia, 2.2% develop chorioretinitis and 6.3% develop endophthalmitis [21, 25]. Ocular candidiasis with only chorioretinitis can be managed with systemic antifungals (fluconazole 400–800 mg by mouth daily or amphotericin B 0.7–1 mg/kg daily plus flucytosine 100 mg/kg by mouth daily in four divided doses), since these achieve therapeutic concentrations in the choroid and retina. When overt endophthalmitis is present, management recommendations include the combination of systemic therapy with fluconazole (400–800 mg by mouth daily), vitrectomy, and intravitreal injection of amphotericin (10 μg). In amphotericin-resistant cases, fluconazole can be used intravitreally; however, fluconazole is usually not preferred because of its retinal toxicity. For fluconazole-resistant *Candida* species (*C. krusei* or *C. glabrata*), voriconazole (6 mg/kg intravenously every 12 h for two loading doses, then 4 mg/kg by mouth twice daily) has shown some success.

36.5.2.2 Mold Endophthalmitis

Endogenous mold endophthalmitis is rare and typically occurs in the setting of relative immunocompromise or intravenous drug use. One review of 86 cases of endogenous *Aspergillus* endophthalmitis from 1949 to 2001 identified associations with intravenous drug use (27% of cases), solid organ transplantation (23%), chronic lung disease (17%), corticosteroid treatment (43%), hematologic malignancy (8%), and other malignancy (1%) [26]. *Aspergillus fumigatus* was the predominant species noted in this study [26].

A study of 23 cancer patients with fungal endophthalmitis confirmed the propensity of mold endophthalmitis in patients with hematologic malignancies—100% of the patients with mold endophthalmitis ($n = 15$) had hematologic malignancies. However, this study revealed *Fusarium* species and *Scedosporium apiospermum* as the most frequent offending organisms, followed by *A. fumigatus* [24].

Studies suggest that endogenous mold endophthalmitis is an often-missed diagnosis. An autopsy study of orthotopic liver transplant recipients revealed that 7% of patients had unrecognized endogenous endophthalmitis [26]. Even patients who are diagnosed have a poor prognosis: studies show that only one-third of patients retain useful vision in an eye affected with endogenous mold endophthalmitis [12].

The treatment of choice for endogenous mold endophthalmitis is oral voriconazole (loading dose of 6 mg/kg intravenously every 12 h for two doses, then 4 mg/kg by mouth twice daily), intravitreal injection of amphotericin (10 μg), and vitrectomy. Studies have indicated that fluconazole is a poor choice for systemic treatment as it has poor activity against molds. Posaconazole has been used for systemic therapy but does not achieve adequate intravitreal levels [14]. Isolated case reports have shown success with caspofungin treatment, but caspofungin is not the mainstay of treatment (Table 36.1) [27].

Table 36.1 Treatment options for endogenous endophthalmitis

Bacterial	Yeast	Mold
Broad-spectrum intravenous antibiotics (vancomycin 1 g IV every 12 h + either ceftazidime 2.2 mg in 0.1 mL IV every 8 h or ciprofloxacin 500–750 mg by mouth twice a day); possibly intravitreal antibiotics and/or vitrectomy	Oral fluconazole (400–800 mg daily), vitrectomy, and intravitreal injection of amphotericin	Oral voriconazole (loading dose of 6 mg/kg IV every 12 h for two doses, then 4 mg/kg by mouth twice daily), intravitreal injection of amphotericin, and vitrectomy

IV, intravenously

36.6 Prognosis

Compared with the outcome of exogenous endophthalmitis, the outcome of endogenous endophthalmitis is disappointing. The three main factors that contribute to a poor prognosis are more virulent organisms, immunocompromised host conditions, and delay in diagnosis. Even with aggressive treatment, useful vision (i.e., ability to count fingers or better) is preserved in only about 40% of patients.

36.7 Summary

Endogenous endophthalmitis is potentially sight-threatening in cancer patients and necessitates emergent diagnosis and management. Etiology includes hematogenous bacterial, yeast, or mold seeding. Recognition of the risk factors is critical to making an early diagnosis. Management includes broad-spectrum intravenous antibiotics and possibly intravitreal antibiotics and vitrectomy.

Although management has improved considerably over the last several decades, limitations persist, and the devastating consequence of visual loss is not always preventable. Thus, our most important management strategy as clinicians should remain vigilance, through close monitoring of immunocompromised cancer patients with systemic infections, which will allow earlier diagnosis and improved prognosis [2].

References

1. Okada AA, Johnson RP, Liles WC, et al. Endogenous bacterial endophthalmitis. Report of a 10-year retrospective study. Ophthalmology 1994;101:832–8.
2. Leibovitch I, Lai T, Raymond G, et al. Endogenous endophthalmitis: a 13-year review at a tertiary hospital in South Australia. Scand J Infect Dis 2005;37(3):184–9.
3. Ness T, Pelz K, Hansen LL. Endogenous endophthalmitis: microorganisms, disposition, and prognosis. Acta Ophthalmol Scand 2007;85(8):852–6.
4. Parke DW 2nd, Jones DB, Gentry LO. Endogenous endophthalmitis among patients with candidemia. Ophthalmology 1982;89(7):789–96.
5. Tanaka M, Kobayashi Y, Takebayashi H, et al. Analysis of predisposing clinical and laboratory findings for the development of endogenous fungal endophthalmitis. A retrospective 12-year study of 79 eyes of 46 patients. Retina 2001;21(3):203–9.
6. Schiedler V, Scott IU, Flynn HW Jr, et al. Culture-proven endogenous endophthalmitis: clinical features and visual acuity outcomes. Am J Ophthalmol 2004;137(4): 725–31.
7. Hawkins AS, Deutsch TA. Infectious endophthalmitis. Curr Infect Dis Rep 1999;1(2):172–7.
8. Godley BF, Folk JC. Retinal hemorrhages as an early sign of acute bacterial endophthalmitis. Am J Ophthalmol 1993;116:246–9.
9. Miailhes P, Labetoulle M, Naas T, et al. Unusual etiology of visual loss in an HIV-infected patient due to endogenous endophthalmitis. Clin Microbiol Infect 2001;7(11):641–5.
10. Perri P, Campa C, Incorvaia C, et al. Endogenous Aspergillus versicolor endophthalmitis in an immuno-competent HIV-positive patient. Mycopathologia 2005;160(3):259–61.
11. Ramakrishnan R, Bharathi MJ, Shivkumar C, et al. Microbiological profile of culture-proven cases of exogenous and endogenous endophthalmitis: a 10-year retrospective study. Eye 2008;23(4):945–56.
12. Essman TF, Flynn HW Jr, Smiddy WE, et al. Treatment outcomes in a 10-year study of endogenous fungal endophthalmitis. Ophthalmic Surg Lasers 1997;28:185–94.
13. Anand A, Madhavan H, Neelam V, et al. Use of polymerase chain reaction in the diagnosis of fungal endophthalmitis. Ophthalmology 2001;108(2):326–30.
14. Durand ML, Kim IK, D'AMico DJ, et al. Successful treatment of fusarium endophthalmitis with voriconazole and Aspergillus endophthalmitis with voriconazole plus caspofungin. Am J Ophthalmol 2005;140:552–4.
15. Kunimoto DY, Kanitkar KD, Makar MS. The Wills Eye Manual, fourth edition. Philadelphia, PA: Lippincott Williams & Wilkins, 2004.

16. Keswani T, Ahua V, Changulani M. Evaluation of outcome of various treatment methods for endogenous endophthalmitis. Indian J Med Sci 2006;60(11):454–60.
17. Desai M, Rapoor R, Gudithi SL, et al. Endophthalmitis: a rare complication of arteriovenous fistula infection. Hemodial Int 2008;12(2):227–9.
18. Hsu KH, Ben RJ, Shiang JC, et al. Pseudomonas aeruginosa endocarditis associated with endophthalmitis caused by arteriovenous fistula and graft infection. J Chin Med Assoc 2003;66(10):617–20.
19. Callegan MC, Cochran DC, Kane ST, et al. Virulence factor profiles and antimicrobial susceptibilities of ocular bacillus isolates. Curr Eye Res 2006;31(9):693–702.
20. Fang CT, Lai SY, Yi WC, et al. Klebsiella pneumoniae genotype K1: an emerging pathogen that causes septic ocular or central nervous system complications from pyogenic liver abscess. Clin Infect Dis 2007;45:284–93.
21. Popovich K, Malani PN, Kauffman CA, et al. Compliance with Infectious Diseases Society of America guidelines for ophthalmologic evaluation of patients with candidemia. Infect Dis Clin Pract 2007;15:254.
22. Edwards JE Jr, Foos RY, Montgomerie JZ, et al. Ocular manifestations of Candida septicemia: review of seventy-six cases of hematogenous candida endophthalmitis. Medicine (Baltimore) 1974;53:47–75.
23. Donahue SP, Greven CM, Zuravleff JJ, et al. Intraocular candidiasis in patients with candidemia. Clinical implications derived from a prospective multicenter study. Ophthalmology 1994;101:1302–9.
24. Lamaris GA, Esmaeli B, Chamilos G, et al. Fungal endophthalmitis in a tertiary care cancer center: a review of 23 cases. Eur J Clin Microbiol Infect Dis 2008;27:343–7.
25. Kannangara S, Shindler D, Kunimoto DY, et al. Candidemia complicated by endophthalmitis: a prospective analysis. Eur J Clin Microbiol Infect Dis 2007;26:839–41.
26. Riddell J, McNeil SA, Johnson TM, et al. Endogenous Aspergillus endophthalmitis: report of three cases and review of the literature. Medicine (Baltimore) 2002;81:311–20.
27. Kramer M, Kramer MR, Blau H, et al. Intravitreal voriconazole for the treatment of endogenous Aspergillus endophthalmitis. Ophthalmology 2006;113:1184–6.

Chapter 37
Viral Retinitis in the Cancer Patient

Gibran S. Khurshid, Garvin H. Davis, Kapil G. Kapoor, and Bernard F. Godley

Abstract Viral retinitis is a vision-threatening infection of the retina that can occur in both immunocompetent and immunocompromised patients and is primarily caused by the human herpesvirus family of viruses. Prompt recognition and treatment are critical for optimal outcomes. This chapter focuses on cytomegalovirus (CMV) retinitis, acute retinal necrosis (ARN), and progressive outer retinal necrosis (PORN). Presentations of CMV retinitis range from an indolent/granular retinitis to a fulminant/edematous retinitis characterized by necrosis and hemorrhage. ARN is a vaso-occlusive necrotizing retinitis that is usually secondary to herpes zoster or HSV. PORN is characterized by primary involvement of the outer retina, minimal to no vitreous inflammation, and extremely rapid progression. Treatment of CMV retinitis consists of improving the patient's immune status and then administering induction and maintenance antiviral therapy. For ARN, intravenous acyclovir is the standard initial treatment; oral acyclovir is then employed for variably prolonged periods. Because of PORN's poor prognosis, a multidisciplinary approach with an infectious disease consultation is favored. In patients with viral retinitis, argon laser photocoagulation posterior to the edge of necrosis may be performed as prophylaxis against retinal detachment, which is the major cause of visual loss after acute manifestations have resolved. Retinal detachments in patients with CMV retinitis have been approached with scleral buckling, gas pneumatic retinopexy, and vitrectomy with either gas or silicone oil tamponade. Visual prognosis is guarded for patients with CMV retinitis or ARN and extremely poor for patients with PORN.

37.1 Introduction

Viral retinitis is a vision-threatening infection of the retina that can occur in both immunocompetent and immunocompromised patients. Viral retinitis is

G.S. Khurshid (✉)
Department of Ophthalmology and Visual Sciences, The University of Texas Medical Branch, Galveston, TX, USA
e-mail: sk.gibran@utmb.edu

B. Esmaeli (ed.), *Ophthalmic Oncology*, M.D. Anderson Solid Tumor Oncology Series 6, DOI 10.1007/978-1-4419-0374-7_37,

primarily caused by the human herpesvirus (HHV) family of viruses, including cytomegalovirus (CMV; HHV 5), varicella-zoster virus (VZV; HHV 3), herpes simplex virus (HSV; HHV 1 and 2), and Epstein–Barr virus (HHV 4) [1]. Host immunoregulation is critical in guarding against viral cytotoxicity and the ocular sequelae of herpetic disease [2]. HHVs are known opportunistic pathogens. They have a notable predilection toward retinal tissue, and the incidence of HHV infection is highest in immunocompromised hosts [3]. Since cancer patients are often both intrinsically immunocompromised because of the cancer itself and iatrogenically immunocompromised because of cancer treatment, they are particularly susceptible to opportunistic infections, including viral retinitis.

Presentations of viral retinitis can range from no symptoms to severe visual loss secondary to aggressive acute retinal necrosis (ARN). Due to this wide range of presentations, routine screening for viral retinitis in cancer patients is of utmost importance. This chapter will focus on CMV retinitis, ARN, and progressive outer retinal necrosis (PORN).

37.2 Epidemiology

The epidemiology of viral retinitis in cancer patients is complicated by the fact that infection can represent a primary infection, reactivation of a latent infection, or reinfection. Reactivation of a latent infection is the most common presentation because of high rates of seropositivity even in the general population, especially for CMV.

Although there has been only limited research on viral retinitis specifically in cancer patients, it is known that CMV is not only the most common opportunistic ocular infection occurring in all immunocompromised hosts but also the most common cause of viral retinitis [4]. Other common causes of viral retinitis include other members of the HHV family, including VZV and HSV. The literature includes case reports of viral retinitis due to rubella, coxsackie virus, Epstein–Barr virus, rubeola, subacute sclerosing panencephalitis virus, Rift Valley fever virus, influenza A virus, mumps virus, and hepatitis B virus in immunocompromised hosts, but not all of these causes have been reported specifically in cancer patients [5–8].

37.3 Clinical Features

37.3.1 CMV Retinitis

Patients with CMV retinitis may be asymptomatic or may present with new floaters, blurred vision, or flashes of light. Although more than 80% of patients present with visual acuity of better than 20/50 [4], central visual loss can occur secondary to retinal necrosis involving the fovea, serous macular exudation, optic nerve involvement, or rhegmatogenous retinal detachment involving the macula [9, 10]. There is an associated mild vitreous inflammation often described as being less than might be expected for the degree of retinal damage. There may be fine, stellate keratic precipitates and posterior synechiae, but there is little overlying vitreous or anterior chamber inflammation [3, 4].

At one end of the spectrum of CMV retinitis is an indolent/granular retinitis, more often seen in the retinal periphery and associated with less dense retinal opacification and little or no hemorrhage or retinal vascular sheathing. At the other end of the spectrum is a fulminant/edematous retinitis, characterized by prominent necrosis and hemorrhage, often along blood vessels in the posterior pole (Fig. 37.1). A striking perivascular sheathing may be present [3]. Although CMV has been associated with ARN, this is not a common presentation [11].

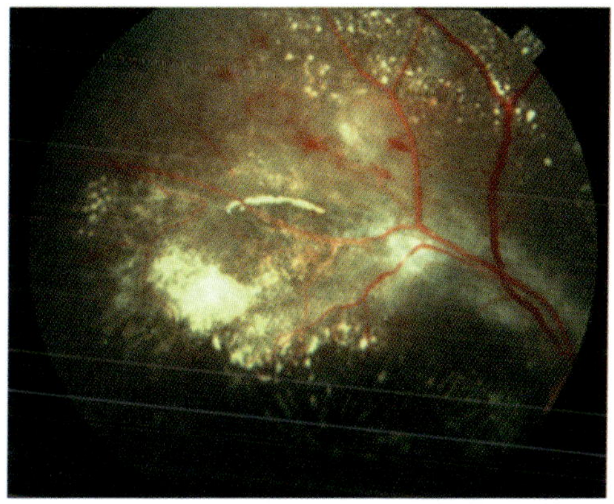

Fig. 37.1 Fulminant retinitis characterized by prominent retinal necrosis and hemorrhage along blood vessels in the posterior pole

A "zone" system is used to classify retinal involvement in CMV retinitis. Zone 1 lesions are present within a circle around the fovea with a radius of 3000 μm or within 1500 μm of the edge of the optic nerve. Zone 2 lesions are located outside zone 1 but posterior to the ampullae of the vortex veins at the equatorial retina. Zone 3 lesions are present between zone 2 and the ora serrata.

CMV retinitis spreads at a rate of approximately 250 μm/week, and there are usually atrophic areas that appear as retinal pigment epithelial pigmentation. Reactivation may begin at the edge of these atrophic scars, expanding outward [3]. Although clinically any area of active retinitis ought to be considered as progression, research studies have defined progression of CMV retinitis as expansion extending from the edge of an atrophic scar by 750 μm along a border at least 750 μm in length, or the appearance of a new area of retinitis greater than one-fourth of the disc diameter [3].

Diagnosis is based on clinical findings, primarily on indirect ophthalmoscopy. Polymerase chain reaction testing of aqueous and/or vitreous samples for CMV is highly specific but rarely clinically necessary. Fundus photography can confirm ophthalmoscopy findings and may be a more sensitive way to monitor response to therapy than clinical examination alone [12]. Fluorescein angiography is not typically indicated but may reveal blocking defects from areas of hemorrhage and leaking or nonperfusion of vessels in involved retinal areas [3].

37.3.2 Acute Retinal Necrosis

ARN is a vaso-occlusive necrotizing retinitis that is usually secondary to herpes zoster or HSV. Even though ARN can result from HSV-1 or HSV-2, herpes zoster is the most frequent culprit, and ARN often develops concurrently with or after zoster dermatitis, ipsilateral facial nerve palsy (Ramsay Hunt syndrome), or herpes zoster ophthalmicus [13, 14]. A bimodal age distribution has been proposed, with HSV-2 affecting younger patients and HSV-1 and herpes zoster affecting older patients. ARN usually presents as unilateral disease, but may involve the second eye (bilateral acute retinal necrosis, BARN) in up to one-third of patients within several months after initial ocular involvement.

ARN is a specific syndrome that is defined by the Executive Committee of the American Uveitis Society [15] as (1) one or more foci of retinal necrosis with discrete borders in peripheral retina, (2) rapid progression of the disease, (3) circumferential spread of the disease, (4) occlusive vasculopathy with arteriolar involvement, and (5) prominent inflammatory reaction in the vitreous and anterior chamber.

ARN is characterized by prominent anterior uveitis with or without keratic precipitates, retinal and choroidal vasculitis, vitritis, and papillitis [4]. The acute phase of ARN lasts 4–12 weeks. ARN begins as a multifocal retinitis with yellowish-white peripheral lesions that gradually enlarge and coalesce 360°, spreading peripherally. The acute phase of ARN may be further characterized by a prominent retinal vasculitis. The junction of necrotic and normal retina can be a site of vitreous traction leading to retinal breaks and subsequent rhegmatogenous retinal detachments, which occur in up to 75% of affected eyes [16].

Rapidly sloughed necrotic retinal debris in the vitreous cavity contributes to a pronounced vitritis that distinguishes ARN from CMV retinitis [3, 4]. ARN also has a more rapid progression and a reduced tendency to hemorrhage compared to CMV retinitis [3].

37.3.3 Progressive Outer Retinal Necrosis

PORN and ARN are considered by some authors to be the same disease process. The umbrella term *necrotizing herpetic retinopathy* has been used to describe a spectrum of infection that includes these two entities. PORN was initially described in patients with advanced HIV infection and typically occurs in immunocompromised patients secondary to herpes zoster [17].

PORN is characterized by primary involvement of the outer retina, minimal to no vitreous inflammation, and extremely rapid progression [4, 18]. Multifocal, peripheral, deep retinal lesions rapidly achieve confluence and posterior progression. A characteristic "cracked mud" perivascular pattern has been described, attributed to early removal of necrotic debris from perivascular retina. PORN can progress to involve the optic nerve, retinal pigment epithelium, and choriocapillaris.

Compared to ARN, PORN may have a greater exclusivity to immunocompromised patients, whereas ARN occurs in immunocompetent and immunocompromised patients. PORN is further characterized by little or no vasculitis, less vitritis than ARN, and early posterior pole involvement.

Compared with progression of CMV retinitis, progression of PORN is markedly accelerated, with a typical absence of intraocular inflammation, vasculitis, or hemorrhage [3].

37.4 Treatment

37.4.1 CMV Retinitis

Treatment for CMV retinitis is complex, requiring collaboration between the ophthalmologist and the infectious disease specialist. Initial antiviral therapy must be individualized based on location and severity of lesions and can involve oral antiviral therapy or intravenous antiviral therapy in combination with intravitreal injection or implant for more sight-threatening lesions. Anti-CMV drugs are virostatic and cannot eliminate the pathogen, which is why, in an immunocompromised patient, the possibility of relapse or progression is important.

The first step is to improve the patient's immune status, if possible. In some patients, particularly cancer patients (but not patients with AIDS), the discontinuation or reduction of immunosuppressive therapy may be sufficient to result in a cure. However, some patients develop active vitritis coinciding with the revitalization of their immune system. This has been described as immune recovery uveitis and should not be interpreted as a relapse [19].

Treatment of CMV retinitis includes an induction phase and a maintenance phase. Induction treatment is directed at halting progression of CMV retinitis lesions and typically lasts for 2–3 weeks. Maintenance therapy is directed at preventing reactivation of the CMV retinitis and generally needs to be maintained throughout the period of immunosuppression. Table 37.1 identifies Food and Drug Administration-approved medications for treatment of CMV retinitis, with appropriate induction and maintenance doses where applicable.

37.4.1.1 Intravitreal Injections

Only fomivirsen has been approved for intravitreal use although the off-label use of intravitreal ganciclovir and foscarnet is relatively common. The off-label use of intravitreal cidofovir has also been reported. However, both the *Physician's Desk Reference* and the drug's package insert specifically prohibit the intraocular use of this drug. Although not approved for initial therapy, fomivirsen is approved for use in patients who are unresponsive to or cannot tolerate other available treatments. The use of fomivirsen is contraindicated within 4 weeks of any use of cidofovir due to reported increased risk of ocular inflammation.

Table 37.1 FDA-approved medications for treatment of CMV retinitis

Medication (brand name)	Approved route and dose
Ganciclovir (Cytovene)	Intravenous. Induction: 5 mg/kg every 12 h for 2 weeks. Maintenance: 5 mg/kg/day
Ganciclovir implant (Vitrasert)	Intraocular. One implant, 4.5 mg, duration of action 8 months
Valganciclovir	Oral. Induction: 900 mg twice daily for 3 weeks. Maintenance: 900 mg daily
Foscarnet (Foscavir)	Intravenous. Induction: 60 mg/kg every 8 h for 2 weeks. Maintenance: 90–120 mg/kg/day
Cidofovir (Vistide)	Intravenous. Induction: 5 mg/kg/week for 2 weeks. Maintenance: 5 mg/kg every 2–3 weeks
Fomivirsen (Vitravene)	Intravitreal. Induction: two injections of 330 μg separated by 2 weeks. Maintenance: one injection of 330 μg/month

The use of the ganciclovir implant is generally felt to be superior to intravitreal injections in patients with sight-threatening lesions. It must also be stressed that implants and intravitreal injections provide local treatment only and that systemic therapy should be maintained in patients in whom these local treatments are employed. Intravitreal injections may be considered if there is a delay in obtaining a ganciclovir implant or operating room time for the implant procedure.

37.4.1.2 Ganciclovir Implant

One treatment option often used for the local treatment of CMV retinitis is the ganciclovir implant. The implant (Vitrasert, Bausch & Lomb Surgical Inc., Claremont, CA) is available in a 4.5-mg size and consists of a pellet of ganciclovir with a polymerized coating through which the drug is released at a rate of 1 μg/hour.

A careful examination of the retina, with scleral depression, is necessary prior to ganciclovir implant placement. Any tears or detachments must be repaired prior to placement of the device.

The implant has a long plastic strut that must be trimmed down to 2 mm. A small hole is fashioned in the strut with a 27-G needle. This hole must be centered on the strut and just under 0.5 mm from the strut's leading edge. A double-armed suture is then passed through the hole. Various sutures have been used in reports on the surgical technique for ganciclovir implants. Both 8-0 nylon and 10-0 Prolene are acceptable, although other similar sutures may also be used. A sectoral conjunctival peritomy is then made in the inferotemporal quadrant. A microvitreoretinal blade is used to make a 5.5-mm sclerotomy parallel to and 4 mm posterior to the limbus over the pars plana. The sclerotomy should be centered at 6:30 in the right eye and 5:30 in the left eye. The implant is then inserted through the sclerotomy and is sutured to the sclera by passing one needle through the anterior edge of sclera and one needle through the posterior edge of sclera. Following this, the sclera is closed with 7.0 Vicryl sutures. After conjunctival closure, subconjunctival antibiotics and steroids are administered. The implant remains suspended within the eye at the surgical incision site overlying the pars plana. Correct placement should be verified with indirect ophthalmoscopy while the patient is still on the operating room table.

The Ganciclovir Implant Study for CMV retinitis demonstrated the efficacy of utilizing ganciclovir implants to treat CMV retinitis [20]. Progression in that study was primarily due to depletion of active drug from the implant and not to the development of viral resistance to ganciclovir. Patients may therefore require the serial placement of multiple implants. Subsequent implants may be placed adjacent to the preexisting implant(s).

37.4.2 Acute Retinal Necrosis

VZV, HSV-1 and HSV-2, and CMV have all been implicated as causes of ARN. Acyclovir is very effective against herpes zoster but not as effective against CMV. Intravenous acyclovir (1500 mg/m^2/day in three divided doses over 10–14 days) is the standard initial treatment for patients with ARN. Oral acyclovir is then employed for variably prolonged periods. Retinal lesions typically dissipate 4–5 days after therapy initiation, which decreases the risk of subsequent development of bilateral acute retinal necrosis (BARN). Palay et al. [21] showed that only 13% of acyclovir-treated patients developed BARN, compared with 70% of untreated patients. Thankfully, most immunocompetent patients with ARN respond to intravenous acyclovir.

In cases of ARN caused by HSV, oral corticosteroids at dosages of 40–60 mg/day may be introduced to limit the inflammatory response following 24–48 hours of antiviral treatment. However, some patients may be infected with HSV strains resistant to conventional therapy; in such patients, intravitreal antiviral therapy may be introduced to improve visual prognosis [22]. Some patients with ARN caused by HSV benefit from intravitreal ganciclovir injection (200 μg/0.05 ml) and intravenous foscarnet (1200 μg/0.05 ml, administered every other day for four doses).

In cases of ARN caused by VZV, brivudine and valganciclovir have shown good results. Valganciclovir is a valyl ester prodrug of ganciclovir, with proven efficacy similar to that of intravenous ganciclovir. Famciclovir has also been used.

In cancer patients, we favor an aggressive multidrug approach and usually start with combination therapy consisting of intravenous acyclovir and ganciclovir. A recent pilot study demonstrated complete resolution of ARN in all patients treated with oral antiviral drugs (valacyclovir and famciclovir) [18]. Low-dose aspirin has been used as an adjuvant antithrombotic treatment, since the majority of patients have occlusive retinal vasculitis. Systemic and topical corticosteroids have also been used to potentiate anti-inflammatory treatment and attempt to minimize optic nerve and retinal vessel damage [23].

Since rhegmatogenous retinal detachment occurs in up to 75% of eyes affected by ARN, therapy for advanced disease focuses on preventing or treating this important sight-threatening complication. If rhegmatogenous retinal detachment does occur, surgical repair may be necessary [23].

37.4.3 Progressive Outer Retinal Necrosis

Treatment regimens for PORN are based largely on small case series of AIDS patients. Due to PORN's poor prognosis, a multidisciplinary approach with an infectious disease consultation is favored. In a small case series, prolonged combination antiviral therapy demonstrated success in arresting progression of PORN, maintaining remission, and preventing involvement of the other eye [24]. For patients not responding to systemic therapy, intravitreal injections of foscarnet and ganciclovir have demonstrated some benefit [25, 26]. Prophylactic laser photocoagulation (described in the next section) is often used to decrease the risk of retinal detachment [25].

37.5 Role of Vitreoretinal Surgery in Viral Retinitis

37.5.1 Argon Laser Photocoagulation

Argon laser photocoagulation posterior to the edge of necrosis may be performed as prophylaxis against retinal detachment, which is the major cause of visual loss after acute manifestations have resolved. Recommendations include three or four rows of 500-μm spots placed posterior to the advancing border of retinitis. The chorioretinal scars produced by the laser burns act as "spot welds," which may hold the retina in place in the event that retinal tears develop in the area of retinal necrosis, leading to subsequent retinal detachment in that area.

37.5.2 Retinal Detachment Repair

Retinal detachments (Fig. 37.2) in patients with CMV retinitis have been approached with scleral buckling, gas pneumatic retinopexy, and vitrectomy with either gas or silicone oil tamponade.

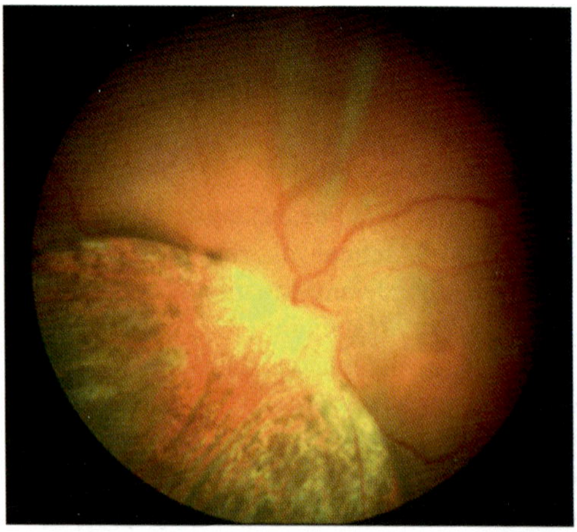

Fig. 37.2 Retinal atrophy and detachment following resolution of acute CMV retinitis

There has been some reluctance to use other approaches to repair retinal detachments related to CMV retinitis because past studies generally showed very limited success when silicone oil was not used. However, this reluctance appears to be lessening with the evolution of vitrectomy techniques and equipment. Pars plana vitrectomy combined with an encircling scleral buckle, complete removal of the posterior hyaloid, and laser retinopexy followed by gas tamponade has produced a total retinal reattachment rate of 83% [27]. Utilizing silicone oil provides an indefinite retinal tamponade and has a high success rate. The progression of inferior detachments not adequately tamponaded by gas may be stabilized with silicone oil use.

Silicone oil can be removed once the period of tamponade has been deemed adequate. Cataract extraction can be performed simultaneously or later if needed. If the silicone oil is well tolerated and the eye is unlikely to have visual improvement, there may be little reason to remove the oil. The use of silicone oil for retinal detachment repair is not contraindicated in patients with a ganciclovir implant, since effective ganciclovir release into the inferior aqueous meniscus continues in eyes filled with silicone oil.

37.6 Prognosis

37.6.1 CMV Retinitis

The visual prognosis for patients with CMV retinitis is guarded, and prompt recognition and treatment of CMV retinitis are critical for optimal outcomes. Frequent follow-up is important in these patients as therapy for CMV retinitis can have systemic and ocular sequelae. Further, patients can develop immune recovery uveitis, as stated previously, with reactivation of previously healed retinitis, rhegmatogenous retinal detachment, macular pucker, and macular edema, often resulting in visual loss [3].

37.6.2 Acute Retinal Necrosis

The visual prognosis for patients with ARN is guarded, particularly for patients with VZV-induced ARN [22]. Major causes of poor visual outcome in ARN include retinal detachment and ischemic vasculopathic involvement of the optic nerve or macula; other causes include macular hole formation, macular pucker, and hypotony [27]. However, some studies have demonstrated improvement in visual outcomes when prompt diagnosis is made and when laser treatment is applied [28].

37.6.3 Progressive Outer Retinal Necrosis

The visual prognosis of patients with PORN remains extremely poor. Blindness is frequent, secondary to progression to optic nerve disease or retinal detachment.

One case series demonstrated that two-thirds of patients had progression to no light perception vision within 1 month of diagnosis [29].

37.7 Conclusion

Both cancer and cancer treatment lead to an immunocompromised state, making cancer patients particularly susceptible to opportunistic viral infections. Appropriate screening for sight-threatening viral retinitis in cancer patients is of utmost importance. Prompt recognition of disease and prompt treatment will help to improve visual outcomes and quality of life for cancer patients.

References

1. Biswas J, Madhavan HN, Gopal L, et al. Clinical features and virologic studies in viral retinitis. Indian J Ophthalmol 1995;43:63–8.
2. Ritterband DC. Virus infections of the eye. Rev Med Virol 1998;8:187–201.
3. Dunn J. Viral retinitis. Ophthalmol Clin North Am 1999;12(1):109–21.
4. Mayo GL, Tolentino MJ. Cytomegalovirus retinitis. Focal Points (educational journal of the American Academy of Ophthalmology) 2007;25(2).
5. Kadrmas EF, Buzney SM. Coxsackievirus B4 as a cause of adult chorioretinitis. Am J Ophthalmol 1999;127(3):347–9.
6. Raymond LA, Wilson CA, Linnemann CC Jr, et al. Punctate outer retinitis in acute Epstein Barr virus infection. Am J Ophthalmol 1987;104:424–6.
7. Weiter JJ, Roh S. Viral infections of the choroid and retina. Infect Dis Clin North Am 1992;6(4):875–91.
8. Yoser SL, Forster DJ, Rao NA. Systemic viral infections and their retinal and choroidal manifestations. Surv Ophthalmol 1993;37:313–52.
9. Freeman WR, Henderly DE, Wan WL, et al. Prevalence, pathophysiology, and treatment of rhegmatogenous retinal detachment in treated cytomegalovirus retinitis. Am J Ophthalmol 1987;103:527–36.
10. Gangan PA, Besen G, Munguia D, et al. Macular serous exudation in patients with acquired immunodeficiency syndrome and cytomegalovirus retinitis. Am J Ophthalmol 1994;118: 212–9.
11. Silverstein BE, Conrad D, Margolis TP, et al. Cytomegalovirus-associated acute retinal necrosis. Am J Ophthalmol 1997;123:257–8.
12. Studies of Ocular Complications of AIDS Research Group and the AIDS Clinical Trials Group. Assessment of cytomegalovirus retinitis: clinical evaluation vs. centralized grading of fundus photographs. Arch Ophthalmol 1996;114:791–805.
13. Culbertson WW, Blumenkranz MS, Pepose JS, et al. Varicella zoster virus is a cause of the acute retinal necrosis syndrome. Ophthalmology 1986;93:559–69.
14. Browning DJ, Blumenkranz MS, Culbertson WW, et al. Association of varicella zoster dermatitis with acute retinal necrosis syndrome. Ophthalmology 1987;94:602–6.
15. Holland GN. Standard diagnostic criteria for the acute retinal necrosis syndrome. Executive Committee of the American Uveitis Society. Am J Ophthalmol 1994;117(5):663–7.
16. Clarkson JG, Blumenkranz MS, Culbertson WW, et al. Retinal detachment following the acute retinal necrosis syndrome. Ophthalmology 1984;91:1665–8.
17. Lewis JM, Nagae Y, Tano Y. Progressive outer retinal necrosis after bone marrow transplantation. Am J Ophthalmol 1996;122:892–5.

18. Aizman A, Johnson MW, Elner SG. Treatment of acute retinal necrosis syndrome with oral antiviral medications. Ophthalmology 2007;114(2):307–12.
19. Schrier RD, Song MK, Smith IL, et al. Intraocular viral and immune pathogenesis of immune recovery uveitis in patients with healed cytomegalovirus retinitis. Retina 2006;26:165–9.
20. Martin DF, Parks DJ, Mellow SD, Ferris III FL, Walton RC, Remaley NA, Chew EY, Ashton P, Davis MD, Nussenblatt RB. Treatment of cytomegalovirus retinitis with an intraocular sustained-release ganciclovir implant: a randomized controlled clinical trial. Arch Ophthalmol 1994;112:1531–9.
21. Palay DA, Sternberg P Jr, Davis J, et al. Decrease in the risk of bilateral acute retinal necrosis by acyclovir therapy. Am J Ophthalmol 1991;112:250–5.
22. Zambarakji HJ, Obi AA, Mitchell SM. Successful treatment of varicella zoster virus retinitis with aggressive intravitreal and systemic antiviral therapy. Ocul Immunol Inflamm 2002;10:41–46.
23. Kawaguchi T, Spencer DB, Mochizuki M. Therapy for acute retinal necrosis. Semin Ophthalmol 2008;23(4):285–90.
24. Ciulla TA, Rutledge BK, Morley MG, et al. The progressive outer retinal necrosis syndrome: successful treatment with combination antiviral therapy. Ophthalmic Surg Lasers 1998;29(3):198–206.
25. Perez-Blazque E, Traspas R, Mendez Marin I, et al. Intravitreal ganciclovir treatment in progressive outer retinal necrosis. Am J Ophthalmol 1997;124(3):418–21.
26. Scott IU, Luu KM, Davis JL. Intravitreal antivirals in the management of patients with acquired immunodeficiency syndrome with progressive outer retinal necrosis. Arch Ophthalmol 2002;120:1219–22.
27. Canzano JC, Morse LS, Wendel RT. Surgical repair of cytomegalovirus-related retinal detachment without silicone oil in patients with AIDS. Retina 1999;19(4):274–80.
28. Lau CH, Salmann J, Lightman SL. Acute retinal necrosis, features, management, and outcomes. Ophthalmology 2007;114:756–62.
29. Engstrom RE Jr, Holland GN, Margolis TP, et al. The progressive outer retinal necrosis syndrome: a variant of necrotizing herpetic retinopathy in patients with AIDS. Ophthalmology 1994;101:1488–502.

Chapter 38
Diagnostic Vitrectomy and the Cancer Patient: Special Considerations

Garvin H. Davis, Gibran S. Khurshid, Kapil G. Kapoor, and Bernard F. Godley

Abstract The term *diagnostic vitrectomy* is used to refer to biopsy of the vitreous or the uvea. In patients with a history of cancer, there is a low clinical threshold for diagnostic vitrectomy as vitritis can represent recurrence of lymphoma or leukemia or an opportunistic infection. The most common clinical scenarios in which diagnostic vitrectomy is performed in cancer patients are new-onset vitreous cellularity in a patient with lymphoma in remission or newly diagnosed lymphoma; vitritis in a patient with recent bone marrow transplantation; atypical retinitis or choroiditis; and atypical iris, ciliary body, or choroidal lesions. In addition, choroidal biopsy is sometimes done to obtain material for cytogenetic studies in patients with uveal melanoma. Vitreous biopsy can be performed successfully with either a two-port or three-port approach; specifics of the technique depend on the vitrector gauge. Uveal biopsy can be performed with fine-needle aspiration biopsy or with transretinal choroidal biopsy with a sutureless vitrectomy system, an approach that is gaining favor. Collaboration and good communication between the ophthalmologist and a pathologist well versed in the handling and analysis of vitreous samples are essential for successful diagnostic vitrectomy.

38.1 Introduction

Diagnostic vitrectomy in cancer patients is used in a wide range of clinical scenarios (Fig. 38.1). Patients with a history of cancer may experience decreased vision or other visual symptoms associated with vitreous hemorrhage, vitritis, retinitis, and/or chorioretinitis. These presentations pose diagnostic challenges, as they can signify a primary intraocular, primary extraocular, or metastatic malignancy; the recurrence of a malignancy; and even a paraneoplastic syndrome or conditions unrelated to

G.H. Davis (✉)
Department of Ophthalmology, The University of Texas at Houston, Houston, TX, USA
e-mail: gdavis@uth.tmc.edu

B. Esmaeli (ed.), *Ophthalmic Oncology*, M.D. Anderson Solid Tumor Oncology Series 6, DOI 10.1007/978-1-4419-0374-7_38,

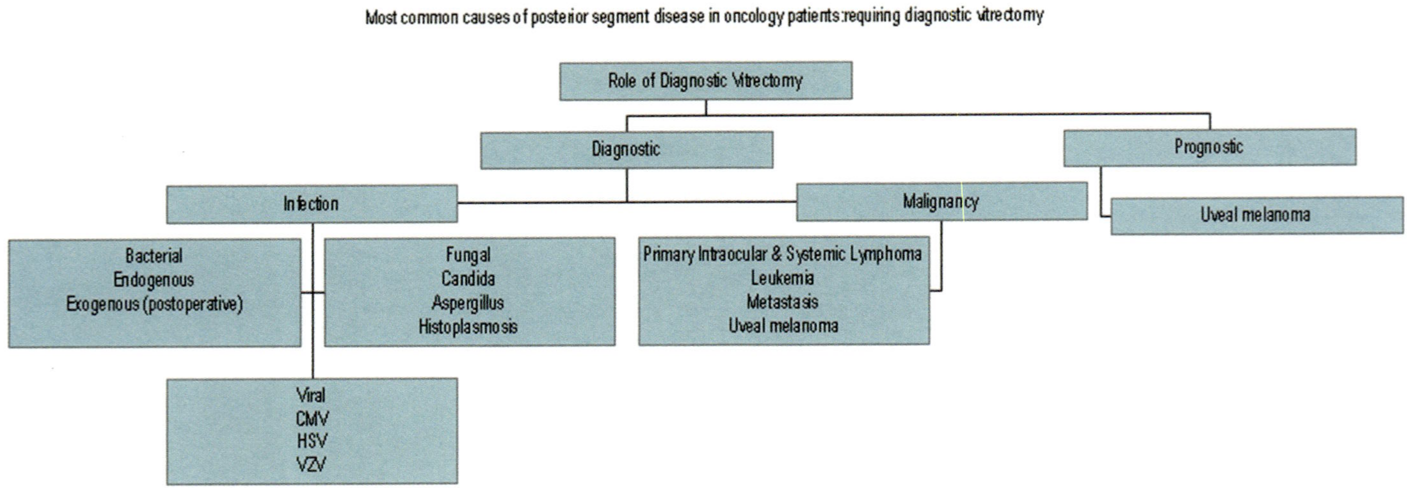

Fig. 38.1 Most common causes of posterior segment disease in cancer patients requiring diagnostic vitrectomy. CMV, cytomegalovirus; HSV, herpes simplex virus; HZV, herpes zoster virus

malignancy [1–3]. The diagnostic challenge is further complicated by iatrogenic immunosuppression from oncologic treatment, which can result in opportunistic fungal, bacterial, and/or viral infections [4–6]. Patients with a history of hematopoietic malignancy in remission may have autoimmune conditions associated with ocular inflammation, such as sarcoidosis or systemic lupus erythematosus.

Often, the etiology of vitreous cells can be determined by careful patient history and clinical examination; however, a tissue diagnosis obtained through vitrectomy is very helpful in many instances. Diagnostic vitrectomy and pathologic analysis of the vitrectomy specimen are well-accepted procedures for the confirmation or exclusion of ocular disorders [7–10].

38.2 Indications for Diagnostic Vitrectomy

The term *diagnostic vitrectomy* is used to refer to biopsy of either of two separate ocular entities, the vitreous and the uvea.

Uncomplicated diagnostic vitrectomy is a low-risk procedure providing valuable clinical benefits. The most common clinical scenarios are new-onset vitreous cellularity in a patient with lymphoma in remission or newly diagnosed lymphoma; vitritis in a patient with recent bone marrow transplantation; atypical retinitis or choroiditis; and atypical iris, ciliary body, or choroidal lesions.

38.2.1 Vitreous Biopsy

The most common indications for vitreous biopsy in cancer patients are vitreous cells or opacities of uncertain nature and vitreous hemorrhage of unknown etiology. In patients with a history of cancer, there is a low clinical threshold for vitrectomy as vitritis can represent recurrence of lymphoma or leukemia or an opportunistic infection. Vitreous hemorrhage can obscure the diagnosis of an ocular neoplasm [11].

38.2.2 Uveal Biopsy

Many tumor types arise in the choroid, each with a variety of clinical manifestations. In almost all patients, a choroidal tumor can be diagnosed readily by performing binocular indirect ophthalmoscopy. Ancillary tests such as echography and angiography can provide confirmatory evidence in some patients. In some instances, it is difficult to establish the diagnosis especially in cases of atypical melanoma or other choroidal lesions, choroidal metastasis, and rare lesions like retinal pigmentary adenoma and neurolemmoma.

Another emerging indication for choroidal biopsy is cytogenetic studies in patients with uveal melanoma. Uveal melanoma is the most common primary cancer of the eye. It often results in vision loss, and in up to half of patients, it results in death due to metastases. For many years, the details of the molecular pathogenesis of uveal melanoma remained elusive. In the past decade, however, many of these details have emerged to reveal a fascinating and complex story of how the primary tumor evolves and progresses. Early events that disrupt cell cycle and apoptotic control lead to malignant transformation and proliferation of uveal melanocytes. Later, the growing tumor encounters a critical bifurcation point, where it progresses along one of two genetic pathways with very distinct genetic signatures (monosomy 3 vs 6p gain) and metastatic propensity. Late genetic events are characterized by increasing aneuploidy, most of which is nonspecific. However, specific chromosomal alterations, such as loss of chromosome 8p, can hasten the onset of metastasis in susceptible tumors. This pathogenetic scheme can be used to construct a molecularly based and prognostically relevant classification of uveal melanomas for personalized patient management, particularly in the setting of metastatic disease [12].

It ought to be noted that biopsy using vitrector instrumentation is being increasingly employed for uveal biopsies.

38.3 Preoperative Considerations

Preoperative considerations in cancer patients scheduled to undergo vitrectomy are similar to those in noncancer patients. Patients should undergo a thorough ocular examination and a general examination to assess anesthetic risk. Cancer patients may be ill and must be stable enough to undergo moderate sedation. Although diagnostic vitrectomy is usually performed with retrobulbar or sub-Tenon injection of local anesthesia and monitored sedation, most anesthesiologists prefer that the patient be medically stable enough for general anesthesia [13]. Most elderly patients require baseline electrocardiography. As cancer patients may have blood cell count abnormalities, e.g., pancytopenia, a complete blood cell count is essential to determine whether transfusions or other precautions may be warranted. Other laboratory tests may be indicated depending on the clinical situation.

38.3.1 Thrombocytopenia

Ocular manifestations of thrombocytopenia include retinal and vitreal hemorrhage, retinal detachment, papilledema, and disc neovascularization. There are no published reports with which to define a minimum safe platelet count for vitrectomy in patients with thrombocytopenia. One study of 11 thrombocytopenic patients undergoing cataract and glaucoma surgery showed that the incidence of hemorrhagic complications was 18% [14]. We generally follow the recommendations of the consensus panel of the British Committee for Standards in Hematology and prefer to have a platelet count above 70,000 per mm^3 of blood (normal is 150,000–400,000 per mm^3 of blood) [15]. In cases of severe thrombocytopenia, frozen platelet transfusion 1–2 hours before surgery is arranged after consulting with a hematologist [15].

38.3.2 Anesthesia

Local anesthesia is commonly obtained with a mixture of bupivacaine (5 mg/ml), lidocaine (10 mg/ml), and hyaluronidase using a retrobulbar, peribulbar, or sub-Tenon insertion technique [16–18]. The block is placed while the patient is under conscious sedation. Recent studies of patients undergoing unilateral ophthalmic surgery with retrobulbar or peribulbar anesthesia showed no difference in patient satisfaction or clinical success between patients who did and those who did not have intravenous sedation [19, 20]. However, given that some cancer patients are critically ill and may have positional discomfort, operative efficiency and patient satisfaction in cancer patients are often enhanced with the use of intravenous sedation. Effective communication and good relationships between the ophthalmologists and the anesthesiologists facilitate excellent patient care.

Despite reports of complications with retrobulbar technique, it is generally accepted that the risk of retrobulbar hemorrhage is low. However, sub-Tenon's anesthetic insertion is occasionally employed, particularly in patients with abnormally functioning platelets or platelet counts below 50×10^9/l. There have been only two published reports of retrobulbar hemorrhage following sub-Tenon's block [19].

38.4 Vitreous Biopsy

38.4.1 Technique

Both two-port and three-port approaches have been successfully employed to obtain vitreous samples. We favor a three-port approach under noncontact wide-angle stereoscopic viewing because of the control and safety that this approach affords the surgeon (Fig. 38.2). There are currently three vitrector gauges available (20, 23, and 25), and all three are used by our surgeons.

Specifics of the technique vary depending on the vitrector gauge. After the patient has been anesthetized and sterile technique applied, an infusion cannula is inserted through the pars plana inferotemporally. Proper cannula placement is confirmed visually, but in order to preserve an undiluted sample, irrigation is not initiated. A second vitrectomy port is created superonasally and is temporarily occluded with a vitrectomy port plug to prevent vitreous prolapse during placement of the final port. A third vitrectomy port is created superotemporally. Instruments in the vitreous cavity are visualized using a binocular indirect ophthalmomicroscope (BIOM). With

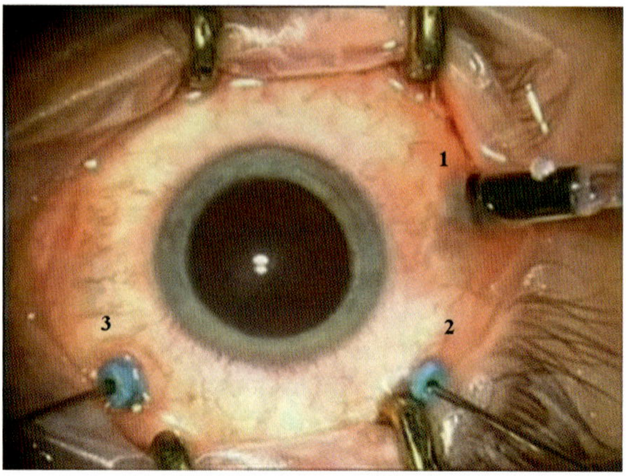

Fig. 38.2 Sutureless 25-G vitrectomy showing (1) infusion, (2) vitrector, and (3) endoilluminator

the infusion occluded, the assistant slowly aspirates undiluted vitreous (through a 3-cc syringe connected to the vacuum tubing from the vitrector) while the surgeon activates the cutter. As the surgeon guides the cutter toward the areas with the densest vitritis, 1.0–1.5 ml of vitreous is collected in the syringe and the eye begins to deflate. The assistant stops aspirating, and the surgeon removes the vitrectomy handpiece from the eye. The assistant can then collect an additional 0.5 ml of undiluted vitreous from the dead space in the tubing into the syringe, which is immediately capped and labeled. The vitreous cavity is then infused with balanced salt solution. If clinically appropriate, an additional core vitrectomy is performed and diluted vitreous in the cassette is sent for cytologic examination. After peripheral examination confirms the absence of peripheral retinal tears, the instrumentation is removed, and the sclerotomy sites either self-seal or are closed with Vicryl sutures.

The amount of undiluted vitreous acquired is limited by hypotony and the risk of suprachoroidal hemorrhage. The risk of suprachoroidal hemorrhage can be minimized by having the assistant perform simultaneous scleral indentation (Fig. 38.3). This maneuver helps to avoid hypotonous complications by stabilizing the intravitreal pressure in the absence of irrigation fluid. Utilizing this technique, we have not encountered any complications in more than 100 vitreous and choroidal biopsies.

Some authors have described a perfluorocarbon-perfused vitrectomy technique that allows an average of 2.24 ml of undiluted vitreous to be removed [21–24]. A syringe of perfluorocarbon liquid is connected to the infusion line. Vitreous is aspirated as the perfluorocarbon is infused. The difference in densities allows separation of the fluids during vitrectomy and processing. However, we do not routinely employ this technique because repeated fluid exchanges add significant complexity to the procedure. The undiluted vitreous is sent to the laboratory for cytologic evaluation, antibody determinations, and polymerase chain reaction (PCR) amplification. The diluted vitreous specimen from the syringe and the vitrectomy cassette can be evaluated with flow cytometry and with bacterial, fungal, and viral cultures.

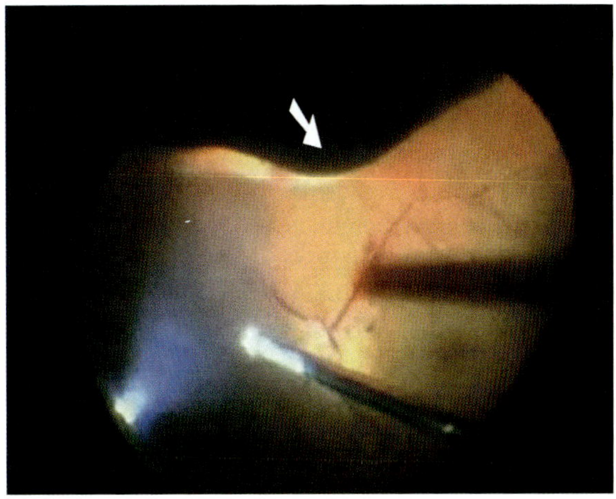

Fig. 38.3 Vitreous biopsy; note scleral indentation (*arrow*) to stabilize intravitreal pressure during dry vitreous sample retrieval

38.4.2 Effect of Vitrector Gauge on Vitreous Sample

Experimental models have shown that obtaining samples by vitrectomy causes minimal damage to human cell structure and should not limit cytologic assessment [25]. Conlon et al. [26] found that suspensions of human leukemic cells that were aspirated through a vitrector could not be distinguished from control cells on cytologic assessment. Vitrectomy had no observable effect on cell preservation using membrane filtration or cytocentrifugation techniques. Various aspiration and guillotine vitrector cutter rates even up to 1500 cuts per minute neither alter the yield of bacterial specimens nor affect the clinical utility of vitreous samples [27]. Higher cut rates mildly reduce the fungal yield and significantly reduce leukocyte viability.

The 25- and 23-G instruments minimize surgically induced trauma from sclerotomy sites, allow for self-sealing (sutureless) sclerotomies, improve operative efficiency, and hasten postoperative recovery. The absence of sutures prevents suture-based complications such as suture irritation, scleral pigmentary changes, and astigmatism induced by tight scleral sutures [28].

38.5 Uveal Biopsy

38.5.1 Technique

Fine-needle aspiration biopsy (FNAB) has traditionally been used for uveal biopsies. For preequatorial tumors, FNAB involves a transscleral approach and a 30-G needle; for postequatorial tumors, FNAB involves a transvitreal approach and a 27-G needle [29]. However, FNAB yields insufficient samples for cytogenetic analysis, and given the recently emphasized importance of cytogenetic testing, transretinal choroidal biopsy (TRCB) with sutureless vitrectomy systems is gaining favor.

TRCB involves insertion of 25-G infusion port, light pipe, and vitreous cutter cannulae 4 mm from the limbus in phakic eyes and 3.5 mm from the limbus in pseudophakic eyes. To separate the conjunctival and scleral openings, the conjunctiva is mobilized toward the corneal limbus with non-toothed forceps as the port is inserted. If a radioactive plaque is inserted during the same operation, the tumor biopsy is performed after these procedures are completed, with the ports passed through undisturbed conjunctiva. The vitreous cutter is advanced across the vitreous cavity and through the retina into the center of the tumor. Tissue samples are taken by rotating the cutter within the tumor. The vitreous cutter is repeatedly withdrawn from the tumor and flushed with a small volume of vitreous to prevent blockage of the aspiration cannula by tumor fragments. A complete vitrectomy is not performed. The specimen is back-flushed into a sterile specimen bottle through the cutter. Tumor fragments are visualized in the specimen bottle under the operating microscope to confirm that an adequate sample has been obtained.

When the scleral ports are removed, cotton-tipped applicators are used to apply pressure to each entry site and stroke the conjunctiva back into position. The aspirate is placed in a sterile container with an equal volume of 10% neutral buffered formalin. This preparation is then centrifuged. The resulting pellet is embedded in agar, and the preparation is processed into paraffin wax. Sections of the resulting wax-embedded cell block are stained with hematoxylin–eosin or periodic acid-Schiff or with immunohistochemical methods.

38.5.2 Complications

One of the authors (GK) observed vitreous hemorrhage in 32 (23%) of 140 cases (personal experience). In most of the patients, vitreous hemorrhage resolved spontaneously over 3–4 weeks, but 25% of affected patients needed vitrectomy to clear the vitreous hemorrhage.

No other intraoperative or postoperative complications were encountered. There are concerns about tumor recurrence or spread after uveal biopsy due to intraocular or extraocular seeding of tumor cells. However, the authors' experience with primary transretinal resection of 60 uveal melanomas over a 5-year period indicates that tumor recurrence from any seeding is rare [30]. The scleral cannula used with the 25-G system should further reduce any chances of implanting tumor cells into the entry sites.

38.5.3 Collaboration with Pathology

Collaboration with a skilled pathologist is essential to successful diagnostic vitrectomy. After a surgical date and time have been set, a pathologist experienced in the analysis of vitreous samples should be contacted and informed of the approximate arrival time of the sample. The likely diagnoses should be discussed with the pathologist, and the pathologist's preference for sample handling should be followed. Lymphoma cells degrade quickly, and some authors recommend placing the sample into a tube containing Roswell Park Memorial Institute culture medium [31]. Placement of the sample into normal saline can be helpful; however, alcohol fixation is not recommended because this can jeopardize identification of lymphoma cells.

We routinely place samples on ice and transport them directly to the laboratory after collection. We prefer immediate processing; samples are not stored overnight.

38.6 Pathologic Processing

There are three classes of laboratory testing for vitreous samples: (1) direct detection of the pathogen, which can be accomplished using cytology, staining and microscopic analysis, and cultures for fungi, bacteria, or viruses; (2) detection of the host response, which is accomplished by measuring interleukin; and (3) indirect detection of the pathogen, which is accomplished by using PCR. The most commonly used techniques at our institution are cytology, microscopic analysis, cultures, and PCR.

38.6.1 Cytology

Cytologic analysis of the vitreous sample is the primary technique for diagnosis of malignancy; however, necrotic cells, debris, and reactive inflammatory cells can pose a diagnostic challenge [32]. When intraocular lymphoma is suspected, characteristic features can be revealed using Giemsa, Papanicolaou, or Diff-Quick staining. A normal population of inflammatory cells would suggest infection or nonmalignant uveitis [33].

Flow cytometry can prove a useful supplement in the diagnosis of primary intraocular lymphoma [34]. Most primary intraocular lymphomas are monoclonal populations of B lymphocytes, and flow cytometry can simultaneously assess several different markers to confirm monoclonality in primary intraocular lymphoma.

38.6.2 Interleukin Measurement

Interleukin-10, a lymphoma cell growth factor, has been found to be elevated in vitreous samples of patients with intraocular lymphoma [35, 36]. Chan et al. [35] analyzed concentrations of five different interleukins (1, 2, 4, 6, and 10) by enzyme-linked immunosorbent assay in vitrectomy specimens from three patients with primary intraocular lymphoma and five patients with uveitis. Interleukin-10 was detected in the patients with lymphoma, and its levels correlated with clinical activity. Other studies have shown that elevated interleukin levels, although helpful, are not always associated with intraocular or central nervous system lymphoma [37]. The specificity of this test is still in doubt, and further studies are needed to ascertain its utility.

38.6.3 Polymerase Chain Reaction

PCR is a technique used to amplify small amounts of genetic material for analysis. The utility of PCR in vitrectomy samples may be particularly great in patients suspected of having infectious endogenous endophthalmitis. In such situations, short sequences of pathogen DNA are combined with the vitreous sample. If the vitreous sample contains matching strands of DNA, the pathogen DNA molecule acts as a primer, allowing the enzyme DNA polymerase to replicate the DNA. PCR has been used to detect many different bacterial, fungal, parasitic, and viral ocular infections. PCR is most commonly used at our institution to detect cytomegalovirus, herpes simplex virus, varicella zoster virus, and *Toxoplasma gondii*. PCR is readily available but may require collaboration with an outside laboratory.

38.6.4 Genetic Analysis

Intraocular lymphoma is often diagnosed by visualization of atypical cells or by flow cytometry. Genetic analysis may be important for determining clinical prognosis. Wallace et al. performed genetic analysis on the vitreous samples of 72 patients with primary intraocular lymphoma [38]. The authors evaluated the presence of the *bcl-2* t(14;18) translocation, the *bcl-10* gene, and the expression of *bcl-6* mRNA in primary intraocular lymphoma cells. The authors attempted to correlate the presence of the *bcl-2* t(14;18) translocation with clinical prognosis.

Although the authors could not correlate the presence of *bc1-2* t(14;18) with clinical prognosis, primary intraocular lymphoma was found to have unique molecular patterns of *bcl-2*, *bcl-10*, and *bcl-6* compared with other systemic lymphomas. This study may lay the foundation for future studies using gene expression profiling to supplement pathologic diagnosis of complex diseases.

38.6.5 Cytogenetic Uveal Melanoma Studies

The details of cytogenetic analysis techniques for uveal melanoma are beyond the scope of this chapter. However, commonly used techniques are fluorescence in situ hybridization (FISH), comparative genomic hybridization, and, most recently, multiplex ligation-dependent probe amplification (MLPA), which is reliable and cost-effective [39].

38.7 Results of Diagnostic Vitrectomy

38.7.1 Common Diagnoses

The clinical utility of diagnostic vitrectomy depends on the nature of the case. The largest series of diagnostic pars plana vitrectomy was published by Palexas et al. [40], who conducted a retrospective study covering 21 years. Pathology samples from 405 consecutive patients at the Wilmer Eye Institute revealed that the breakdown of results was as follows: posttraumatic infections, 8.4%; postoperative endophthalmitis, 38.5%; endogenous endophthalmitis, 6.2%; idiopathic inflammation, 25.4%; intraocular neoplasm, 14.3%; and miscellaneous, 7.2%. Palexas et al. [40] found that when the clinician suspected ocular lymphoma, 42 of 87 patients (48%) had positive biopsies. When the clinician suspected endogenous endophthalmitis, 23 of 25 biopsies (92%) were positive.

38.7.2 Diagnostic Utility

The vast majority of vitreous biopsies performed at The University of Texas M. D. Anderson Cancer Center are done to confirm or exclude intraocular malignancy or infection.

Davis et al. [9] reviewed cases to assess the utility of diagnostic tests performed on vitrectomy specimens from patients with suspected lymphoma or infection. Seventy-eight consecutive patients (84 eyes) underwent pars plana vitrectomy with cytologic, cytofluorographic, or microbiologic analysis. There were 33 eyes (28 patients) with suspected intraocular lymphoma and 51 eyes (50 patients) with suspected infection. Diagnostic vitrectomy led to the diagnosis in 48 of the 78 patients (61.5%). The biopsies for 14 patients were positive for lymphoma or leukemia and for 34 patients were positive for infection.

In this study, diagnostic vitrectomy for two of the most common indications at M. D. Anderson, lymphoma and infection, revealed a positive predictive value of 100%, and negative predictive values of 70 and 95%, respectively [9].

In contrast to the 70% negative predictive value for lymphoma reported by Davis et al. [9], a 98% negative predictive value was reported by Zhai et al. [41]. These authors reviewed the clinical records of 54 patients whose vitreous fluid samples were reported as "negative for malignancy" by an experienced pathologist. The main indication for vitrectomy was confirmation of intraocular inflammation. There was only 1 false-negative case identified among 54 cytologically benign vitreous samples. The negative predictive value of diagnostic vitrectomy in this study was 98%.

38.8 Postoperative Considerations

Patients are prescribed a combination of a topical steroid and an antibiotic to be taken for 2–3 weeks following diagnostic vitrectomy. Patients are understandably concerned about the results of the procedure and should have the results communicated as soon as possible. Verbal communication with the cytopathologist confirming the presence or absence of malignant cells on cytology is expected promptly, and the patient is usually notified of the preliminary results on the first postoperative visit. Usually the cytology result is available within 24 hours. Final results from PCR and fungal, bacterial, and/or viral cultures often require a week.

Postoperative complications include cataract, glaucoma, hypotony, infection, and retinal tear or detachment. Fortunately, the complication rate following vitrectomy is low. Palexas et al. and Scott et al. reported an overall incidence of endophthalmitis of 0.03% for 20-G vitrectomy and 0.84% for 25-G vitrectomy [40, 42].

38.9 Conclusion

Diagnostic vitrectomy in a patient with a known or suspected history of cancer is a useful tool in the diagnosis and management of ocular inflammation of unknown etiology. Generally, a low threshold for biopsy is required in patients with a history of cancer. Collaboration and good communication between the ophthalmologist and a pathologist well versed in the handling and analysis of vitreous samples are essential.

References

1. Robertson DM, Wilkinson CP, Murray JL, et al. Metastatic tumor to the retina and vitreous cavity from primary melanoma of the skin: treatment with systemic and subconjunctival chemotherapy. Ophthalmology 1981;88(12):1296–1301.
2. Jaissle GB, Szurman P, Rohrbach JM, et al. A case of cutaneous melanoma metastatic to the vitreous cavity: possible pathomechanism and review of the literature. Graefes Arch Clin Exp Ophthalmol 2007;245(5):733–40.
3. Soheilian M, Mirbabai F, Shahsavari M, et al. Metastatic cutaneous melanoma to the vitreous cavity masquerading as intermediate uveitis. Eur J Ophthalmol 2002;12(4):324–7.
4. Greene WH, Wiernik PH. Candida endophthalmitis. Successful treatment in a patient with acute leukemia. Am J Ophthalmol 1972;74(6):1100–4.
5. Rogers SJ, Johnson BL. Endogenous Nocardia endophthalmitis: report of a case in a patient treated for lymphocytic lymphoma. Ann Ophthalmol 1977;9(9):1123–31.
6. Lamaris GA, Esmaeli B, Chamilos G, et al. Fungal endophthalmitis in a tertiary care cancer center: a review of 23 cases. Eur J Clin Microbiol Infect Dis 2008;27(5):343–7.
7. Engel HM, Green WR, Michels RG, et al. Diagnostic vitrectomy. Retina 1981;1(2):121–49.

8. Green WR. Diagnostic cytopathology of ocular fluid specimens. Ophthalmology 1984;91(6):726–49.
9. Davis JL, Miller DM, Ruiz P. Diagnostic testing of vitrectomy specimens. Am J Ophthalmol 2005;140(5):822–9.
10. Foulds WS. The uses and limitations of intraocular biopsy. Eye 1992;6(Pt 1):11–27.
11. Saro F, Clua A, Esteva E, et al. Cytologic diagnosis of ocular melanocytoma: a case report. Acta Cytol 2008;52(1):87–90.
12. Landreville S, Agapova OA, Harbour JW. Emerging insights into the molecular pathogenesis of uveal melanoma. Future Oncol 2008;4:629–36.
13. Rosenfeld SI, Litinsky SM, Snyder DA, et al. Effectiveness of monitored anesthesia care in cataract surgery. Ophthalmology 1999;106(7):1256–60; discussion 1261.
14. Papamatheakis DG, Demers P, Vachon A, et al. Thrombocytopenia and the risks of intraocular surgery. Ophthalmic Surg Lasers Imaging 2005;36(2):103–7.
15. Saeed MU, Wong D, Heimann H, et al. Spontaneous progressive supra-choroidal haemorrhage in a patient undergoing haemodialysis. Graefes Arch Clin Exp Ophthalmol 2007;245(11):1741–2.
16. Hamilton RC. Retrobulbar block revisited and revised. J Cataract Refract Surg 1996;22(9):1147–50.
17. Duker JS. Retrobulbar injections: standards of care. Surv Ophthalmol 1995;39(4):344–5.
18. Demediuk OM, Dhaliwal RS, Papworth DP, et al. A comparison of peribulbar and retrobulbar anesthesia for vitreoretinal surgical procedures. Arch Ophthalmol 1995;113(7):908–13.
19. Kallio H, Uusitalo RJ, Maunuksela EL. Topical anesthesia with or without propofol sedation versus retrobulbar/peribulbar anesthesia for cataract extraction: prospective randomized trial. J Cataract Refract Surg 2001;27(9):1372–9.
20. Lim TH, Humayun MS, Yoon YH, et al. The efficacy of retrobulbar block anesthesia only in pars plana vitrectomy and transconjunctival sutureless vitrectomy. Ophthalmic Surg Lasers Imaging 2008;39(3):191–5.
21. Quiroz-Mercado H, Garcia-Aguirre G, Ustariz-Gonzalez O, et al. Perfluorocarbon-perfused vitrectomy using a transconjunctival 25-gauge system. Retina 2007;27(7):926–31.
22. Quiroz-Mercado H, Rivera-Sempertegui J, Macky TA, et al. Performing vitreous biopsy by perfluorocarbon-perfused vitrectomy. Am J Ophthalmol 2005;140(6):1161–3.
23. Quiroz-Mercado H, Guerrero-Naranjo J, Agurto-Rivera R, et al. Perfluorocarbon-perfused vitrectomy: a new method for vitrectomy—a safety and feasibility study. Graefes Arch Clin Exp Ophthalmol 2005;243(6):551–62.
24. Quiroz Mercado H, Suarez-Tata L, Magdalenic R, et al. Perfluorocarbon perfused vitrectomy: animal studies. Am J Ophthalmol 2004;137(2):287–93.
25. Huang JS, Russack V, Flores-Aguilar M, et al. Evaluation of cytologic specimens obtained during experimental vitreous biopsy. Retina 1993;13(2):160–5.
26. Conlon MR, Craig I, Harris JF, et al. Effect of vitrectomy and cytopreparatory techniques on cell survival and preservation. Can J Ophthalmol 1992;27(4):168–71.
27. Ratanapojnard T, Roy CR, Gariano RF. Effect of vitrector cutting rate on vitreous biopsy yield. Retina 2005;25(6):795–7.
28. Van Kuijk FJ, Uwaydatt S, Godley BF. Self-sealing sclerotomies in pars plana vitrectomy. Retina 2001;21:547–50.
29. Shields CL, Ganguly A, Materin MA, et al. Chromosome 3 analysis of uveal melanoma using fine-needle aspiration biopsy at the time of plaque radiotherapy in 140 consecutive cases. Trans Am Ophthalmol Soc 2007;105:43–53.
30. Damato B, Groenewald C, McGalliard J, et al. Endoresection of choroidal melanoma. Br J Ophthalmol 1998;82:213–8.
31. Whitcup SM, Chan CC, Buggage RR, et al. Improving the diagnostic yield of vitrectomy for intraocular lymphoma. Arch Ophthalmol 2000;118(3):446.
32. Margolis R. Diagnostic vitrectomy for the diagnosis and management of posterior uveitis of unknown etiology. Curr Opin Ophthalmol 2008;19(3):218–24.

33. Intzedy L, Teoh SC, Hogan A, et al. Cytopathological analysis of vitreous in intraocular lymphoma. Eye 2008;22(2):289–93.
34. Stacchini A, Demurtas A, Godio L, et al. Flow cytometry in the bone marrow staging of mature B-cell neoplasms. Cytometry B Clin Cytom 2003;54:10–8.
35. Chan CC, Whitcup SM, Solomon D, et al. Interleukin-10 in the vitreous of patients with primary intraocular lymphoma. Am J Ophthalmol 1995;120(5):671–3.
36. Tritten JJ, Haefliger JM, Delouche D, et al. Interleukin 10 and chronic vitritis in a case of ocular lymphoma [in German]. Klin Monatsbl Augenheilkd 1998;212(5):416–7.
37. Akpek EK, Maca SM, Christen WG, et al. Elevated vitreous interleukin-10 level is not diagnostic of intraocular-central nervous system lymphoma. Ophthalmology 1999;106(12): 2291–5.
38. Wallace DJ, Shen D, Reed GF, et al. Detection of the bcl-2 t(14;18) translocation and proto-oncogene expression in primary intraocular lymphoma. Invest Ophthalmol Vis Sci 2006;47(7):2750–6.
39. van Dijk MC, Rombout PD, Boots-Sprenger SH, et al. Multiplex ligation-dependent probe amplification for the detection of chromosomal gains and losses in formalin-fixed tissue. Diagn Mol Pathol 2005;14(1):9–16.
40. Palcxas GN, Green WR, Goldberg MF, et al. Diagnostic pars plana vitrectomy report of a 21-year retrospective study. Trans Am Ophthalmol Soc 1995;93:281–308; discussion 308–14.
41. Zhai J, Harbour JW, Smith ME, et al. Correlation study of benign cytomorphology and final clinical diagnosis. Acta Cytol 2008;52(2):196–200.
42. Scott IU, Flynn HW Jr, Dev S, et al. Endophthalmitis after 25-gauge and 20-gauge pars plana vitrectomy: incidence and outcomes. Retina 2008;28(1):138–42.

Chapter 39
Intraocular Lymphoma: Current Therapy and Future Trends

Christopher J. Calvano, Stella K. Kim, and Dan S. Gombos

Abstract Intraocular lymphoma is a rare non-Hodgkin's lymphoma with three main presentations: primary retinal lymphoma, primary uveal lymphoma, and secondary uveal lymphoma in a patient with known central nervous system lymphoma. Primary intraocular lymphomas are usually diffuse large B-cell lymphomas and generally are associated with a poor prognosis. Patients present with recurrent vitritis or uveitis that may initially respond to topical steroids. Some complain of increased floaters or generalized blurry vision. Cytologic evaluation is the mainstay of accurate diagnosis of primary intraocular lymphoma; genetic information from flow cytometry evaluation may also be useful. There is no clear consensus on treatment, but generally whole-eye radiotherapy should be considered, possibly after administration of systemic high-dose methotrexate.

39.1 Introduction and Epidemiology

Lymphomas account for about 5% of cancer cases in the United States. There are two general categories of lymphoma: Hodgkin's lymphoma and non-Hodgkin's lymphoma (NHL). The majority of lymphomas are NHL. Over the past 25 years, there has been a significant improvement in mortality from Hodgkin's lymphoma, but both the incidence of NHL and mortality from NHL have increased.

Intraocular lymphoma is a rare NHL and is considered a subtype of primary central nervous system (CNS) lymphoma. Intraocular lymphoma has three main presentations: primary retinal lymphoma, primary uveal lymphoma, and secondary uveal lymphoma in a patient with known CNS lymphoma. Primary intraocular lymphomas are usually diffuse large B-cell lymphomas and generally are associated

C.J. Calvano (✉)
Division of Ophthalmic Plastic Surgery, Kresge Eye Institute, Wayne State University, Detroit, MI, USA
e-mail: chris_calvano@yahoo.com

B. Esmaeli (ed.), *Ophthalmic Oncology*, M.D. Anderson Solid Tumor Oncology Series 6, DOI 10.1007/978-1-4419-0374-7_39,

with a poor prognosis. This chapter will focus on patients presenting with primary intraocular lymphoma with no history of CNS involvement.

The most recent World Health Organization Classification of Lymphoma [1] is based on the Revised European American Lymphoma classification. The World Health Organization classification employs clinical as well as pathologic, immunologic, and genetic parameters.

A key lymphoma risk factor is increased age; the majority of patients present in their sixth or seventh decades. The elderly population is increasing, especially in western Europe and the United States. The incidence of NHL is also increasing in this growing population, which represents both a challenge and an opportunity for clinicians and researchers to effectively serve this expanding cohort [2].

39.2 Presentation and Diagnosis

Several recently published reviews have summarized the natural history and standard diagnostic and treatment strategies for intraocular lymphoma [3–8]. In primary intraocular lymphoma, patients present with recurrent vitritis or uveitis that may initially respond to topical steroids. Some complain of increased floaters or generalized blurry vision. The lack of other ocular findings and the initial response to topical anti-inflammatory drops often lead to a delayed diagnosis.

In patients with primary uveal lymphoma, clinicians may detect choroidal or subretinal infiltration. The differential diagnosis of vitritis is beyond the scope of this chapter, but other causes should be entertained and ruled out before lymphoma is considered; in particular, infectious etiologies should be ruled out. Pathologic assessment of the vitreous plays a key role in arriving at the correct diagnosis. While some clinicians advocate fine needle aspiration, most centers proceed with a pars plana vitrectomy. The surgeon should first confirm that there is enough cellular material in the vitreous to justify biopsy. A scant specimen is unlikely to yield enough tissue for the pathologist to arrive at a definitive diagnosis. It cannot be overemphasized how critical it is to coordinate such a procedure in advance with an ocular pathologist experienced in processing vitreous and choroidal specimens.

The core vitrectomy specimen should be obtained with the cutter on slow speed to minimize damage to the cells (please see Chapter 38). This specimen should be sent off separately from the rest of the tissue, which can be obtained from the vitrectomy cassette. A fresh specimen should be supplied to the pathologist, who can also perform appropriate stains to rule out infectious etiologies. Cytospin and liquid-based cytology studies are generally employed to increase the sensitivity of the testing. In some cases, the core vitrectomy specimen may demonstrate only reactive lymphocytes. It is the authors' experience that in such patients, additional tissue from a choroidal infiltrate (if present) is very helpful in arriving at the correct diagnosis. The uveal biopsy may be performed using either an ab interno approach (via retinotomy) or an ab externo approach (with scleral flap). Both approaches can yield a significant amount of monoclonal cells.

Cytologic evaluation remains the mainstay of accurate diagnosis of primary intraocular lymphoma, but flow cytometry may contribute important additional genetic information allowing targeted treatment strategies. Flow cytometry is useful for immunophenotyping but may require multiple biopsies to achieve a correct diagnosis [9].

The advent of 25-G vitrectomy may further minimize the risk of vitreous biopsy. A comparison of cytology and flow cytometry results obtained via 25- and 20-G vitrectomy techniques was recently performed in an animal model using lymphoma cells obtained from human enucleation specimens [10]. In samples obtained with 25-G vitrectomy, cytology and immunophenotypic features were described as adequate for diagnosis, but overall cellularity was significantly reduced compared with cellularity in 20-G vitrectomy samples.

39.3 Management

Once primary retinal or uveal lymphoma is pathologically confirmed, it is often best to coordinate treatment with an oncologist experienced in the management of systemic and CNS lymphomas. A workup should be performed to ensure that there is no lymphoma elsewhere in the body. Generally, this workup includes a bone marrow biopsy, multiple lumbar punctures, and whole-body computed tomography and/or positron emission tomography.

There is no single consensus on the management of localized primary intraocular lymphoma without CNS involvement. At a minimum, whole-eye radiotherapy should be considered [3]. Given the high propensity of intraocular lymphoma for ocular and CNS recurrence, many clinicians at our institution administer systemic chemotherapy with high-dose methotrexate prior to radiotherapy. In general, the initial response is excellent and includes a reduction in vitritis and resolution of choroidal infiltrates.

If ocular disease recurs, additional radiotherapy or intraocular methotrexate is generally employed. The challenge with methotrexate is that numerous and frequent injections must be administered initially and continued later to maintain remission. It is the authors' experience that subsequent ocular relapse is not infrequent. Relapse involving the CNS is associated with high patient morbidity and mortality. High-dose chemotherapy with autologous stem cell transplantation may prove successful in refractory or recurrent cases [4].

39.4 Future Considerations

As the optimal management of primary intraocular lymphoma remains elusive [6, 11], the use of intrathecal, intraventricular, and intravitreal rituximab (anti-CD20 antibody) for the treatment of CNS lymphoma with and without ocular involvement has been investigated. One study showed that for recurrent primary CNS lymphoma ($n = 4$) and for NHL with leptomeningeal involvement ($n = 2$), systemic administration of rituximab via a combination of intravenous and intraventricular injections, intraventricular injections alone, or intrathecal injections alone had some benefit in terms of clearing the leptomeningeal process but was less efficacious for solid parenchymal disease [12].

Given the blood–brain barrier, the efficacy of intravenous administration of immunotherapy is limited. Intrathecal administration of rituximab appears to overcome the penetration limitation of intravenous administration, as shown in a recent phase I trial in which intrathecal administration of rituximab at a dose ranging from 10 to 25 mg via an Ommaya reservoir over 5 weeks resulted in cytologic response in 6 of 10 patients with non-Hodgkin's CNS lymphoma [13].

Some believe that intravitreal treatment of primary intraocular lymphoma with rituximab is ideal given the specificity of CD20-positive cells for primary intraocular lymphoma and the lack of CD20-positive cells in the normal eye, in particular in the neurons and glial tissues [14]. Intravitreal injection of rituximab has been studied in animals and in humans [15–18]. In rabbit studies, the half-life of rituximab 1 mg delivered by intravitreal injection was 4.7 days, and the drug was detectable up to 72 days, although the threshold dose needed for clinical efficacy is unclear [16]. In a small number of patients, no obvious toxicity was observed with intravitreal rituximab at a dose of 1 mg/0.1 ml, although longer term data from histologic and electrophysiologic studies are lacking [15, 16, 19, 20]. Further studies are warranted to evaluate the optimal conditions under which intravitreal rituximab may be of benefit to patients with primary intraocular lymphoma.

Other local therapies currently being considered include treatment with siRNA, anti-adhesion molecule therapy, anti-CD22 constructs, anti-angiogenic agents, and anti-interleukin-10 therapy [21]. Other broad areas for further research include identifying better prognostic factors, improving the sensitivity of diagnostic tools and imaging modalities, and increasing the use of animal models in testing preclinical local and systemic treatments [21].

39.5 Conclusions

At present, intraocular lymphoma remains a challenging disease to diagnose and cure. Early clinical recognition, core vitreous biopsy, and expert cytologic assessment are critical components in achieving improved clinical outcomes. Multidisciplinary treatment in consultation with experts on CNS lymphoma is the standard approach at our institution. Intensive systemic chemotherapy and ocular radiotherapy are often considered initially. Future studies using anti-CD20 monoclonal antibodies, such as rituximab, appear promising.

References

1. Jaffe ES, et al. World Health Organization Classification of Tumors. Tumors of Hematopoietic and Lymphoid Tissues. Pathology and Genetics. Lyons: IARC Press, 2001.
2. Moslehi R, Devesa SS, Schairer C, et al. Rapidly increasing incidence of ocular non-Hodgkin lymphoma. J Natl Cancer Inst 2006;98:936–9.
3. Gunduz K, Pulido JS, McCannel CA, et al. Ocular manifestations and treatment of central nervous system lymphoma. Neurosurg Focus 2006;21:E9.
4. Chan CC, Wallace DJ. Intraocular lymphoma: update on diagnosis and management. Cancer Control 2004;11:285–95.
5. Coupland SE, Heimann H, Bechrakis NE. Primary intraocular lymphoma: a review of the clinical histopathological and molecular biological features. Graefes Arch Clin Exp Ophthalmol 2004;242:901–13.
6. Kim SK, Chan CC, Wallace DJ. Management of primary intraocular lymphoma. Curr Oncol Rep 2005;7:74–9.
7. Chan CC, Buggage RR, Nussenblatt RB. Intraocular lymphoma. Curr Opin Ophthalmol 2002;13:411–8.
8. Coupland SE, Damato B. Lymphoma involving the eye and ocular adnexa. Curr Opin Ophthalmol 2006;17:523–31.
9. Zaldivar RA, Martin DF, Holden JT, et al. Primary intraocular lymphoma: clinical, cytologic, and flow cytometric analysis. Ophthalmology 2004;111:1762–7.
10. Fortun JA, Carvounis PE, Albini TA, et al. Comparison of cytologic and flow cytometry features of vitreous samples obtained using 20- or 25-gauge vitrectomy for the diagnosis of lymphoma. Poster presented at Association for Research in Vision and Ophthalmology. 2007, Ft. Lauderdale, FL.
11. Karma A, von Willebrand EO, Tommila PV, et al. Primary intraocular lymphoma: improving the diagnostic procedure. Ophthalmology 2007;114:1372–7.
12. Schulz H, Pels H, Schmidt-Wolf I, et al. Intraventricular treatment of relapsed central nervous system lymphoma with the anti-CD20 antibody rituximab. Haematologica 2004;89(6):753–4.
13. Rubenstein JL, Fridlyand J, Abrey L, et al. Phase I study of intraventricular administration of rituximab in patients with recurrent CNS and intraocular lymphoma. J Clin Oncol 2007;25(11):1350–6.
14. Maloney DG, Smith B, Rose A. Rituximab: mechanism of action and resistance. Semin Oncol 2002;29(1 Suppl 2):2–9.
15. Kitzmann AS, Pulido JS, Mohney BG, et al. Intraocular use of rituximab. Eye 2007;21(12):1524–7.
16. Kim H, Csaky KG, Chan CC, et al. The pharmacokinetics of rituximab following an intravitreal injection. Exp Eye Res 2006;82(5):760–6.
17. Mineo JF, Scheffer A, Karkoutly C, et al. Using human CD20-transfected murine lymphomatous B cells to evaluate the efficacy of intravitreal and intracerebral rituximab injections in mice. Invest Ophthalmol Vis Sci 2008;49(11):4738–45.
18. Ohguro N, Hashida N, Tano Y. Effect of intravitreous rituximab injections in patients with recurrent ocular lesions associated with central nervous system lymphoma. Arch Ophthalmol 2008;126(7):1002–3.
19. Bakri SJ, Cameron JD, McCannel CA, et al. Absence of histologic retinal toxicity of intravitreal bevacizumab in a rabbit model. Am J Ophthalmol 2006;142(1):162–4.
20. Itty S, Pulido JS. Rituximab for intraocular lymphoma. Retina 2009;29(2):129–32.
21. Nussenblatt RB, Chan CC, Wilson WH, et al. International Central Nervous System and Ocular Lymphoma Workshop: recommendations for the future. Ocul Immunol Inflamm 2006;14(3):139–44.

Index

B. Esmaeli (ed.), *Ophthalmic Oncology,* M.D. Anderson Solid Tumor Oncology Series 6, DOI 10.1007/978-1-4419-0374-7,

D

R

Printed in the United States of America